GERONTOLOGIC PALLIATIVE CARE NURSING

GERONTOLOGIC PALLIATIVE CARE NURSING

MARIANNE LAPORTE MATZO, PhD, APRN, GNP, BC, FAAN
Associate Professor, Graduate School of Nursing
University of Massachusetts, Worcester, Massachusetts;
Graduate Faculty, The Union Institute and University
Cincinnati, Ohio;
Professor of Nursing, New Hampshire Community Technical College
Manchester, New Hampshire;
Hospice Nurse, Visiting Nurses Association
Manchester, New Hampshire
Project on Death in America Faculty Scholar
New York, New York

DEBORAH WITT SHERMAN, PhD, APRN, ANP, BC, FAAN, BC-PCM
Associate Professor of Nursing
New York University;
Program Coordinator, Advanced Practice Palliative Care
Master's and Post-Master's Programs
Project on Death in America Faculty Scholar
New York, New York
Associate Director, Interdisciplinary Palliative Care
Fellowship Program
Bronx Veterans Medical Center
Bronx, New York

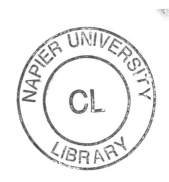
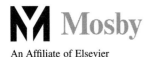
Mosby
An Affiliate of Elsevier

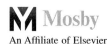
Mosby

An Affiliate of Elsevier

11830 Westline Industrial Drive
St. Louis, Missouri 63146

GERONTOLOGIC PALLIATIVE CARE NURSING   ISBN 0-323-01990-0

NOTICE

Nursing is an ever-changing field. Standard safety precautions must be followed, but as new research and clinical experience broaden our knowledge, changes in treatment and drug therapy may become necessary or appropriate. Readers are advised to check the most current product information provided by the manufacturer of each drug to be administered to verify the recommended dose, the method and duration of administration, and contraindications. It is the responsibility of the licensed prescriber, relying on experience and knowledge of the patient, to determine dosages and the best treatment for each individual patient. Neither the publisher nor the author assumes any liability for any injury and/or damage to persons or property arising from this publication.

International Standard Book Number 0-323-01990-0

Executive Editor: Michael S. Ledbetter
Senior Developmental Editor: Laurie K. Gower
Publishing Services Manager: Catherine Albright Jackson
Project Manager: Celeste Clingan
Design Manager: Gail Morcy Hudson

Printed in United States of America

Last digit is the print number: 9 8 7 6 5 4 3 2 1

CONTRIBUTORS

Janet L. Abrahm, MD
Associate Professor, Medicine & Anesthesia
Harvard Medical School
Director, Pain & Palliative Care Program
Dana-Farber Cancer Institute
Boston, Massachusetts

Robert L. Arnold, EdD, MA
Professional Development Coordinator
The Hospice Institute of the Florida Suncoast
Largo, Florida

Elizabeth A. Ayello, PhD, RN, CS, CWOCN
Clinical Associate Professor, Division of Nursing
Director of Adult Nursing Science
Senior Advisor, The John A. Hartford Institute for
    Geriatric Nursing, New York University
New York, New York

Cynthia R. Balkstra, MS, APRN, BC
Pulmonary Clinical Nurse Specialist
St. Joseph's/Candler Health System
Savannah, Georgia

Patricia H. Berry, PhD, APRN, BC-PCM, CHPN
Assistant Professor, College of Nursing
University of Utah
Salt Lake City, Utah

Kathleen T. Cumming, MS, APRN, BC
Geriatric Nurse Practitioner
Hospice and Palliative Care of Cape Cod, Inc.
Hyannis, Massachusetts

Constance Dahlin, MS, APRN, BC, PCM
Advanced Practice Nurse—Palliative Care Service
Massachusetts General Hospital
Boston, Massachusetts

Robert B. Davis, RN, FNP
Family Nurse Practitioner, University of Virginia
Charlottesville, Virginia

Susan A. Derby, RN, MA, CGNP
Geriatric Nurse Practitioner
Pain and Palliative Care Service
Memorial Sloan-Kettering Cancer Center
New York, New York

Judith B. Dyne, MS, RN, APRN, BC
Adult Nurse Practitioner—Cardiology
New York Heart Center
Syracuse, New York

Kathleen A. Egan, MA, BSN, CHPN
Vice President
The Hospice Institute of the Florida Suncoast
Largo, Florida

Barbara Duffy Evans, MS, RN, GNP
Geriatric Nurse Practitioner
Palliative Care Consultant
Home and Hospice Care of Rhode Island
Pawtucket, Rhode Island

Amy E. Guthrie, MSN, APRN, CHPN
Hospital Services Liaison
Hospice of Wayne County, Ohio
Wooster, Ohio

Patricia Hess, PhD, APRN, BC, NAP
Professor Emeritus, San Francisco State University
San Francisco, California

Nichole M. Irish, MSN, RN, ANP-BC
Adult Nurse Practitioner
Carolinas Heathcare System, The MS Center
Charlotte, North Carolina

Christine R. Kovach, PhD, RN
Professor, University of Wisconsin, Milwaukee
Milwaukee, Wisconsin

Pamala D. Larsen, PhD, CRRN
Director, School of Nursing
University of North Carolina at Charlotte
Charlotte, North Carolina

Polly Mazanec, MSN, APRN, BC, AOCN
Palliative Care Advanced Practice Nurse
Hospice of the Western Reserve
Cleveland, Ohio

Sue E. Meiner, EdD, APRN, BC, GNP
Assistant Professor, University of Nevada, Las Vegas
Las Vegas, Nevada

Mathy D. Mezey, EdD, RN, FAAN
Director, The John A. Hartford Foundation
Institute for Geriatric Nursing
New York University—Division of Nursing
New York, New York

Ethel L. Mitty, EdD, RN
Adjunct Clinical Professor
New York University—Division of Nursing
New York, New York

Bridget J. Montana, MSN, APRN, MBA
Chief Operating Officer
Hospice of the Western Reserve
Cleveland, Ohio

Lynn R. Noland, PhD, FNP
Assistant Professor, School of Nursing
University of Virginia;
Nurse Practitioner, Division of Nephrology
University of Virginia Medical Center
Charlottesville, Virginia

Sally Neylan Okun, BSN, RN, MMHS
Independent Consultant, CAReTOGRAPHY
Barnstable, Massachusetts

Karen Parr-Day, MS, RN, CCRN
Professor of Nursing
New Hampshire Community Technical College
Manchester, New Hampshire

Kathleen Ouimet Perrin, PhD, RN, CCRN
Interim Director, Department of Nursing,
    St. Anselm College
Manchester, New Hampshire

Elizabeth Ford Pitorak, MSN, APRN, CHPN
Director of the Hospice Institute
Hospice of the Western Reserve
Cleveland, Ohio

Judith Kennedy Schwarz, RN, PhD
Nurse Ethicist, Consultant—End of Life Care
New York, New York

Lynn H. Simpkins, RN, MSN, FNP, CDE
Family Nurse Practitioner, Informed Care, Inc.
Charlottesville, Virginia

Valerie Swigart, PhD, MSN, MEd, CRNP
Assistant Professor of Nursing
University of Pittsburgh
Pittsburgh, Pennsylvania

Anita J. Tarzian, PhD, RN
Independent Consultant/Research Associate
University of Maryland School of Law
Law and Health Care Program
Baltimore, Maryland

Shirley S. Travis, PhD, APRN, BC
Professor, University of North Carolina at Charlotte
Charlotte, North Carolina

Reviewers

Barbara Daniel, RN, MEd, MS, GNP
Professor of Nursing
Cecil Community College
North East, Maryland

Laurie Dazarow, MSN, RN
Director of Senior Services
Saginaw Cooperative Hospitals, Inc.
Saginaw, Michigan

Winifred Guariglia, MS, APRN, BC, GNP
Associate Professor of Nursing
Bergen Community College
Paramus, New Jersey

Katherine Howard, MS, APRN, BC
Instructor, Charles E. Gregory School of Nursing
Raritan Bay Medical Center
Old Bridge, New Jersey

Patricia Moran Woodbery, APRN, BC
Professor of Nursing
Valencia Community College
Orlando, Florida

This book is dedicated to my sisters,
Joan Ellen Matzo and **Kathleen Enderton**.
During Joan's life, I learned the meaning of courage and optimism;
her dying and death taught me the value of hope.
Kathleen made it possible for me to learn these lessons,
nurturing both my children and myself during the process.
MLM

To my loving **family**, **friends**, and **colleagues**
who have helped heal my body and nurtured my spirit
through their consistent, loving care during my recent illness.

With great love to my father, **Lothar Witt**, who taught me dignity
and grace in living with and dying from a life-threatening illness and to
my mother, **Mary Witt**, who have always been a source of strength, courage
and love.

To my dearest husband, **Neal**, and our children, **Ben**, **Rachael**, and **Joe**
who are the joys of my life and who make every day a precious gift and a
blessing.

To my **nursing students** and my **patients** who continuously teach me
resilience of the spirit and who reinforce the importance of coupling the
science and art of nursing—

To all of you I send my love and thanks always.
DWS

FOREWORD

Some would say this text is long overdue, but timing is everything in human events, and this is the time. The post-modern era has ushered in a greater concern for life-meanings because we have discovered that our scientific era may have produced more harm for humans than good. We have discovered that viruses and bacteria can outwit us, and that the medicalization of the "developed" countries can extend life in many circumstances, but economically is terribly costly and often at the sacrifice of quality of life. Some researchers now seriously examine the phenomenology of experience rather than simple demographics.

The American Geriatrics Society, the American Medical Association, and the American Association of the Colleges of Nursing (AACN) have published guidelines for end-of-life care, and the JCAHO Accreditation Board recently published standards to measure such care. This text addresses 15 very specific and measurable competencies (AACN) necessary for quality care of the dying.

Appropriate end-of-life care, a progeny of the hospice movement, acknowledges the uniqueness of each person in the dying process: no pattern is to be expected but support is to be given for whatever the dying person can muster from self, family, friends, cultural rituals, and professionals. Spiritual aspects of dying are also of great concern.

The experience of dying is of universal consequence. In so many ways, it is akin to that of giving birth. We are aware that the body carries out its own processes, quite physiologically apart from the control of the dying or birthing person. There is a profound loneliness in the experience, which cries out for the presence of caring others. We do not tread the path with the dying person but carefully attend as he or she goes through the door that we all must enter. For several decades the medical management of the birthing process has become more humane, but only recently has dying received similar attention it so badly needed. Entry into life and departure from it are universal experiences that are heavily influenced by custom and culture. The unique needs of each individual during the dying process must be given the utmost attention. Nurses are in a sacred role when planning the care of and attending to a dying person.

Nurses and doctors have been taught to preserve life, and sometimes preserving vital function, regardless of the life-quality, has become the priority. The "rectangularization" of life is a hope that we have entertained for two or three decades. Simply, this means that a long and healthy life would be maintained until just before death, at which point, one would then quickly succumb to "old age," whatever that may be. However, this is not presently the case. In Oregon, where physician-assisted suicide has been available, very few terminally ill people have taken that option. The life force, even in the most extenuating circumstances, is persistent.

One of the major concerns in end-of-life care is to provide as much comfort and freedom from pain as possible. Excruciating pain that has so often accompanied one's last hours prevents attention to the good-byes one might wish to say and torments the intimates standing by, often heightening their desire to flee and not remain with the person at a time when they are so desperately needed. Nurses, themselves, are not immune to these same reactions.

Although nurses are most often with the dying and their families, this textbook is of value not only to nurses but also to all professionals and paraprofessionals who care for the seriously ill older adult. This palliative care text is especially valuable because it deals with specific disorders and symptoms, as well as the universal requirements in the care of dying persons. Psychosocial symptoms and problems are discussed in detail. Dealing with families appropriately and compassionately is integral to end-of-life care, and these are thoroughly addressed. This work has been needed for a very long time and should be a requirement in every nursing program.

In this text, the caring professional is first challenged to examine personal biases, feelings, and attitudes that may complicate the care of diverse elders, because they require sensitivity to their unique cultural and spiritual beliefs and customs. The in-depth, practical, and humane considerations that form the fundamentals of holistic care comprise the first section of the text and form the essential background necessary for comprehensive end-of-life care. These are not simply called into play on the deathbed. Providers are given specific knowledge and behaviors to guide them in formulating care plans that will ease the passage of the client through the various stages of decline and the underlying influence of aging changes.

The uniqueness of this text, in contrast to many of the publications now addressing palliative care, is that it demonstrates a trajectory of caring that follows the physical and mental decline of individuals with certain specific chronic disorders. The scope and sophistication of the text is particularly exceptional because it presents case studies drawn from real situations and briefly reviews the pathophysiology of conditions to prepare the reader for addressing the broad range of physical and emotional needs from beginning to end of the continuum of these disorders. Throughout, there is an emphasis on methods and recognition of the need for holistic interventions in the care of the aged.

I believe this text has the potential for profoundly influencing palliative care of the elders in our society and the satisfaction of nurses in providing this care.

Priscilla Ebersole, PhD, RN, FAAN
Editor, *Geriatric Nursing*

CONTENTS

I PROMOTING QUALITY OF LIFE DURING THE DYING PROCESS

Patricia H. Berry

The changing demographics in the United States population and the marked increase in numbers of older persons create an urgent need for nurses who have knowledge and skill in the care of older adults and their families. Older persons by nature of their extensive life histories bring unique needs with them into the health care setting. Understanding and striving to meet these needs becomes especially critical at the end of life. End of life care, unlike other kinds of care usually offers one chance to "get it right." Put another way, there is no "dress rehearsal" in end of life care; careful planning and understanding the context of care ensures the least stressful and best possible quality of life outcome for all involved.

The purpose of this section is to introduce and discuss the important contexts surrounding the older adult during end of life transition. These include cultural and spiritual aspects of care; the impact of the aging population on end of life care; palliative care in communities and across healthcare settings; ethics and legal issues; resource allocation; advance care planning; including special considerations with persons with dementia; family caregiving; and suffering, loss, grief, and bereavement.

Consideration of cultural competence and spirituality should include the perspectives of African-Americans, Chinese, Asian Indians, Native Americans, and Latinos and Hispanics. However, increasing one's cultural awareness, conducting a spiritual assessment, and providing spiritual caregiving is an integral part of truly comprehensive care for the older adult and his/her family. Additionally, the changing demographics, economics, health status and expenditures, social interaction, culture and historical aspects of death must be also be considered. Current trends and statistics suggest the nature of the challenges posed for caregivers of the aged in the coming decades.

The barriers to providing palliative care, however many, are not insurmountable. The need to include palliative care in hospice programs and beyond is driven in part by the new, involved consumer concerned with issues of quality of care and quality of life as well as advance care planning, and the burdens of caregiving.

When offered within settings such as nursing homes or assisted living facilities, palliative care must adjust to expectations of patients, caregivers, and health professionals as traditional views of dying are replaced with contemporary attitudes. Central to this process is creation of "seamless" care with interdisciplinary collaboration and assurance of reasonable reimbursement regardless of care setting. The often difficult issues of what is moral, or "right," end-of-life care and how patient wishes can be honored, while considering legal aspects, constitute the legal and ethical aspects of dying. Individual decisions such as withholding vs. withdrawing medical treatments, patient requests for hastened death, and assisted suicide must be considered, particularly within the context of allocating health care resources and health care rationing.

Communication is especially important when discussing the desirability of advance care planning and the issues involved as family elders, physicians, and nurses participate in the process. These issues may include cultural barriers or a deep-seated reluctance to confront an end-of-life situation. The ideal approach is interdisciplinary, but the nurse should facilitate informed decision making for the patient and family. This process can be especially difficult for older adults with dementia in its various manifestations; the introduction of an advance directive and the special issues involved when decision-making capacity has been compromised, provide formidable challenges. The ethics of this type of advance planning and proxy (surrogate) decision making, including mediating differences of opinion, must be part of the process. Placing the family, rather than the patient, as the focus of palliative care creates certain burdens but opens the door to substantial rewards for caregiver, family, and patient. The health care professional is called on to facilitate this process with sensitivity to cultural issues and the ability to integrate concepts such as self-transcendence as the family transitions through the loss of a loved one.

Grief, which may be assessed by the nurse as anticipatory, normal, complicated, or disenfranchised, may persist long after death of the family member. Implicit in successful nursing care for these families is cultural sensitivity and a "team" approach; nurses should also be aware of the emotional strain they themselves may undergo and of the support services available to them.

Caring for elderly patients and their families at the end of life is an honor and privilege. Nowhere else in nursing is one invited to be a companion with older patients and their family and to celebrate their life. Likewise, nowhere else in the practice of nursing is our attention to the important contexts of care and thus, our words, actions, and guidance more remembered and cherished. Ensuring quality of life for older persons and their families is important from both a professional and personal perspective—as most of us will, sooner or later, find ourselves in need of such care.

1

CULTURAL AND SPIRITUAL BACKGROUNDS OF OLDER ADULTS

Deborah Witt Sherman

Case Study

Mrs. M. is an 84-year-old Latino woman who has progressive pain and weakness as a result of sensory neuropathy, secondary to diabetes and arthritis. During the course of her illness, she has maintained her independence and good spirits. Mrs. M. believes that her faith in God has enabled her to endure her chronic pain. She states, "Sometimes I pray when I am in deep, serious pain. I pray and all at once the pain gets easy. I feel it has helped me more than the medication. I believe in God. He is my guide and protector." Mrs. M. lives with her daughter, son-in-law, and grandchildren. They are a source of comfort and support and are very concerned about her well-being.

Unfortunately, Mrs. M. recently had a stroke, which resulted in left hemiplegia. After an initial hospital stay, her family insisted that they care for her at home. On a visit to their home, the health care professional observes a shrine to Mary in the front yard, as well as crucifixes and pictures of Jesus in every room. In addition to traditional medications prescribed by her physician, Mrs. M. takes herbal remedies in an attempt to restore her health. The health care professional acknowledges the cultural and spiritual values and beliefs of Mrs. M. as considerations in providing quality palliative care.

INTRODUCTION

Palliative care strives to meet the physical, emotional, social, and spiritual expectations and needs of patients and families experiencing chronic, life-limiting or life-threatening illness, while remaining sensitive to cultural and religious beliefs and practices (Ferris & Cummings, 1995). The culture and spirituality of older adults are often sources of connection with others because they provide a lens through which older adults interpret their world and a context in which to share life experiences (Sherman, 2001). Culture and spirituality are among the most important factors that structure human experience, values, beliefs, attitudes, and behaviors, and they influence practices related to health and illness. As a system of shared symbols and beliefs, culture supports a person's sense of security, integrity, and belonging and provides a prescription for how to conduct life and approach death (End of Life Nursing Education Consortium [ELNEC], 2001). Spirituality can be understood as dynamic principles developed throughout the life span that guide a person's view of the world, and influence one's perception of a higher power or relationship with God, as well as a sense of hope, moral conviction, faith, love, and trust (Hicks, 1999). Spirituality plays a vital role in the lives of elders in times of crisis and chronic illness because it provides a sense of connection to self, others, nature, and God and is a means to cope with loss, grief, and death (Weaver, Flannelly, & Flannelly, 2001). The cultural and spiritual backgrounds of older adults are important aspects of assessment and intervention in providing quality palliative care.

UNDERSTANDING THE CULTURAL BACKGROUND OF OLDER ADULTS

Culture is defined as a way of life that provides a worldview, which is fundamental in defining and creating a person's reality, determining their meaning and purpose in life, and providing guidelines for living (Ersek, Kagawa-Singer, Barnes, Blackhall, & Koenig, 1998). As cultural perspectives evolve, changes are evident in the beliefs, values, and attitudes of a cultural group or its members. Cultures are not monolithic; rather, there is a range of potential responses to each issue in every cultural group. Thus there may be within-group variations, such as those attributed to acculturation differences as well as to differences related to age, education, geographic location, and social context (Kagawa-Singer & Blackhall, 2001). It is important to inquire whether an individual patient adheres to the beliefs and practices of his or her cultural group, rather than assuming that he or she holds the same values and beliefs (Crawley, Marshall, Lo, & Koenig, 2002).

Although culture is often identified with ethnicity, it is a far broader concept that encompasses the components of gender, age, sexual orientation, differing abilities, educational level, employment, and place of residency (ELNEC, 2001). As examples, cultures may value male children more than female; the young more than the old; heterosexuals rather than homosexuals; the educated and employed more than the uneducated or unemployed; individuals with stable domiciles more than the homeless; and the healthy more than the physically, emotionally, or intellectually challenged. The diversity of the older population with regard to many of these factors may increase their vulnerability in terms of perceived cultural status. Concepts of culture and ethnicity may be useful for making generalizations about populations; however, if they limit appreciation of the unique differences of people and are used to predict individual behavior, they may lead to stereotyping (La Vera, Marshall, Lo, & Koenig, 2002). This is also true regarding stereotyping of older adults.

Cultural background also relates to issues of gender and power, decision making, language and communication, sources of support within the community, degree of fatalism or activism in accepting or controlling death, maintaining hope, and even views of the patient and family about death (Sherman, 2001). Cultural differences are further evident in terms of the relationship between the older adult and his or her family. In certain cultures, the older person is viewed as the patriarch or matriarch of the family who has the final word in personal and family matters. In other cultures, the older person defers decision making to members of the family because interdependence among the family and community members is more valued than individual autonomy (Ersek et al., 1998). Depending on cultural expectations, families may believe that it is their duty to protect the older person from bad news, which is believed to burden the individual or cause emotional distress or harm. Other cultures, with great reverence toward their elders, may view full disclosure of information as disrespectful and rude. As the cultural diversity of patients and practitioners in the United States continues to increase, there is a risk for cross-cultural misunderstanding surrounding care at the end of life. Cross-cultural understanding and communication techniques increase the likelihood that both the process and outcome of health care are satisfactory for all involved (Kagawa-Singer & Blackhall, 2001).

Recognizing Cultural Diversity

Cultural diversity refers to differences between people based on treasured beliefs, shared teachings, norms, customs, language, and meaning that influence the individual's and family's response to illness, treatment, death, and bereavement (Showalter, 1998). Cultural diversity is evident in the perception of pain, ways of coping with life-threatening illness, and the behavioral manifestations of grief, mourning, and funeral customs (DeSpelder & Strickland, 1999). The acknowledgment of such concepts and their relationships may provide a framework for cultural assessment and an opportunity to provide quality care respectful of differences with regard to cultural expectations and needs. Failure to take culture seriously means that health professionals elevate their values above the values of others, which is culturally destructive rather than culturally skilled (Kagawa-Singer & Blackhall, 2001). Therefore, it is important to support trusting and effective patient and provider interactions through respect and acknowledgment of cultural diversity and avoidance of misperceptions.

For the older adult and for individuals experiencing life-threatening illness, several issues are relevant with respect to culture. One such issue is patient autonomy, which emphasizes the rights of patients to be informed about their condition, its treatments, and the right to choose or refuse life-prolonging care. However, an emphasis on autonomy reflects American beliefs regarding independence and individual rights, which may not be shared by patients and families from other cultures (Kagawa-Singer & Blackhall, 2001). For example, those from Asian cultures may believe that the family as a whole should make decisions regarding the aged individual.

Another issue influenced by culture is response to inequities in care. When not addressed, this issue may lead to feelings of mistrust regarding the intentions of health care providers and a lack of cooperation and collaboration between the patient, family, and health care provider. Discussions of the cost of technology and the ineffectiveness of treatment may be perceived by patients as a devaluation of their life (Crawley et al., 2002). As a result, there may be an increased desire for futile aggressive care at the end of life, and dissatisfaction with care. This issue is relevant to the care of African American patients and families, who are more likely to want aggressive medical care at the end of life and less likely to have do-not-resuscitate orders. To address this issue, practitioners can ask directly if the individual trusts someone who is not from their same background. Practitioners can work toward addressing inequities in care, or can attempt to understand and accommodate desires for more aggressive care (Kagawa-Singer & Blackhall, 2001).

Furthermore, communication or language barriers may lead to bidirectional misunderstanding and unnecessary physical, emotional, social, or spiritual suffering. It is therefore important to avoid medical jargon, make language simple, and check for understanding or hire a trained interpreter. The use of family or untrained interpreters should be avoided because they may misinterpret phrases, censor sensitive or taboo topics, or filter and summarize discussions rather than translating them completely (Crawley et al., 2002).

There may also be differences in religion and spirituality, which may create a lack of trust between patients and professionals from different backgrounds. To create a sense of connection, health care professionals need to ask about religious or spiritual beliefs and practices and how the patient could be supported in addressing religious or spiritual needs.

Another issue that may need to be negotiated is truth-telling. Individuals from certain cultures

may develop mistrust or anger if the health care team insists on informing the patient about his or her diagnosis or prognosis against the wishes of the family. Families often believe that such knowledge will result in a sense of hopelessness for the patient, which contributes to his or her suffering. In this situation, it would be appropriate for the health care provider to ask whether the patient would want to know everything about his or her illness, and to be cognizant of nonverbal communication when discussing serious information (Kagawa-Singer & Blackhall, 2001).

Consideration should also be given to the issue of family involvement in decision making. Disagreement and conflict between family and health care professionals may occur when the family insists on making decisions for patients who have decisional capacity. It is important for health care professionals to identify the key members of the family and involve them in the discussions as desired by the patient. If the patient is capable of making decisions for him- or herself, yet the family requests that information be withheld from the patient and that they make the decisions, it is helpful to conduct a family meeting in which the patient, family members, and health care professionals are present. This may provide an opportunity to clarify issues, address conflicts, and provide clarity about the decisions and preferences of the patient.

At the end of life, cultural differences may also exist regarding the desire to enroll in hospice care. Health professionals need to understand the feelings and perceptions of patients and families from varying cultural perspectives, and emphasize that hospice is not a replacement for the family, but rather a way of providing resources to support quality of life for patients and families (Kagawa-Singer & Blackhall, 2001).

Although there may be diversity in terms of desires, preferences, and expectations across cultures, there are also similarities. In a study of the needs and experiences of non—English-speaking hospice patients and families in an English-speaking country, McGrath, Vun, and McLeod (2001) found, based on focus groups that included Indian, Filipino, Chinese, and Italian cultural groups and their caregivers, that participants from all groups expressed the same concerns. These included the importance of support from families, the pressures on family members to care for relatives at the end of life, lack of knowledge about hospice and palliative care services, lack of choice in how they wished to care for their family member, difficulty in talking about dying, and desire to care for a family member at home.

Cultural Perspectives in Health Care

Understanding the cultural backgrounds of older adults is fundamental to the development of a trusting and supportive relationship between patient, family, and health care professionals, and essential in developing a plan for health care that is consistent with their cultural expectations and health beliefs. Andrews and Boyle (1995) discussed three types of health belief systems: magico-religious, biomedical, and holistic. In the magico-religious paradigm, a person believes that God or supernatural forces control health and illness. In the biomedical paradigm, to which most Americans subscribe, illness is believed to be caused by a disruption in physical or biochemical processes that can be manipulated by health care. In the holistic paradigm, health results from a balance or harmony among the elements of nature and illness is produced by disharmony. Examples of the magico-religious system include a Haitian patient who believes that his symptoms are caused by spirits, or the Mexican American who uses herbs, oils, incense, or religious figurines to drive away evil spirits or to relieve gastric pains. In the biomedical system, Americans or Europeans seek cure of illness through advanced medical technology and pharmacologic management. Based on the holistic belief system, a Chinese woman may attribute her headache to a stagnation of Qi, believing in the need for balance between yin and yang, while a Native American patient may wear a bag of herbs blessed by the medicine man around his neck to maintain his strength (Grossman, 1996).

Recognition of these health belief systems is evident in the health care practices of many cultures. The health beliefs of the African American, Chinese, Asian Indian, Latino and Hispanic, and Native American cultures are discussed based on recent studies or cultural inquiries and provide a framework for offering culturally competent hospice and palliative care to members of these cultural groups. The only truly accurate way to know what individuals believe in or the effect that their culture or religion plays in their lives is to ask them. The following information will guide the nurse regarding areas to be assessed.

Cultural Perspectives of African Americans

Within the African American culture, there is a strong sense of community and of the importance of family, friends, and the church community as sources of support. The extended African American family consists of mother, father, children, grandparents, aunts, uncles, nieces, nephews, and cousins, with a willingness to accept all relatives regardless of their circumstances (McDavis, Parker, & Parker, 1995). Older adults are prized in the African American family, and they play key roles in the family, church, and community. Many grandparents accept the responsibility for rearing their grandchildren, while the parents of those children work or receive higher education. Children are taught to take care of their parents and to be devoted to them. In addition, older African American family members play a significant role in passing on cultural values, customs, and traditions to the children (McDavis et al., 1995).

With respect to health care, African Americans are often distrustful of the health care system, given a history of oppression from slavery and racism. Common themes of justice and respect have reinforced the importance of self-determination. As a result of these factors, there has been a lack of interest among African Americans in hospice care (DeSpelder & Strickland, 1999). Because family is central to the care of the dying, and with the assistance and supportive relationships established with church members and neighbors, there is a decreased need for outside support (Sherman, 2001). Given strong family loyalty, there is reluctance to hospitalize family members. As a measure of respect and devotion, elder African Americans are placed in nursing homes only as a last resort (McDavis et al., 1995).

In the African American culture, death is integrated into the totality of life. Ancestor worship involves the communion with the living dead through memories, and the deceased are remembered by name. When the deceased are no longer remembered by people who are alive, they become part of the anonymous dead, but by this time their spirit has been reborn in a new child (Sherman, 2001).

To explore the meaning of death and the experience of grieving, Abrums (2000) conducted life history interviews of nine church-going women, ranging in age from 19 to 82 years, from a small black storefront Baptist church in the Pacific Northwest. The findings indicated that the women in the church had been taught to be strong in the face of death and to handle their grief "head on." The women believed that they would one day be reunited with their loved ones. The terminology of dying included use of the words "passed on," "passed away," or "died." Participants described many visits from spirits for the purpose of offering warnings or as direct messages. Belief in an afterlife was sustained by day-to-day experiences of visions or messages from another world. It was believed that God spoke to them in many ways through premonitions, perceived as the voice of God. There was strong perception of the journey of life, in which there was a job to do on earth and a purpose to one's life. No life was in vain. Time was needed to prepare for death and to make peace with God as dying individuals prepared physically, finished up emotionally, looked forward and backward, and got set to move in one direction. Participants also described the importance of hope, acceptance, and responsibility to comfort the dying and the bereaved.

Abrums (2000) concluded that health professionals should learn to value the spiritual beliefs and grieving behaviors of members of other cultures, rather than viewing them as maladaptive. The people in this storefront church were often comforted by the recognition that God sustained them in times of adversity and that God would protect their loved ones. Supporting the dying elder and his or her family in their beliefs is important in providing spiritual care. Verbal recognition of specific actions taken by the family to support the dying provided a sense of comfort and support to the family in their grief. This acknowledgment of the family's belief system by health professionals can augment the healing process during times of loss and grief.

Cultural Perspectives of Chinese

In the Chinese culture, the primary theme related to social structure is the centrality of the family. From the centrality of the family arise many cultural expectations, such as (1) duty to family, manifested by respect and reverence for parents; (2) conformance to family and societal norms, and especially not bringing shame to the family; (3) family recognition through achievement; (4) emotional self-control, manifested through reserved and formal public verbal and nonverbal communications; (5) family disagreement or demands kept to a minimum; (6) collectivism, evidenced by people keeping a focus on the family and community over self; and (7) humility, manifested by a lack of striving for individual achievement except achievement that is related to the family (Kemp & Chang, 2002).

Given the traditionally hierarchical and patriarchal family structure of the Chinese, the oldest adult male is the primary decision maker. In family matters, there is significant influence of elders. Health decisions may be made by the family, and are based on what is best not only for the elder patient, but for the family. In general, yes-and-no questions should be avoided because "yes" is considered to be the polite answer and is nearly always given.

In China, the primary religion is Buddhism. The essence of Buddhism is the Four Noble Truths, specifically that (1) all sentient beings suffer; (2) the cause of suffering is desire manifested by attachment to life, to security, and to others; (3) the way to end suffering is to cease to desire; and (4) the way to cease desire is to follow the Eightfold Path of knowledge of the Four Noble Truths, right intent, right speech, right action, right endeavor, right mindfulness, and right meditation. It is believed that following the Eightfold Path leads to emancipation from rebirth (Kemp & Chang, 2002).

In the Chinese culture, it is also important to understand the importance of balance of yin and yang, which are complementary forces. A second important concept is that of traditional Chinese medicine (TCM), which is based on channel (meridian) systems, in which various body channels carry vital or life energy, called *chi*. Imbalance or disruption of channels leads to illness, and the treatment goal of TCM is to restore balance. A third important concept in understanding Chinese approaches to health and illness is the use of allopathic medicine, as well as TCM.

Issues central to the care of the Chinese patient at the end of life center around family and communications (Kemp & Chang, 2002). Symptom management may be complicated by patient and family reluctance to complain because of respect for others in positions of authority. Concerns also center around fears of addiction, desire to be a good patient, and fear of distracting the physician from treating the disease. In some cases, elders may even deny symptoms when asked directly; however, a visual analogue scale and numeric rating scale can be used to assess pain. Patients may want to keep warm during illness by wearing sweaters or socks in bed and drinking warm liquids and avoiding cold drinks. As death nears, the family may wish to call monks or nuns for ritual prayers (Kemp & Chang, 2002).

Communications at the end of life are also complicated by reluctance to discuss prognosis and diagnosis. Chinese families often withhold information from the older adult, and the elder may pretend that he or she does not know what is happening. Families believe that discussing end-of-life issues is like wishing death upon the elder, or may lead to hopelessness, especially since terminal illness is not socially accepted. As death approaches, it is believed that a person's final days should be characterized by calm and that the elder patient should not be involved in decision making. The best way to handle the conspiracy of silence is to ask the patient to whom the information should be given and who should make decisions. Families often feel it is their cultural obligation to care for the person who is dying, and therefore hospice services are often refused (Kemp & Chang, 2002).

Cultural Perspectives of Asian Indians

Among Asian Indians, extended families are prevalent and elders are highly respected. The husband's parents often move in with the family after retirement, when the family decides to have children, or if there is illness. Elders are highly valued, as is their role as grandparents in raising children. Value is placed on independence and privacy in Indian culture, and family issues are discussed within the immediate family before outside help is sought (Bhungalia & Kemp, 2002). Health care decisions usually require family input.

Many Indians are of the Hindu faith. The goal of Hinduism is to free the soul from endless incarnation and the suffering inherent in existence. The endless reincarnations of the soul are the result of *karma*, or actions of the individual in this present life and the accumulation of actions from past lives.

The caste system is part of Hinduism. In this system, society is divided into four social classes: the highest class is the priest class, or Brahmans, and the lowest class is the laborer class, or Sudras. A person's class is inherited at birth based on his or her karma. Hindu beliefs that may affect patient care include
- Karma, or the consequences of one's actions or behaviors, which influences the circumstances of life and may have caused an illness
- The importance of meditation and prayer
- The practice of vegetarianism, in which Hindus pray a specific prayer before eating to ask forgiveness for eating a plant or vegetable in which a soul may dwell

Most Indians eat two to three meals a day, eating with the fingers of their right hand, and avoiding distractions while eating, such as watching television or excessive talking. Some foods are considered hot and others cold, and these should not be eaten in combination because this is believed to affect bodily functions.

The Indian system of medicine is known as Ayurveda, which means "knowledge of life." Indian medicine mixes religion and secular medicine, with more than 80% of people in India relying on herbal remedies to cure or prevent illness. In this system, the root of disease is not always inside the body, but may be related to the environment or other factors. In the Ayurveda system, the body comprises three primary forces, called *dosha*, specifically the Vata, Pitta, and Kapha. Each represents characteristics derived from the five elements of space, air, fire, water, and earth; the balance between these forces is essential to health. Once there is imbalance between the forces, balance is sought using different therapies, which include approximately 1400 plants used in Ayurvedic medicine.

Cultural Perspectives of Latinos and Hispanics

The cultural group referred to as Latinos comprises individuals of Hispanic background. By conducting 10 focus groups and interviews with 17 gatekeepers in Latino communities, Sullivan (2001) identified Latino views regarding end-of-life care. The results indicated that many Latinos felt that they could not communicate effectively with health care providers because of language barriers, and were not able to understand the concept of informed consent even when interpreters were used. None of the Latino participants wanted to die in a nursing home, believing that it is the family's responsibility to care for their relative. Most participants were also not aware of hospice services or had false information. Although participants expressed diverse views, one third of participants were against the use of life support, particularly if it prolonged the suffering of the patient. Participants also believed that their religious beliefs, especially fatalism and reliance on God, were central to their decision making regarding end-of-life care. There was division among the participants regarding the extent to which they wanted to be informed about a fatal diagnosis, with some fearing that being informed may accelerate the illness. Many Latinos also perceived racial discrimination and cultural insensitivity as barriers to quality care and healing (Sullivan, 2001).

Given that cultural values profoundly influence the experience of health and illness for individuals, Martinez (1995) conducted a qualitative study of 14 Hispanic participants, ranging in age from 60 to 89, along with 6 health professionals and 2 clergy who practiced in the community. They perceived health as creating balance in life and as faith that one will be cared for by God, family, and community. Participants held holistic views of self and emphasized the spiritual aspects of life in relation to health. Mental health was described as knowing what is right, living a life consistent with one's beliefs and values, trusting that life will work out, and maintaining faith in God. Caring for self was through caring for others for whom one had responsibility. In dealing with illness, there was a blending of modern medicine and traditional healing remedies. It was also appropriate to include family members in making health decisions.

In the Hispanic culture, there are several considerations that relate to quality care at the end of life (Sherman, 2001). It is recognized that, in Hispanic culture, there is strong family support and a belief that the dying elder should be protected from his or her prognosis. The family often assume responsibility for their dying family members and prefer to care for them at home. Although death is viewed as an adversity, references to dying and death are common in the culture: children play with toys symbolizing death, and the funeral is an important family ceremony. Given the strong Catholic background of many Hispanics and a belief in an afterlife, the Day of the Dead, which coincides with All Soul's Day, is celebrated in November. This is a day that celebrates of the life of the dead, with music, food, and the decoration of graves.

Cultural Perspectives of Native Americans

For Native Americans, the focus of identity is on the tribe, rather than having simply Native American ancestry. This is important because values and beliefs vary among tribes and among the different bands in the "First Nations." There may be similarities in nations originating in the same region, but there are also tribal distinctions (Brokenleg & Middleton, 1993). For many Native Americans, however, life and death are viewed as a natural part of the life cycle as and a part of human existence. Time is considered as a recurring cycle, rather than a linear process. Native Americans are concerned with how this cycle affects people in this life, and death is viewed as a motivation to treat people kindly and lead a good life (Brokenleg & Middleton, 1993; Sherman, 2001).

From a cultural perspective, Native Americans avoid eye contact and are stoic regarding the expression of pain and suffering, and traditional tribal medicines are used (Sherman, 2001). Prayer is a medium through which one might come to accept the outcome of a situation, and it is not appropriate to question "why" something is happening because there is an acceptance of the natural order of things (Brokenleg & Middleton, 1993). There is also enormous reverence for the body both in life and death; autopsies and cremation are not acceptable. Death may be forecast by unusual spiritual or physical events. As examples, the sighting of an owl may signify that someone close will soon die, and a blue light seen coming from the direction of a relative's home or room indicates death (Brokenleg & Middleton, 1993).

Based on focus groups representing many Native American tribes and conducted by Native American nurses, Lowe and Struthers (2001) identified seven themes representing core principles relevant to health care:

1. Caring, which embodies characteristics of health, relationships, holism, and knowledge and is characterized as a "partnership in healing"
2. Tradition, which refers to the characteristics of respect, wisdom, and values and refers to the valuing of and connection with heritage
3. Respect, which includes characteristics of honor, identity, and strength and refers to the components of presence and compassion
4. Connection, which honors all people, harmony with nature, and the past, present, and future, and explores differences and similarities
5. Holism, which includes balance and culture
6. Trust, which is characterized through relationship, presence, and respect
7. Spirituality, which includes unity, honor, balance, and healing and also includes components of touching, learning, and utilizing traditions to recognize oneness and unity

Developing Cultural Competence

Given the diverse cultural and spiritual perspectives of older adult patients, there is a need for the development of cultural competency by health professionals. Cultural competency refers to a set of academic and personal skills that allow practitioners to increase understanding and appreciation of cultural differences between groups (American Medical Student Association, 2001). Practitioners need to appreciate and accept cultural differences, to learn to culturally assess a patient to avoid stereotyping, and to explain an issue from another's cultural perspective. Areas of dissonance between patients and health care providers include historical distrust, varying interpretations regarding disability, the influence of family structure on decision making, and differences in willingness to treat diseases without symptoms, such as high cholesterol, or appreciating illness even when there are no observable manifestations.

Cultural competence entails listening with sympathy and understanding, acknowledging and discussing differences and similarities between perceptions of illness and its treatment, recommending treatments while remembering the patient's cultural perspectives, and negotiating and compromising when worldviews are in conflict (American Medical Student Association, 2001; Crawley et al., 2002). In improving the relationship between the health professional and the patient across cultures, it is important to maintain nonjudgmental attitudes toward unfamiliar beliefs and practices, and to determine what is appropriate and polite caring behavior. It is respectful to begin by being more formal with older adult patients, addressing them by their surname rather than first name. It may be a sign of disrespect to look directly into another's eye or to ask questions regarding treatment. Shaking of the hands as a form of introduction, although valued in American culture, may be inappropriate by a female when introducing herself to an Orthodox Jewish or Muslim male (Grossman, 1996). Furthermore, a firm handshake may be interpreted by members of Native American tribes as aggressive or rude.

Asian Americans may tend to have subtle and indirect communication styles that rely heavily on nonverbal cues, such as facial expression, body movements, use of physical space, and tone of voice. For example, a patient may bow his or her head or may disengage from the health care professional if he or she is in disagreement with the plan of care (Grossman, 1996). Nodding of the head in Asian or Hispanic populations may be merely a social custom, showing politeness and respect for a person in authority rather than representing a sign of agreement. Given this possibility, the health care provider may need to ask specific questions that require the patient to express his or her feelings and wishes (Crawley et al., 2002).

It is important to ask questions to explore the older adult's beliefs about health, illness, and prevention. Health care professionals must accept the fact that many patients use complementary therapies as well as Western medicine, and not discount the possible effects of the supernatural on health. It is important for health professionals to have knowledge of the patient's family and kinship structure to help ascertain the values, differing gender roles, and issues concerning authority and decision making within a household, as well as the value of involving the family in the treatment (Grossman, 1996). Discussion with elders and their families may also involve the importance of food and eating as potentially enhancing a sense of community and as a way of supporting customs and heritage. Such information can assist the health care team in providing appropriate dietary instructions. For examples, Islamic law forbids Muslim patients to ingest alcohol, pork, or meat from an animal that is not appropriately slaughtered. Jewish patients may observe the laws of *kashrut*, which prescribe specific ways of food preparation and prohibit the eating of pork, shellfish, and wild birds. Individuals from Cuban backgrounds may prefer a diet that is high in calories, starches, and saturated fats, and modification of such a diet may mean just adhering to a modest serving size (Grossman, 1996).

Principles of Culturally Sensitive Care

In providing quality palliative care for older patients and their families, consideration should also be given to the principles of culturally sensitive care (CSWE Faculty Development Institute, 2001). As previously discussed, the first principle is to *be knowledgeable about cultural values and attitudes*. Health care professionals should attend to a patient's needs in a sensitive, understanding, and nonjudgmental way, and respond with flexibility as much as possible. The second principle is for health care practitioners to *attend to diverse communication styles*, including spending time listening to the older person's needs, views, and concerns. The third principle is to *ask the older patient for his or her preferences for decision making* early in the care process. As a fourth principle, it is important to *recognize cultural differences and varying comfort levels* with regard to personal space, eye contact, touch, time orientation, learning styles, and conversation styles.

The fifth principle is to *use a cultural guide from the elder's ethnic or religious background* to clarify cultural problems or concerns if communication with the patient or family is unclear. If necessary, ask the older adult to identify a spokesperson and respect the appointment made by the elder, even if the person is not a family member or does not live nearby. If the elder's preference is for family involvement, family meetings are opportunities to identify family's needs and concerns, and an opportunity for the family to understand the patient's goals of care and end-of-life wishes.

A sixth principle is to *get to know the community, its people, and its resources* to identify the availability of social support and resource needs. Health care professionals may establish relationships with key community resources to assist the seriously ill older adult and his or her family. As a seventh principle, health practitioners should *create a culturally friendly physical environment* by designing facilities with artwork or pictures valued by the cultural groups to whom care is most commonly provided. Written materials should be available in the language of patients to enhance their understanding of their disease and treatment options and provide them with a sense of partnership in making health care decisions.

As an eighth principle, it is appropriate for health professionals to *determine the acceptability of patients' being physically examined by a practitioner of a different gender*. Older patients should also be asked if they would want to have a family member present during the physical examination. Symptom recognition, as well as its reporting and meaning, may vary based on the elder patient's cultural background. A ninth principle is for health professionals to *advocate for availability of services, accessibility in terms of cost and location, and acceptability of services* that are compatible with cultural values and practices of the older adult.

A final principle is for each health professional to *conduct a self-assessment of his or her own beliefs* about illness and death and how they influence his or her attitudes; determine how significant culture and religion are in his or her personal attitudes toward death; and examine his or her feelings regarding what kind of death he or she would prefer, what efforts should be made to keep a seriously ill person alive, the disposition of his or her body, and his or her experience of participating in rituals to remember the dead (DeSpelder, 1998).

Cultural Assessment

Cultural assessment is important to determine beliefs, values, and perceptions regarding health and illness. Much can be learned about an elder's cultural beliefs and values by observing for symbols that are often the first sign of cultural identity (Grossman, 1996). For example, does the older adult or family place cultural or religious pictures, statues, or shrines in his or her room? If health practitioners are unfamiliar with such symbols, a polite inquiry about their significance can enhance one's understanding of the patient's cultural beliefs and needs. Recognition of cultural influences on the behavioral expressions of pain and the meaning of pain and suffering are also important considerations in pain assessment. Health professionals can also address cultural values at the end of life by asking open-ended questions, such as "What do you think is going on with your illness?", "What does your illness mean to you?", and "What is the meaning of pain and suffering?" The answers to such questions may indicate what the elder patient believes about the causation of his or her illness and the type of treatment he or she will seek or accept (Grossman, 1996).

It is important that health professionals not use shortcuts when asking about patients' care preferences and be explicit about what the patient and family members want in terms of care. Communication at the patient's level, without the use of medical jargon, is important in avoiding problems related to language barriers (Beckwith, 2001). In conducting a cultural assessment, there are several areas to be addressed, as noted in Box 1-1.

Having considered the importance of a comprehensive cultural assessment, it is also valuable for health professionals to have knowledge of the principles of culturally sensitive care. With this knowledge and understanding, health professionals are able to develop a culturally appropriate plan of care that addresses the cultural needs and expectations of older patients and their families and supports their trust of health professionals and satisfaction with health care.

Box 1-1 Cultural Assessment

- Identify the patient's birthplace.
- Ask the patient about his or her immigration experience.
- Determine the level of ethnic identity.
- Assess the primary and secondary language.
- Determine the person's verbal and nonverbal communication patterns.
- Evaluate the degree of acculturation as evidenced by the use of the English language, the length of time in the United States, and adaptation.
- Determine the family structure.
- Identify who makes decisions, such as the individual patient, the family, or another social unit.
- Identify the use of informal networks and sources of support within the community.
- Consider gender and power issues within relationships.
- Evaluate the patient's sense of self-esteem.
- Identify the influence of religion or spirituality on the patient's and family's expectations and behaviors.
- Identify cooking and dining traditions and the meaning of food.
- Determine the patient's educational level and socioeconomic status.
- Assess attitudes, beliefs, and practices related to health, illness, suffering, and death.
- Determine the patient's and family's preferences regarding location of death.
- Discuss expectations regarding health care.
- Determine the degree of fatalism or activism in accepting or controlling care and death.
- Evaluate the patient's knowledge and trust regarding the health care system.
- Ascertain the patient's perceptions regarding discrimination or racism.
- Assess the value and use of pharmacologic, nonpharmacologic, and complementary therapies.
- Discuss how hope is maintained.

Data from American Medical Student Association. (2001). Cultural competency in medicine. [http://www.amsa.org/pro grams/gpit/cultural); End of Life Nursing Education Consortium (2001). *Module 5: Cultural considerations*. City of Hope Medical Center and American Association of Colleges of Nursing. Retrieved from the American Association of Colleges of Nursing Web sites: www.aacn.nche.edu/elnec; and Ersek, M., Kagawa-Singer, M., Barnes, D., Blackhall, L., & Koenig, B. (1998). Multicultural considerations in the use of advance directives. *Oncology Nursing Forum, 25*(10), 1683-1689.

UNDERSTANDING SPIRITUALITY OR RELIGIOSITY OF OLDER ADULTS

Spirituality and religiosity are often fundamental to the way elder patients face chronic illness, suffering, loss, dying, and death. Spirituality and religiosity are integral to holistic care and are important considerations, particularly since spirituality may be a dynamic in the patient's understanding of his or her disease and way of coping, and religious convictions may affect health care decision making (Puchalski, 2001a). Spiritual ideas are fundamental to palliative care because both are concerned with nonabandonment and the value of interpersonal relationships, and recognize the value of transcendent support (Purdy, 2002).

Although spirituality and religion are often used interchangeably in common conversations, spirituality is a more broad concept than religiosity. Religiosity is one means of expressing spirituality, as are prayer and meditation (Puchalski, 1998). Spirituality comes from the Latin word *spiritus*, which refers to breath, air, and wind. Spirituality refers to the energy in the deepest core of the individual. It is the integrating life force that allows us to transcend our physical being and gives us ultimate meaning and purpose in life (Conrad, 1985). Spirituality represents the harmonious interconnectedness with self, others, nature, and God, and can also be communicated through, art, music, and relationships with family or the community (Puchalski & Romer, 2000). Spirituality further involves a melding of the individual's past, present, and future (Hicks, 1999). Even individuals who have no specific religion or faith background are spiritual beings and can have spiritual needs.

Religiosity refers to beliefs and practices of different faiths and an acceptance of their traditions, such as Catholicism, Eastern perspectives, Islam, Judaism, and Protestantism (Table 1-1). For many people, religion forms a basis for meaning and purpose in life, and provides the moral codes by which to live. Because illness can call into question the person's purpose in life and work, spiritual and religious issues often arise. Seventy-eight percent of Americans indicate that they receive comfort and support through religious beliefs and have greater trust in health professionals who ask them about their spiritual or religious needs (Ehman, Ott, Short, Ciampa, & Hanson-Flaschen, 1999; Koenig, 2002).

Spirituality, as a concept, also includes references to the soul as well as spiritual needs, perspectives, and spiritual well-being. Moberg (1984) conceptualized spiritual well-being as encompassing a horizontal dimension that refers to a sense of purpose and mission in life and life satisfaction, and a vertical dimension that refers to a sense of well-being in relation to God. Downey (1997, p. 16) described spirituality as "an awareness that there are levels of reality not immediately apparent and that there is a quest for personal integration in the face of forces of fragmentation and depersonalization." Therefore, spirituality is that aspect of human beings that seeks to heal or be whole (Puchalski, 2001b).

Moore (1992) has discussed the individual's spiritual quest, which is a process of "re-sacralization" of the self and the world in which we live. Individuals are embarking on spiritual journeys to discover the transcendent in daily life and in interpersonal relationships. The spiritual need is one of finding the mystery and sacredness of daily existence. Wink (1999) believes that individuals are searching for meaning outside of the confines of their religion. This is particularly important for individuals who are aging and who may be experiencing a chronic, debilitating, or life-threatening illness and who are questioning the meaning of not only their life, but of their suffering. Within this context, the spirit of the person seeks to transcend suffering through the virtues of love, hope, faith, courage, acceptance, and a sense of meaning in the encounter with death (Arnold, 1989).

Throughout a person's lifetime, and particularly as people age, religion and spirituality assist them to confront their finitude and vulnerability; to uncover meaning, value, and dignity in illness and death; to establish connection with others and a higher life force; and to find hope, love, and forgiveness in the midst of fear and despair. Thus spirituality engenders serenity and transcendence, thereby buffering stress (Doka, 1993).

As a chaplain, Ryan (1997) emphasized the five fundamental spiritual needs of all people, which include (1) finding meaning in life, particularly during adverse circumstances; (2) the need for a relationship with a higher life force or transcendent being; (3) the need to transcend the sources of suffering; (4) the need for hope no matter how

Table 1-1 **Perspectives of Major Religious Faiths**	
Religious Faith	**Perspectives**
Catholicism	• Catholics believe that Jesus was the messiah and that his death was a means of atonement for the sins of mankind. • Jesus experienced suffering, grief, and death, as do human beings. • Human beings experience the tragedy of death but are beneficiaries of its forgiveness and liberation. Emphasis is on the risen life. • Catholics follow Jesus into the mystery of death. • Faith will allow Catholics to see death as an entry into life with God. • God is viewed as a forgiving and loving God. • Confession and communion are important rituals conducted by priests. • The Sacrament of Anointing the Sick provides bodily and spiritual renewal, and this term has replaced the term *Last Rites*, which was viewed as a harbinger of death.
Eastern perspectives	• **Hinduism** originated in India with belief in the cycle of being born and dying in an infinite series of lives or successive creations. • There is a belief in karma—that every act of a human being, even an internal act such as a desire, has an effect on who that person becomes. • Most Hindus are vegetarians, including not eating eggs. • Hindus accept death philosophically, and a Hindu priest assists with the process. • Hindu rituals include tying a thread around the neck or wrist of the dying patient, and sprinkling him or her with water from the Ganges River. After death, the thread is removed and the body is bathed. • **Buddhism** is another religious perspective from India in which there is also a belief in karma and rebirth. The way to attain the truth is through the path of enlightenment or changed state of awareness, known as Nirvana. • Those practicing Buddhism are also vegetarians. • At the end of life, Buddhists monks should be consulted to offer spiritual support. After death, the monk may recite prayers for 1 hour. • A shrine of Buddha may be placed at the bedside of a ill or dying person. • Mindfulness is an important state of being and may be why patients may refuse opioids. • Most Buddhists have their body cremated. • A new incarnation is believed to occur immediately after a person's death. • **Confucianism** has its origins in China and stresses the importance of improving human relationships. The proper relationship between the living and the dead is one of continual remembrance and affection. • **Taoism** also originated in China and focuses on nature and remedying society's disorder and lack of harmony. Nature is looked toward to discover the principles of life.
Islam	• Islam means *submission*; Muslim means *one who submits*. • A Muslim is one who submits to Allah, the Arabic word for God. • Muslims, Jews, and Christians worship the same God. • The founder of Islam is Mohammed, who received a vision while meditating, which later became the Koran. • The five pillars of Islam are confession of faith daily in front of witnesses; prayer five times a day, fasting during the month of Ramadan, almsgiving, and a pilgrimage to Mecca.

Table 1-1 **Perspectives of Major Religious Faiths—cont'd**

Religious Faith	Perspectives
Islam—cont'd	• In diet and fasting, pork, bacon, and ham are forbidden, as well as alcohol. Beef, mutton, and poultry must be *halal* (killed and prepared under Islamic law). Fasting during Ramadan is not required of the sick. • Second-degree male relatives (e.g., cousins or uncles) should be contacted when a person is sick. They determine if a person or family should be told the diagnosis or prognosis. • Patients may choose to face Mecca (east), and the head should be elevated above the body. • Discussions about death are not usually welcomed. • Grief may be expressed by slapping or hitting the body. • Same-sex Muslims should handle the body after death; otherwise, the individual should wear gloves so as not to touch the body.
Judaism	• Judaism began when the descendants of Abraham's grandson Israel were enslaved in Egypt. Moses led them to Palestine. During this time, Jewish law was divinely revealed to Moses. The law is known as the Torah. • The Sabbath is celebrated from sunset on Friday to sunset on Saturday evening. The Sabbath is the day of rest. • The degree to which a Jew observes the Sabbath and other rituals depends on whether he or she is Orthodox, Conservative, or Reformed. • Observant Jews will eat only kosher foods that have been prepared under strict guidelines and monitoring by a rabbi. Meat and milk are eaten separately, and seafood and pork are prohibited. A vegetarian diet is acceptable if a kosher meal is not available. • Focus is on life and its preservation, and on the fostering and establishing of religion in the life of people on earth. • Everything must be done to prolong life and no actions taken to hasten death. • Illness and death are neither punishment nor reward. • Death is considered inevitable. • A dying person should never be left alone. • Autopsy, embalming, and cremation are not acceptable. • The memory of the deceased must be perpetuated. • The funeral is a rite of separation. • *Shiva* refers to the 7-day intensive mourning period beginning right after the funeral.
Protestantism	• Spirituality is viewed as a dimension of humanness, a process of interaction, and an awareness of relationship. • Spirituality is lived through one's religion, which is regarded as a cultural institution. • God protects but judges. Each Protestant has a direct and personal relationship with God unmediated by a priest or sacrament. • Suffering and overcoming evil are the core of Protestant teaching. The focus is on salvation. • The issue is not how the individual can participate in Jesus's suffering, but rather the individual accepting the gift of God's grace through Jesus's death. • Some groups accept anointing the sick. • There are no Last Rites, but prayers are given to offer support.

Data from Sherman, D. W. (2001). Spiritual and cultural competence in palliative care. In M. Matzo & D. W. Sherman (Eds.), *Palliative care nursing: Quality care to the end of life* (pp. 3–47). New York: Springer Publishers; and Kirkwood, N. (1993). *A hospital handbook on multiculturalism and religion: Practical guidelines for health care workers.* Newtown, NW: Millennium Books.

difficult life can be; and (5) the need to have others who share our life journey and care for us. As one example, a 68-year-old woman with advanced breast cancer revealed her spiritual need when she stated "I only wish there was one person in this world who could tell me that they love me."

Benefits of Religiosity and Spirituality for Older Adults

In a study of religiosity, Bergan and McConatha (2000) reported that religious affiliation and private religious devotion increased with age across the life span. Based on a sample of 2025 community-dwelling elder residents, it was found that religious attendance provided a persistent protective effect against mortality, even after controlling for most potential confounders, such as social support, health status, and physical functioning (Oman & Reed, 1998).

Based on a sample of community-residing and institutionalized older adults, Fry (2000) found that personal meaning, involvement in formal religion, sense of inner peace with self, and accessibility to religious resources were significant predictors of well-being. Religiosity and spirituality contributed more significantly to the variance in well-being than did demographic variables, social resources, physical health, or negative life events. These results support the findings of Mull, Cox, and Sullivan (1987), based on a random sample of 380 older adults in specialized housing units, that as more symptoms were reported, personal religious practices increased, including the frequency of prayer and listening to religious programs, as well as the importance of religious beliefs. Religious beliefs and practices served as a coping mechanism to deal with life's problems and as a source of social support.

Interested in religiosity and spirituality, Heintz and Baruss (2001) conducted a study based on a sample of 30 people whose mean age was 72.6 years. Although some religious behaviors, such as frequent religious practice, prayer, and church attendance, were correlated with some dimensions of spirituality, many of the scores on the Expressions of Spirituality Inventory were independent of self-reported religious behaviors. These results reinforced the differences between the concepts of religiosity and spirituality.

In a qualitative study of 41 male and female residents ages 66 to 92 years, most of the older adults believed that a higher power was present in their lives, which supported them constantly and was perceived as protecting, guiding, helping, teaching, and healing them (Mackenzie, Rajogopal, Meibohm, & Lavizzo-Mourey, 2000). God was perceived to work through the mundane world, such as through the work of physicians, loving friends, and helpful strangers. Many felt that their relationship with God formed the foundation of their psychological well-being. The authors concluded that the subjective experience of spiritual support may form the core of the spirituality-health connection for older adults.

Hyland (1996) examined the influence of religiosity on an older person's adjustment to the nursing home environment. A total of 60 nursing home residents, ages 65 to 108, completed the Index of Religiosity, the Religious Orientation Scale—Revised, and the Geriatric Depression Scale. Results indicated that the residents were highly religious and that intrinsic religious motivation was a significant predictor of adjustment to the nursing home, as measured by the Geriatric Depression Scale.

In a study of homebound elders, Brennan (1994) found that spirituality became more important and meaningful to them over the years and that personal prayer was the most common expression of spirituality. Sharing their personal beliefs with another person was an important aspect of their spirituality.

Spirituality and Health Care

Physicians, psychologists, and other professionals are researching the role of spirituality in health care. Research indicates that spirituality is related to mortality, coping, and recovery, because people with regular spiritual practices tend to live longer; utilize health beliefs in coping with illness, pain, and life stress; and have enhanced recovery from illness and surgery (Puchalski, 2001a). A systematic review of the literature published during the 20th century revealed, based on 724 quantitative studies, a significant relationship between religious involvement and better mental health, greater social support, and less substance abuse (Koenig, Cohen, & Blazer, 1992). In a study of religious coping in 850 hospitalized patients, a significant inverse correlation ($p < .001$) was found between religious coping and depressive symptoms (Koenig et al., 1992).

In another study examining the speed of recovery from depression of 87 medical inpatients, Koenig, George, and Peterson (1998) reported that, of nearly 30 baseline characteristics, intrinsic religiosity was one of only five independent predictors of the speed of recovery.

In terms of health consequences, religious involvement has been associated with improved attendance at medical appointments, greater adherence to medical regimens, and improved medical outcomes. Studies indicate that those who are religious or spiritual have lower blood pressure, fewer cardiac events, better results following heart surgery, and longer survival in general (Koenig, 2002). Furthermore, religious or spiritual practices are believed to influence sympathetic and parasympathetic nerve pathways connecting thoughts and emotions to circulatory and immune system changes, counteracting stress-related physiologic states that impair healing (Koenig, 2002).

Religion or spirituality also facilitates coping with chronic pain, disability, and serious illness by providing an indirect form of control that helps to interrupt the cycle of anxiety and depression. For some individuals, prayer provides a form of control by believing that, through prayer, they can influence their medical outcome; in contrast, others deliberately turn over to God their health situation (Koenig, 2002). The belief that God is with them provides relief from loneliness and isolation. Individuals who attend religious services also have an opportunity for socialization and support from others, and praying for others in need often provides a distraction from one's own pain (Koenig, 2002).

Role of Religiosity and Spirituality in Coping with Serious Illness

As older adults are faced with chronic or serious illness and eventually near death, they may experience despair, with spiritual and religious concerns intensified or awakened (Lo et al., 2002). The elder may struggle with the physical aspects of the disease, as well as the pain related to mental and spiritual suffering. He or she may ask "Why did this happen to me?", "Why is God allowing me to suffer?", "What will happen after I die?", "Will I be remembered or missed?", or "Will I be able to finish my life's work?" (Puchalski, 2002). True healing requires an answer to these questions because healing can be experienced as acceptance of illness and peace with one's life (Puchalski, 2001a).

It is through spirituality that people find meaning in illness and suffering and are liberated from their despair. Spiritual care changes chaos to order, and seeks to discern what, if any, blessings might be revealed in spite of and even through tragedy (Purdy, 2002). As people are dying, they want to be listened to, to have someone share their fears, to be forgiven by God or by others, and to believe that they will live on in the hearts of others or through their good works (Puchalski, 2002).

Taylor and Outlaw (2002) conducted a qualitative study to understand the use of prayer among persons with cancer ($N = 30$) and recognized that individuals with cancer use prayer to cope with their illness. Participants viewed prayer as personal communication involving or allowing transcendence. The communication or prayer was initiative and receptive. The initiative aspect of praying was to talk to God, get in touch with God, or beseech God, while the receptive aspect of prayer was characterized by phrases such as "being quiet," "being accessible," and "listening to God." For these individuals, prayer meant being constantly conscious of God and coming into that higher intention in life. Participants' illnesses increased their awareness of the inadequacy of relying on self and the need to rely on a greater power. Some described prayer as an active cognitive process, while others described prayer as a more passive process or as "prayer of the heart." Assistive strategies for praying included constructing a prayer, writing a prayer, relaxing, and reading religious material, and how one prayed depended on the purpose of the prayer. Some individuals prayed about healing, or that "God's will be done." Many prayed for forgiveness or to be a better person. Most prayed for family and friends who needed peace and support, and also included thanks and praise in their prayers that they were given another day to live. Through the process of prayer, many individuals believed that they benefited, whether their prayer was answered or not. From prayer, they expected that the "best will happen," or that they would receive comfort, forgiveness, or salvation. For health professionals, the implications for prayer are that clinicians can help by fostering a

EVIDENCE-BASED PRACTICE

Reference: Pargament, K., Koenig, H., Tatakeshwar, N., & Hanh, J. (2001). Religious struggle as a predictor of mortality among medically ill elder patients: A two-year longitudinal study. *Archives of Internal Medicine, 161,* 1881-1885.

Research Problem: To investigate longitudinally the relationship between positive religious coping and religious struggle with an illness and mortality.

Design: A longitudinal cohort study from 1996 to 1997.

Sample and Setting: 596 patients, ages 55 and older, on the medical inpatient services of a Veterans Affairs Medical Center in North Carolina.

Methods: T test and chi-square test statistics were used to compare survivors and deceased with respect to their demographic characteristics, physical health, mental health, positive religious coping, religious struggle, and global religiousness. To determine whether religious coping was a significant predictor of mortality, Cox regression analyses were used.

Results: Compared with the deceased, survivors were significantly younger, more educated, and white, with fewer medical diagnoses, less severe illness, better subjective health, more independent functional status, better cognitive functioning, and better mood and quality of life at baseline. With respect to positive religious coping and religious struggle, both groups reported low religious struggle; however, the survivors reported lower levels of religious struggle at baseline and attended church more frequently. Based on Cox regression analyses, religious struggle was a significant predictor of increased risk for mortality in the model and remained significant after controlling for the demographic variables and the variables of physical and mental heath. The items that were the most significant predictors of increased risk for mortality were "Has God abandoned me?", "Does God love me?", and "God is punishing me."

Implications for Nursing Practice: The results suggest that spiritual assessment is important in identifying individuals who have religious struggle and that interventions that support positive religious coping and church attendance may improve health outcomes.

Conclusion: Certain forms of religiousness may increase the risk of death. Ill elder men and women who experience religious struggle with their illness appear to be at increased risk of death, even after controlling for baseline health, mental health status, and demographic factors.

condition and environment conducive to prayer and can facilitate patient's use of prayer, which is unique to individuals.

In a study of 19 individuals with advanced cancer, Thomas and Retsas (1999) learned through in-depth interviews that people with cancer developed a spiritual perspective that strengthened their approach to life and death. As cancer progressed, participants described the transaction of self-preservation by discovering deeper levels of understanding self, which incorporated a higher level of spiritual growth, spiritual awareness, and spiritual experiences.

Individuals at the end of life also express spiritual needs. Based on a qualitative study of nine hospice patients, Hermann (2001) reported their need for religion, companionship, involvement, and control; the need to finish business; the need to experience nature; and the need for a positive outlook. Participants perceived spirituality as a broad concept that may or may not involve religion and believed that spiritual needs were closely linked to the purpose and meaning in life. In studying older patients approaching the end of life from advanced heart disease, it was found that 24% of the variance in their global quality of life was predicted by their spirituality (Berry, Baas, Fowler, & Allen, 2002).

Spirituality and Palliative Care
Even as the physical body declines, healing, which means to make whole, can occur as

spiritual needs are identified and spiritual care is given to restore a person to wholeness. Healing can be accomplished through the spiritual journey of remembering, assessing, searching for meaning, forgiving, reconciling, loving, and maintaining hope (Puchalski, 1998a). Holistic care, including care of the soul or spirit, is important to quality palliative care, whose goal is to enhance a person's quality of life across the illness trajectory. People do want their spiritual needs addressed at the end of life and feel that health professionals should speak to patients about their spiritual concerns (Gallop, 1997). Furthermore, elder individuals who are dying express the need for companionship and spiritual support, particularly human contact, and to have the opportunity to pray alone or with others (Nathan Cummings Foundation, 1999).

When providing palliative care for older adults and their families, it is important to remember the principles outlined in Box 1-2.

Spirituality or Religiosity During the Dying Process

The attitudes an elder individual holds regarding the dying process and death are embedded in his or her cultural and religious values. Values affect the way individuals conceptualize death and behave in relation to death (Meagher & Bell,

---

Box 1-2 Principles for Providing Palliative Care

- Each person has a spiritual dimension.
- Illness and death can be opportunities for spiritual growth.
- Spiritual care may be different for each individual depending on his or her religious or cultural background.
- Spirituality is supported through formal and informal ways, such as religious practices, secular practices, symbols, rituals, art forms, prayer and meditation.
- Care should be offered in settings that accommodate the needs of religious or spiritual practices and rituals, and promote spiritual work.

From Morgan, J. D. (1993). The existential quest for meaning. In K. Doka & J. Morgan (Eds.), *Death and spirituality* (pp. 12-13). Amityville, NY: Baywood Publishing Company.

1993). Many people return to the religious legacies of their childhood during the dying process because it may have been the first time that they heard about death and learned about Christian resurrection (Satterly, 2001).

At this time, it would be important for the health care professional to explore guilt as central to the older adult's religious pain, as well as the concept of forgiveness from his or her religious perspective. Religious rituals for cleansing or religious doctrine may allay feelings of remorse and guilt, providing for renewal of the soul and redemption. In supporting elders in spiritual pain, it may also be helpful to consider the concept of love. Most religious traditions provide a hopeful belief in the unconditional love of God, as well as reinforcing how unconditional love can be allowed for the self, especially when an individual may have previously engaged in self-criticism or self-hatred (Satterly, 2001).

Doka (1993) identified the spiritual need of individuals to die in a way that is consistent with their self-identity as they approach death. For example, if a person's approach to life has also been to remain in control and "not give up the fight," then it would be expected that he or she may not want to forego aggressive therapies, even if the chances of cure or remission are low. The person's spiritual need may be to continue to fight the disease. For those who are dying, Doka (1993) also emphasizes the spiritual task of finding hope that extends beyond the grave, as one seeks a sense of symbolic immortality. Individuals often need to feel that they are leaving a legacy, whether through having children or being remembered through their contributions to community, or through artwork, music, or their writings.

Role of Hope in Spiritual Well-Being

Cousins (1979) reminded us that death is not the ultimate tragedy of life, but rather being separated from our connection with others, and separated from a desire to experience the things that make life worth living, separated from hope. Spirituality may help people to cope with their dying because it may offer hope. In early illness, the hope may be for the cure of the disease, for treatment, and later on for the hope of prolongation of life. When cure is not possible, hope may be to see a loved one, to have a day without pain, to celebrate a certain life event, or have the time to travel or complete unfinished business. Eventually, hope may be for a peaceful death. It may be hope that allows seriously ill individuals to find courage and strength to transcend their suffering, and teach others how to die with dignity.

In redefining hope for the seriously ill or the dying, Corr (1991) distinguished between hope and a "wish," stating that hope is grounded in reality, while wishing is not. Mitchell (1997) offered a definition that hope is not a belief that something is going to go well, but rather that whatever happens will make sense, no matter how it turns out. For elders who are dying, hope may be defined as "an inner life force that helps each dying person to live life until the moment of death" (Parker-Oliver, p. 116, 2002). Indeed, hope may be defined as the positive expectation for meaning attached to an event, recognizing that individuals shape their hopes by finding new meanings for living (Parker-Oliver, 2002). Hope allows for a sense of control and promotes active rather than passive participation in life's events. Even in dying, people have the hope to discover new meanings.

The challenge for health care professionals is therefore to help individuals find hope as they search for meaning in their illness, suffering, and death. This can happen as professionals assist individuals to identify key relationships, facilitate caring relationships, and encourage the opportunity to heal relationships and complete unfinished business. Byock (1997) encouraged the completion of relationships by saying "I forgive you," "Forgive me," "I love you," "Thank you," and "Goodbye." Through the encouragement of short-term, attainable goals, hope can also be promoted by recognizing and encouraging a sense of determination and courage in the face of adversity.

Hope can also be found within the context of spirituality, because spiritual beliefs systems hold hope for happiness, and a promise of an afterlife. Spirituality offers hope for living on in the world through a connection with others, traditions, and rituals and through establishing legacies. Hope can also be easily discovered by just asking elders what is meaningful to them and what they want to do with the remainder of their lives. Based on a study of 69 participants age 65 or older, Theris

(2001) reported a significant difference in hope based on the religion of participants. According to the results of a one-way analysis of variance and Scheffe tests, Catholic participants expressed greater hope than those of the Jewish faith, and another significant difference existed between participants of the Protestant and Jewish faiths. There was also a significant, positive correlation between spirituality and level of hope ($r = .73$, $p = .000$). In a multiple regression analysis used to test for the combined contribution of spirituality and connectedness with others to levels of hope, only spirituality emerged as a significant predictor of hope. The author concluded that connection with oneself and connection with a higher being were especially important in the maintenance of hope in nursing home residents. Such results are consistent with the findings of Buchanan (1993), who reported, based on a sample of 160 older adults who were depressed and nondepressed, that higher levels of spirituality, hope, health, and social support were positively correlated with meaning in life, and that there was an inverse relationship between meaning in life and depression.

For those who are dying, the focus of hope changes from a hope in the future, or a redefinition of the future, to a hope in living day to day. The focus of hope for those with advanced disease is also hope for no more suffering, hope for life after death, and hope that their families will not suffer when they are gone (Duggleby, 2001). At times, the most important way to provide hope is by listening attentively and being physically present, which convey a sense of value and affirmation of worth. The individual then gains hope that he or she will not be abandoned and isolated (Duggleby, 2000).

Based on qualitative studies of elder hospice patients, Herth (1992) found that hope facilitated the transcendence of the present situation and movement toward new awareness and enrichment of being, while Duggleby (2000) found that hope was a process of enduring suffering through a trust in a higher power and making meaning of one's life.

Conversations about Spiritual or Religious Issues

Conversations regarding spiritual needs often begin with the use of open-ended questions, such as "Do you have any thoughts about why this is happening to you?" Practitioners can also encourage the patient to say more by such statements as "Tell me more about that." When exploring spiritual concerns, practitioners should acknowledge and normalize patient's concerns by comments such as "Many patients ask the same question," and responding with empathetic comments, such as "That sounds like a painful situation" (Lo et al., 2002).

Pitfalls in discussions about spiritual or religious issues near the end of life often occur by trying to solve the elder patient's problems or resolve unanswerable questions; going beyond the practitioner's expertise or role in providing spiritual care; imposing one's beliefs on the patient; or providing premature reassurance, which may appear superficial or deter the disclosure of other important issues or emotions (Lo et al., 2002). When patients inquire about the religious background of the practitioner, they may be inquiring to determine whether it is safe to talk about spiritual or religious issues, or they may prefer to talk to someone who shares the same religious faith. The practitioner may answer the question regarding his or her religious background, but need not explicate his or her religious or spiritual beliefs (Lo et al., 2002). If the patient asks for details, it is appropriate to refocus the conversation back to the patient.

In addition to clarifying the elder patient's spiritual concerns and needs by following spiritual cues and exploring emotions with emphatic support, health care professionals may also

- Make wish statements, such as "I also wish you were not ill"
- Identify common goals for care and reach agreement on clinical decisions
- Mobilize support for the patient and family from family, church members, or the community (Lo et al., 2002)

When the older adult or his or her family is praying for a miracle even in medically futile situations, the role of health professionals is to respect their beliefs and remain supportive by trying to understand their worldview and the role their beliefs have in coping. Criticism or confrontation will lead to distrust and close the dialogue between health care professionals and the elder. When older patients and their families feel that they can talk to health professionals about their religious or spiritual beliefs, there is a greater chance that they will accept what the professional is saying. A response may be that "Sometimes God answers our prayers for healing in interpersonal ways that may ultimately be more important than physical healing" (Koenig, 2002, p. 492.)

Conducting a Spiritual Assessment

Holistic care involves assessment not only of physical, emotional, and social needs, but also of spiritual needs and expectations. A spiritual history is a history about a person's values or beliefs that explicitly opens the door to conversations about the role of spirituality and religion in the person's life (Puchalski & Romer, 2000). Although it is not the health professional's responsibility to solve spiritual problems or provide answers, health practitioners need to conduct a spiritual assessment to identify when a older adult or family member is experiencing spiritual distress. It is important to create an environment that nurtures the patient's exploration of spiritual needs and concerns, and supports him or her in the search for answers. A spiritual history or assessment should be completed with each new patient visit and on annual examinations, as a part of routine history taking (Puchalski, 2001b). A spiritual history inquires about the role religion or spirituality plays in the elder patient's ability to cope with illness. Affiliation with a religious or spiritual community is important for many individuals, and such communities often serves as an extended family for many older adults, especially those who live alone or have limited family support (Koenig, 2002). In taking a spiritual history, Puchalski (1999) suggested that the mnemonic FICA (faith, influence, community, and addressing spiritual concerns) be used (Box 1-3).

A spiritual history is important not only in identifying ways older adults may cope with adverse life circumstances, but also to examine potential negative effects in elders for whom religious beliefs are a source of distress and emotional turmoil (Koenig, 2002). Religious pain is a condition in which the patient feels guilty over the violation of the moral codes or values of his or her religious tradition. This may arise as a result of major transgressions such as abortion,

Box 1-3 **Taking a Spiritual History**
<ul><li>**F:** Faith, as identified by the question, "What is your faith or beliefs and do you consider yourself religious or spiritual?"</li><li>**I:** Influence, which is assessed by the question, "How does your faith or spirituality influence your medical decisions?"</li><li>**C:** Community, which is related to the question, "Are you a part of a spiritual or religious community?"</li><li>**A:** Addressing spiritual concerns, as exemplified by the question, "Would you like someone to address your spiritual needs or concerns?"</li></ul>

From Puchalski, C. M. (1999). Taking a Spiritual history: FICA. *Spirituality & Medicine Connection*, 3, 1.

Box 1-4 **Conducting a Spiritual Interview**
S Spiritual belief system (religious affiliation)
P Personal spirituality (beliefs and practices of affiliation that the patient and family accept)
I Integration with a spiritual community (role of the religious/spiritual group; individual's role in the group)
R Ritualized practices and restrictions (beliefs that health care providers should remember during care)
I Implications for medical care
T Terminal events planning (impact of beliefs on advance directives; contacting the clergy)

From Highfield, M. (2000). Providing spiritual care to patients with cancer. *Clinical Journal of Oncology Nursing*, 4(3), 115-120.

adultery, or overt cruelty, or from minor transgressions such as not seeking a second opinion or failing to take better care of one's self. As a result, the patient may feel that that God is disappointed in his or her past or present behaviors, actions, or thoughts (Satterly, 2001). Feelings of guilt are often accompanied by a fear of punishment from God, or a fear that God does not love them or has abandoned them in their time of need.

Individuals may believe that future punishment from God can be avoided if enough self-pain is endured in the here and now (Satterly, 2001). Such may be the case for individuals who refuse pain medications, and may warrant spiritual exploration by members of the palliative care team. Chaplains have the knowledge and skills to discuss spiritual issues related to a patient's perceived need for pain and suffering, and they may provide an alternative perspective concerning the patient's perception of either a punishing or a forgiving God. In some cases, a patient may refuse to speak with the chaplain or clergy because he or she is angry with God, thereby rejecting religion or his or her spirituality as a source of comfort. It is important for health care professionals to recognize that religious or spiritual pain is highly personal and deeply subjective, and does not have to make "sense" to the professional in order for a patient to experience it (Satterly, 2001).

Religious beliefs may also influence an individual's decisions about medical treatments, particularly if he or she becomes seriously ill, such as decisions related to cardiopulmonary resuscitation or withholding or withdrawal of life-prolonging treatments. Medical therapies may also be refused if a patient is a Jehovah's Witness or Christian Scientist; in such situations, health professionals need to understand the patient's viewpoint and show respect for his or her beliefs (Koenig, 2002).

As an approach to spiritual assessment, Highfield (2000) used the letters from the word "SPIRIT" to remember questions appropriate to a spiritual interview (Box 1-4). Spiritual assessment further includes assessment of personal beliefs, sources of meaning and hope, values, belief in an afterlife, and sense of connection to self, others, nature, and God. Health practitioners can begin to address spirituality by asking such questions as "How are your spirits?", "How do you define your spirit?", "What nourishes your spirit?", or "How have you relieved your spiritual pain in the past?" (O'Connor, 1993). For older adults with life-limiting or life-threatening illness, there are valuable questions to explore (Box 1-5).

Hermann (2000) suggested asking in a spiritual assessment such additional questions as

Box 1-5 **Spiritual Assessment**

- Are you suffering in physical, emotional, social, or spiritual ways?
- What is the meaning of illness and suffering?
- Do you see purpose in your suffering?
- Are you able to transcend your suffering?
- Are you at peace, or feeling hope and despair?
- Do your personal beliefs help you to cope with anxiety about pain and death and provide a way for achieving peace?

From Puchalski, C. M. (1999). Taking a Spiritual history: FICA. *Spirituality & Medicine Connection, 3,* 1.

"What gives your life meaning and purpose?", "Do you have goals you would still like to achieve?", "How has your diagnosis changed the meaning of your life?", "What kinds of things do you hope for?", and "To whom do you turn to for help?" Practitioners should also observe for objective data such as signs of depression, flat affect, or refusal of treatment, as well as the presence of religious, spiritual, or inspirational books or other literature, or jewelry (Hermann, 2000).

Health professionals may recognize spiritual pain as the older adult expresses sorrow or grief or verbalizes a sense of meaninglessness or emptiness to life, fear and avoidance of the future, a sense of hopelessness and despair, anger toward God, and a sense of isolation of self and others (Matthews, 1999). It is important to realize that indications of spiritual pain can be both verbal and nonverbal, and that, just as physical pain may change in nature and intensity over time, so too can spiritual pain change over time. As death approaches, new spiritual issues may arise that may or may not be accompanied by spiritual pain (O'Connor, 1993). Furthermore, although health professionals may wish to alleviate spiritual pain, it is important to recognize the meaning and value of experiencing pain from the patient's perspective. Some individuals may believe that pain will lead to salvation or is a way of coming closer to God.

The assessment of spiritual needs is important in determining meaningful ways of providing spiritual care. Spiritual care, in the form of listening, presence, and nonabandonment, can provide the encouragement, nonjudgmental support, and connection important to finding meaning in life, suffering, and death, and can support older adults in ways that allow them to actualize their human potential and experience personal growth even as death approaches.

Instruments to Measure Spirituality

In the past several years there has been a focus on the role of spirituality, as distinct from religion, in coping with illness. However, there remains a dearth of well-validated, psychometrically sound instruments to measure aspects of spirituality (Peterman, Fitchett, Brady, Hernandez, & Cella, 2002). One instrument that is a psychometrically sound measure of spiritual well-being is the Functional Assessment of Chronic Illness Therapy–Spiritual Well-Being (FACIT-Sp). This instrument comprises two subscales, one measuring a sense of meaning and peace and the other assessing the role of faith in illness. The FACIT-Sp has convergent validity with five other measures of spirituality and religion in samples of early-stage and metastatic cancer diagnoses, as well as documented reliability. A total score can be obtained.

A second spirituality assessment instrument with clinical utility is Paloutzian and Ellison's Spiritual Well-Being Scale, which has also been administered to 70 family members caring for a relative with life-limiting illness. This 20-item instrument yields three scores: a total score of spiritual well-being (overall score); an existential well-being score, which relates to feelings about meaning and purpose in life, feelings about the future, and sense of well-being; and a religious well-being score that represents a sense of support and connection with God (Kirschling & Pittman, 1989).

Such instruments are of value in conducting research studies that explore the relationships of spirituality and quality of life for palliative-care patients. By identifying a patient or family member's sense of spiritual well-being or spiritual distress, spiritual interventions may be provided to maintain or improve spiritual well-being and hopefully the quality of life and quality of dying as perceived by patients and family members.

EVIDENCE-BASED PRACTICE

Reference: Walsh, K., King, M., Jones, L., Tookman, A., & Blizard, R. (2002). Spiritual beliefs may affect outcome of bereavement: A prospective study. *British Medical Journal, 324,* 1551-1559.

Research Problem: To explore the relation between spiritual beliefs and resolution of bereavement.

Design: Prospective cohort study of people about to be bereaved with follow-up continuing for 14 months after death.

Sample and Setting: 135 relatives and close friends of patients admitted to the Marie Curie Centre for palliative care in London.

Methods: Using a priori basis, the sample was divided into three groups on the basis of their beliefs: no spiritual belief, low spiritual belief, and high spiritual belief. Using a one-way analysis of variance, the three groups were compared on core bereavement items and on a measure of grief at 1, 9, and 14 months after the patient's death. A repeated measures analysis compared the groups on the outcomes at the three time points, and the interaction of time and strength of belief was also tested.

Results: People reporting no spiritual belief had not resolved their grief by 14 months after the death. Participants with strong spiritual beliefs resolved their grief progressively over the same period. People with low levels of belief showed little change in the first 9 months, but their grief lessened thereafter. These differences approached significance in a repeated-measures analysis of variance ($F = 2.42, p = .058$). Strength of spiritual belief remained an important predictor after controlling for confounding variables (age and sex). At 14 months, the difference between the group with no beliefs and the groups with low and high beliefs combined was 7.30 (95% confidence interval, 0.86 to 13.73) on the core bereavement item scale.

Implications for Nursing Practice: Spiritual beliefs may provide an existential framework in which grief is resolved more readily, with the strength of belief having an effect on resolution of bereavement. The focus on spiritual matters may be important for both the dying person and his or her family members. The absence of spiritual beliefs may be a risk factor for complicated grief.

Conclusion: People who profess stronger spiritual beliefs seem to resolve their grief more rapidly and completely after the death of a close person than do people with no spiritual beliefs. Most palliative care units involve the family and friends of the person dying; attention to spiritual matters is an important component of this work.

Spiritual Caregiving

"Spiritual care is so much more than religious care. Spiritual care discovers, reverences, and tends the spirit—that is the energy or place of meaning and values—of another human being" (Driscoll, 2001, p. 334). In providing spiritual care to the older adult, health professionals express the capacity to enter the world of others; to respond to fears, concerns, and feelings with compassion; and to bear witness to the physical, emotional, social, and spiritual dimensions of their suffering. As adults age, health care professionals can provide an opportunity for elders to find intrinsic dignity, which is the dignity that comes from being a human being with inherent value and worth. By reviewing past life experiences, health professionals can assist elders to reflect on their life accomplishments and the value of their relationships with others; to forgive or be forgiven by others; and to say goodbye. Support can be given to older adults to complete unfinished tasks or goals, and to make peace with themselves or with God.

During hospitalizations, health professionals may ask if the person would like to speak with the clergy or chaplain or have the opportunity to attend a hospital worship service. Patients may also be asked if they would like someone to pray with or for them or have spiritual reading materials. Prayer has been identified as the most frequently reported alternative treatment modality of elders, with women and blacks using prayer as a coping strategy significantly more than men and whites (Dunn & Horgas, 2000). At times, if the older adult is of the same faith background as the health professional, the patient may request joint prayer. However, prayer is appropriate only when the patient wants it and will be comforted by it (Koenig, 2002). Prayer should not be prescribed because the risk is that the intention is not patient centered but provider centered, and in that context prayers offered by health professionals may be viewed as coercive (Koenig, 2002). The existing religious or spiritual beliefs of the older adult should be supported and encouraged, yet the end of life is not the appropriate time to introduce new or unfamiliar spiritual beliefs or practices (Koenig, 2002). In a study of 30 individuals with cancer, Taylor, Outlaw, Bernardo, and Roy (1999) reported that several individuals described hesitancies about petitionary prayers for particular things, for cure, or for themselves, and described inner conflicts about releasing control to God.

If a person is not religious or does not want a health professional to address religious issues, spiritual conversations around hope, love, courage, and forgiveness can occur in the provider–patient relationship (Koenig, 2002). Patients and health professionals of different faith backgrounds can appreciate the commonalities of basic human needs, such as love and hope, and can explore issues of coping and what it means to live with an illness. Although health professionals can assess spiritual needs and address uncomplicated spiritual issues, caring and listening is the intervention, not giving advice or trying to address spiritual problems (Koenig, 2002).

Addressing spiritual problems is the role of the chaplain or clergy, as a member of the interdisciplinary team. The chaplain is a health care professional who has been trained to offer spiritual care to all people of any or no religious tradition and whose primary focus is the spiritual needs of patients, families, and staff (Driscoll, 2001). Like other members of the palliative care team, chaplains are alert to the expressed needs of the patient. As counselors, they take time to listen, discern the significance of the words spoken, intuit what is the importance of what is unspoken, and affirm the value of shared silence

(Purdy, 2002). Often spiritual support involves listening to rhetorical questions, in cases in which the patient wants an honest hearing of the question rather than an answer. Patients may want to explore with chaplains whether God exists, the meaning of mortality, what Heaven is like, who goes to Hell, the integrity of doubt, the possibility of a miracle, the need to forgive, or the loneliness of suffering (Purdy, 2002). Patients and their families experience spiritual support when interdisciplinary team members actively listen to their anxiety and allow discussion of the question, "Are we doing the right thing here?" (Purdy, 2002). Health professionals can also provide support by silent witnessing and being present, as well as serving as a liaison with other health professionals in addressing physical, emotional, and spiritual needs (Hicks, 1999).

Humor also has an effect on the spiritual aspect of healing, because many patients find humor "spiritually uplifting." As an element of spirituality and a coping method for spiritual growth and healing, humor can be transcendent, momentarily removing one from an isolated state to join in surprise at ludicrous human situations (Johnson, 2002). In a study of nine women with breast cancer, participants stated that they looked for meaning in their lives through spirituality and humor, because humor helped them to laugh at themselves and life. For some, it appeared that God had a sense of humor and that finding humorous moments was a step to recovery because humor heals and gives hope to survive the moment (Johnson, 2002).

Health professionals can also encourage older patients to socialize with friends, family, and children, as well as encouraging them to help others, even if only by active listening. Supporting others often preserves an older person's meaning in life and sense of usefulness. Older adults can also pass on their legacy to others by recording personal histories, telling stories, and reminiscing about the past. If the older adult is isolated, the health practitioner can suggest that he or she watch spiritual or religious television programs or provide an opportunity for the elder to enjoy his or her favorite sacred or secular music, or other forms of art (Hermann, 2000). Practitioners may encourage opportunities for patients to experience nature in whatever ways they can, such as a walk or wheelchair ride in the garden or courtyard so that they can sit outside feeling the air and warmth of the sun.

Spiritual uplifting in the present moment can also occur as the practitioner attempts to create meaning and a source of pleasure in the moment. This can be done by encouraging, through story telling, the reliving of a pleasurable experience in the patient's past while making plans to experience a physical or emotional pleasure in the near future. As one example, a bed-bound patient with Parkinsonism found a moment of meaning and pleasure in the day by retelling to the nurse practitioner a story from his childhood, while anticipating a favorite meal to brought in by his family the following day. Spiritual care can also involve "making meaning" through other forms of life review, such as looking at old photographs or personal memorabilia, or reading old letters or diary entries. By such efforts, health care professionals can acknowledge the individuality of older adults and promote their sense of connection to self, others, and nature, thereby supporting their spirits and sense of well-being.

Spiritual support for elders may also be available through parish nursing, which expands home health and public health provider roles. Parish nursing uses the faith community as a cooperative means of successful health promotion and maintenance for the older adult (Boland, 1998). In a survey of parish, oncology, and hospice nurses, the most frequently identified spiritual interventions were referral, prayer, active listening, facilitation and validation of patients' thoughts and feelings, conveying acceptance, and instilling hope (Sellers & Haag, 1998).

Learning about Spiritual Assessment and Caregiving

Health professionals need to be attuned to their own spirituality before participating in spiritual care of older adults. Personal preparation for spiritual caregiving includes the professional's self-evaluation of personal spirituality; reviewing personal beliefs, opinions, and biases; understanding the meaning of spirituality; becoming aware of how one's own cultural and religious beliefs influence caregiving; and establishing a trusting patient–provider relationship (Hermann, 2000).

As in the care of all patients and families, health professionals caring for older adults and their families must learn the specific techniques for addressing spirituality in clinical practice, including how to conduct a spiritual assessment. This also requires that the health professional be totally present and open by listening actively to spiritual issues (Hermann, 2000). Learning spiritual assessment and caregiving can also occur through a combination of teaching/learning strategies, including small group discussions; reflective writing, storytelling, and use of poetry; case presentation and discussion; panel discussions with chaplains, patients, and health care practitioners; role playing with standardized patients; and attending lectures on the role of spirituality in health care (Puchalski, 2001b).

In providing spiritual care, health care professionals must remember that religion is only one way of enhancing spiritual well-being. Conversations about life, love, hope, trust, and forgiveness may renew the spirit of both patients and health care providers. Although the perspective of health professionals is one of personal value in one's role as a health practitioner, it is important to be nonjudgmental, never imposing one's own beliefs and values on the patient or family, and always remembering that it is the spiritual or religious perspective of the patient or family that is important. Indeed, the therapeutic value of the self will be recognized through listening, presence, and nonabandonment.

Case Study Conclusion

Mrs. M.'s weakness and fatigue progressed, with only a slight improvement in her left-sided weakness. She spent the last 6 months of her life in the loving care of her family with the support of hospice. The nurse continued to address Mrs. M.'s physical needs, which were increasing pain, constipation, and nausea, while recognizing the multidimensional aspects of her suffering. Mrs. M. enjoyed her visits with the hospice chaplain, who was a Catholic priest. He prayed with her at her request, administered weekly Holy Communion, and administered the Sacrament of the Anointing of the Sick. Like Mrs. M., the family expressed its appreciation for the chaplain's spiritual sensitivity and care.

Spiritual support was further offered by the nurse practitioner, who recognized the value of life review and sat with Mrs. M. and the family as they watched family videotapes and reminisced about special occasions. With help from the nurse, the daughter would take her mother in a wheelchair to sit for short periods in the yard. Mrs. M.'s face relaxed as she listened to the birds and enjoyed her watching grandchildren.

Till the very last days of her life, Mrs. M. experienced the love and support of her family. Sips of herbal teas were encouraged to give her strength or relieve her nausea. Latino music was played, reminding her of her cultural connection. Members of her church visited, and prayer novenas were conducted. Mrs. M. died in her own room with her family and the hospice nurse at her side. The nurse and family discussed the cultural and spiritual practices of the family in preparing for Mrs. M.'s funeral and plans to celebrate her life.

During a follow-up bereavement visit, Mrs. M.'s family acknowledged their appreciation for the culturally and spiritually sensitive care received by the hospice team. Mrs. M.'s daughter told the nurse that they considered her a member of their family. This comment reveals the depth of connection that can be established with older patients and their families, and the importance of cultural and spiritual sensitivity in providing quality palliative care.

CONCLUSION

"Although aging changes can affect the body and the mind, there is no evidence that the spirit succumbs to the aging process, even in the presence of debilitating physical and emotional illness" (Heriot, 1992, p. 25). Limiting care to the physical needs of the elder denies the opportunity for the older adult to live out his or her life with meaning, purpose, and hope (Theris, 2001). Frankl (1988) reminded us that man is not destroyed by suffering, but by suffering without meaning.

Cultural and spiritual values, beliefs, and practices profoundly influence life and living and death and dying. Identifying cultural and spiritual factors pertinent to an older patient's health is critical to the development of a successful plan of care that supports an elder's sense of worth and integrity and the continued actualization of his or her potentials. Within the context of culturally and spiritually diverse beliefs and practices, health professionals should preserve beliefs and practices of individuals that have beneficial effects on health, encourage the adaptation or adjustment of practices that are neutral or indifferent, and suggest the repatterning of those practices that are potentially harmful to health (Leininger, 1995).

Culturally and spiritually competent care requires self-reflection and self-care if health care professionals are to be therapeutic. Therefore, health care professionals need to replenish their own vessels in culturally and spiritually renewing ways to actualize their caregiving potential (Sherman, 2001). In doing so, health care practitioners can offer a strong healing presence, true compassion, and sensitivity to the cultural and spiritual needs of older patients and their families.

Consideration of the cultural and spiritual backgrounds of older adults and attention to their cultural and spiritual needs often enables older patients to live as fully as possible until death, and to maintain or restore quality to their lives. Byock (1997) reminded us that, through competent and compassionate end-of-life care, older adults and all other patients can achieve a sense of inner well-being even as death approaches, and that "when the human dimension of dying is nurtured, for many the transition from life can be as profound, intimate, and precious as the miracle of death" (p. 57).

REFERENCES

Abrums, M. (2000). Death and meaning in a storefront church. *Public Health Nursing, 17*(2), 132-142.

American Medical Student Association. (2001). Cultural competency in medicine. Retrieved from http://www.amsa.org/programs/gpit/cultural.cfm.

Andrews, M., & Boyle J. (1995). *Transcultural concepts in nursing care.* Philadelphia: Lippincott.

Arnold, E. (1989). Burnout as a spiritual issue: Rediscovering meaning in nursing practice. In V. Carson (Ed.), *Spiritual dimensions of nursing practice* (pp. 320-353). Philadelphia: Saunders.

Beckwith, S. (2001). The connection between spirituality and cultural diversity. Retrieved from http://www.lastacts. org/statsite/4774la_eln_newsletter.html

Beery, T., Baas, L., Fowler, C., & Allen, G. (2002). Spirituality in persons with heart failure. *Journal of Holistic Nursing, 20*(1), 5-25.

Bergan, A., & McConatha, J. (2000). Religiosity and life satisfaction. *Activities Adapt Aging, 24*(3), 23-24.

Bhungalia, S., & Kemp, C. (2002). (Asian) Indian health beliefs and practices related to end of life. *Journal of Hospice and Palliative Nursing, 4*(1), 54-58.

Boland, C. (1998). Parish nursing: Addressing the significance of social support and spirituality for sustained health-promoting behaviors in the elderly. *Journal of Holistic Nursing, 16*(3), 355-368.

Brennan, M. R. (1994). *Spirituality in the homebound elderly.* Unpublished doctoral dissertation, Catholic University of America.

Brokenleg, M., & Middleton, D. (1993). Native Americans: Adapting, yet retaining. In D. Irish, K. Lundquist, & V. Nelsen (Eds.), *Ethnic variations in dying, death, and grief* (pp. 101-112). Philadelphia: Taylor & Francis.

Buchanan, D. (1993). *Meaning in life, depression, suicide in older adults: A comparative survey study.* Unpublished doctoral dissertation, Rush University.

Byock, I. (1997). *Dying well: The prospect for growth at the end of life.* New York: Riverhead Books.

Conrad, N. L. (1985). Spiritual support for the dying. *Nursing Clinics of North America, 20,* 415-425.

Corr, C. (1991). A task-based approach to coping with dying. *Omega—Journal of Death and Dying, 24*(2), 81-94.

Cousins, N. (1979). *Anatomy of an illness.* New York: Norton.

Crawley, L., Marshall, PL, Lo, B., & Koenig, B. (2002). Strategies for culturally effective end of life care. *Annals of Internal Medicine, 136,* 673-679.

Council on Social Work Education (CSWE). Jan 5-8, 2002. Virginia.

DeSpelder, L. (1998). Developing cultural competency. In K. Doka & J. Davidson (Eds.), *Living with grief* (pp. 97-106). Washington, DC: Hospice Foundation of America.

DeSpelder, L., & Strickland, A. (1999). *The last dance: Encountering death and dying.* California: Mayfield Publishing Company.

Downey, M. (1997). *Understanding Christian spirituality.* Mahwah, NJ: Paulist Press.

Driscoll, J. (2001). Spirituality and religion in end of life care. *Journal of Palliative Medicine, 4*(3), 333-335.

Duggleby, W. (2000). Enduring suffering: A grounded theory analysis of the pain experience of elderly hospice patients with cancer. *Oncology Nursing Forum, 27,* 825-830.

Duggleby, W. (2001). Hope at the end of life. *Journal of Hospice and Palliative Nursing, 3*(2), 51-57.

Dunn, K., & Horgas, A. (2000). The prevalence of prayer as a spiritual self-care modality of elders. *Journal of Holistic Nursing, 18*(4), 337-351.

Ehman, J. W., Ott, B. B., Short, T. H., Ciampa, R. C., & Hansen-Flaschen, J. (1999). Do patients want physicians to inquire about their spiritual or religious beliefs when they become gravely ill? *Archive of Internal Medicine, 159,* 1803-1806.

End of Life Nursing Education Consortium. (2001). *Module 5: Cultural considerations in EOL care.* City of Hope Medical Center and American Association of Colleges of Nursing. Retrieved from http://www.aacn.nche.edu/elnec

Ersek, M., Kagawa-Singer, M., Barnes, D., Blackhall, L., & Koenig, B. (1998). Multicultural considerations in the use of advance directives. *Oncology Nursing Forum, 25,* 1683-1689.

Ferris, F., & Cummings, I. (1995). *Palliative care: Towards a consensus in standardized principles of practice.* Ottawa, ON: Canadian Palliative Care Association.

Frankl, V. E. (1988). *Man's search for meaning.* New York: Simon and Schuster.

Fry, P. S. (2000). Religious involvement, spirituality, and personal meaning in life: Existential predictors of psychological well-being in community-residing and institutional care elders. *Aging & Mental Health, 4*(4), 375-387.

Gallop, G. (1997). *Spiritual beliefs and the dying process: A national survey conducted for the Nathan Cummings Foundation and the Fetzer Institute.* New York: The Nathan Cummings Foundation.

Grossman, D. (1996). Cultural dimensions in home health nursing. *American Journal of Nursing, 96*(7), 33-36.

Heintz, L., & Baruss. L. (2001). Spirituality in late adulthood. *Psychological Reports, 88,* 651-654.

Heriot, C. (1992). Spirituality and aging. *Holistic Nursing Practice, 7,* 22-31.

Hermann, C. (2000). A guide to the spiritual needs of elderly cancer patients. *Geriatric Nursing, 21*(6), 324-325.

Hermann, C. (2001). Spiritual needs of dying patients: A qualitative study. *Oncology Nursing Forum, 28,* 67-72.

Herth, K. (1992). Fostering hope in terminally ill people. *Journal of Advanced Nursing, 15,* 1250-1259.

Hicks, T. (1999). Spirituality and the elderly: Nursing implications with nursing home residents. *Geriatric Nursing, 20*(3), 144-146.

Highfield, M. (2000). Providing spiritual care to patients with cancer. *Clinical Journal of Oncology Nursing, 4*(3), 115-120.

Hyland, K. (1996). *The influence of religiosity on an older person's adjustment to the nursing home environment.* Unpublished doctoral dissertation, Long Island University.

Johnson, P. (2002). The use of humor and its influences on spirituality and coping in breast cancer survivors. *Oncology Nursing Forum, 29*(4), 691-695.

Kagawa-Singer, M., & Blackhall, L. (2001). Negotiating cross-cultural issues at the end of life. *Journal of the American Medical Association, 286,* 2993-3001.

Kirschling, J., & Pittman, J. (1989). Measurement of spiritual well-being: A hospice caregiver sample. *Hospice Journal, 5*(2), 1-11.

Koenig, H. G. (2002). An 83-year old woman with chronic illness and strong religious beliefs. *Journal of the American Medical Association, 288,* 487-493.

Koenig, H. G., Cohen, H. J., & Blazer, D. G (1992). Religious coping and depression in elderly hospitalized medically ill men. *American Journal of Psychiatry, 149*, 1693-1700.

Koenig, H. G., George, L. K., & Peterson, B. L. (1998). Religiosity and remission from depression in medically ill older patients. *American Journal of Psychiatry, 155*, 536-542.

La Vera, C., Marshall, P. A., Lo, B., & Koenig, B. A. (2002). Strategies for culturally effective end-of-life care. *Annals of Internal Medicine, 136*(9) suppl:673-679.

Leininger, M. (1995). *Transcultural nursing: Concepts, theories, research, and practice.* New York: McGraw-Hill.

Lo, B., Ruston, D., Kates, L., Arnold, R., Cohen, C., Faber-Langendoen, K., et al. (2002). Discussing religious and spiritual issues at the end of life: a practical guide for physicians. *Journal of the American Medical Association, 287*, 749-754.

Lowe, J., & Struthers, R. (2001). A conceptual framework of nursing in Native American culture. *Journal of Nursing Scholarship, 33*(3), 279-283.

Mackenzie, E., Rajogopal, D., Meibohm, M., & Lavizzo-Mourey, R. (2000). Spiritual support and psychological well-being: Older adults' perceptions of the religion and health connection. *Alternative Therapies in Health & Medicine, 6*(6), 37-45.

Martinez, R. (1995). *Close friends of God: An ethnography of health of older Hispanic people.* Unpublished doctoral dissertation, University of Colorado Health Sciences Center.

Matthews, D. (1999). *The faith factor: Is religion good for your health?* Paper presented at the Harvard University Spirituality and Healing Conference, Denver, CO.

McDavis, R., Parker, W., & Parker, W. (1995). Counseling African Americans. In N. Vace, S. DeVaney, & J. Wittmer (Eds.), *Experiencing and counseling multicultural and diverse populations* (pp. 217-248.). Bristol, PA: Accelerated Development.

McGrath, P., Vun, M., & McLeod, L. (2001). Needs and experiences of non-English speaking hospice patients and families in an English-speaking country. *American Journal of Hospice and Palliative Care, 18*(5), 305-312.

Meagher, D., & Bell, C. (1993). Perspectives on death in the African-American community. In K. Doka, & J. D. Morgan (Eds.), *Death and spirituality* (pp. 113-130. Amityville, NY: Baywood Publishing Company.

Mitchell, D. (1997). The good death: Three promises to make at the bedside. *Geriatrics, 52*(8), 91-92.

Moberg, D. O. (1984). Subjective measures for spiritual well-being. *Review of Religious Research, 25*(4), 351-364.

Moore, T. (1992). *Care of the soul: A guide for cultivating depth and sacredness in everyday life.* New York: Harper-Collins.

Morgan, J. D. (1993). The Existential quest for meaning. In K. Doka & J. Morgan (Eds.), *Death and spirituality* (pp. 1-18). Amityville, NY: Baywood Publishing Company.

Mull, C., Cox, C., & Sullivan, J. (1987). Religion's role in the health and well-being of well elders. *Public Health Nursing, 4*(3), 151-159.

Nathan Cummings Foundation. (1999). Spiritual beliefs and the dying process: Key findings. Retrieved 12/06/2002 from http://www.ncf.org/ncf/publications/reports/fetzer/fetzer_keyfindings.html

O'Connor, P. (1993). A clinical paradigm for exploring spiritual concerns. In K. Doka & J. Morgan (Eds.), *Death and spirituality* (pp.133-150). Amityville, NY: Baywood Publishing Company.

Oman, D., & Reed, D. (1998). Religion and mortality among the community-dwelling elderly. *American Journal of Public Health, 88*, 1469-1475.

Parker-Oliver, D. (2002). Redefining hope for the terminally ill. *American Journal of Hospice and Palliative Care, 19*(2), 115-120.

Peterman, A., Fitchett, G., Brady, M., Hernandez, L., & Cella, D. (2002). Measuring spiritual well-being in people with cancer: The Functional Assessment of Chronic Illness Therapy–Spiritual Well-Being Scale (FACIT-Sp). *Annals of Behavioral Medicine, 24*(1), 49-58.

Puchalski, C. (1998). Facing death with dignity. *The World and I, 3*, 34-39.

Puchalski, C. M. (1999). Taking a Spiritual history: FICA. *Spirituality & Medicine Connection, 3*, 1.

Puchalski, C. M. (2001). Spirituality and health: the art of compassionate medicine. *Hospital Physician, 37*(3), 30-36.

Puchalski, C. (2001b). Spirituality and health: The art of compassionate medicine. *Hospital Physician, 37*(3), 30-36.

Puchalski, C. (2002). Spirituality and end of life care: A time for listening and caring. *Journal of Palliative Medicine, 5*(2), 289-294.

Puchalski, C., & Romer, A. (2000). Taking a spiritual history allows clinicians to understand patients more fully. *Journal of Palliative Medicine, 3*(1), 129-137.

Purdy, W. (2002). Spiritual discernment in palliative care. *Journal of Palliative Medicine, 5*(1), 139-141.

Ryan, S. (1997). Chaplains are more than what chaplains do. *Visions, 7*, 8-9.

Satterly, L. (2001). Guilt, shame, and religious and spiritual pain. *Holistic Nursing Practice, 15*(2), 30-39.

Sellers, S., & Haag, B. (1998). Spiritual nursing interventions. *Journal of Holistic Nursing, 16*(3), 338-354.

Sherman, D. W. (2001). Spiritual and cultural competence in palliative care. In M. Matzo & D. W. Sherman (Eds.), *Palliative care nursing: Quality care to the end of life* (pp. 3-47). New York: Springer.

Showalter, S. (1998). Looking through different eyes: Beyond cultural diversity. In K. Doka & J. Davidson (Eds.), *Living with grief when illness is prolonged* (pp. 71-82). Washington, DC: Hospice Foundation of America.

Sullivan, M. (2001). Lost in translation: How Latinos view end of life care. Retrieved from http://www.lastacts.org/statsite/4907la_eln_newsletter.html

Taylor, E., & Outlaw, F. (2002). Use of prayer among persons with cancer. *Holistic Nursing Practice, 16*(3), 46-60.

Taylor, E. J., Outlaw, F. H., Bernardo, T. T., & Roy, A. (1991). Spiritual conflicts associated with praying about cancer. *Psycho-oncology*, 8(5), 386-394.

Theris, T. (2001). Nurturing hope and spirituality in the nursing home. *Holistic Nursing Practice*, 15(4), 45-56.

Thomas, J., & Retsas, A. (1999). Transacting self-preservation: A grounded theory of the spiritual dimensions of people with terminal cancer. *International Journal of Nursing Studies*, 36(3), 191-201.

Weaver, J. Flannelly, L., & Flannelly, K. (2001). A review of research on religious and spiritual values in two primary gerontological journals. *Journal of Gerontological Nursing*, 27(9), 47-54.

Wink, P. (1999). Addressing end of life issues: Spirituality and inner life. *Generations*, 23(1), 75-80.

2 DEATH AND AN AGING SOCIETY

Patricia H. Berry and Marianne L. Matzo

Case Study

Mrs. E. is an 87-year-old fiercely independent, widow who recently relocated far away from her original home to be closer to her daughter, her only child. She settled into an independent retirement apartment community and began busying herself with volunteering, visiting other residents who were ill, and becoming active in a center for older adults. Because she reached young adulthood during the Depression, she worries about money and wears her clothes until they literally fall apart, saves and eats every food leftover, and carefully cleans and saves every plastic bag and Styrofoam food container. She is appalled at how much everything costs and is worried she may not have enough money to care for herself. Being independent, however, she has always contended that she never wants to live with or be dependent on her daughter and her daughter's family.

Her daughter is a professional with a demanding job and three teenage boys who are active in sports, band, and other school activities. Her husband also works full time and is often out of town on business. Her daughter feels pulled between the needs of her mother and those of her children and husband. She does realize, however, that she is all the family her mother has, so she makes every effort to visit, be available, and offer assistance.

On the day that her grandson severely injured his eye during football practice, Mrs. E. fell outside her apartment and fractured both her right wrist and hip; her daughter received the call from the apartment manager just as she and her son were arriving home from the emergency room. She then went to her mother's apartment, arranged transportation to the emergency room, and stayed with her mother until she was admitted to the hospital for a hip replacement and fixation of her wrist the following day. Soon after surgery, Mrs. E. experienced a grand mal seizure, the cause of which was determined to be a mass in her brain representing an inoperable tumor. After 3 weeks in a rehabilitation facility, Mrs. E. was ready to go home, but her daughter did not think her mother should live alone, with her increased risk of seizures and falls.

INTRODUCTION

In 1900, living to age 70 was considered a result of luck or grace; living that long in 2000 is commonplace and anticipated (Matzo & Lynn, 2000). The usual causes of death have changed from accidents and infections to chronic illnesses. The "end of life" has also changed from a period of minutes to days with overwhelming illness to a period of months to years with slowly worsening disability. Nurses need to be prepared not only to address issues related to dying and death with older adult patients, but at the same time to care for problems associated with chronic medical conditions. The five most common chronic conditions for people age 75 and older are arthritis, hypertension, hearing impairments, heart disease, and cataracts (Summer, O'Neill, & Shirey, 1999).

Human development and aging also occur in a particular cultural and historical context. This is often referred in social psychology as the "cohort" effect. When taking a cohort perspective of the life course and aging, how persons age is largely defined by the time in which they live. The era in which persons live largely shapes how members of the cohort ascribe meaning to life events resulting in sometimes radical social change. Indeed, social change implies that successive cohort groups will act in a different fashion than their predecessors (Uhlenberg & Miner, 1996). Several factors create the climate of change and thus can produce significant differences in the experience of aging for cohorts separated by several decades. These factors, a brief definition, and some ques-tions for reflection regarding end-of-life care are found in Table 2-1. As you review them, think of yourself and your grandparents and how different your life experiences and aging are in the context of these factors.

Consider the natural birth movement, an outgrowth of the then-younger "baby boom" generation's desire for fewer interventions during

Table 2-1 Cohort Differences: Factors Working against Stability in the Aging Process

Cohort Factor	Definition	Questions to Consider
Differences in composition and history	Differences in size, racial and ethnic composition, educational background, commitment to religious beliefs, war experiences, wealth, and major world events. The larger the differences within a given cohort, the more significant the changes in the aging process.	• How will the rapid increases in the very old affect the aging process of the aging group as a whole? • How does a national milestone event (such as the terrorist attacks of September 11, 2001) affect attitudes toward aging and hope?
Organization of society	Opportunities and constraints imposed upon major social institutions (i.e., government) radically affect the experience of aging through the allocation of resources and the protection of rights. Rapid social change produces rapid changes in the meaning of old age.	• How will existing government programs meet the needs of the rapidly growing old-old population?
Technological development	Changes in medical and public health technology, including housing, adaptive equipment for disabled people, communications, monitors, and emergency care. Rapid changes in technology can influence the ability of persons to live independently. Rapid changes in technology can significantly impact upon the experience of aging.	• Could older people need less assistance because of technology? (i.e., Will assisted-living centers become obsolete?) • Will people expect to live forever?
Structure of linkages with cohorts in other life stages	Every cohort is linked with other cohorts through family, kinship, economic, political, and social bonds. The size, composition, and behavior of younger cohorts influence the aging experience of those in the older cohort groups.	• How will the expectations of "generation X" affect how the "baby boom" generation ages and approaches death?

From Uhlenberg, P., & Miner, S. (1996). Life course and aging: A cohort perspective. In R. H. Binstock & L. K. George (Eds.), *Handbook of aging and the social sciences* (4th ed., pp. 208–228). San Diego: Academic Press.

childbirth. Hospice, also a grassroots movement by persons concerned that their own death might be "medicalized," in part set the stage for improvements in pain and symptom management. Consider also what the long-term care environment will be like in the year 2030. What will be the living arrangements? What resources will be available related to health care? What technologies will be developed to cure or control disease?

This chapter explores how the changing milieu affects the way older adults are living with chronic illness and dying in what can be considered an unpredictable and protracted manner. We also explore how the cohort one is born into in large part shapes one's aging experience. Differences in cohorts are the primary forces that demand and drive social change. What is appropriate for one cohort may not be at all appropriate for another. As you read through this chapter, consider how much the aging population is changing, because it is indeed a rapid and radical process.

DEMOGRAPHICS
Demographics in the United States changed dramatically during the 20th century. Those hundred years brought remarkable shifts in patterns of aging, mortality, and the nature and degree of illness in the population.

Population
Life expectancy at birth in 1900 was about 49 years. This increased to 70 years by 1960, and to 74 and 79 years for men and women, respectively, by the end of the century. Additionally, life expectancies for older persons increased; men who reach 85 may expect an additional 6 years of life while women reaching the same age may anticipate living 7 more years (Federal Interagency Forum on Aging-Related Statistics, 2002).

As a result of these changes, the proportion of older Americans increased dramatically in this century. In 1900 just over 4% of the population was over age 65; as of 2000, an estimated 35 million Americans were 65 or older, representing almost 13% of the total population. In the last half of the century, the number of persons 85 years and older increased over 300%. Projecting these trends leads to a fifth of the population

being older than 65 by 2030 and a quadrupling of those 85 and older by 2040 (Federal Interagency Forum on Aging-Related Statistics, 2002).

The segment of the population that is 85 and older totaled only 2% in 2000, but is the fastest growing of all categories and is expected to reach 5% in 2050, which, by some studies, is a conservative estimate. Women comprise 58% of those 65 years and older and 70% of those 85 years and older (Federal Interagency Forum on Aging-Related Statistics, 2002). The largest increase in older adults will occur between 2010 and 2030, when baby boomers reach age 65. These data reflect an increase of nearly 25 years in life expectancy in the United States as a result of progress in living and working conditions; advances in sanitation, nutrition, and immunization; decreased infant and maternal mortality; and heightened efforts in disease prevention (Administration on Aging, 2001).

Implicit in this aging population is the growing incidence of chronic disease, with degenerative diseases supplanting communicable diseases as the leading cause of death (Table 2-2). Five of the six leading causes of death of older Americans are chronic diseases, which are often protracted and often involve chronic disabilities. These chronic or terminal illnesses have corresponding needs for assistance, symptom management, and hospice and palliative care services that may be taxing to the health care system and financially burdensome. Older adults are at an increased risk for developing multiple chronic or life-threatening diseases: heart disease, cancer, stroke, respiratory diseases, and other terminal illnesses, such as Alzheimer's disease. As a result of these chronic diseases, both direct and indirect health care costs can increase. For example, adults may live with chronic obstructive pulmonary disease for as long as 20 years before they die, at a cost of $8 billion to the economy through lost productivity caused by morbidity and death from this disease (Burke & Walsh, 1997).

The four leading causes of death in the United States for people over the age of 65 are heart disease (44%), cancer (29%), cerebrovascular disease (11%), and chronic respiratory disease (8%). The remaining causes of death are accounted for by influenza and pneumonia (4%) and diabetes 4% (Centers for Disease Control

Table 2-2 Cause of Death and Demographic/Social Trends

	Early 1900s	Current
Medicine's focus	Comfort	Cure
Cause of death	Infectious diseases/ communicable diseases	Chronic illnesses
Age-adjusted death rate	1720 per 100,000 (1900)	865 per 100,000 (1997)
Average life expectancy	50	76
Number of persons >65 years old	3.1 million	~35 million (estimate for 2000)
Site of death	Home	Institutions
Caregiver	Family	Strangers/health care providers
Disease/dying trajectory	Relatively short	Prolonged

Data from Field, M. J., & Cassel, C. K. (Eds.) (1997). *Approaching death: Improving care at the end of life* (Committee on Care at the End of Life, Division of Health Care Services, Institute of Medicine). Washington, DC: National Academy Press; Ventura, S. J., Anderson, R. N., Martin, J. A., & Smith, B. L. (1998). Births and deaths: Preliminary data for 1997. *National Vital Statistics Reports, 47*(4); and Administration on Aging. (2000). *Older population by Age: 1900 to 2050.* Retrieved from http://www.aoa.dhhs.gov./aoa/stats/AgePop2050Chart-numbers.html.

and Prevention, unpublished statistics, 1999). In the years from 1984 to 1995, the incidence of stroke increased by 1%, diabetes by 2%, arthritis by 3%, heart disease by 5%, and cancer by 7%. Approximately one third of those 85 years and older demonstrate some form of memory impairment, and over one fifth of this age group experience severe symptoms of depression (Federal Interagency Forum on Aging-Related Statistics, 2002). Thus the agenda of the National Institute on Aging (2000) for the years 2001 to 2005 targets three areas for research: (1) preventing or reducing age-related diseases, disorders, and disability; (2) maintaining physical health and function; and (3) enhancing older adults' societal roles and interpersonal support, and reducing social isolation.

For the older adult, many different trajectories ultimately lead to death (Corr, 1998; Emanuel, von Gunten, & Ferris, 1999; Field & Cassel, 1997). Elders with chronic, progressive diseases (e.g., heart disease, diabetes, chronic obstructive pulmonary disease) may not see themselves, or be perceived by their families and friends, to be dying. The report of the Institute of Medicine (IOM) Committee on Care at the End of Life (Field & Cassel, 1997) identified three illness/ dying trajectories (Fig. 2-1). The first trajectory is that of a sudden and unexpected death (e.g., accidents). The second trajectory encompasses those people who are terminally ill and experi-

ence a steady decline in their physical health and a relatively short terminal phase. The last trajectory is that most often experienced by older adults. Their life expectancy is that of an unpredictable number of years with a prolonged decline in health punctuated by periodic crises that ultimately result in their death. Older adults in this group carry out their activities of daily living while coping with the possibility of death.

The symptom burden related to chronic illness is much higher for older adults than for younger people. Looking at all symptoms that are common at the end of life, the number of symptoms experienced increases with age from 5.7 for those under age 65 to 7.4 for those over age 85. The symptoms more commonly seen in older adults at the end of their lives are mental confusion, incontinence, difficulty hearing and seeing, and dizziness (American Board of Internal Medicine [ABIM], 1998). Dying at an older age also means that the symptom burden is carried for much a longer period of time; 39% of persons under age 65 reported symptoms for a year or more before death, compared to 52% of those ages 65 to 84 and 69% of elders over the age of 85 (ABIM, 1998). Quality of life and independence may be decreased for the terminally ill older adult by weakness, falls, delirium, urinary incontinence, sleep disturbances, and serious depression.

a. Sudden death, unexpected cause
• < 10% (MI, accident, etc.)

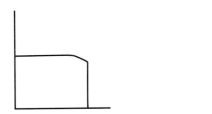

b. Steady decline, short terminal phase

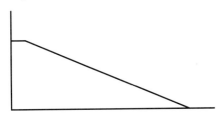

c. Slow decline, periodic crises, and death

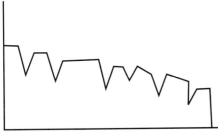

Fig. 2-1 Illness/dying trajectories. MI, myocardial infarction. (From Field, M. J., & Cassel, C. K. (1997). *Approaching death: Improving care at the end of life* [Committee on Care at the End of Life, Division of Health Care Services, Institute of Medicine) [p. 29]. Washington, DC: National Academy Press)

Racial and Ethnic Composition

Presently, the population of older Americans includes 84% non-Hispanic white, 8% non-Hispanic black, 2% non-Hispanic Asian and Pacific Islander, 6% Hispanic, and less than 1% non-Hispanic American Indian/Alaska Native. The Hispanic segment is expected to grow most rapidly, from 2 million today to over 13 million by 2050 (Federal Interagency Forum on Aging-Related Statistics, 2002). Data from 1995 show that black women can expect to live to 74 years, in contrast to 79.6 years for white women; black men can expect to live 65.4 years, contrasted to

73.4 years for white males (Field & Cassel, 1997). Age-adjusted mortality rates for black women are 1.5 times those of white women, and black males have nearly twice the mortality of white men (Federal Interagency Forum on Aging-Related Statistics, 2002).

Marital Status

Marital status in the older segment of the population has extra significance because of its role in emotional and economic well-being, as well as caregiving. In 1998, nearly 80% of men ages 65 to 74 were married, compared to 55% of women. For those 85 years and older, 50% of the men, but only 13% of the women, were married. Older women are much more likely to be widowed than men because of gender differences in life expectancy, the tendency for women to marry older men, and higher remarriage rates for older widowed men than women. Currently, about 77% of women 85 or older are widowed, compared with 42% of men, and only 4% of men and 5% of woman have never married (Federal Interagency Forum on Aging-Related Statistics, 2002).

Education

Educational status is often reflective of general well-being in older Americans, with higher levels of attainment usually allowing a better standard of living and more favorable health status. At mid-century, less than one fifth of older Americans had finished high school, but this increased to 75% by 1998. Those who had earned a bachelor's degree increased from 4% in 1950 to nearly 15% in 1998. Disparities continue in educational achievement among racial and ethnic groups; 72% of the non-Hispanic white elder population finished high school, compared to 29% of the Hispanic elder population (Federal Interagency Forum on Aging-Related Statistics, 2002).

Living Arrangements/Family

Living arrangements also impact greatly on the general well-being of the older population because of the link to income, health status, and caregiver availability. Those older persons living alone are much more likely to be poor than those who are living with spouses. In 1998, 73% of older men lived with spouses, 7% with other relatives, and 3% with nonrelatives, and 17% lived alone.

Women were equally likely to live with a spouse as alone, about 41% each. A higher proportion of older white and black women (41%) lived alone, compared with 27% of older Hispanic women. About 19% of older white women who lived alone were in poverty, while approximately 50% of older black and Hispanic women who lived alone lived in poverty (Federal Interagency Forum on Aging-Related Statistics, 2002).

ECONOMICS

As with education and martial status, one's economic security impacts upon quality and quantity of life in old age. Analysis of Medicare data regarding beneficiaries age 65 and older with incomes less than or equal to 175% of the federal poverty level shows a very different demographic profile from those with income above this level (Table 2-3). These data show that beneficiaries below this poverty level are more than twice as likely to be widowed, divorced, or separated; they are less likely to be white or to have finished high school; and a larger proportion report their health to be either fair or poor (National Institute on Aging, 1998).

Poverty

Poverty, which is measured based on a family's annual income compared to a set of thresholds that indicate a risk of inadequate resources, has decreased for older Americans in recent decades. In 1966, one of three persons ages 65 and older could be defined as living in poverty, but this declined to about 10% by 1998, an improvement double that of other age groups. Currently, the poverty rate is 9.7% for older Americans, equaling that of working-age persons (Administration on Aging, 2001). The degree of poverty increases with age, from 9% for those ages 65 to 74 to 14% for those 85 years and older. Also, poverty rates are higher for women (13%) than for men (7%) and for the nonmarried (17%) than the married (5%) (Federal Interagency Forum on Aging-Related Statistics, 2002).

Income Distribution, Sources of Income, and Net Worth

Examining income distribution provides an additional perspective on the economic status of the older population. Using five categories (high,

Table 2-3 Characteristics of Medicare Beneficiaries Age 65 and Older

	Income at or below 175% of the Federal Poverty Level	Income Greater than 175% of the Federal Poverty Level
Mean age	76	74
Female	70%	52%
Marital status		
Married	32%	67%
Divorced/separated	13%	6%
Widowed	51%	24%
Never married	4%	3%
Race		
Black	16%	5%
White	79%	94%
Other	5%	2%
Graduated from high school	41%	78%
Self-reported health status		
Very good to excellent	23%	39%
Good	28%	33%
Fair	28%	20%
Poor	21%	8%

Data from National Institute on Aging. (1998). Center on an Aging Society analysis of data from the 1998 Health and Retirement Study, sponsored by the National Institute on Aging. Washington, DC: Author.

Reference: Humphrey, L: *Americans' changing lives: longitudinal survey.* Portland, OR: Portland Veterans Affairs Medical Center.

Research Problem: To explore the relationships of health behaviors to increased mortality in poorer persons.

Design: 7.5-year longitudinal cohort study of community-dwelling adults.

Sample and Setting: 3617 community-living adults (age 25 years or older) in the United States; 33% were age 65 years or older, 32% of the total sample were black.

Methods: Risk factors such as total years of education, income, and health behaviors (cigarette smoking, alcohol drinking, body weight, and level of physical activity) were assessed. Age, sex, race, and residence were also assessed for potential confounding effects. All-cause mortality data were obtained from the National Death Index and informants.

Results: Poorer and less educated people were more likely to be smokers, sedentary, and overweight. After adjusting for age, sex, and urban residence, the lowest income level (<$10,000/yr) relative to the highest (≥$30,000/yr) showed an odds ratio of 3.13 (95% confidence interval [CI], 1.97 to 4.95) for death in men and 3.82 (95% CI, 1.86 to 7.85) in women. With further adjustment for smoking, alcohol, phys-

ical activity, and weight, the association with income remained statistically significant. Other factors associated with mortality after adjustment for all other variables were age, sex, urban residence, being underweight, and low levels of physical activity.

Implications for Nursing Practice: The investigators, however, did not explore the factors associated with poverty that might explain the association with poor health, which include malnutrition, depression, chronic stress, poor housing, overcrowding, hostility, social isolation and lack of social support, and poor access to health care. The public health implications of the study findings are that interventions aimed at improving health behaviors among persons with low SES will have only a modest effect in reducing mortality, and efforts should be directed toward other factors that may be more successful in improving health outcomes. This study also suggests that, in addition to addressing lifestyle factors with patients, psychosocial factors such as depression, loneliness, and social isolation should be addressed when possible.

Conclusion: Lower socioeconomic status (SES) is one of the most powerful predictors of poor health and early death worldwide. High-risk health behaviors are more common in persons of lower SES. Low income remained a risk factor for premature death even after adjustment for the health behaviors of smoking, alcohol use, physical activity, and body weight.

medium, and low income; poverty; and extreme poverty), shifts can be noted between categories in recent years. Although a constant 2% of the population has remained in extreme poverty since 1974, the proportion in poverty declined from 13% to 8% in 1998. Those in the low-income category declined from 35% to 27%. The proportion of medium- and high-income persons increased from 50% to 75% over this time span, and the medium-income group

emerged as the largest single category at 35% (Federal Interagency Forum on Aging-Related Statistics, 2002).

The sources of income for older Americans have also changed proportionally in recent years. Social Security has provided an increasing percentage of income, accounting for about 40% on average in 1998, with the remainder coming in equal proportions from asset income, pensions, and personal earnings. Pensions have provided a consistent 50% of income for retired workers since the 1970s, though their nature has shifted from defined-benefit, such as an annuity, to defined-contribution, in which income depends on investment results. Those in the lowest fifth of income depend on Social Security for over 80% of their income, while those in the upper fifth find it totals only about 20%.

In addition to income, net worth (the value of real estate and other assets minus debts) is an important measure of well-being and the ability to weather stressors such as illness. The net worth of households headed by people ages 65 and older increased by 69% from 1984 to 1999; however, most of this is represented by increases in home equity. If home equity is excluded from determining net worth for the bottom fifth of older Americans, the total drops from over $30,000 to less than $3000. Noteworthy as well is the disparity in net worth between black and white households of older persons, ranging from about $13,000 for blacks to $181,000 for whites.

Educational status is a considerable factor as well. Those household heads 65 and older with at least some college education reported a net worth four times that of those lacking a high school diploma (Federal Interagency Forum on Aging-Related Statistics, 2002).

Participation in the Labor Force

Many older Americans work or seek work. Following the lowering of the Social Security age of eligibility in 1960, this participation dropped significantly for men until 1980, when the law changed again. Since then, elimination of mandatory retirement laws and modification of the Social Security "earnings test," which allows one to keep more benefits while working, have likely produced a halt in this trend toward less work participation for men. Women have tended to participate in the workforce in greater numbers as they age, partly because many married women took jobs after their husbands had retired and because of the influence of the Civil Rights Act of 1965, which outlawed discrimination on the basis of gender. These factors have narrowed the gap between the rates of participation of men and women ages 65 to 69 from 24% in 1963 to 10% in 1999 (Federal Interagency Forum on Aging-Related Statistics, 2002).

Housing

Housing, while adequate for most older Americans, may demand a considerably higher portion of resources, depending on income status. That is, for those 65 and older in the bottom 20% of income distribution, housing required 36% of expenditures. For those in the top 20% of income, it required 26%. Specifically, those in the lowest level of income spent $4686 annually on housing, while those in the highest level of income spent $10,119 (Federal Interagency Forum on Aging-Related Statistics, 2002).

In 1999, approximately $90 billion was spent on nursing home care ($55,900 per resident) in the United States; 60% of this cost was paid for by Medicare or Medicaid (Walshe, 2001). One in every five older adults in the United States dies in a nursing home (Miller, Gozalo, & Mor, 2001).

HEALTH STATUS, HEALTH CARE EXPENDITURES, AND MEDICARE

Another major expense for many older Americans is health care: those funds spent on physician services, hospitalization, home health care, nursing home care, medications, and the like. In 1996, those ages 65 to 69 spent $5864 annually on health care, while those ages 75 to 79 spent $9414, and those living in institutions incurred $38,906 annually in health care expenses. Spending is concentrated within a small segment of the older population. In 1996, the 5% of Medicare enrollees with the highest expenditures incurred 37% of total spending (Federal Interagency Forum on Aging-Related Statistics, 2002).

Components of health care expenditures include type of service (e.g., nursing home and hospital settings), variations of spending with age group or income level, and types of insurance. In 1996, inpatient hospital care incurred 29% of expenditures, while skilled nursing facility care incurred 10%, and prescription drug costs totaled 7%. For those 85 and older, 46% of health care expenditures were spent on nursing home care compared to 7% for those ages 65 to 69. Lower-income older Americans used proportionately more skilled nursing home care, but less outpatient care and prescription medications. In 1996, 69% of noninstitutionalized Medicare beneficiaries had prescription drug coverage of some nature (e.g., from health maintenance organizations), while those with no coverage found their expenditures to be 83% higher than those of the insured (Federal Interagency Forum on Aging-Related Statistics, 2002).

National programs such as Medicare provide health insurance for older adults and certain disabled persons. In 2001, the program covered an estimated 39 million people, approximately 34 million of whom were over the age of 65 (Maxwell, Moon, & Segal, 2000). The Medicare program has a significant cost-sharing requirement in the form of premiums, co-insurance, and deductibles. For those Medicare beneficiaries over the age of 65, this amounts to 22% of their incomes in out-of-pocket costs. More vulnerable elders, such as low-income women in poor health, are estimated to spend 50% of their incomes on out-of-pocket medical care (Maxwell et al., 2001).

The proportion of out-of-pocket expenditures for health care may reflect the degree of burden on older individuals, depending on income category. Lower-income older Americans averaged $1654 yearly in out-of-pocket costs for health care, while the upper 20% in income averaged $3614 in 1998. These amounts represent 16% to 9% of total out-of-pocket expenditures, respectively. This type of expense has increased somewhat for all income categories in the past decade (Federal Interagency Forum on Aging-Related Statistics, 2002).

Six to 8% of Medicare enrollees die annually, and 83% of these people are over the age of 65; these deaths account for 27% to 30% of annual Medicare expenses, an amount unchanged from 20 years ago (Gornick, McMillan, & Lubitz, 1993). Thirty-eight percent of Medicare patients have some nursing home use in the year of their death (Hogan, Lunney, Gabel, & Lynn, 2001). In the year 2001, more than 50% of all deaths of Medicare recipients occurred in the hospital, often after days or weeks in critical care settings (Clark, 2002).

Access to health care varies according to cost, quality, and availability of services. Over 96% of older Americans are covered by Medicare, and, although access can be problematic, only 2% of those enrolled reported difficulty in obtaining care in 1996. Across the age spectrum of older persons, 3% to 7% reported delaying seeking health care because of cost. When categorized by race, non-Hispanic black persons reported a 10% level of delay, Hispanics a 7% level, and non-Hispanic whites a 5% level of delay (Federal Interagency Forum on Aging-Related Statistics, 2002).

Medicare still does not cover the majority of outpatient prescription drug expenditures. The exceptions are primarily certain immunosuppressive and oncology medicines and antinausea drugs for chemotherapy patients (Pharmaceutical Research and Manufacturers of America, 2000). Concerns about the long-term solvency of the program have prompted calls to restructure the Medicare program for the needs of the 21st century; issues being raised include the advantages and feasibility of a prescription drug benefit. Many drug companies offer medication-assistance programs to pay for prescription drugs, and a number of other resources are available for nurses to help patients access these programs (Table 2-4).

The use of health care services, while guaranteed by Medicare, has varied in type of service demanded over the years. From 1990 to 1998, physician visits and consultations increased from 10,800 to 13,100 per 1000 beneficiaries, and home health visits per 1000 enrollees increased from 2141 to 8227 in 1997, but this number dropped to 5058 in 1998 due to a change in Medicare payment policies for home health services. From 1990 to 1998, skilled nursing facility admissions increased from 23 to 69 per 1000 enrollees, and, when categorized by age, ranged from 27 per 1000 for those ages 65 to 74 to 200 per 1000 for those age 85 and older. The oldest Americans utilize proportionately more home health services. In 1996, the program covered an estimated 38 million people, with approximately 87% being over the age of 65 (Federal Interagency Forum on Aging-Related Statistics, 2002).

Another important consideration is the lack of specialists in gerontology as well as the even smaller number of specialists with combined credentials in both gerontology and palliative care. Few geriatric specialty programs in nursing and medicine address palliative care as an emphasis. There are fewer than 10,000 certified geriatricians and only 4200 advanced practice nurses certified as clinical nurse specialists or

Table 2-4 Medication Assistance Programs

Agency	Description
THE MEDICINE PROGRAM 1-573-996-7300 *www.themedicineprogram.com* e-mail: *help@themedicineprogram.com*	Helps people (for a $5 fee per drug) to apply for enrollment in one of more of the many patient assistance programs that are available. The majority of these programs provide prescription medication free of charge to individuals in need, regardless of age, if they meet the sponsor's criteria. Enrollment requirements: • No insurance coverage for outpatient prescription drugs • Income at a level that causes a hardship when the patient is required to purchase medications at retail prices • Not qualified for a government or third-party program that provides for prescription medication
HARSONHILL 1-818-716-4100 *www.prescriptions4free.com*	Sells a booklet ($20) with information on the prescription drug programs offered by drug manufacturers, including each company's eligibility requirements.
PHARMACEUTICAL RESEARCH AND MANUFACTURERS OF AMERICA 1-800-762-4636 *www.phrma.org* *www.helpingpatients.org*	The research-based pharmaceutical industry has had a long-standing tradition of providing prescription medicines free of charge to physicians whose patients might not otherwise have access to necessary medicines. To make it easier for physicians to identify the growing number of programs available for needy patients, member companies of the Pharmaceutical Research and Manufacturers of America (PhRMA) created a Patient Assistance Programs directory listing company programs that provide drugs to physicians whose patients could not otherwise afford them. The programs are listed alphabetically by company. Under the entry for each program is information about how to make a request for assistance, what prescription medicines are covered, and basic eligibility criteria
DEPARTMENT OF HEALTH & HUMAN SERVICES Financial Aid—Federal Hill-Burton Free Care Program Rockville, MD 20857 1-800-638-0742 *www.hrsa.dhhs.gov/osp/dfcr/index.htm*	Assists eligible persons in obtaining free medical care, technically assisting obligated facilities concerning provision of free or reduced-cost medical care.
AVON FOUNDATION BREAST CARE FUND 1-212-244-5638 *www.avonbreastcare.org*	Provides limited financial assistance for women with breast, cervical, ovarian, and uterine cancers for transportation, child care, or escort services. Also provides grants for women needing help paying for prediagnostic testing for these cancers.
THE LIFELINE PROGRAM 2810 E. Oakland Park Blvd. Suite 300 Fort Lauderdale, FL 33306 1-800-572-4346 *www.thelifeline.com*	Provides financial options for people with a life-threatening illness who own a life insurance policy. Will pay lump sum percentage of face value of policy. The Lifeline Program is rated #1 in the highest financial payments to the terminally ill in the state of Florida.

Table 2-4 Medication Assistance Programs—cont'd

Agency	Description
NOVARTIS PROGRAM FOR MEN WITH CANCER Contact Cancer Care: 1-800-813-Hope (4673)	Limited financial assistance for men with all types of cancer for transportation, home care, and child care services.
MARY KAY ASH CHARITABLE FOUNDATION GRANTS 1-877-652-2737	Limited financial assistance for women with all types of cancer for transportation, home care, and child care services
THE LEUKEMIA & LYMPHOMA SOCIETY—CENTRAL FLORIDA 3319 Maguire Blvd. #101 Orlando, FL 32803 1-407-898-0733 1-800-955-4572 *www.leukemia.org*	Provides supplementary financial assistance to patients in significant financial need, up to $500 per year. The program pays for specific approved drugs; processing; typing, screening, and cross-matching blood, etc.; and radiation therapy.
H. LEE MOFFITT CANCER CENTER AND RESEARCH INSTITUTE UNIVERSITY OF SOUTH FLORIDA 12902 Magnolia Drive Tampa, FL 333612 1-800-456-7121 *www.moffitt.usf.edu*	Entitlement and benefits assistance. Offers direct financial assistance and health insurance information.
ELDER HELPLINE Information Clearinghouse Florida Dept. of Elder Affairs 1371 Winewood Blvd., Bldg. E Tallahassee, FL 32399 1-800-677-1116	An information clearinghouse for senior citizens. Provides entitlement and benefits assistance and health insurance information.
AMERICAN KIDNEY FUND 6110 Executive Blvd. Suite 1010 Rockville, Md. 20852 Help Line: 1-800-638-8299 *www.akflinc.org*	Provides financial aid for the urgent needs of people with chronic kidney disease. Also offers free vitamin supplements for renal patients and a prescription drug discount card for anyone.
AMERICAN CANCER SOCIETY (See local phone book) National phone: 1-800-227-2345 *www.cancercare.org*	Local office may offer reimbursement for expenses related to cancer treatment, including transportation, medicine, and medical supplies.
MEDICAID *www.cms.gov/medicaid*	Jointly funded, federal–state health insurance program for people who need financial assistance for medical expenses. Coordinated by the Health Care Financing Administration (now called the Centers for Medicare & Medicaid Services [CMS]). Includes part-time nursing, home care aide services, and medical supplies and equipment.

Table 2-4 **Medication Assistance Programs—cont'd**	
Agency	Description
MEDICARE 1-800-633-4227 *www.medicare.gov*	Federal health insurance program administered by the CMS. Eligible individuals include those 65 and over, anyone with permanent kidney failure, and disabled people under 65. Cancer patients may also be eligible for hospice care.
SOCIAL SECURITY ADMINISTRATION 1-800-772-1213 *www.ssa.gov*	The government agency that oversees Social Security and Supplemental Security Income. Provides a monthly income for eligible elders and disabled individuals.
VETERANS ADMINISTRATION 1-800-827-1000 1-800-822-Vets Visit website for local information: *www.va.gov/vbs*	Veterans and their dependents may receive cancer treatment at a Veterans Affairs Medical Center
AIR CARE ALLIANCE *www.aircareall.org*	Nationwide league of humanitarian flying organizations dedicated to community service. Provides links to nationwide organizations that provide transport for patients and sometimes family members needing to get treatment.
ANGEL FLIGHT SOUTHEAST Lee Johnson, Exec. Director Bob Reymount, Mission coordinator 8747 Airport Blvd, #1 Leesburg, FL 34788 1-800-FLA-HALO *www.angelflightse.org*	Nonprofit volunteer pilot organization involved in "public benefit flying." Coordinates travel to distant health facilities when commercial service is not available, impractical, or not affordable.
BLOOD AND BONE MARROW TRANSPLANT INFORMATION NETWORK *www.bmtnews.org*	If your health insurance plan has refused to pay for all or part of your treatment, the *Blood and Marrow Transplant Newsletter* can refer you to not-for-profit organizations and attorneys who may be able to help you. All the attorneys on their referral list have successfully persuaded insurers to pay for transplant-related expenses, usually without resorting to litigation.
NEEDY MEDS *www.needymeds.com*	Lists pharmaceutical manufacturers who provide drugs free of charge to patients with limited financial resources.
NIELSEN ORGAN TRANSPLANT FOUNDATION 580 W. 8th Street Jacksonville, FL 32209 1-904-244-9823	Financial aid for some Florida residents

gerontologic nurse practitioners (Mezey & Fulmer, 2002).

SOCIAL INTERACTION AND LIFESTYLE ISSUES

Older persons can influence their health status through their own risk-taking and health promotion behaviors and social activities. Most persons 70 and older report some social interaction in any 2-week period, most often with family (92%) or friends or neighbors (88%), and many attend religious services (50%). These types of social activities decline with age; attendance at a social event declines from about 33% among those ages 70 to 74 to less than 14% among those 85 and older. Avoiding a sedentary lifestyle usually improves quality of life and resistance to disease (Federal Interagency Forum on Aging-Related Statistics, 2002).

CULTURAL ASPECTS OF ADVANCED AGE

When references are made to culture, typically what comes to mind are issues related to race and ethnicity. Age itself is also a function of culture; each age cohort has its own identity and subculture (e.g., "Depression babies," baby boomers, "generation X"). These cultural aspects are characterized by labor force participation, consumer behaviors, leisure and religious activities, education, values, and attitudes (Matteson, McConnell, & Linton, 1997). The status of older adults in American society might be characterized as "double jeopardy" in that they may have diminished status as a result of both their age and their ethnic status.

The dying elder may also experience "triple jeopardy"; dying older adults represent two stigmatized fears to society at large: fear of aging and fear of death. They can feel the societal discomfort that is associated with aging and death (Kastenbaum, 1996). Converging negative attitudes toward aging and death have potentially negative consequences for the older adult. These negative views make it easier for society to restrict resources to this population, allow the death of an older adult to seem unimportant, and justify minimal interactions with elders (Kastenbaum, 1996). The conventional wisdom holds that, because a person is of advanced age, he or she has fulfilled his or her life's work and therefore should be ready to die. These attitudes

are presumptive and "ageist"; many elders feel there is much they would still like to do.

Awareness of the cultural aspects of advanced age in the United States has importance in relation to service delivery and plans of care. For example, research studies indicate that elders over age 75 have less desire to be informed of a cancer diagnosis than do those under age 75 (Ajaj, Singh, & Abdulla, 2001). Ageist approaches by institutions and caregivers may result in erosion of the older adult's self-esteem and a loss of privacy and dignity. The lowered self-esteem can intensify feelings of psychological and physical pain and aloneness. Consequently, elders may feel their energy has been depleted, may feel hopeless, and may believe that they are a burden to others.

DEATH AND THE AGING PERSON
Historical Aspects

Death in the 19th century was an event that occurred in the home, and poor sanitation, famine, and infectious diseases killed large numbers in the population. Dying and death became less of a household event during the 20th century, and hospitals began to be seen as offering the hope of a cure; death occurred more frequently in the hospital milieu. As the century progressed, the family was no longer solely responsible for the care of sick relatives and the burial of deceased family members, chronically ill persons were hospitalized, and dependent elders had an increased likelihood of ending their years in life-care communities or nursing homes (Fulton & Owen, 1988).

Older adults are now often away from their usual surroundings when they die; between 55% and 66% of persons older than age 65 die in a hospital or nursing home (Ebersole & Hess, 2001; Kaufman, 1998). Approximately 17% to 22% of all deaths in this country occur in nursing homes (National Center for Health Statistics, 1996). This number might in fact be higher were it not for the trend to transfer nursing home residents to the hospital in the period immediately prior to death (Mezey et al., 2002). Levy, Eilertsen, and Kramer (2002) conducted a national review of nursing home resident records ($N = 1,381,729$) and documented that 25% of these elders died within 24 hours of transfer to the hospital. In this same sample, 50% of elders transferred died within 4 days. These researchers estimated that the additional cost per patient was $10,759 when the death occurred in the hospital rather than the nursing home.

Findings from the Study to Understand Prognoses and Preferences for Outcomes and Risks of Treatments (SUPPORT) investigators (Pritchard et al., 1998) corroborate national polls reporting that, although most people prefer to die at home, their deaths usually take place in the hospital. The number of patients dying in the hospital varied between 29% and 66% in the five SUPPORT national research hospitals, with 23% to 54% of these cases being Medicare beneficiaries. However, a retrospective cohort study of residents of nursing homes in five states who enrolled in hospice between 1992 and 1996 (N = 9202) was conducted by Miller et al. (2001). The researchers compared hospice and nonhospice residents' rate of hospitalization prior to death and found that 24% of the hospice and 44% of the nonhospice residents were hospitalized in the last 30 days of life. They concluded that, when hospice care was integrated into the processes of the nursing home, there is an associated lower rate of hospitalization for Medicare hospice patients.

Institutional care of the dying person often results in the dominance of medical science over the individual and family's beliefs and needs and the institutionalization of death. Patients and families may give over their personal power and autonomy in deference to the paternalism and authority of the health care system. The transfer of the control of natural processes to the health care system was prompted by two social/historical factors. First, with industrialization and more adults working outside of the home, the extended family was less available to care for the elders in the family and the sick or dying. The second factor was the belief in the hegemony of science and the evolution of medical care. As persons had less contact with death in their families and homes, they began to fear it more.

The way that older adults will respond to the experience of dying will be influenced by their background, past experiences, and religious and philosophical orientation and by how involved they were in life prior to their illness (Ebersole &

Hess, 1998). Death anxiety scores on standard questionnaires suggest that older adults experience a decrease in death anxiety rather than an increase with advanced age. This is thought to be due to the elders' perception that they have been able to "live their life" and the fact that they have had experience with cumulative losses and limitations (Kastenbaum, 1996).

Dying older adults may have addressed their own mortality prior to their impending death, but one should not assume this is true. Factors thought to positively influence the elder facing death include whether they are philosophically accepting of what life has to offer; their encounters with death and how they have learned to cope with it; personal loss of parents, friends, spouse, or children; if they perceive death as developmentally appropriate; and support that they perceive from religious beliefs and if they have a concept of life after death (Burke & Walsh, 1997). Factors that negatively impact the acceptance of death are the experience of multiple losses in rapid succession, which may have left the elder emotionally exhausted. The deaths of significant others can result in fewer support people to be available to the elder, and, finally, the incorrect societal assumption that older adults easily accept death (Burke & Walsh, 1997).

The institutionalization of death raised new questions and problems for society to consider. These issues included questions regarding decision making; the utilization of aggressive treatments; support and competent professional care for the dying; issues regarding isolation and depersonalization in institutional settings; and how to best meet the nonphysical but critically important sociologic, spiritual, and emotional needs of patients and family members. Policies imposed on institutions from managed care organizations often result in earlier discharges, shortened lengths of stay, and follow-up home care needs that are far greater than previously experienced (Bookbinder & Kiss, 2001). This is validated by data from 1987 through 1997, in which use of Medicare-covered home health care services tripled for almost all ages, with the most use and fastest growth among the oldest group of beneficiaries (85 years and older). In that same period, Medicare home health expenditures increased at an annual average rate of 21%, reaching $16.7 billion dollars in 1997 (Health Care Financing Administration, 1999).

Insurance programs such as Medicare and Medicaid make it possible for health care providers to be reimbursed for the technology associated with dying. No limits are put on the use of this technology, and it is considered an individual's "right" to have all possible life-saving interventions available to him or her. The threat of malpractice suits rationalized the use of heroic efforts to maintain life. According to the National Center for Policy Analysis, the average cost of death for persons over 65 is $50,000, including the health cost for the 2 years prior to death, private medical insurance, and out-of-pocket expenses (Kellog, 2002). Medicare, however, only covers 65% of the total, leaving the average family with, on average, a $22,500 bill.

Research

Two major research studies in the last 10 years have documented the dismal state of affairs related to dying and death in this country: SUPPORT (SUPPORT Principal Investigators, 1995) and the report of the IOM Committee on Care at the End of Life (Field & Cassel, 1997). SUPPORT was a $29 million multiyear, multisite research project funded by the Robert Wood Johnson Foundation to study the process of dying in American hospitals. The main objective was to improve end-of-life decision making and reduce the frequency of painful, mechanically supported, prolonged patterns of dying. The goal of the project was the development of a model intervention that would enhance the frequency and effectiveness of patient-physician communication about medical decisions.

The support study was designed to include a 2-year prospective observational study (phase I) of 4301 patients followed by a 2-year controlled clinical trial (phase II) in which 4804 patients and their physicians were randomized by specialty group to an intervention group ($n = 2652$) or a control group ($n = 2152$). The "intervention" was a specially trained nurse who had multiple contacts with patient, family, physician, and hospital staff. The purpose of these interactions was to discuss preferences regarding end-of-life care, encourage attention to pain control, assist with advance care planning, and facilitate physician-patient communication.

Findings in general were very disappointing; in fact, patient care remained unchanged. What the researchers were able to document was considerable suffering and inappropriate use of resources; many patients died in pain and with high symptom burdens, and doctors proved no better than chance in judging whether their patients wanted cardiopulmonary resuscitation (CPR). It was found that 46% of do-not-resuscitate orders were written within 2 days of death, only 47% of physicians knew when their patient did not want CPR, 38% of patients who died spent at least 10 days in the intensive care unit, 50% of the patients who died in the hospital experienced moderate to severe pain (as reported by families) at least half the time, and there was a high use of hospital resources.

The findings indicated that, despite well-planned, comprehensive interventions to improve study outcomes, clients in the intervention group fared no better than those in the control group. A major conclusion of this intervention study was that efforts to improve communication about patients' preferences for end-of-life care to physicians by nurses did not have a significant impact on the care that was provided in hospitals. The findings from SUPPORT have provided the data for leaders in all aspects of health care delivery to develop and implement initiatives in research, education, and practice with the goal of changing the culture of death and dying in this country.

The second major landmark report, *Approaching Death: Improving Care at the End of Life,* was produced by the IOM Committee on Care at the End of Life (Field & Cassel, 1997). This report came from the shared efforts of 12 authorities in medicine and nursing with expertise in providing care to chronically and terminally ill patients. The IOM report summarized priority issues regarding end-of-life care that should be addressed in order to facilitate change: (1) the state of the knowledge in end-of-life care, (2) evaluation methods for measuring outcomes, (3) factors impeding high-quality care, and (4) steps toward agreement on what constitutes "appropriate care" at the end of life. Four major

EVIDENCE-BASED PRACTICE

Reference: Fried, T.R., van Doorn, C., O'Leary, J. R., Tinetti, M. E., & Drickamer, M. A. (1999). Older persons' preferences for site of terminal care. *Annals of Internal Medicine, 313,* 109-112.

Research Problem: To describe older persons' preferences for home or hospital as the site for terminal care and explore their perspectives regarding their preferences.

Design: Cross-sectional quantitative design with qualitative interviews.

Setting and Sample: Community-dwelling persons over the age of 65 years who had been recently hospitalized with congestive heart failure, chronic obstructive pulmonary disease, or pneumonia without regard to life expectancy; 246 participated in the quantitative interviews; 29 participated in the qualitative interviews.

Methods: The participants were interviewed 2 months after their hospitalizations, and asked to consider if the hospital or home would be their preferred place for terminal care. The qualitative interviews were conducted within 6 months of the hospitalization. Open-ended questions elicited preferences for

the site of care and the reasons for their preferences. Interview data were analyzed by the constant comparative method.

Results: 118 participants (48%) preferred terminal care in the hospital, 106 (43%) preferred home, and 22 (9%) did not know. Reasons for the preference identified during the qualitative interviews were the desire to be close to family, concerns about being a burden, and doubts that family could handle the care demands. Concern about long-term care needs resulted in preference for a nursing home when the choice was broadened to include other sites for care.

Implications for Nursing Practice: The majority of the persons with a preference only slightly preferred the hospital as the site for terminal care. The issue of slow decline and worsening health—not often part of the discussion regarding site of care—was a concern of many of the qualitative interview participants.

Conclusion: Although the preference for terminal care in the home is higher than the actual incidence, a characteristic of older persons—disability and illnesses that often precede death for months and years—may be a more salient issue in the most appropriate site of terminal care for older persons.

---

findings from the committee offered the health care community succinct issues to be addressed in relation to patient care, organizations, education, and research:
- Too many people suffer endlessly at the end of life both from errors of omission (when caregivers fail to provide palliative and supportive care known to be effective) and from errors of commission (when caregivers do what is known to be ineffective and even harmful).
- Legal, organizational, and economic obstacles conspire to obstruct reliably excellent care at the end of life.
- The education and training of physicians and other health care professionals fail to provide them with knowledge, skills, and attitudes required to care for the dying patient.

- Current knowledge and understanding are inadequate to guide and support consistent practice of evidence-based medicine at the end of life (Field & Cassel, 1997).

Recommendations from the IOM Committee on Care at the End of Life are listed in Box 2-1.

The IOM's report defined a "good death" as one free from avoidable stress and suffering for patients, families, and caregivers; in general accord with patients' and families' wishes; and reasonably consistent with clinical, cultural, and ethical standards. In contrast, a "bad death" is one in which there is needless suffering, disregard for patients or family's wishes or values, and a sense among participants or observers that the norms of decency have been offended.

Box 2-1 Recommendations from the IOM Committee on Care at the End of Life

1. People with advanced, potentially fatal illnesses and those close to them should be able to expect and receive reliable, skillful, and supportive care.
2. Physicians, nurses, social workers, and other health professionals must commit themselves to improving care for dying patients and to using existing knowledge effectively to prevent and relieve pain and other symptoms.
3. Because many deficiencies in care reflect system problems, policy makers, consumer groups, and purchasers of health care should work with health care providers and researchers to:
   a. strengthen methods for measuring the quality of life and other outcomes of care for dying patients and those close to them;
   b. develop better tools and strategies for improving the quality of care and holding health care organizations accountable for care at the end of life;
   c. revise mechanisms for financing care so that they encourage rather than impede good end-of-life care and sustain rather than

frustrate coordinated systems of excellent care; and
   d. reform drug prescription laws, burdensome regulations, and state medical board policies and practices that impede effective use of opioids to relieve pain and suffering.
4. Educators and other health professionals should initiate changes in undergraduate, graduate, and continuing education to ensure that practitioners have the relevant attitudes, knowledge, and skills to care well for dying patients.
5. Palliative care should become, if not a medical specialty, at least a defined area of expertise, education, and research.
6. The nation's research establishment should define and implement priorities for strengthening the knowledge base for end-of-life care.
7. A continuing public discussion is essential to develop a better understanding of the modern experience of dying, the options available to dying patients and families, and the obligations of communities to those approaching death.

Adapted from Field, M. J., & Cassel, C. K. (Eds.) (1997). *Approaching death: Improving care at the end of life* (Committee on Care at the End of Life, Division of Health Care Services, Institute of Medicine). Washington, DC: National Academy Press.

Other studies document the need to improve care of the oldest and frail elders, in particular those who are residents in a nursing home. It is estimated that 40% of deaths will occur in long-term care settings in the United States by the year 2040. The older a person is, the more likely he or she will spend his or her final days in a long-term care facility. In addition, the percentage of older adults who use long-term care, either as a place to recover or rehabilitate after illness or surgery or as a permanent residence to live out the rest of their lives, continues to rise (Teno, Bird, & Mor, 2000). The oldest of old often experience deaths with untreated pain and other symptoms resulting from their chronic conditions, as well as an increasing functional dependency, often unpredictable disease course, and extensive family and caregiver needs (Covinsky et al., 1999; SUPPORT Principal Investigators, 1995).

End-of-life care in the long-term care setting presents special challenges in the areas of pain

and symptom management. Overall, the symptom profiles of long-term care residents are different from those reported for cancer patients, who are reported to have more pain and less dyspnea. This is not surprising given the wide variety of noncancer diagnoses found in long-term care, including cognitive impairment, cardiovascular disease, respiratory disease, neurologic disease, musculoskeletal disease, and renal failure (Hall, Schroder, & Weaver, 2002). Although dying in long-term care is less technologically oriented than a hospital setting, it comes with its special issues, including isolation from and lack of involvement of family; roommates the resident may not know well; the general lack of attention to the spiritual needs of the resident; and often unclear goals of care, including unnecessary transfer to an acute care hospital (Field & Cassel, 1997; Lewis, 2001). The need to improve care of the dying is well documented, especially for society's oldest citizens.

For each resident, complete the chart below and tabulate a total score:

Resident: Date:

Resident Characteristic	Scoring Chart	Score
Functional Ability Score*	If summary functional ability score is greater than 4, score 2.50. If summary functional ability score is 4 or less, score 0.	
Weight Loss	If lost 5 or more pounds in last 30 days 10 *or* more pounds in last 180 days, score 2.26. If not, score 0.	
Shortness of Breath	If has shortness of breath, score 2.08. If not, score 0.	
Swallowing Problems	If has swallowing problems, score 1.81. If not, score 0.	
Male Sex	If male, score 1.76. If female, score 0.	
Body Mass Index	If BMI is less than 22 kg/m^2; score 1.75. If BMI is 22+ kg/m^2, score 0.	
Congestive Heart Failure	If has CHF, score 1.57. If not, score 0.	
Age >88 years	If age greater than 88, score 1.48. If 88 or younger, score 0.	
	TOTAL SCORE:	

*To derive functional ability score, use MDS data for the following 7 items: bed mobility, transferring, eating, toileting, hygiene, locomotion on unit, and dressing. Each item is scored on a scale of 0 (no impairment) to 4 (high impairment), for a summary scale score ranging from 0-28.

If total score is:	Probability of dying within 1 year is approximately:
0-2	7.1%
3-6	19.2%
7-10	50.5%
11+	85.7%

Fig. 2-2 Using the Flacker Mortality Score and Resident Assessment Instrument to identify residents at high risk for dying within 1 year. BMI, body mass index; CHF, congestive heart failure; MDS, minimum data set. (Modified from Flacker, J. M., & Kiely, D. K. (1998). A practical approach to identifying mortality-related factors in established long-term care residents. *Journal of the American Geriatrics Society, 46,* 1012-1015.)

The responsibility falls squarely in the realm of nursing.

Prognostication

A significant barrier to the provision of excellent end-of-life care for older adults is the inability to prognosticate the course that the elder's disease will take and, ultimately, when death will occur. In a study of physicians' ($N = 343$) estimates of survival of terminally ill patients, Christakis and Lamont (2000) found that only 20% of predictions were accurate (within 33% of actual survival). Most physicians were found to be systematically overly optimistic (63%), with 17% overly pessimistic. In response to this study, Smith's (2000) commentary acknowledges that physicians are reluctant to concede that patients they know well are close to death.

Defining transition points in the condition of older adults helps the elder, his or her family, and

Risk Factors for Post-Discharge Death	Point(s)	Patient's Score
Male Gender	1	
Limitations of ADLs: 1–4 ADLs ALL 5 ADLs	2 5	
Congestive Heart Failure	2	
Cancer: Solitary Metastatic	3 8	
Creatinine Level >3.0 g/dL (indicative of renal dysfunction)	2	
Low Albumin Level: 3.0–3.4 g/dL <3.0 g/dL (marker for both malnutrition and general disease severity)	1 2	
	Total Risk Score	
0–1 Point = Lowest risk of death in one year (13% chance of death)		
2–3 Points = Low risk (20% chance of death)		
4–5 Points = Moderate risk (37% chance of death)		
>6 points = High risk of death (68% chance of death)		

Fig. 2-3 Risk index for older adults (age 70+). ADLs, activities of daily living. (From Walter, L. C., Vrand, R. J., Counsell, S. R., Palmer, R. M., Landefeld, C. S., Fortinsky, R. H., et al. (2001). Development and validation of a prognostic index for 1-year mortality in older adults after hospitalization. *Journal of the American Medical Association, 285,* 2987-2994.)

health care providers themselves prepare for the final stage of life. Prognostication in the form of a risk index or scale can help clinicians working with older adults begin to plan clinical strategies with elders and their families and help them consider their needs regarding home care, long-term care, hospice, or other supportive services. Flacker and Kiely (1998) developed a model for identifying factors associated with 1-year mortality by conducting a retrospective cohort study using minimum data set information from residents in a 725-bed long-term care facility. Figure 2-2 presents the risk index developed from those findings; this scale allows the clinician to assess the elder and approximate the probability of death within the next year. Figure 2-3 provides a risk index based on the correlation of medical factors with death 1 year after discharge from an acute care hospital ($N = 2922$) (Walter et al., 2001).

The researchers concluded that, for predicting 1-year mortality, this index performed better than other prognostic indexes that focus only on coexisting illnesses or physiologic measures.

Case Study Conclusion

Mrs. E.'s daughter decided that an assisted living facility would work the best for her mother's care needs at the present time, promising her mom she would take a leave from work to care for her as she died. They looked at several assisted living facilities together and decided on one where an old friend of Mrs. E.'s had recently moved. Mrs. E.'s family packed up her belongings and moved her into the assisted living facility. Mrs. E. happily remained there for several months under the care of a local hospice program and with her good friend until her cancer progressed and she became weaker and experienced increased pain and seizure activity. Her daughter then took family leave from her job with support from her co-workers and her family, moved her mom into her home, and cared for her until she died. The experience was growth-producing for Mrs. E.'s grandsons as they watched their mom care for her and even participated in her care. Her daughter was proud that she was able to care for her mother as she promised and expressed gratitude for the flexibility to be able to care for her mother at this special time in both of their lives.

CONCLUSION

The need to improve end-of-life care is well documented. However, older persons can be some of society's most frail and vulnerable members. Over two decades ago, Robert Kastenbaum, a gerontologist, shared the following words with one of the authors. Even though time has passed and the demographics of our population have dramatically changed, there is wisdom in these lines. To effectively care for dying persons and their families, one needs to understand and appreciate the historical and social context in which they live, as well as individual desires and motivations. Indeed, the need to improve end of life care is urgent . . . for the patients and families for whom we care, for our families, and even for ourselves.

If we are convinced it is right for older persons to die, we may be making it extraordinarily difficult for them to live. We may fail to bolster their chances of remaining in good health; we may fail to recognize when, in fact, their pre-terminal process has begun, and we may remain so closeted in our own assumptions that we do not bother to find out what it is they really need in their last hours.

And then, one of these days, there is somebody standing over us with the same ignorant benevolence we have taught them. . . .

Robert Kastenbaum, 1983

REFERENCES

Administration on Aging. (2000). *Older population by Age: 1900 to 2050.* Retrieved from http://www.aoa.dhhs.gov./aoa/stats/AgePop2050Chart-numbers.html.

Administration on Aging. (2001). *Fact for features from the Census Bureau.* Retrieved February 6, 2002 from http://www.aoa.dhhs.gov/aoa/stats/2001pop/factsforfeatures2001.html.

Ajaj, A., Singh, M. P., & Abdulla, A. J. J. (2001). Should elderly patients be told they have cancer? Questionnaire survey of older people. *British Medical Journal, 323,* 1169.

American Board of Internal Medicine. (1998). *Caring for the dying: Identification and promotion of physician competency.* Philadelphia: Author.

Bookbinder, M., & Kiss, M. (2001). Death and society. In M. Matzo & D. W. Sherman (Eds.), *Palliative care nursing: Quality care to the end of life* (pp. 89-117). New York: Springer.

Burke, M. M., & Walsh, M. B. (1997). *Gerontologic nursing: Wholistic care of the older adult.* St. Louis: Mosby.

Christakis, N., & Lamont, E. B. (2000). Extent and determinants of error in doctors' prognoses in terminally ill patients: prospective cohort study. *BMJ, 320,* 469-473.

Clark, A. P. (2002). Can we improve the quality of dying in hospitals? *Clinical Nurse Specialist,. 16*(4), 180-181.

Corr, C. A. (1998). Death in modern society. In D. Doyle, G. W. C. Hanks, & N. MacDonald (Eds.), *Oxford textbook of palliative medicine* (2nd ed., pp. 31-40). New York: Oxford University Press.

Covinsky, K. E., Goldman, L., Cook, E. F., Oye, R., Desbiens, N., Reding, D., et al. (1999). The impact of serious illness on patients' families. *Journal of the American Medical Association, 272,* 1839-1844.

Ebersole, P., & Hess, P. (2001). *Toward healthy aging: Human needs and nursing response* (6th ed.). St. Louis: Mosby.

Emanuel, L. L., von Gunten, C. F., & Ferris, F. D. (Eds.). (1999). *The Education for physicians on end-of-life care (EPEC) curriculum.* Princeton, NJ: The Robert Wood Johnson Foundation. [For information on the EPEC Project, go to www.EPEC.net]

Federal Interagency Forum on Aging-Related Statistics. (2002). *Older Americans 2000: Key indicators of well-being.* Washington, DC: Author.

Field, M. J., & Cassel, C. K. (Eds.). (1997). *Approaching death: Improving care at the end of life* (Committee on Care at the End of Life, Division of Health Care Services, Institute of Medicine). Washington, DC: National Academy Press.

Flacker, J. M., & Kiely, D. K. (1998). A practical approach to identifying mortality-related factors in established long-term care residents. *Journal of the American Geriatrics Society, 46,* 1012-1015.

Fulton, R., & Owen, G. (1988). Death and society in twentieth century America. *Omega—Journal of Death and Dying, 18*(4), 379-395.

Gornick, M., McMillan, A., & Lubitz, J. (1993). A longitudinal perspective on patterns of Medicare payments. *Health Affairs, 12*(2), 140-150.

Hall, P., Schroder, C., & Weaver, L. (2002). The last 48 hours of life in long-term care: A focused chart audit. *Journal of the American Geriatrics Society, 50,* 501-506.

Health Care Financing Administration (HCFA). (1999). A *profile of medicare home health chart book.* Produced by the Office of Strategic Planning and HCFA. Baltimore: Author.

Hogan, C., Lunney, J., Gabel, J., & Lynn, J. (2001). Medicare beneficiaries' costs of care in the last year of life. *Health Affairs, 20*(4), 188-195.

Kastenbaum, R. (1996). Death and dying. In J. E. Birren (Ed.), *Encyclopedia of gerontology* (pp. 361-372). San Diego: Academic Press.

Kaufman, S. (1998). Intensive care, old age, and the problem in America. *The Gerontologist, 38,* 715-725.

Kellog, B. (2002). Cost of dying is high. *Family News in Focus.* Retrieved January 2, 2003 from http://www.family.org/cforum/fnif/news/a0022673.html

Levy, C., Eilertsen, T., & Kramer, A. (2002). Hospital versus nursing home: A comparison of nursing home residents who die in the hospital rather than the nursing home. *Journal of the American Geriatrics Society, 50,* 41.

Lewis, L. (2001). Toward a good death in the nursing home: Pain management and hospice are key. *Caring for the Ages, 2*(7), 24-26.

Matteson, M. A., McConnell, E. S., & Linton, A. D. (1997). *Gerontological nursing concepts and practice.* Philadelphia: Saunders.

Matzo, M., & Lynn, J. (Eds.). (2000). Death and dying. *Clinics in Geriatric Medicine, 16*(2).

Maxwell, S., Moon, M., & Segal, M. (2000). *Growth in Medicare and out of pocket spending: impact on vulnerable beneficiaries.* The Urban Institute research paper. URL: http://www.urban.org/url.cfm?ID=410253.

Mezey, M., & Fulmer, T. (2002). The future history of gerontological nursing. *Journals of Gerontology, Series A, Biological Sciences and Medical Sciences, 57,* 438-441.

Mezey, M., Dubler, N. N., Bottrell, M., Mitty, E., Ramsey, G., Post, L. F., et al. (2002). *Guidelines for end-of-life care in nursing facilities: Principles and recommendations.* New York: John A. Hartford Foundation Institute for Geriatric Nursing.

Miller, S. C., Gozalo, P., & Mor, V. (2001). Hospice enrollment and hospitalization of dying nursing home patients. *American Journal of Medicine, 111,* 38-44.

National Center for Health Statistics. (1996). *Vital statistics of the United States, 1992. Vol 2: Mortality. Part A, Section 1.* Washington, DC: Department of Health and Human Services.

National Institute on Aging. (1998). Center on an Aging Society analysis of data from the 1998 Health and Retirement Study, sponsored by the National Institute on Aging. Washington, DC: Author.

National Institute on Aging. (2000). Research goal A: Improve health and quality of life of older people. Retrieved June 5, 2002 from http://www.nia.nih.gov/plan/goal-a.htm.

Pharmaceutical Research and Manufacturers of America. (2000). The myth of rising drug prices exposed. Retrieved June 5, 2002 from http://www.phrma.org/press/print/phtml?article=333

Pritchard, R. S., Fisher, E. S., Teno, J. M., Sharp, S. M., Reding, D. J., Knaus, W. A., et al. (1998). Influence of patient preferences and local health system characteristics on place of death. *Journal of the American Geriatrics Society, 46,* 1242-1250.

Smith, J. L. (2000). Commentary: Why do doctors overestimate? *British Medical Journal, 320,* 469-473.

Summer, L., O'Neill, G., & Shirey, L., for the National Academy on an Aging Society. (1999). *Chronic conditions: A challenge for the 21st century.* Washington, DC: Gerontological Society of America.

SUPPORT Principal Investigators. (1995). A controlled trial to improve care for seriously ill, hospitalized patients: The Study to Understand Prognoses and Preferences for Outcomes and Risks of Treatments (SUPPORT). *Journal of the American Medical Association, 274,* 1591-1598.

Teno, J., Bird, C., & Mor, V. (2001). *The prevalence and treatment of pain in US nursing homes.* Unpublished manuscript, University of Michigan.

Uhlenberg, P., & Miner, S. (1996). Life course and aging: A cohort perspective. In R. H. Binstock & L. K. George (Eds.). *Handbook of aging and the social sciences* (4th ed., pp. 208-228). San Diego: Academic Press.

Ventura, S. J., Anderson, R. N., Martin, J. A., & Smith, B. L. (1998). Births and deaths: Preliminary data for 1997. *National Vital Statistics. Reports, 47*(4).

Walshe, K. (2001). Nursing home regulation: Lessons learned for reform. *Health Affairs, 20*(6), 128-144.

Walter, L. C., Vrand, R. J., Counsell, S. R., Palmer, R. M., Landefeld, C. S., Fortinsky, R. H., et al. (2001). Development and validation of a prognostic index for 1-year mortality in older adults after hospitalization. *Journal of the American Medical Association, 285,* 2987-2994.

3 COMMUNITY-BASED PALLIATIVE CARE FOR OLDER ADULTS

Kathleen T. Cumming and Sally Neylan Okun

Mr. J. is 73-year-old married man who was diagnosed with multiple myeloma and chronic renal failure. Mr. J. received his diagnosis 3 months prior to the time he and his wife requested a consultation from the Community Palliative Care Project. With the onset of kidney failure secondary to oncologic treatment for his cancer, Mr. J. and his wife proceeded with hemodialysis. Prior to their request for consultation, he was physically stable and enjoying life with his wife and family. He was able to be independent, and especially proud that he could transport himself to and from his home to a dialysis center for treatment three times a week without burdening his wife.

After a few months, Mr. J. began to experience subtle changes in his physical condition. He had less energy to do the activities he enjoyed, especially woodworking in his shop. Instead, Joe required more time resting in his recliner; his appetite lessened in spite of his wife preparing his favorite meals, and he was experiencing changes in his comfort level, requiring use of additional medication and experimenting with different positions for comfort. These changes were beginning to affect the caregiving harmony that he and his wife had been successfully managing until this time.

Mr. J. and his wife agreed that it was time to have additional help in the home, and they were prepared for discussion of end-of-life planning and care. His wife called the local hospice organization and was declined admission because Mr. J. was a dialysis patient. Although Mr. J. and his wife were ready to work on end-of-life issues, he was not ready to stop dialysis treatments. His needs were not appropriate for hospice care at this time, but he and his wife had specific care needs regarding his life-limiting condition.

INTRODUCTION

In the last decade, considerable attention has been paid to the need to incorporate palliative care into nursing education and practice. Palliative care services are emerging rapidly from hospitals and health systems, as evidenced by the more than 25% of academic medical centers that have begun palliative care practice and training programs in the last 5 years (Center to Advance Palliative Care, 2002). There is tremendous potential for advance practice nurses (APNs) and nurse practitioners (NPs) to be in the community providing palliative care; however, currently few models exist in this setting. As palliative care begins its evolution within community-based environments, the exploration of innovative programs, including primary palliative care, palliative care consultation, and emergency palliative response mechanisms, will be essential to assure that end-of-life interventions are effective, efficacious, and in keeping with the elder's preferences, values, and wishes.

Kaplan, Urbina, and Koren (n.d.), in a background paper for the Fan Fox and Leslie R. Samuels Foundation, suggested that palliative care be initiated at the time of diagnosis of a debilitating or life-threatening disease. Ideally, palliative care would be woven into the elder's primary care, and, as the disease progresses, palliative care interventions would become more prominent. It is thought that this approach to providing palliative care would prevent abrupt changes in the delivery of care from curative to palliative, and would be supportive to the elder's and his or her family's spiritual and emotional end-of-life philosophy.

A novel program in Cape Cod, Massachusetts, Hospice & Palliative Care of Cape Cod, Inc. (H&PCCC), supports a Community Palliative Care Project within the organizational structure of a community-based hospice program. Led by a physician and a nurse practitioner (NP), interdisciplinary consultations are available across all care settings for persons living with illness, their loved ones, and their health care providers. In just under 2 years, the team has provided over 200 community-based consultations. Unlike the experience of hospital-based palliative care providers, who receive most of their referrals from professional sources, community-based referrals are generated primarily from family, friends, and the patients themselves (Okun, 2001).

Data from this experience indicate that elders living in the community with life-limiting illness benefit from targeted palliative care interventions earlier in the disease trajectory. The consultations provide an opportunity for elders and their families to explore in a setting of their choice the management of care provision issues, what to expect as the disease progresses, and end-of-life concerns. From these consultations, interventions are discussed to prevent unnecessary hospitalizations. This would include anticipatory guidance about the disease trajectory and what choices for care are available for the specific scenarios that might occur. Many elders and their families have found knowing how to use the right "medical language" when discussing issues with their providers to be very helpful, further empowering their ability to make informed choices about their health care.

Living with a chronic and life-limiting illness in the community setting is challenging, even under the best of circumstances. For older adults, these challenges become more complex, especially when the goals of care are palliative. In communities across this country, we have created a sophisticated emergency response system that is just a three-digit phone call away, known as 911. This system, designed for acute medical events and trauma, is essential to the well-being of thousands of people every day. Yet this response, as currently employed, is inappropriate to address a variety of emergency palliative care needs associated with chronic and life-limiting illness.

NPs are well positioned to initiate individualized advance care planning discussions with their patients and families. These discussions, as a routine component of care, will provide ongoing opportunities for anticipatory guidance along the illness continuum of their patients.

HOSPICE: A WELL-REGULATED PALLIATIVE CARE PROGRAM

Community-based palliative care, known as hospice, is not a new phenomenon. In fact, for nearly three decades in communities across the United States, hospice programs have provided comprehensive and interdisciplinary palliative care to persons and their loved ones living with advancing life-limiting illnesses. Yet, only about 25% of all Medicare beneficiaries who die each year receive services from hospice. In 2000, of those who did receive hospice, 33% died in 7 days or less. In that same year, the median length of service for all hospice patients nationwide was 25 days (National Hospice and Palliative Care Organization, 2001). Today, many programs are experiencing a median length of stay as low as 14 to 16 days. These data suggest that many older adults living in the community with life-limiting illness are not likely to receive community-based palliative care at all. If they and their loved ones do find their way to a hospice program, it will likely be in the last days and sometimes even hours of life.

In the early days of hospice, reimbursement was unavailable. Despite the financial challenge this presented, programs were able to exercise greater flexibility in admission policies. In the early 1980s, Congress added a comprehensive hospice benefit to the Medicare program for persons eligible for Medicare Part A. Reimbursement provided an environment for growth and, as other payer sources followed suit, hospice programs grew rapidly in number. Yet constraints came with reimbursement. Today, hospice is largely defined by the Medicare hospice benefit and its conditions of participation as a program of palliative care for persons certified by their physician to be terminally ill with an expected prognosis of 6 months or less if the disease runs its usual course (Hospice Care, 1986). This eligibility criterion has significantly impacted hospice's ability to respond to the changing profile of illness that has occurred

EVIDENCE-BASED PRACTICE

Reference: Schwartz, C. E., Wheeler, H. B., Hammes, B., Basque, N., Edmunds, J., Reed, G., et al. (2002). Early intervention in planning end-of-life care with ambulatory geriatric patients. *Archives of Internal Medicine 162*, 1611-1618.

Research Problem: To examine the effect of facilitated discussion with elders and their health care agents about describing and implementation of their end-of-life care wishes.

Design: Specifically studied outcomes were (1) patient–agent congruence as to patient wishes for end-of-life care, (2) patient knowledge about the legal and practical aspects of advance care planning (ACP), and (3) the agent's comfort with his/her role.

Sample and Setting: Two groups of ambulatory geriatric patients (*N* = 61).

Methods: The authors introduced their hypothesis by reflecting and contrasting two existing studies, the Study to Understand Prognoses and Preferences for Outcomes and Risks for Treatment (SUPPORT) in 1995 and the Respecting Choices study, from Gunderson Lutheran Medical Foundation, La Crosse, Wisconsin, in 1999. The former study examined compliance with end-of-life care wishes for hospitalized patients, and the latter, a community-based educational effort to transform the culturally reluctant approach to death and dying to an educated and open

forum among patients, families, and providers. The SUPPORT study provided evidence of end-of-life care not being optimal in hospital settings, but the Respecting Choices 2-year program had elicited a positive effect toward desired change to improved compliance and communication about end-of-life wishes. The hypothesis tested was: Are facilitated interviews used in the La Crosse intervention effective in improving short-term outcomes in end-of-life care? One group was given a health care proxy to complete, the other group discussed ACP with a trained nurse facilitator.

Results: The intervention group achieved higher congruence with understanding of and agreement on preferences and increased patient knowledge about ACP, leading to more informed and better defined choices for end-of-life care.

Implications for Nursing Practice: This study has demonstrated that nurses trained in facilitating conversations about end-of-life planning can be instrumental in improving an elder's opportunity to obtain compliance with his or her end-of-life care wishes. This study provides the framework for nurses to capture this opportunity to assist their patients in end-of-life care planning.

Conclusion: Facilitated discussions among facilitator, patient, and health care agent about end-of-life care help define and document a patient's wishes for end-of-life care.

over the last century (SUPPORT Principle Investigators, 1995) As described by Okun (2001), palliative interventions for incurable conditions such as cancer and cardiac disease have dramatically changed the profile of terminal illness. For example, whereas nearly 50% of persons with cancer will eventually die of their disease, many patients have long-term survival not previously seen as a result of new treatments and other advances.

The introduction of effective pharmacologic and procedural interventions for cardiac disease

has altered how older adults live with these conditions over time as well. Many people now experience long periods of chronicity associated with insidious decline and acute exacerbations that can extend for years. This is also true for older adults living with Alzheimer's disease, neurodegenerative conditions, chronic obstructive pulmonary disease, and other noncancer diagnoses that directly or indirectly cause death over time. The trajectories of these diseases can span many years, sometimes even decades. People living with these illnesses often experience dramatic declines followed by periods of relative stability, yet their caregiving needs will escalate with every exacerbation.

For most of this decline, these elders are living in familiar community settings with intermittent episodes of hospitalization. Each time illness comes, home care needs change and grow more challenging and demanding. Yet, even with increasing needs, many older adults do not meet the eligibility requirements for traditional home health care and may not be considered "terminal enough" for hospice care. This shift from acute fatal illness to chronic fatal illness challenges the time-limited parameter of the Medicare hospice benefit and has resulted in the need for further study and innovative thinking to assure access to an expanded model of community-based palliative care.

A Framework for Community Palliative Care Emerges

In 1990, the World Health Organization defined palliative care as

the active total care of patients whose disease is not responsive to curative treatment. Control of pain, of other symptoms, and of psychological, social and spiritual problems is paramount. The goal of palliative care is achievement of the best quality of life for patients and their families. (p. 11)

This definition was created in response to a need for improvement in care for persons with a cancer diagnosis. In 1997, the Last Acts Palliative Care Task Force recognized the need to reformulate the palliative care approach to include all persons with a serious or life-threatening disease. The Last Acts Palliative Care Task Force formulated five palliative care precepts, or principles of care, to be incorporated into the practice of providers, including NPs, in caring for patients and families dealing with a serious or life-threatening illness (Box 3-1).

Advance practice clinicians who traditionally view their practice as curative could challenge this established paradigm by acknowledging patient's needs for ongoing active treatment for a life-limiting illness. However, palliative care is currently not restricted by prognosis and can be initiated at the time of diagnosis. It does not exclude those who continue to seek aggressive, potentially curative treatment for management of

---

Box 3-1 Precepts of Palliative Care

- Respecting patient goals, preferences, and choices
- Providing comprehensive caring
- Utilizing the strengths of interdisciplinary resources
- Acknowledging and addressing caregiver concerns
- Building systems and mechanisms of support

From Lomax, K. J., & Scanlon, C. (1997). *Precepts of palliative care* (Last Acts Task Force on Palliative Care). Princeton, NJ: The Robert Wood Johnson Foundation/Last Acts.

Box 3-2 Precepts of Palliative Care for Acute Care

- Integration of care for body, mind, and spirit
- Communication about needs and proposed solutions
- Ongoing meaningful conversations about advance care planning
- Prevention and management of complications due to advancing disease
- Timely introduction to hospice and end-of-life care

From LeGrand, S. B. (2002). *Integrating palliative care into the acute care setting.* Cleveland, OH: Cleveland. Clinic Foundation, The Harry Horvitz Center for Palliative Medicine.

---

symptoms related to their disease, especially when prognosis is uncertain (Lomax & Scanlon, 1997). Hospice, which is always palliative and often considered as the "gold standard" in end-of-life care, is available only when the trajectory of disease is expected to be 6 months or less (Billings, 1998).

When integrated into practice, the Last Acts precepts offer the clinician an opportunity to provide a continuum of care typically unavailable for the patient and family as they proceed along the trajectory of advancing illness. LeGrand (2002) proposed suggestions to integrate palliative care precepts into the acute care setting for providers, their patients, and families (Box 3-2).

Operational Definition Emerges

Community-based palliative care, as proposed here, is a new practice model grounded in the philosophical and structural framework of hospice. This model is designed to support interdisciplinary collaboration across the multiple communities involved in the lives of older persons living with illness. Figure 3-1 illustrates the various communities and connections that constitute the fabric of a person's life. In the absence of illness, the health care community plays a relatively small part in one's daily life, while other communities assume positions of priority. For example, a person's intimate community may include his or her church, neighbors, book club, employer, and so forth. When illness comes home, each of these communities becomes a potential resource for both formal and informal support that depends heavily upon the coordinated involvement of the health care community.

The community-based palliative plan of care considers these communities in the context of their contribution to an elder's quality of life and quality of care across the illness trajectory. Coordination of care in these communities is particularly challenging, especially within the health care delivery system. Too often, elders living with illness and their caregivers are left to sort through this fragmented system at a time when their need for coordinated care is greatest.

Recent literature suggests that palliative care be made available within clinical care settings, including long-term care environments where many elders live out the end of their lives (Kaplan et al., n.d.). Little research is available to support the integration of palliative care precepts into community-based environments, such as primary care practices, community health centers, home health care, and other locations where people with illness and those who care for them experience most of their daily living. Opportunities exist for advance practice clinicians to support the ongoing and ever-changing needs of persons living in the community with serious and complex illnesses by developing clinical expertise in palliative care practice and consultation. These services can be provided in various community-based settings, including the home, long-term care facilities, and alternative living environments such as assisted living.

Any new model of care requires operational definitions if the model is to be replicable and useful to other practitioners. In considering a theoretical framework for community-based palliative care, it is essential to look for practice models that provide a structure for interorganizational collaboration. The experience of the H&PCCC with community-based advance care planning and palliative care consultation provides an interesting backdrop for suggesting the use of a theoretical construct known as *relational coordination*, described by Gittell and colleagues (2000) as follows:

[R]ecent research has shown that *relational coordination*—coordination carried out in the context of shared goals, shared knowledge and mutual respect among those caring for a particular patient—has a strong positive effect on the quality and efficiency of care (pp. 807-808).

Most of this research has been conducted within hospital settings and does not encompass the whole episode of care for individual patients, who upon discharge are likely to receive follow-up care from a variety of unrelated care providers. Creating processes and mechanisms to support relational coordination for community-based palliative care requires further study.

Increasingly, elders are returning home with chronic and advancing illness to informal caregivers ill-prepared for the task of coordinating care for their loved one. Care is more complex than before as pressure to discharge patients from institutional settings grows (Gittell & Weiss, 2002). As these situations become more common, the need for relational coordination and creative collaboration across multiple providers and community resources grows. Yet the obstacles to interorganizational coordination are significant as a result of various issues such as reimbursement, competition, staffing demands, and effective communication mechanisms. Studies done by Provan and Milward (1995) and Gittell and Fairfield (2002) indicate that successful relational coordination across organizations correlates with higher levels of patient satisfaction, improved clinical outcomes, and more efficient utilization of resources. These findings are consistent with the outcomes of the Palliative Care Consultation Service at H&PCCC. This program employs the principles of relational coordination through the

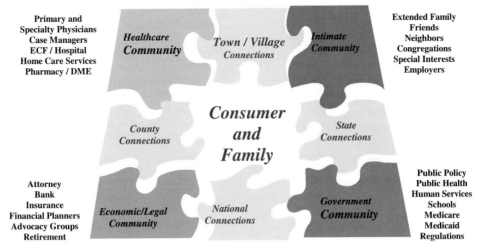

Healthcare Community
Primary and
Specialty Physicians
Case Managers
ECF / Hospital
Home Care Services
Pharmacy / DME

Town / Village Connections

Intimate Community
Extended Family
Friends
Neighbors
Congregations
Special Interests
Employers

Consumer and Family

County Connections

State Connections

Economic/Legal Community
Attorney
Bank
Insurance
Financial Planners
Advocacy Groups
Retirement

National Connections

Government Community
Public Policy
Public Health
Human Services
Schools
Medicare
Medicaid
Regulations

Fig. 3-1 CAReTOGRAPHY model for patient-centered, family focused care. (Developed by Sally Neylan Okun, 1999.)

development of a cross-provider interdisciplinary plan of care for persons living in the community with chronic, complex, or advancing illness. Although such a plan is ideal in practice and well suited to support the ongoing and changing needs of older adults and their loved ones, reimbursement continues to present challenges and barriers. Further study is essential as more and more care is provided in the community setting. APNs and NPs in community-based settings are well positioned to contribute to both research and practice in exploring the applicability of relational coordination in the field of palliative care.

PREPARING FOR THE NEW CONSUMER

The population is aging rapidly. As the "baby boomer" generation reaches retirement, a collaborative practice model will be needed to respond to changes in the profile of illness and its impact on caregiving while supporting the expectations of the "new consumer." Sanstad (2001) in her foreword to the text *Transforming Death in America: A State of the Nation Report,* describes the new consumers as

those with at least one year of college, an annual household income of at least $53,000 in 1998 dollars, and a computer. *New consumers* want choices, control, information, and service. *New consumers* will be the majority of health care consumers by 2005, and

patients who don't take an active role in their own care will be a thing of the past. (p. v)

This phenomenon is emerging as a catalyst for community-based palliative care by facilitating a person's ability to live well with serious illness in the place where he or she resides.

Astute planning and creative collaboration are required for an elder with a life-threatening illness to live well in the community. In the fragmented U.S. health care delivery system, no one provider can meet the complex and ever-changing needs of persons living with serious illness. A community-based palliative care program that offers the full palliative care experience, ranging from consultation early in the diagnostic process through hospice and bereavement counseling, provides specialized support across the diverse communities that make up a person's life. These services provide anticipatory guidance to all involved, including those individuals important to the person with serious illness and his or her health care providers (Okun, 2001).

Giving Voice to Consumer Needs

Palliative care involves various domains of care and caregiving that require collaboration among many disciplines and resources, both formal and informal. Institutionally based palliative care engages multiple disciplines from within the facility setting. In contrast, community-based palliative care looks into the community to create this interdisciplinary approach to care to meet the identified needs of the elder and his or her loved ones. Findings from the field in the Community Palliative Care Project pilot study conducted at H&PCCC identified serious gaps in how the health care delivery system fails to address the stated needs of persons living in the community with chronic and advancing illness (Okun, 2001).

A study done by Hanson, Danis, and Garrett (1997) supports the findings of the H&PCCC pilot study. The purpose of their study was to better understand and improve end-of-life care. The methodology was to interview surviving family members of a cohort of elders who had died of chronic diseases commonly seen in practice. Diseases experienced by this cohort included chronic lung disease, cancer, hepatic cirrhosis, congestive heart failure, and stroke. These conditions lend themselves to anticipation of and planning for treatment decisions. The family members were asked, from their experience, what was wrong with end-of-life care. Communication among patient, family, and provider was identified as being very important—but noted to be ineffective. Information about disease trajectory and expected outcomes was identified as lacking, and skilled communication (e.g., compassion, sensitivity to the humanness of the situation) was rarely evident.

Hanson et al. (1997) cited in their study research conducted by Guyatt (1995) that identified factors that are highly valued by elders with life-limiting illnesses receiving care in an outpatient setting. These factors were excellent communication skills from their providers, information about anticipated disease symptom management, and participation in decision making about their treatment options. Teno, Byock, and Field (1999), in the White Paper from the Conference on Excellent Care at the End of Life, identified additional factors important to consumers at the end of life (Box 3-3).

The new paradigm of palliative care delivery allows coordination of care and services and advance care planning as part of a clinician's practice to improve end-of-life care. In this clinical environment, advance practice clinicians empower new consumers to have their voices heard.

Box 3-3 Factors Important at the End of Life

- Importance of spirituality and transcendence
- Communication to understand present as well as what to expect in future
- Autonomy in care decisions
- Choice in site of death
- Expert symptom management
- Acknowledgment of burden of caregiving

From Teno, J. M., Byock, I., & Field, M. J. (1999). Research agenda for developing measures to examine quality of care and quality of life of patients diagnosed with life-limiting illness. *Journal of Pain and Symptom Management, 17,* 75-82.

LINKING QUALITY OF CARE AND QUALITY OF LIFE

Americans now experience improved health and longer lives as a result of the advances in the science and technology of health care. This advancement brings with it the need to consider how to assist in the guidance of managing the important quality-of-care and quality-of-life issues for elders who are living longer, but often with chronic and life-limiting diseases. Nurses need guidance not only on what constitutes quality of care and its impact on quality of life for their patients, but also on what quality of life means for their elder patients. How does this get measured and validated for the science of nursing and the art of health care delivery? How does it get actualized into practice?

For elders, the actualization of their quality of life is partially derived from receipt of good-quality care that is both coordinated and collaborative among providers caring for them. Quality care is identified as care that enhances functioning, enables control, avoids impoverishment, encourages relationships, supports family, assuages pain, respects spiritual growth, and otherwise generally supports having a good life despite the shadow of death (Lynn, 1997). Quality of life is the individual's measurement of his or her actual situation against his or her expectations. This measurement is often subjective, and influenced by the individual's culture (Clinch, Dudgeon, & Schipper, 1999). Components of quality of life generally include physical, psychological, and social function;

Box 3-4 Barriers to Providing Palliative Care

- Identification of available community resources
- Alignment of the interest of the community to this philosophy (changing attitudes)
- Costs of implementation and maintenance of a community-based program
- Potential for cultural distrust
- The need for education not only to providers, but to potential patients and the public at large

From Kaplan, O. K., Urbina, J., Koren, M. J. (n.d.) *Moving palliative care upstream: integrating curing and caring paradigms in long term care*. Background paper for Partnership for Caring, Inc. & The Fan Fox and Leslie R. Samuels Foundation. Washington, DC: Partnership for caring, Inc.

Box 3-5 Processes for Improving Quality of Life

- Tool development to implement rapid quality improvement strategies
- Conferences and seminars to mentor improvement and foster awareness
- Lead and direct nationwide improvement forums and action projects
- Provide technical support to groups engaged in end of life improvement efforts

From RAND Center to Improve Care of the Dying & Institute for Healthcare Improvement (n.d.). *Initiative to improve quality of care at the end of life* [Brochure]. Boston: Institute for Healthcare Improvement.

---

symptoms of disease and its treatment; spirituality; sexual function; financial impact; and body image concerns (Clinch et al., 1999).

Elders with chronic and life-limiting diseases experience a longer trajectory of illness to death, and may become vulnerable and frail as a result of comorbid illnesses and disabilities. They are confronted with the costs of health care, the difficulty in accessing both informal and formal systems of health care, and the threat of isolation, and are witness to the debate over assisted suicide (Rudberg, Teno, & Lynn, 1997). Kaplan et al. (n.d.) identified additional barriers to providing palliative care (Box 3-4).

Improving the clinical connection between meeting an individual's quality-of-life needs and good quality of care requires diligent testing of interventions used and outcomes achieved. National initiatives have identified various process and assessment domains to measure the impact of quality of life and quality of care at the end of life (Boxes 3-5 and 3-6). Good measurement tools to assess the impact of community-based palliative care should be easy to use, with easy application to practice and record keeping. They should be applicable and relevant to scientific, clinical, and patient and family arenas, and have the ability to convert measurements to processes to improve care at the end of life across community settings. Additionally, they should be able to address the demands of regulations and payer sources (Rudberg et al., 1997).

Box 3-6 Assessment Domains

- Symptom management—both physical and emotional
- Support of function and autonomy
- Advance care planning
- Aggressive care near death—CPR, site of death and hospitalization
- Patient and family satisfaction
- Global quality of life
- Family burden
- Survival time
- Provider continuity and skill
- Bereavement

From Lynn, J. (1997). Measuring quality of care at the end of life: a statement of principles. *Journal of the American Geriatrics Society, 45*(4), 526-527.

Finding the way to have quality care delivery be in sync with expectations about quality of life from elder consumers requires a means of validating the effort. It is suggested that measurement of this intervention be longitudinal, include the patient's and family members' perspective; describe a continuum of care, include the array of care sites; and, importantly, acknowledge the homogeneity of the dying—that is, their different diseases and spiritual and cultural backgrounds (Rudberg et al., 1997).

The development and use of a measurement tool to measure the impact of quality of care on an individual's quality of life will require time, money, bold innovation, and commitment to continuous quality improvement as standards of performance and reporting are developed (Rudberg et al., 1997). Additionally, more research is needed to measure the impact of cross-provider relational coordination on quality of care and quality of life. Recent studies indicate that relational coordination among care providers strengthens the patient–caregiver relationship and inspires patient confidence in all involved providers (Gittell & Weiss, 2002).

ADVANCE CARE PLANNING AND ANTICIPATORY GUIDANCE

With the expansion of technology, there has been growing attention to the acceptability of limiting treatment interventions and focusing on the comprehensive, ignoring holistic needs of the person with life-threatening illness. Recent decades have witnessed the affirmation of the decisional authority of the individual, the dominance of self-determination, the acceptability of do-not-resuscitate decisions, the use of advance directives, and the acceptance of the withdrawal of life-sustaining therapies (Scanlon, 2001, p. 682).

Advance directives have been used as a vehicle for directing decision making about end-of-life care for nearly 30 years. However, as acknowledged by Teno and Lynn (1996) and Gabany (2000), advance directives too often fail to supply health care providers with adequate information to support patient preferences and wishes for medical decision making. Advance care planning is an organized approach to initiating discussion, reflection, and understanding regarding an individual's current state of health, goals, values, and preferences for medical treatment decisions (Hammes & Briggs, 2000).

Advance care planning allows the actualization of patient preferences that may be part of the solution to achieving quality of care at the end of life. It may also be a format to develop meaningful measurement tools to assist in the standardization of best practices in end-of-life care. The goal of advance care planning is to shape an individual's care by the elder's articulated values, beliefs, and preferences in the event that he or she is not able to participate in the decision-making process. The advance care planning process provides an important basis for a cooperative effort between health care providers, patients, and their families to ensure that wishes are known, respected, and honored. According to Byock (2001), "advance care planning is a distinct process that is carefully charted and guides the therapeutic plan of care" (p. 7a).

Initial conversations about advance care planning may culminate in completion of an advance directive. Subsequent advance care planning sessions should take place at planned intervals, during episodes of complications or exacerbation, and when there is noted functional decline. Advance care planning is fluid—it is important to revisit goals of care, discuss treatment options, understand preferences for care, and make care plan revisions as needed (Byock, 2001). Fried, Bradley, Towle, and Allore (2002) concluded that "advance care planning should take into account patients' attitudes toward the burden of treatment, the possible outcomes, and their likelihood. The likelihood of adverse functional and cognitive outcomes of treatment requires explicit consideration" (p. 1066).

New thinking about advance care planning was initiated by the use of the "surprise" question. The IHI Breakthrough Series Team of the Franciscan Health Systems of Tacoma, Washington, asked providers, "Would you be surprised if this patient died within the year?" (Lynn, Schuster, & Kabcenell, 2000). This question did in fact improve access to supportive services for the patients of these providers. Engaging in advance care planning with a patient and his or her family not only represents quality care but respects their perception of quality of life as they define it. Discussions about disease trajectory, including anticipatory guidance, takes the "surprise" out of this question for elders living with a chronic or serious illness. As nurses, the normative response that we hear after a patient's death should be "We [patient, loved ones, and practitioner] were prepared for the eventuality of this death. Together we worked to identify and honor this person's wishes for care from the onset of the disease."

THE BURDEN OF CAREGIVING

The impact of caregiving responsibilities effects major life changes for caregivers. Specifically, loss of monetary savings and the potential for loss of

EVIDENCE-BASED PRACTICE

Reference: Fried, T. R., Bradley, E. H., Towle, V. R., & Allore, H. (2002). Understanding the treatment preferences of seriously ill patients. *New England Journal of Medicine 346*, 1061-1066.

Research Problem: Seriously ill patients articulate different treatment preferences when provided information about likely outcomes of specific life-sustaining interventions.

Design: Questionnaire about treatment preferences.

Sample and Setting: Eligibility requirements
- Full-time residents of Connecticut with no cognitive impairment
- 60 years of age or older with a limited life expectancy as a result of a primary diagnosis of cancer, congestive heart failure, or chronic obstructive pulmonary disease
- Require assistance with at least one instrumental activity of daily living

Participants were identified from six cardiology, four oncology, and three pulmonary practices in southeastern Connecticut and outpatient clinics at two Veterans Affairs hospitals. Inpatients in a university teaching hospital, a community hospital, and a Veterans Affairs hospital were also screened.

Methods: A questionnaire about treatment preferences was administered to 226 persons who met the eligibility criterion. Participants were asked whether they would want to receive a given treatment, first when the outcome was known with certainty and then with different likelihood of an adverse outcome.

The outcome without treatment was specified as death from the underlying disease.

Results: The burden of treatment, the outcome, and the likelihood of the outcome all influenced treatment preferences. The number of participants who said they would choose treatment declined as the likelihood of an adverse outcome increased, with fewer participants choosing treatment when the possible outcome was functional or cognitive impairment than when it was death.

Implications for Nursing Practice: APNs are ideally situated to explore the outcomes of specific interventions over the trajectory of illnesses such as cancer, congestive heart disease, and chronic obstructive pulmonary disease. Advance care planning provides a wonderful opportunity to keep patients informed about the progression of their disease and the changing implications the progression will have on the outcomes of specific life-sustaining interventions. Most patients with cancer, congestive heart failure, and chronic obstructive pulmonary disease can be active participants in the evolving discussion of the benefits and burdens of specific interventions, thus avoiding the crisis-focused decision making so often associated with serious and advancing illness.

Conclusion: Advance care planning should take into account a patient's attitudes toward the burden of treatment, the possible outcomes, and their likelihood. The likelihood of adverse functional and cognitive outcomes of treatment requires explicit consideration.

function significantly add to the stress of caregiving (Covinsky et al., 1994). Some older adults have savings, are more eligible for social support, and may have guaranteed income such as Social Security, pensions, and Medicare (Covinsky et al., 1994). What they often discover is that these resources are inadequate to meet their health care needs. This implies an opportunity for nurses to influence policy development that includes the voice of the consumer.

Informal caregiving responsibilities increasingly fall to the friends and family, especially the wives and daughters, of older adults with serious illness. This is due in large part to the changes in the health care delivery system, availability of advanced technologies, and demographic shifts in the population. The need to support caregivers, both formal and informal, has moved ahead of our ability to effectively respond. Direction is needed on how to manage and organize the complexities of caregiving now superimposed on one's daily life (Arno, Levine, & Memmott, 1999; Covinsky et al., 1994; Glajchen, in press).

Caregiving, for some people, is viewed as a rewarding and fulfilling experience. For many others it can have unexpected negative effects on physical and psychological health. Chronic stress, emotional strain, fatigue, depression, alterations in quality of life, isolation, and anxiety can lead to lower levels of a caregiver's health, in turn leading to his or her utilization of medical services along with the person for whom he or she is caring (Arno et al., 1999).

As illness progresses, the burden of caregiving increases to accommodate the sick person's increased dependency and decreased functioning (Glajchen, in press). The study by Schulz and Beach (1999) demonstrated a 63% increased risk of mortality for elders within 5 years as a result of caregiver strain, and those elders who live with the patient experience higher levels of caregiver strain and burden. The spouses of persons with Alzheimer's disease reported poorer health, both mentally and physically, than the general population (Covinsky et al., 1994). These findings underscore the need for advance practice clinicians to give attention to the caregiver burden imposed on the spouse or family member responsible for care interventions in the home. It is suggested by Covinsky et al. (1994) that strategies to lessen the impact of this burden be tested to assure they are useful, and that research continue so as to enhance provider understanding of how serious illness affects the delivery of care in the home.

MODELS FROM PRACTICE

The Center for Life Care, Planning & Support was created within the structure of the H&PCCC in 1999 to assist the organization in developing a community-based response to the emerging field of palliative care. In collaboration with consumers, professionals, systems, and communities, the Center for Life Care, Planning & Support fostered supportive environments for living well with serious and complex illness through program development, interdisciplinary education, consumer engagement, and research.

A physician/nurse consultation model evolved quickly as consumers and their loved ones living

with illness began to more fully explore their options and understand their choices for living well with serious illness. The pilot data suggested that consumers and their caregivers living with the daily challenges of serious illness were able to identify specific needs when asked. The consultations are completed in the home, which offers the patient an opportunity for comfortable and nonthreatening validation of his or her issues and the provider additional clarity regarding the patient's circumstances by observing them firsthand. Often these needs require a collaborative approach across more than one community-based and possibly faith-based provider. Prior to the introduction of the Community Palliative Care Project, these needs often were not articulated because they did not quite fit the array of services offered through traditional programs and services (see Box 3-7 for three practice models).

Although palliative care services continue to emerge rapidly in hospitals and health systems, relatively few models are available in the community-based setting. Avoiding duplication and redundancy in health care programs is essential if we are to rein in our ever-expanding health care expenditures and foster a higher quality of care for the consumer. This is not just policy wisdom but also the sentiment expressed by the majority of consumers reached through the outreach efforts of LifeCare Conversations and in consultations through the Community Palliative Care Project.

Consumers report a high degree of dissatisfaction with the fragmented health care delivery system, and data from the Community Palliative Care Project pilot study support the need for coordination, planning, and advocacy when one is faced with a serious and complex illness. Yet these kinds of interventions are time consuming and reimbursement is limited, if available at all. Further study is needed to demonstrate the impact of community-based palliative care consultation across various domains, including clinical outcomes, quality of life, consumer satisfaction, and associated fiscal and policy implications (Okun, 2001).

Case Study Conclusion

The hospice organization that Mr. J.'s wife called recognized their needs and referred them to the

---

Box 3-7 Nurse Practitioners and Palliative Care: Three Models from the Field

HOSPITAL-BASED MODEL

Massachusetts General Hospital Palliative Care Service, an early pioneer in palliative care, offers inpatient consultation with some primary care services. An interdisciplinary team, including three physicians, two physician fellows, a nurse practitioner, a social worker, and a volunteer/bereavement coordinator, provides services.

Advanced Practice Nurse Contact:
Connie Dahlin, RNCS, MSN, ANP
MGH Palliative Care
Founders House 600
55 Fruit Street
Boston, MA 02114-2966
www.massgeneral.org/palliativecare

GROUP PRACTICE MODEL

Harvard Vanguard Medical Associates' Palliative and Supportive Medicine Program is uniquely positioned in a multispecialty medical practice setting. The palliative care team includes two physicians, a nurse practitioner, a social worker, and a pastoral care intern. Patients are seen in hospitals, nursing facilities, outpatient clinics, and home settings.

Advanced Practice Nurse Contact:
Rose Cain, NP, JD
Harvard Vanguard Medical Associates
Palliative & Supportive Medicine
133 Brookline Avenue
Boston, MA 02215-3904
1-617-421-6760
www.harvardvanguard.org/feature20.html

PRACTICE MODEL

In 2002, Montgomery Hospice launched the first palliative medicine practice in the Washington, DC, area. Palliative Medicine Consultants (PMCs) offer services to patients, physicians, and family members of those suffering from serious illness at home and in hospitals, nursing facilities, and clinics. Staff includes a physician, a nurse practitioner, and a social worker.

Advanced Practice Nurse Contact:
Anna Moretti, NP, JD
Palliative Medicine Consultants
600 South Frederick Avenue
Suite 200
Gaithersburg, MD 20877
1-301-926-1675
www.montgomeryhospice.org

---

newly established Community Palliative Care Project. This referral allowed the hospice organization to assist in meeting his needs, rather than refusing to provide requested care, by connecting Mr. J. and his wife to an innovative consultative program that would guide, honor, and support their wishes for care along his disease trajectory.

A home visit was arranged and Mr. J.'s first question to the community palliative care NP was, "When I die, will I be able to be buried in the National Cemetery?" That question was researched for Mr. J., and from that point the NP had regular visits with him and his wife. Most often the visits were to discuss end-of-life concerns and questions, but they also included conversations about what it meant to Mr. J. and his wife to be living as well as possible with his

serious illness. Mr. J. felt his physician and his wife were providing him the emotional support he needed. Mr. J. declined an offer of spiritual support, but his wife requested support for herself. She sought and received chaplain services, which were arranged by the NP.

Over the summer and into the fall, Mr. J. experienced two episodes of pneumonia. He was hospitalized for treatment for the first pneumonia. He appreciated the convenience of receiving dialysis while hospitalized, but his wish was to not have to be hospitalized again. Mr. J., his wife, and the community palliative care NP discussed how this would be possible, and a plan was put forward and shared with his physician. When Mr. J. contracted pneumonia again, he was able to stay at home.

Periodically Mr. J. would exclaim, "I can't live like this anymore—it is no kind of life!" and would ask what stopping dialysis would be like and who would be involved. Mr. J. also asked these questions of his primary care provider, who consistently provided him with empathic support and guidance. Over this time, Mr. J.'s symptoms continued to worsen, but for him they were tolerable.

One day, Mr. J.'s questions stopped. Presumably, he had the answers he needed. He and his wife decided that it was now time to stop dialysis. However, the NP and Mr. J.'s wife recognized her need for ongoing support through his death and into her bereavement. Contact was made with the organization's bereavement team for future follow-up. Mr. J. was referred to hospice after 8 months on the community palliative care service. He was now appropriate for hospice care. Mr. J. died in his home within the week of his decision to terminate his dialysis treatments. Mr. J. was buried, as he had wished, in the National Cemetery.

Mr. J.'s end-of-life care wishes and preferences were honored during the 8-month relationship with palliative care. This is in contrast to what is usually available under current hospice guidelines regarding a dialysis patient and his or her family attempting to come to terms with end-of-life issues. After Mr. J.'s death, his wife submitted her evaluation of the Community Palliative Care Project. Her comments were, "People don't know what's available. This has been a life-changing experience for my husband and me. Palliative care helped take the fear out of it."

CONCLUSION

Mr. J.'s case illustrates the complexity of not only managing illness but working with a patient and his or her family about perceptions of illness, goals for managing care, and the need for collaboration across providers to achieve the patient's and family's desired outcomes. There are risks for APNs and NPs entering into palliative care practice at this time because of the scarcity of practice models available. However, inclusion of palliative care precepts into one's practice invites an APN or NP to transcend the traditional approach of providing care to elders.

Palliative care practice presents numerous opportunities for an APN or NP to assume leadership within this emerging field. Some include

- Creating new practice paradigms in the care of elders in community-based environments
- Conducting research to lead and define standards for community-based palliative care
- Developing policy to support access to and reimbursement for palliative care
- Developing curriculum for advance practice educational programs
- Developing collaborative practice skills in the care management of elders across the trajectory of aging, illness, and caregiving

Incorporating palliative care precepts and skills into your practice will create an environment for patient- and family-centered care across the trajectory of aging, illness, and caregiving, supporting collaborative practice when illness comes home.

REFERENCES

Arno, P., Levine, C., & Memmott, M. M. (1999). The economic value of informal caregiving. *Health Affairs, 18*(2), 182-188.

Billings, J. A. (1998). What is palliative care? *Journal of Palliative Medicine, 1*(1), 73-81.

Byock, I. R. (2001). End of life care: A public health crisis and an opportunity for managed care. *American Journal of Managed Care, 7*, 1a-10a.

Center to Advance Palliative Care. (2002). *Call for proposals: Palliative care leadership centers* [Brochure]. Princeton, NJ: Center to Advance Palliative Care & The Robert Wood Johnson Foundation.

Clinch, J. J., Dudgeon, D., & Schipper, H. (1999). Quality of life assessment in palliative care. In D. Doyle, G. W. C. Hanks, & N. MacDonald (Eds.), *Oxford textbook of palliative medicine* (pp. 83-94). New York: Oxford University Press.

Covinsky, K. E., Goldman, L., Cook, E. E., Oye, R., Desbiens, N., & Reding, D. (1994). The impact of serious illness on patients' families. *JAMA, 272*(23), 1839-1844.

Fried, T. R., Bradley, E. H., Towle, V. R., & Allore, H. (2002). Understanding the treatment preferences of seriously ill patients. *New England Journal of Medicine, 346*(14), 1061-1066.

Gabany, J. M. (2000). Factors contributing to the quality of end-of-life care. *Journal of the Academy of Nurse Practitioners, 12*(11), 472-474.

Gittell, J. H., Fairfield, K. M., Bierbaum, B., Head, W., Jackson, R., Kelly, M., et al. (2000). Impact of relational coordination on quality care, post operative pain and functioning and the length of stay: a nine hospital study. *Medical Care, 38*, 807-808.

Gittell, J. H., & Weiss, L. (2002). *Linking intra and interorganizational networks through organizational design: The case of patient care coordination.* Manuscript submitted for publication.

Glajchen, M. (in press). Role of family caregivers in cancer pain management. In *Cancer pain.* Cambridge, UK: Cambridge University Press.

Guyatt, G. H., Mitchell, A., & Molloy, D. W. (1995). Measuring patient and relative satisfaction with level of aggressiveness of care and involvement in care decisions in the context of life threatening illness. *Journal of Clinical Epidemiology, 48,* 1215-1224.

Hammes, B. J., & Briggs, L. (2000). *Respecting choices: Advance care planning.* La Crosse, WI: Gunderson Lutheran Medical Foundation.

Hanson, L. C., Danis, M., & Garrett, J. (1997). What is wrong with end-of-life care? Opinions of bereaved family members. *Journal of the American Geriatrics Society, 45*(11), 1339-1344.

Hospice Care, 42 C.F.R. 418 (1986).

Kaplan, O. K., Urbina, J., & Koren, M. J. (n.d.). *Moving palliative care upstream: integrating curing and caring paradigms in long term care.* Background paper for Partnership for Caring, Inc. & The Fan Fox and Leslie R. Samuels Foundation. Washington, DC: Partnership for Caring, Inc.

LeGrand, S. B. (2002). *Integrating palliative care into the acute care setting.* Cleveland, OH: Cleveland Clinic Foundation, The Harry Horvitz Center for Palliative Medicine.

Lomax, K. J., & Scanlon, C. (1997). *Precepts of palliative care* (Last Acts Task Force on Palliative Care). Princeton, NJ: The Robert Wood Johnson Foundation/Last Acts.

Lynn, J. (1997). Measuring quality of care at the end of life: a statement of principles. *Journal of the American Geriatrics Society, 45*(4), 526-527.

Lynn, J., Schuster, J. L., & Kabcenell, A. (2000). *Improving care for the end of life.* New York: Oxford University Press.

National Hospice and Palliative Care Organization. (2001). *National data set 2000.* Arlington, VA: Author.

Okun, S. N. (2001). *Community Palliative Care Project overview.* Unpublished report.

Okun, S. N. (1999). *CAReTOGRAPHY model for patient-centered, family focused care*

Provan, K. G., & Milward, H. B. (1995). A preliminary theory of inter-organizational network effectiveness: A comparative study of four community mental health systems. *Administrative Science Quarterly, 40,* 1-33.

RAND Center to Improve Care of the Dying & Institute for Healthcare Improvement (n.d.). *Initiative to improve quality of care at the end of life* [Brochure]. Boston: Institute for Healthcare Improvement.

Rudberg, M. A., Teno, J. M., & Lynn, J. (1997). Developing and implementing measures of quality of care at the end of life: A call to action. *Journal of the American Geriatrics Society, 45*(4), 528-530.

Sanstad, K. H. (2001). Foreword. In M. Metzger, O. K. Kaplan, & K. H. Sanstad, *Transforming death in America: A state of the nation report.* Washington, DC: Partnership for Caring, Inc./Last Acts.

Scanlon, C. (2001). Public policy and end-of-life care: The nurse's role. In B. R. Ferrell & N. Coyle (Eds.), *Textbook of palliative nursing* (pp. 682-689). New York: Oxford University Press.

Schulz, R., & Beach, S. R. (1999). Caregiving as a risk factor for mortality: The caregiver health effects study. *Journal of the American Medical Association, 282,* 2215-2219.

SUPPORT Principle Investigators. (1995). A controlled trial to improve care for seriously ill hospitalized patients: The Study to Understand Prognosis and Preferences for Outcomes and Risks of Treatment. *Journal of the American Medical Association, 274,* 1591-1598.

Teno, J. M., Byock, I., & Field, M. J. (1999). Research agenda for developing measures to examine quality of care and quality of life of patients diagnosed with life-limiting illness. *Journal of Pain and Symptom Management, 17,* 75-82.

Teno, J. M., & Lynn, J. (1996). Putting advance-care planning into action. *Journal of Clinical Ethics, 7*(3), 205-213.

World Health Organization. (1990). *Cancer pain relief and palliative care* (Technical Report Series 804) (p. 11). Geneva, Switzerland: World Health Organization.

4 PALLIATION AND END OF LIFE CARE ACROSS HEALTH CARE SETTINGS

Shirley S. Travis and Pamala D. Larsen

Case Study

Writing this chapter reminded us of an elder woman in a nursing facility whose situation, unfortunately, was not atypical. During the course of her stay, her family members clearly documented their mother's care-limiting decisions for the medical record and were consistently in agreement regarding her palliative mode of care. Very early one morning, after all interventions to treat the woman's dyspnea failed, she was transferred to the hospital. After her mother returned to the nursing facility, the woman's daughter appeared at her mother's care planning conference to express her frustration. The daughter was frustrated not with the need for the transfer, but with the number of questions she was asked by the hospital staff regarding her mother's preferences for care and decisions about the goals of care, all of which had already been documented on the nursing facility's medical record. Her question was simple: "Don't you people talk to each other?"

INTRODUCTION

For professionals who advocated continuity of care in the 1990s, the barriers and challenges associated with having different health professionals within one organization collaboratively share information and develop an interdisciplinary plan of care responsive to patient care issues and goals are well known (Hutchens, 1994; Porter-O'Grady, 1994; Sorrells-Jones, 1997). Creating a "seamless" health care delivery system to provide effective palliation and end-of-life care across health care settings for a diverse and rapidly aging society is an imperative for ensuring quality of life even as death approaches.

Collaboration, coordination, and continuity of care across health care settings are challenges to be addressed by palliative care practitioners.

This chapter addresses traditional views of aging and dying that must be replaced with contemporary models of living and dying with chronic illness, as well as the need to bring existing service delivery models and reimbursement streams for palliation and end-of-life care in line with patient's right to determine his or her care. Finally, the need for team models and practice paradigms that will change the ways that professional health care providers and elder patients think about, plan for, and select palliation and end-of-life care across care settings is discussed.

DYING TRAJECTORIES

Older adults are a heterogeneous group of individuals in the ways they live, as well as the ways they die, given differences in their dying trajectories. The living–dying intervals and the types and places of care that seem to be most appropriate for each interval are important to consider, particularly because individuals are living much longer and dying from chronic versus acute illness conditions. These "dying trajectories," as they have been labeled (Field & Cassel, 1997; Glaser & Strauss, 1965), include two considerations: duration of illness and shape of the pattern of decline. These two properties are plotted on two axes: health status on the vertical axis and time on the horizontal axis.

For example, an older adult who is in a state of good health and is killed suddenly in an automobile accident will have a steady line high on the health axis across time until the accident, which would be signified by a straight decline in health status at the moment of death. In contrast, an elder who enters a nursing facility in the middle stages of dementia would be categorized at the moderate level of health status on admission. During the course of the next 5 years or so, intermittent illnesses such as respiratory infections or falls with injury may temporarily diminish the elder's health status. Rather than a rapid and steady decline over a short period of time, as described in the first example, this older adult will experience progressive decline from his or her dementia that is punctuated by sharp temporary declines for acute illness or injury and full or partial recovery to his or her "usual" preillness or preinjury health status. This "sawtooth" trajectory (see Chapter 2, Fig. 2-1) is a classic pattern for older residents who are permanently placed in long-term care, including institutional, home, or community-based situations. Therefore, sawtooth trajectories will be very familiar to nurses who work with older adults in home health care, adult day services, assisted living communities, and nursing facilities.

CONCEPTUAL MODEL FOR LIVING AND DYING WITH CHRONIC ILLNESS

A model that originated in the 1970s addresses some of the issues that professional providers need to consider when caring for elder individuals who are living and dying with debilitating chronic illnesses (Pattison, 1977). As individuals advance toward end-stage disease, several transitions in care are usually needed to deliver the "right kind of care" at the "right time" (Ackermann & Kemle, 1999).

Pattison (1977) initially conceptualized a living–dying trajectory that included transitions in care with intervals for living, living–dying, and death. Subsequent applications of this trajectory to long-term care settings include the suggestion that nearly all permanently placed nursing facility residents enter care during the living–dying interval, at a point at which they experience a need for blended care (a mix of long-term, acute, and palliative care) (Engle, 1998; Lawhorne, 1999). The most recent refinements to the model include descriptions of the treatment modalities associated with each interval on the continuum (Travis, Loving, McClanahan, & Bernard, 2001). Added to this model is the concept of late-life

long-term care (LLC) (McAuley & Travis, 2001; Travis, 2001), which describes an important transitional period in long-term care.

The term *late-life long-term care* is used to describe the care delivered expressly to individuals age 65 and over who are in permanent long-term care situations and are transitioning from blended care to palliative/hospice care as they approach the end stage of their disease and are about to begin a terminal decline (Travis, 2001; Travis et al., 2002). Referring back to the previous discussion of dying trajectories, LLC should commence at about the time that the sawtooth pattern becomes steeper and straightens toward decline. LLC highlights the complex care decisions that are required as dying elders transition out of blended care toward hospice care. The updated living–dying continuum is presented in Figure 4-1.

Palliation, as used in Figure 4-1, is the term for care that is no longer aimed at cure or active treatment of medical conditions. Instead, the goals of palliation are patient comfort and symptom management (Mann & Welk, 1997; Post & Dubler, 1997). Hospice care is a subset of palliative care that occurs at the end of life. Hospice care, which is generally defined as care given during the last 6 months of life, is reimbursable under the current federal entitlement Medicare program, whereas care delivered under the more general concept of palliative care is not. Therefore, "end-of-life care" has become synonymous with "reimbursable hospice care." This is unfortunate for older people who are dying over extended periods of time from chronic illness, because thinking of end-of-life care in such a restrictive way seriously limits the care and preparation that are available to these individuals and their families. For some individuals with chronic illness, such as congestive heart failure on diabetes; blended care (active curative treatment with certain elements of palliation) may last for years with relatively short periods dedicated solely to palliation (Boling & Lynn, 1998). For others, such as those with Alzheimer's disease, it has been argued that palliative care should be the dominant mode of care for the long term (Solomon & Jennings, 1998), with the specialized knowledge of hospice teams available for the final transition from dying to death (Mann & Welk, 1997).

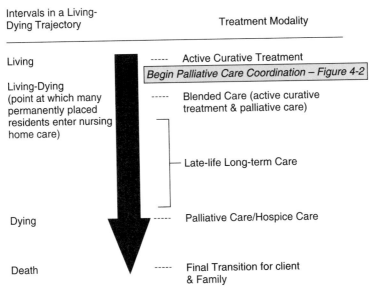

Fig. 4-1 Living–dying trajectory. (Adapted from Travis, S. S., Loving, G., McClanahan, L., & Bernard, M. [2001]. Hospitalization patterns and palliation in the last year of life among residents in long-term care. *The Gerontologist, 41*, 153-160.)

An advantage of using models such as the living–dying model in Figure 4-1 is that this enables patients, their families, and their professional health care teams to share a common understanding of the patient's chronic course of care, even when sawtooth decline is present. Understanding a person's dying trajectory highlights the need to discuss care options and clarify plans of care as he or she moves through the various intervals (McAuley & Travis, 2001). Lack of understanding of the progressive nature of chronic care, as is often seen in the end-of-life care of older people, can lead to chaotic and inconsistent decision making (Travis et al., 2001).

WHERE PEOPLE DIE AND WHERE PEOPLE PREFER TO DIE

Preferences for place of death are determined by very personal ideals and beliefs about the death and dying experience. Although the majority of deaths now occur in institutional settings, this is not where most people report that they would prefer to die (Hays, Galanos, Palmer, McQuoid, & Flint, 2001; Schonwetter, 1996). A Gallup poll commissioned by the National Hospice and Palliative Care Organization found that 88% of

those individuals polled stated that they preferred to die at home (cited in Egan & Labyak, 2001).

At first glance, this discrepancy seems alarming and suggests that people are being forced into end-of-life situations that they do not want. Recently, Steinhauser and colleagues (2000) reported that freedom from pain was most important to their cross-sectional, stratified random national sample of seriously ill patients, and dying at home was least important, among nine major attributes of end-of-life care. So, although the home is often reported as "preferred" over other places to die, place of death may take on less importance than other aspects of control over one's dying experience. With this additional information, it is less surprising to find that 60% of persons age 65 and over who die in the United States die in hospital settings (Brock & Foley, 1996).

Unfortunately, the end-of-life care that consumers think they will receive in hospitals, and the reason so many families agree to hospital admissions for dying family members, is not what patients and their families actually experience. Acute care environments are designed and organized to provide efficient, cost-effective, aggressive

Reference: Hays, J. C., Galanos, A. N., Palmer, T. A., McQuoid, D. R., & Flint, E. P. (2001). Preference for place of death in a continuing care retirement community. *The Gerontologist, 41*, 123-128.

Research Problem: Study designed to understand death-related motivation to enter a continuing care retirement community (CCRC), preferences for place of death, importance placed on communication with clinicians about place of death.

Design: Cross-sectional prevalence survey design.

Sample and Setting: 219 residents of a CCRC.

Methods: Written questionnaire (closed- and open-ended questions) distributed to all independent living residents of a CCRC (response rate of 67.1%).

Results: Forty percent of respondents reported that death-related planning played a role in their decision to move to a CCRC. Most residents preferred to die on the CCRC campus. Most respondents indicated an interest in discussing their preferences for place of death with their health care provider.

Implications for Nursing Practice: Nurses who work in CCRC settings should be aware that many residents are ready and willing to discuss their end-of-life care concerns and wishes while they are still independent and able to make their own decisions. These practice settings are important environments for end-of-life research and practice.

Conclusion: Many older adults wish to die in low-intervention settings.

---

curative care. Death in these settings may represent to some practitioners the ultimate failure of the medical treatment plan. Very often, providing effective end-of-life care does not fit well with the philosophy, policies, operating procedures, and care offered in acute care settings.

For example, the new "hospitalist" model actually builds on and promotes discontinuity of care between inpatients and their primary care physicians (PCPs) (Pantilant, Alpers, & Wachter, 1999). In this model of care, the hospitalist literally replaces the PCP during a patient's inpatient hospital stay. Proponents of the model cite improved outcomes and efficiencies in inpatient care (Wachter & Goldman, 1996), while critics argue that the model "imposes complete. . .disruption when patients most need the protection provided by a long standing relationship [with the PCP]" (Pantilant et al., 1999, p. 171). At a time when care-limiting decisions are often required, the older patient and his or her family members may be forced to receive care from a physician who does not know about end-of-life discussions that may have occurred at another place and time (Gambert, 2002).

Even when hospitals seek to find means to support patients' preferences for comfort care, disappointing results occur. The best example comes from the results of the multisite Study to Understand Prognoses and Preferences for Outcomes and Risk of Treatment Protocols, most often referred to by the acronym SUPPORT. The SUPPORT project demonstrated that medical center hospitals in the study failed to follow patients' preferences for comfort care at alarmingly high rates (Teno, Fisher, Hamel, Coppola, & Dawson, 2002). Contrary to the perceived advantages of being in an acute care, medical center environment for symptom management at the end of life, the reality is that dying well is not always compatible with acute care (Lynn et al., 1997).

The inconsistency between where people die and where they say they prefer to die and the confusion surrounding preferred plans of care has created a great deal of debate and discussion among health care professionals and payer sources (Table 4-1). On the one hand, most providers would agree that an individual has a right to determine his or her end-of-life care. On the other hand, the policies, programs, and services that adequately support patients' preferences

Table 4-1 **Dissonance between Patient Needs/Wishes and Available Health and Human Services for Effective Palliative Care**	
Patient Needs/Wishes	**Available Health & Human Services**
Control over treatment decisions	Care driven by external regulations and incompatible quality indicators across care settings
Informal support for personal care	Inadequate resources for formal/informal care coordination
Appropriate symptom management	Routine care versus patient-centered care
Freedom to choose place of death	Inflexible systems of care and/or few reimbursement options for care

for care, allay their fears about adequate pain control and other symptom management, or offer adequate information to help patients and their families stay a course of palliative care are not always available.

SETTINGS FOR HOSPICE AND PALLIATIVE CARE

The settings where palliative care can be provided continue to change as caregivers and society in general wrestle with old paradigms of death and dying and end-of-life care. In the past, the concept of palliative care has been restricted for those that are in the active dying process; palliative care was equivalent to hospice care. A newer paradigm from the Institute of Medicine study (Field & Cassel, 1997) suggests that palliative care should be defined in a broader sense and not mean merely care restricted to those who are dying or those enrolled only in hospice programs. In fact, as the living–dying model in Figure 4-1 shows, palliative care may be an adjunct to the curative care received by certain older patients, and therefore can and should be provided in a variety of settings.

What Is Hospice Care?

Hospice care was originally conceptualized by Dame Cicely Saunders, who envisioned care that offered modern medical innovations at the end of life and provided the emotional, social, and spiritual aspects of care for patients and their families (Egan & Labyak, 2001). The hospice philosophy focuses on quality of life and patient/family choices and uses the concepts of autonomy and self-determination as cornerstones of hospice care.

Hospice programs may be organized as community-based independent programs (not associated with a hospital, home health agency, other formal service) or as part of a corporation, such as a health care system. Approximately 90% of hospice care is provided in a home setting (Egan & Labyak, 2001) through community-based, freestanding programs. Many of these organizations also contract with nursing facilities, assisted living communities, and hospice units in acute care settings to provide end-of-life care. Typically, patients admitted to hospice care die within 10 to 14 days of their admission, and most are in great need of pain and symptom management at the time of admission (Super, 2001). Some hospice programs report that as many as 9% of their referred patients die before admission to hospice can be completed (Super, 2001). These trends are alarming to many in the health care field, and highly coordinated efforts will be needed to overcome the multifactorial causes for short lengths of stay (U.S. General Accounting Office, 2000). As described below, several of the common care settings used by older people as they approach the end of life have both unique and shared roles to play in improving access to and delivery of palliative care, including hospice care.

Common Care Settings for the Older Adult

Nursing Homes

For many older adults who are in a permanent long-term care arrangement, the probability that the nursing home will be their place of death has steadily increased from 18.7% in 1986 to 20% by 1993 (Zerzan, Stearns, & Hanson, 2000). Often, these older residents are frail and dependent on others for their daily care. As mentioned above in the discussion of the living–dying trajectory, most permanently placed residents enter nursing facilities during the blended care interval. It follows that fluid and dynamic palliative plans of care should offer explicit guidance for their care and should follow them across care settings, as needed, for the remainder of their lives.

With regard to hospice intervention, there appears to be "value-added" care in nursing facilities when hospice care is provided. The enhancements include reports of increased quality of life for residents at the end of life, reduced hospitalization patterns, improved pain control, and reduced restraint use (Miller, Gozalo, & Mor, 2000a). The weak penetration and duration of hospice care for older adults in general, and for those in nursing homes in particular, is an ongoing matter of concern for many groups involved in end-of-life care (National Hospice and Palliative Care Organization, 2000). Refined benchmarks for hospice lengths of stay in long-term care are sorely needed to know what benefits are gained and when the beneficial effects of hospice care typically begin.

Assisted Living Facilities

For newer generations of older persons who are opting for less restrictive long-term care settings, such as assisted living communities, the ability of these communities to support people in place as they age and die is still unclear. What is known is that older adults who anticipate the need for assistance as they age are moving to assisted living settings with expectations of remaining in those communities until death. At the same time, the assisted living industry is struggling to put in place the financial and human resources that will be required to meet these consumer expectations (Dixon, Fortner, & Travis, 2002). The lack of professional staff in these settings suggests that some type of contractual arrangement with case management services and hospice organizations may be one solution for their current staffing barriers to effective planning and management of palliative care plans.

Home Health Care

The provision of palliative care without hospice intervention by home health care agencies does not occur as a primary focus of the plan of care, although subtle, largely invisible, palliative care probably exists. In countries other than the United States, there have been positive outcomes from palliative home care programs (Milone-Nuzzo & McCorkle, 2001). These programs include "hospice-like" services, but most are focused on symptom management in general rather than end-of-life palliative care. Although hospice care is a logical component of home care for elders with end-stage disease, regulatory and reimbursement barriers have eliminated all providers except certified hospices from providing reimbursable palliative care. In order for palliative care to be provided through home care organizations, the structure of home care and the reimbursement mechanisms to pay for such care would need to change (Milone-Nuzzo & McCorkle, 2001).

CHARACTERISTICS OF PATIENTS WITH CHRONIC, FATAL, PROGRESSIVE ILLNESS

As previously noted, being comfortable and being allowed to maintain a self-defined quality of life at the end of life are priorities for most individuals (Ganzini et al., 2002). Having relief of physical symptoms and emotional distress is paramount so that the client can focus on life and other priorities. If clients at the end of life have unrelieved pain, nausea, vomiting, diarrhea, and/or dyspnea, the quality of their lives suffers significantly. If they are unable to receive the existential support they need, quality of life also suffers.

Research from the Committee on Care at the End of Life, completed thorough the Institute of Medicine, characterized "good" deaths versus "bad" deaths. This study suggested that clients, families, and caregivers want to avoid a "bad" death (Field & Cassel, 1997). The committee's definition of a "good" death is "one that is free from avoidable distress suffering for patients, families, and caregivers; in general accord with patients and families' wishes; and reasonably consistent with clinical, cultural, and ethical standards" (p. 4).

Obviously, much work remains to be done before the principles of care in this definition are achieved. Portenoy et al. (1994) reported that the mean number of symptoms experienced per patient at end of life was 11, and that these were highly related to poor quality of life. Lynn et al. (1997) examined 9105 seriously ill patients in acute care and concluded that pain and other symptoms were commonplace, reporting moderate to high rates of dyspnea, confusion, and severe pain at the end of life, with 4 of 10 patients reporting severe unrelieved pain most of the time. Most alarming about these and other findings is the fact that most end-of-life symptoms can be effectively treated. In addition to the management of physical needs, persistent problems with short lengths of stay also suggest that adequate time for much-needed existential support at the end of life is also severely limited and inadequate for high-quality care.

INTERDISCIPLINARY VERSUS MULTIDISCIPLINARY TEAM MODELS

The chronic care of most older patients typically involves interactions among the patient, at least one responsible party (guardian, individual with health care power of attorney, and/or family member), and formal providers (physician, nurse, social worker, dietitian, therapists, chaplain). Often referred to as the "caregiver coalition" in the health care literature (Caplow, 1968; Coe & Pendergast, 1985), these coalition members are responsible for giving and receiving information among themselves, planning care, and making choices and decisions about various aspects of the patient's plan of care.

Historically, the norm was a noncollaborative approach to care in which the physician wrote medical orders and others carried them out (Coyle, 1997), often without active involvement of the patient and his or her family. Since the early 1990s, health care settings have largely accepted collaborative models as the better approach to care (Joint Commission on Accreditation of Healthcare Organizations, 1994). These models are particularly well suited to care for oncology, gerontology, and palliative/hospice patients whose plans of care (1) involve complex care regimens requiring input from multiple disciplines; (2) rely heavily on informal and formal care for the long term; (3) span months or years; (4) cut across multiple levels, stages, or phases of care; (5) may not end in cure; and (6) are grossly ineffective without coordinated attention to the wholeness of the person being treated (Fisher & Ross, 2000;

Marrelli, 1999; Travis & Duer, 2000). Contemporary health care delivery teams range in size from a core team structure consisting of a physician, nurse, and social worker to large teams with 10 or more members.

There are two major collaborative team models used in health care settings: multidisciplinary and interdisciplinary teams. Although the terms are often used interchangeably, they are different collaborative models and can have very different effects on patient outcomes and end-of-life care.

Multidisciplinary Teams

Members from several different disciplines who share common patient care goals but work independently from one another to propose and implement interventions for the older adult are called multidisciplinary teams (Robertson, 1992; Tuchman, 1996). Members of this team model usually have strong discipline-specific identities and attachments to traditional roles and responsibilities for patient care. These teams operate with little or no integrated effort across disciplines (Krammer, Ring, Martinez, Jacobs, & Williams, 2001; Tuchman, 1996).

Interdisciplinary Teams

In contrast, interdisciplinary teams work together to identify and analyze problems, plan actions and interventions, and monitor results of the plan of care (Travis & Duer, 2000). One striking characteristic of these teams is the openness of communication among team members and the intentional blurring of disciplinary boundaries (Krammer et al., 2001; Robertson, 1992; Tuchman, 1996). Because of the nature of the care provided, interdisciplinary teams are the more desirable team model for palliative/hospice care (Robbins, 1998). Many of the problems, needs, and concerns of the dying patient, such as comfort, quality of life, and meaning and purpose in life, require complex understanding of the human experience. Interventions require creative, artful, and skillful applications of knowledge that cut across disciplinary areas of expertise.

The core interdisciplinary team in health care settings most often consists of the primary physician, a nurse, and a social worker. As the needs of the elder patient change, consultation with

EVIDENCE-BASED PRACTICE

Reference: Silba, D., Kington, R., Buchanan, J., Bell, R., Wang, M., Lee, M., et al. (2000). Appropriateness of the decision to transfer nursing facility residents to the hospital. *Journal of the American Geriatrics Society, 48,* 154-163.

Research Problem: Study designed to assess, using a new standardized instrument, whether physician reviewers can agree on the appropriateness of decisions to transfer from skilled nursing facilities (SNF) to emergency departments (EDs) or hospitals, how many of the transfers and hospital admissions reviewed are assessed as "inappropriate" (when patient care that could have been managed safely in a nursing facility was provided in EDs or hospital settings), and what factors affect physicians' assessments of appropriateness.

Design: Multiphase project consisting of phases for (1) development of the assessment conceptual framework and development and testing of the Structured Implicit Review (SIR) instrument, (2) panel validation of the SIR, and (3) retrospective chart reviews of SNF residents transferred to ED or hospital care.

Sample and Setting: 100 medical records (including ED records and/or records for the first two days of hospital care) of residents in eight participating SNFs.

Methods: Chart review and data collection using the SIR instrument, with separate assessments for the appropriateness of ED transfer and/or hospital admission.

Results: When resident advance directives were considered, 44% of ED transfers and 45% of admissions were judged inappropriate. Factors associated with "inappropriate transfers" included (1) poor quality of care in the facility, necessitating a transfer; (2) needed services would be available in outpatient settings; and (3) chief complaint did not warrant hospital care.

Implications for Nursing Practice: Persistent problems in maintaining high-quality care in nursing facilities (e.g., staffing, salaries, work environments) are having serious effects on patient care. Well-trained professional staff available on site to monitor residents' needs and care and other innovative staffing solutions are needed for improved care of seriously ill residents in SNF environments.

Conclusion: Unnecessary ED and hospital transfers impose stress and risk on residents, interrupt care, and represent unnecessary expense for patient care.

---

other disciplines is required. Thus the core is often expanded in palliative/hospice care to include, at a minimum, a chaplain, a pharmacist, and lay volunteers. One major advantage of small teams is that the members learn to work well with each other and have fewer interpersonal issues to overcome.

In order to be successful in interdisciplinary team models, nurses must be secure enough with their nursing knowledge and professional identity to relax the boundaries surrounding their care. Successful team members are able to give suggestions to others and to accept suggestions about care with ease and comfort. Interdisciplinary teams are not about telling someone else what to do, they are about the team deciding what needs

to be done to achieve patient-focused, patient-driven goals for the older adult at the end of life, and designating team members to set the plans into action.

CREATING SEAMLESS CARE AT THE END OF LIFE

Older people tend to access care from multiple care settings (e.g., hospitals, outpatient clinics, nursing homes, adult day service centers, home health care, assisted living facilities) at the end of life; as a result, several interdisciplinary teams may be simultaneously involved in an individual's care (Field & Cassel, 1997). Unless a hospice team is involved for overall care coordination, which is generally the case only at the very end of life, the older adult who is transitioning from active curative treatment to blended care or blended care to palliative care can expect to face many communication and coordination barriers to seamless care under current service delivery practices.

Most authors recognize the need to study the whole system from which older persons receive care (Ledbetter-Stone, 1999; Shidler, 1999), but few researchers and clinicians have been able to suggest coordination solutions when multiple systems of care are simultaneously involved. Even integrated systems of care, such as the highly acclaimed Programs of All-Inclusive Care for the Elderly (PACE), have met with mixed results in their efforts to define and stay a course of end-of-life care for older persons in their care (Lee, Brummel-Smith, Meyer, Drew, & London, 2000). In their study at an Oregon PACE site, Lee and colleagues (2000) found that a preprinted physician order form called Physician Orders for Life-Sustaining Treatment (POLST) resulted in appropriate care at the end of life for such instructions as cardiopulmonary resuscitation, antibiotics, intravenous fluids, and feeding tubes. However, the level of medical intervention was consistent with POLST instructions for less than half of the participants in the program. Many questions remain regarding the factors that lead physicians to deviate from patients' stated preferences for end-of-life care (Lee et al., 2000). These include the possibility that discussions about hypothetical situations in a doctor's office or in a home setting do not have the same meaning to elder individuals, their families, or professional providers as they do in "real-time" acute situations, when limiting care can produce an irreversible outcome.

CHALLENGES FOR NEW PRACTICE MODELS AND CARING PARADIGMS

One of the unexpected benefits of interdisciplinary models is the opportunity for team members to create "new" knowledge at the points where existing knowledge from individual disciplinary perspectives converges on patient problems and needs (Travis & Duer, 2000). In addition to offering new perspectives, merging interdisciplinary teams across various care settings also has the potential to create new practice models and caring paradigms for palliative/hospice care.

Box 4-1 Questions to Be Answered for Seamless Models of Palliation and End-of-Life Care Across Care Settings

- Who is accountable for coordinating seamless palliation and end-of-life care for older adults dying with chronic illness and being cared for across multiple care settings?
- Who will be paid for the coordination work, and what reimbursement streams will be used for this care?
- How will confidential information be shared among all care providers?
- How will standards of palliation and end-of-life care be defined when many organizations and individuals are involved? By whom?
- How will new benchmarks be established? By whom?

From a review of the literature, the most pressing issues for seamless models of care for older people at the end of life across care settings include (1) defined provider accountability, (2) reimbursement mechanisms for coordinated care, (3) processes for client information sharing, and (4) as yet undefined universal standards of palliative and hospice care. Box 4-1 poses these issues as questions that remain to be answered before effective palliative/hospice care can be a reality for older adults who are dying with chronic illnesses over the long term and across care settings.

In addition to these system-level issues, there is a set of patient–practitioner-level issues that need to be addressed for effective palliative/hospice care within and across health care settings.

BARRIERS TO EFFECTIVE PALLIATION AND END-OF-LIFE CARE

The literature points to four major barriers to palliative/hospice care (Box 4-2). These obstacles are (1) failure to recognize that treatment futility has commenced; (2) lack of communication among decision makers; (3) no agreement on the goals of care and treatment for end-of-life care; and (4) failure to implement a timely end-of-life plan of care (Travis et al., 2002).

Box 4-2 Barriers to Palliation and End-of-Life Care

Failure to recognize that treatment futility has commenced

Lack of communication among decision makers

No agreement on course of care

Failure to implement timely end-of-life plan of care

Failure to Recognize Treatment Futility

Prognosticating time until death, when older adults present with multiple comorbid conditions and advanced age, is not an easy task for clinicians (Gage & Dao, 2000). One of the problems is that prognostication must consider both quantitative and qualitative dimensions of decline (Shelton, 1998; Wiener, Eton, Gibbons, Goldner, & Johnson, 1998). The quantitative dimension is most often associated with what the client, family, and physician understand as the probability of successful treatment (rehabilitation, weight gain, behavioral management, etc.). In contrast, the qualitative dimension includes various parties' levels of perceived quality of life for the resident, their personal values and individual preferences for care, and families' wishes for treatment. In combination, these two dimensions strongly affect the clinical care of an individual. Failure to address and document treatment futility can keep the resident from the "right" kind of care (Rowe, 1996). Competing qualitative and quantitative realities may result in difficulties in determining the point in time when medical treatment becomes futile. Moreover, choices for a person on a trajectory of steep decline are logically different from those choices for someone on a slower sawtooth pattern of decline (Field & Cassel, 1997).

Lack of Communication among Decision Makers

Caregiver coalitions are important for understanding the complex decision-making process that occurs in chronic illness and long-term care situations, and for identifying who must communicate with whom about care decisions and care transitions (Ackermann & Kemle, 1999; Quill, 2000; Travis et al., 2001). A fundamental element of effective caregiver coalitions is that the older person and his or her family members are known by and have an established relationship with the physician (VonGunten, Ferris, Frank, & Emanuel, 2000) and other providers in the health care organization (Travis et al., 2001), and that all of the coalition members are committed to open communication about end-of-life treatment plans.

Problems in communication can and often do occur within the coalition. In cancer care, for example, a form of patient–physician collusion has been reported in which the doctor does not want to deliver futility news and the older adult and/or family members do not want to hear it (The, Hak, Koeter, & van der Wal, 2000). Long-term care settings have their own unique barriers to communication. Kayser-Jones (1995) described the "practice of medicine by telephone," in which physicians and family members never or rarely meet each other face to face. This type of arrangement can lead to serious barriers to effective communication among the key decision makers (Kayser-Jones, 1995), especially when decisions are as emotionally charged as are those at the end of life.

It is widely understood that families have a difficult time discussing end-of-life and care-limiting issues for a loved one (Basile, 1998; Roberto, 1999). Even when elder residents in long-term care report discussing preferences for care with family members, it is not known how specific those discussions are with regard to the many care and treatment decisions that are required as end-stage disease approaches (Cicircelli, 2000). Physicians may never be made aware of those wishes (Lurie, Pheley, Miles, & Bannick-Mohrland, 1992). If members of the coalition are not sharing information, problems with agreeing on and implementing an effective treatment plan are inevitable (Brechtelsbauer, 2000; Forbes, Bern-Klug, & Gessert, 2000).

No Agreements on Course of Treatment for End-of-Life Care

Family members often either will not or cannot choose to forgo aggressive curative care, such as hospitalization or tube feedings, for an older relative because they want to limit the likelihood that they may later feel regret or guilt that they withheld potentially effective treatment. "Do

---

EVIDENCE-BASED PRACTICE

Reference: Forbes, S., Bern-Klug, M., & Gessert, C. (2000). End-of-life decision making for nursing home residents with dementia. *Journal of Nursing Scholarship, 32,* 251-258.

Research Problem: Study designed to describe both cognitive and affective decision-making processes used by families regarding end-of-life treatments for nursing home residents with moderately severe to very severe dementia.

Design: Naturalistic inquiry for a descriptive, qualitative study.

Sample and Setting: 28 family members of residents in one of four participating nursing facilities.

Methods: Focus groups, with qualitative content analysis of group transcripts.

Results: Family members experience significant emotional burden as decision makers. The dementing

disease process robs the resident of a complete life and the family members of their life plans. Death of the resident is both a tragedy and a blessing. Family members make decisions that will preserve their own peace of mind. The dying trajectory of individuals living and dying with a chronic illness was invisible to family caregivers.

Implications for Nursing Practice: Family decision makers experience a great deal of anguish, especially in the late stages of dementing disease as end of life approaches. Help for families and residents to plan ahead for inevitable end-of-life decisions is needed.

Conclusion: Many nurses are not adequately trained or prepared to help families with their end-of-life needs. Improving end-of-life care in long-term care environments requires that health care providers become much more knowledgeable about these issues.

---

everything possible" is a common response to discussions about limiting certain types of aggressive/curative care (Travis et al., 2001).

Regret theory, which holds that decision makers worry about making decisions that in hindsight might prove to be "incorrect" and that they will regret (Djulbegovic, Hozo, Schwartz, & McMasters, 1999), is a useful orientation for understanding why families may act as they do. Most people seek to avoid regret in medical decision making. The health care team must be vigilant in enabling decision makers to access information, understand possible treatment outcomes, and clarify the net benefit of a treatment (Forbes et al., 2000). Failure to do so can result in serious disagreement about a plan of care at the end of life.

Failure to Implement Timely End-of-Life Care Plan

Nationally, only about 1% of a nursing facility's residents receive hospice services (Gage & Dao,

2000), or hospice enrollment is delayed until very late in the course of care. Hospice enrollment occurs less than a week before death for almost 25% and 30 days or less for 52% of hospice residents in nursing homes across the United States (Miller, Gozalo, & Mor, 2000b). It should be noted that there is no clear evidence about what the "right" time and "right" length of hospice care should be for persons of advanced age with noncancer, end-stage chronic illness (American Medical Directors Association, 2000; Miller, Gozalo, & Mor, 2000a; U.S. General Accounting Office, 2000). In addition, many individuals will not opt for formal hospice care, even if it is offered.

What seems to be important is that the nursing facility or any other provider of health care to an older person at the end of life accept responsibility for creating an environment that supports appropriate care, maintains ongoing communication among all decision makers, supports client and family decisions, and provides high-quality care and symptom management for the dying older person (Mezey et al., 2000). These are important considerations for quality palliative/hospice care.

Obstacles Hierarchy

In a recent analysis of obstacles to palliative care in a long-term care population, Travis and colleagues (2002) found that the four obstacles described above form a hierarchy in 93% of the cases studied. The hierarchy, as depicted in Box 4-2, begins with the lack of recognition of treatment futility; failure to prognosticate futility is the most powerful obstacle to effective palliative/hospice care. For example, if this obstacle is present, it is almost inevitable that the other obstacles will follow. However, according to Travis and colleagues (2002), the two most prevalent obstacles involve agreeing on and implementing a course of care. The challenge to health professionals is to remove obstacles so that continuity of care can emerge across care settings for older persons at the end of life.

CONTINUITY OF CARE ACROSS HEALTH CARE SETTINGS

Much has been written about the changing paradigms of health care and how the system, or "nonsystem," does not address societal needs. The current system continues to be one primarily dedicated to acute care and illness. Although there has been progress in identifying the needs of individuals with chronic illness and disability, much work remains to be done to improve care for older clients with chronic illnesses who are at the end of life.

For those professionals, policy makers, and advocates who call for reforming the current situation in health and human services, continuity of care is a recurrent theme and a cornerstone of reform plans (Lynn, Schuster, & Kabcenell, 2000). Unfortunately, continuity of care is a difficult concept to define. Sparbel and Anderson (2000), in their integrative research review, concluded that, although there is no consensus as to the definition of continuity, it is widely understood that communication patterns and system issues are involved. Communication includes information sharing between organizations, between provider and patient/family, and between providers within the same organization

(Sparbel & Anderson, 2000). System issues are the philosophy, values, policies, and procedures that directly impact on care and treatment decisions.

Drawing from the work of Lynn and colleagues (2000), improving continuity of end-of-life care across care settings will most likely be guided by five principles. First, communities that wish to improve continuity of care must set goals that promote coordinated care across care settings. Second, public promises for improved care coordination and continuity must be kept. Organizations must be held accountable to follow through on promises, and penalized if they do not. Third, patient transfers for the sake of better reimbursement streams, staff convenience, or any number of other factors unrelated to quality patient care must be reduced, especially when individuals are very near death. Fourth, the elder client's preferences must be known and accessible to all health care providers who will intervene in his or her end-of-life care. It is simply not acceptable to have elder patients' wishes ignored or to plead ignorance of those wishes when a system commits to continuity of care. Fifth, communication procedures for sharing information across care settings must be established and mechanisms for quickly sharing information must be maintained. The traditional problems associated with creating procedures for sharing information with other providers also apply at the end of life. However, this is no excuse for allowing "bad" deaths to continue across care settings for older adults.

To the above list is added the need to educate health professionals to provide care that is consistently at an acceptable and defensible standard. One of the recommendations of the Institute of Medicine's study is that all future health professionals and all current practitioners must receive education regarding end-of-life care (Field & Cassel, 1997). The evidence is very clear that adequate content on end-of-life care is missing from professional textbooks and that continuing education opportunities have been sorely deficient (Ferrell, Virani, & Grant, 1999a, 1999b; Meier, Morrison, & Cassel, 1997). National initiatives by the American Association of Colleges of Nursing and City of Hope Medical Center to educate nurses through the End of Life Nursing Education Consortium (American

Association of Colleges of Nursing, 2003) and the American Medical Association (2003) to educate physicians through the Education for Physicians on End-of-life Care [EPEC] Project are beginning to make an impact. The resulting "train the trainer" programs from these Robert Wood Johnson Foundation–funded projects for faculty members in medical and nursing schools should begin to have an impact on the ability of key health care professionals to affect change in end-of-life care in the United States.

STRATEGIES TO OVERCOMING OBSTACLES TO EFFECTIVE PALLIATIVE/HOSPICE CARE

Figure 4-2 represents the dilemma facing those who want to provide effective palliative/hospice care across care settings. The goals of care on the outside of the model are clear and well documented in the literature. What is not clear is who will occupy the coordinating hub of the model. This is an important question because we have placed the "need to begin palliative care coordination," as described in Figure 4-2, at the top of

the living–dying trajectory in Figure 4-1. In other words, palliative care plans should begin as soon as the client transitions to blended care, the point at which an array of care decisions begin. Unfortunately, there are no funding streams available for this type of care coordination in the general older adult population.

For those older adults and their families who can afford to pay out of pocket for services and for those older adults who are receiving Medicaid, case management services can be helpful. Geriatric case managers (GCMs) specialize in serving adults ages 65 and over and, according to Cress (2001), differ from other case managers in several important ways. First, their case loads tend to be smaller than usual case manager loads so that the GCM can deliver highly personalized services to the senior client. Second, GCMs operate 24 hours a day, 7 days a week, 365 days a year in order to be responsive to the changing needs of the elder client. Finally, the GCM tends to develop a long-standing and personal relationship with the elder client and his

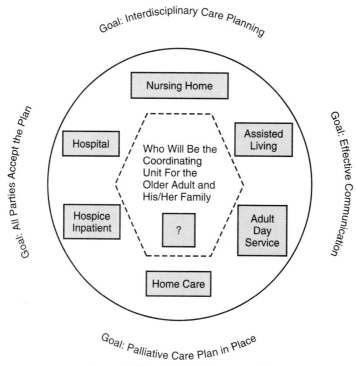

Fig. 4-2 Palliative care coordination model.

or her family members, many of whom live out of town or out of state. Unfortunately, older adults who are neither sufficiently financially well off to afford this private care nor impoverished enough for Medicaid benefits have no such option to help them navigate the health care system and to help them make informed decisions regarding their end-of-life care.

Case Study Conclusion

In the case of the client's story that began this chapter, having a GCM who followed the client between nursing facility and hospital may have helped with the coordination of her care. A case manager with whom the family could communicate might have reduced their levels of stress and frustration at dealing with two separate care settings. As is described in Figure 4-2, the question is not whether coordination is needed, but who will provide the coordinating function for older people who frequently move between health care settings.

CONCLUSION

This chapter has documented the difficulty providers face in providing continuity of palliative care for the older adult at the end of life. Clearly the issue remains that palliative care needs to "follow" the patient rather than such care being dependent on the care setting. Timely communication among the elder patient, his or her family, and care providers will allow an appropriate plan of care to be developed across the illness/dying trajectory. Perhaps the plan should be transported with the patient from setting to setting, much like one's insurance or Medicare card. The problem remains as to whether or not anyone will pay attention. For years, long-term care facilities have sent "transfer summaries" with elder residents when they were admitted to an acute care setting. Salient information was contained in such summaries, but rarely did acute care providers take the time to read it. Palliative care plans may suffer from the same predicament.

Providing continuity of palliative care for the older adult will require the development of a new paradigm and a health care system that acts as a system. Currently, programs and services do little to promote continuity of care and a unified plan of care. Different care settings and goals of care

for the older adult will only be unified when we answer the difficult delivery and reimbursement question, who will coordinate the care of the older client who is approaching end-stage disease and death?

REFERENCES

Ackermann, R. J., & Kemle, K. A. (1999). Death in a nursing home with active medical management. *Annals of Long Term Care, 7,* 313-319.

American Association of Colleges of Nursing. (2003). *End of Life Nursing Education Consortium.* Retrieved from http://www.aacn.nche.edu/elnec

American Medical Association. (2003). *Education for Physicians on End-of-life Care [EPEC] Project.* Retrieved from http://www.ama-assn.org/ama/pub/category/2910.html

American Medical Directors Association. (2000). *White paper on hospice in long term care.* Columbia, MD: American Medical Directors Association.

Basile, C. M. (1998). Advance directives and advocacy in end of life decisions. *The Nurse Practitioner, 23,* 44, 46, 54, 57-60.

Boling, A., & Lynn J. (1998). Hospice: Current practice, future possibilities. *The Hospice Journal, 13*(1/2), 29-32.

Brechtelsbauer, D. A. (2000). Care of dying patients in the nursing home: A call for excellence. *Caring for the Ages, 1*(8), 3-4, 7.

Brock, D. B., & Foley, D. J. (1996). Demography and epidemiology of the dying in the U.S. with emphasis on deaths of older persons. *The Hospice Journal, 13*(1/2), 49-60.

Caplow, T. (1968). *Two against one: Coalitions in triads.* Englewood Cliffs, NJ: Prentice Hall.

Cicircelli, V. G. (2000). Healthy elders' early decisions for end of life living and dying. In M. P. Lawton (Ed.), *Focus on the end of life: Scientific and social issues* (pp. 163-192). New York: Springer.

Coe, R., & Pendergast, C. (1985). The formation of coalitions: Interaction strategies in triads. *Sociology of Health and Illness, 7,* 236-247.

Coyle, N. (1997). Interdisciplinary collaboration in hospital palliative care: Chimera or goal? *Palliative Medicine, 11,* 265-266.

Cress, C. (2001). *Handbook of geriatric care management.* Gaithersburg, MD: Aspen.

Dixon, S., Fortner, J., & Travis, S. S. (2002). Barriers, challenges, and opportunities related to the provision of hospice care in assisted-living communities. *American Journal of Hospice & Palliative Care, 19,* 187-192.

Djulbegovic, B., Hozo, I., Schwartz, A., & McMasters, K. M. (1999). Acceptable regret in medical decision making. *Medical Hypotheses, 53,* 253-259.

Egan, K., & Labyak, M. (2001). Hospice care: A model for quality end-of-life care. In B. Ferrell & N. Coyle (eds.) *Textbook of palliative nursing* (pp. 7-26). New York: Oxford University Press.

Engle, V. F. (1998). Care of the living, care of the dying: Reconceptualization of nursing home care. *Journal of the American Geriatrics Society, 46,* 1172-1174.

Ferrell, B., Virani, R., & Grant, M. (1999a). Analysis of end-of-life content in nursing textbooks. *Oncology Nursing Forum, 26,* 869-876.

Ferrell, B., Virani, R., & Grant, M. (1999b). Analysis of symptom assessment and management content in nursing textbooks. *Journal of Palliative Medicine, 2,* 161-172.

Field, M. J., & Cassel, C. K. (Eds.). (1997). *Approaching death: Improving care at the end of life* (Committee on Care at the End of Life, Division of Health Care Services, Institute of Medicine). Washington, DC: National Academy Press.

Fisher, R., & Ross, M. M. (Eds.). (2000). *A guide to end-of-life care for seniors.* Toronto, ON: University of Toronto and University of Ottawa.

Forbes, S., Bern-Klug, M., & Gessert, C. (2000). End of life decision making for nursing home residents with dementia. *Journal of Nursing Scholarship, 32,* 251-258.

Gage, B., & Dao, T. (2000). *Medicare's hospice benefit: Use and expenditures.* Washington, DC: U.S. Department of Health and Human Services, Office of Disability, Aging and Long-Term Care Policy.

Gambert, S. R. (2000). Is the hospitalist program compromising our quality of care? *Clinical Geriatrics, 10,* 15-16.

Ganzini, L., Harvath, T. A., Jackson, A., Goy, E. R., Miller, L. L., & Delorit, M. A. (2002). Experiences of Oregon nurses and social workers with hospice patients who requested assistance with suicide. *New England Journal of Medicine, 347,* 582-588.

Glaser, B. G., & Strauss, A. L. (1965). *Awareness of dying.* Chicago: Aldine Publishing.

Hays, J. C., Galanos, A. N., Palmer, T. A., McQuoid, D. R., & Flint, E. P. (2001). Preference for place of death in a continuing care retirement community. *The Gerontologist, 41,* 123-128.

Hutchens, G. C. (1994). Differentiated interdisciplinary practice. *Journal of Nursing Administration, 24,* 52-58.

Joint Commission on the Accreditation of Healthcare Organizations. (1994). *Accreditation manual for hospitals.* Chicago: Author.

Kayser-Jones, J. (1995). Decision making in the treatment of acute illness in nursing homes: Framing the decision problem, treatment plan, and outcome. *Medical Anthropology Quarterly, 9,* 236-256.

Krammer, L. M., Ring, A. A., Martinez, J., Jacobs, M. J., & Williams, M. B. (2001). The nurse's role in interdisciplinary and palliative care. In M. L. Matzo & D. W. Sherman (Eds.), *Palliative care nursing: Quality care to the end of life* (pp. 118-139). New York: Springer.

Lawhorne, L. W. (1999). Avoidable and unavoidable decline and the naturalness of dying: The nursing home dilemma. *Annals of Long-Term Care, 7,* 309-312.

Ledbetter-Stone, M. (1999). Family intervention strategies when dealing with futility of treatment issues: A case study. *Critical Care Nursing Quarterly, 22,* 45-50.

Lee, M. A., Brummel-Smith, K., Meyer, J., Drew, N., & London, M. R. (2000). Physician orders for life-sustaining treatment (POLST): Outcomes in a PACE program. *Journal of the American Geriatrics Society, 48,* 1219-1225.

Lurie, N., Pheley, A. M., Miles, S. H., & Bannick-Mohrland, S. (1992). Attitudes toward discussing life-sustaining treatments in extended care facility residents. *Journal of the American Geriatrics Society, 40,* 1205-1208.

Lynn, J., Schuster, J., & Kabcenell, A. (2000). *Improving care for the end of life: A sourcebook for health care managers and clinicians.* New York: Oxford University Press.

Lynn, J., Teno, J. M., Phillips, R. S., Wu, A. W., Desbiens, N., Harrold, J., et al. (1997). Perceptions by family members of the dying experience of older and seriously ill patients. *Annals of Internal Medicine, 126,* 97-107.

Mann, S. M., & Welk, T. A. (1997). Hospice and/or palliative care? *American Journal of Hospice and Palliative Care, 14,* 314-315.

Marrelli, T. M. (1999). *Hospice and palliative care handbook: Quality, compliance, and reimbursement.* St. Louis: Mosby.

McAuley, W. J., & Travis, S. S. (2001, July). Advance care planning among residents in a national sample of U.S. nursing home residents. Presentation at the 17th World Congress of the International Association of Gerontology, Vancouver, BC.

Meier D., Morrison, R. S., & Cassel, C. (1997). Improving palliative care. *Annals of Internal Medicine, 127,* 225-230.

Mezey, M. D., Dubler, N. N., Bottrell, M., Mitty, E., Ramsey, G., Post, L. F., et al. (2000). *Guidelines for end-of-life care in nursing facilities: Principles and recommendations.* New York: John A. Hartford Foundation Institute for Geriatric Nursing.

Miller, S. C., Gozalo, P., & Mor, V. (2000a). *Outcomes and utilization for hospice and non-hospice nursing facility decedents.* Washington, DC: U.S. Department of Health and Human Services, Office of Disability, Aging and Long-Term Care Policy.

Miller, S. C., Gozalo, P., & Mor, V. (2000b). *Use of Medicare's hospice benefit by nursing facility residents.* Washington, DC: U.S. Department of Health and Human Services, Office of Disability, Aging and Long-Term Care Policy.

Milone-Nuzzo, P., & McCorkle, R. (2001). Home care. In B. Ferrell, & N. Coyle (Eds.), *Textbook of palliative nursing* (pp. 543-555). New York: Oxford University Press.

National Hospice and Palliative Care Organization. (2000). *News release: Summary of key findings of synthesis and analysis of Medicare's hospice benefit.* Alexandria, VA: Author.

Pantilant, S. Z., Alpers, A., & Wachter, R. M. (1999). A new doctor in the house: Ethical issues in hospitalist systems. *Journal of the American Medical Association, 282,* 171-174.

Pattison, E. M. (1977). *The experience of dying.* Englewood Cliffs, NJ: Prentice Hall.

Portenoy, R. K., Thaler, H. T., Kornblith, A. B., Lepore, J. M., Friedlander-Klar, B., Coyle, N., et al. (1994). Symptom prevalence, characteristics and distress in a cancer population. *Quality of Life Research, 3*(3), 183-189.

Porter-O'Grady, T. (1994). Whole systems shared governance: Creating the seamless organization. *Nursing Economics, 12,* 187-195.

Post, L. F., & Dubler, N. N. (1997). Palliative care: A bioethical definition, principles, and clinical guidelines. *Bioethics Forum, 13*(3), 17-24.

Quill, T. E. (2000). Initiating end of life discussions with seriously ill residents: Addressing the elephant in the room. *Journal of the American Medical Association, 284,* 2502-2507.

Roberto, K. A. (1999). Making critical health care decisions for older adults: Consensus among family members. *Family Relations, 49,* 167-175.

Robertson, D. (1992). The roles of health care teams in care of the elderly. *Family Medicine, 24,* 136-141.

Robbins, M. (1998). *Evaluating palliative care: Establishing the evidence base.* New York: Oxford University Press.

Rowe, J. W. (1996). Health care myths at the end of life. *Bulletin of the American College of Surgeons, 81*(6), 11-18.

Schonwetter, R. S. (1996). Care of the dying geriatric patient. *Clinics in Geriatric Medicine, 12,* 253-265.

Shelton, W. (1998). A broader look at medical futility. *Theoretical Medicine and Bioethics, 19,* 383-400.

Shidler, S. (1999). Effective communication of the long-term care resident's life prolonging treatment wishes: A systematic perspective. In B. de Vries (Ed.), *End of life issues: Interdisciplinary and multidimensional perspectives* (pp. 185-204). New York: Springer.

Solomon, M. Z., & Jennings, B. (1998). Palliative care for Alzheimer's patients: Implications for institutions, caregivers, and families. In L. Volicer & A. Hurley (Eds.), *Hospice care for patients with advanced progressive dementia* (pp. 132-154). New York: Springer.

Sorrells-Jones, J. (1997). The challenge of making it real: Interdisciplinary practice in a "seamless" organization. *Nursing Administration Quarterly, 21,* 20-30.

Sparbel, K., & Anderson, M. A. (2000). Integrated literature review of continuity of care: Part 1, Conceptual issues. *Journal of Nursing Scholarship, 32*(1), 17-24.

Steinhauser, K. E., Christakis, N. A., Clipp, E. C., McNeilly, M., McIntyre, L., & Tulsky, J. A. (2000). Factors considered important at the end of life by patients, family, physicians, and other care providers. *Journal of the American Medical Association, 248,* 2476-2482.

Super, A. (2001). The context of palliative care in progressive illness. In B. Ferrell & N. Coyle (Eds.), *Textbook of palliative nursing* (pp. 27-36). New York: Oxford University Press.

Teno, J. M., Fisher, E. S., Hamel, M. B., Coppola, K., & Dawson, N. V. (2002). Medical care inconsistent with patients' treatment goals: Association with 1-year medicare resource use and survival. *Journal of the American Geriatrics Society, 50,* 496-500.

The, A., Hak, T., Koeter, G., & van der Wal, G. (2000). Collusion in doctor-residents communication about imminent death: An ethnographic study. *British Medical Journal, 321,* 1376-1381.

Travis, S. S. (2001). Palliative care: A way of thinking, a prescription for doing. *Geriatric Nursing, 22,* 284-285.

Travis, S. S., Bernard, M. A., Dixon, S., McAuley, W. J., Loving, G., & McClanahan, L. (2002). Obstacles to palliation and end-of-life care in a long-term care facility. *The Gerontologist, 42,* 342-349.

Travis, S. S., & Duer, B. (2000). Interdisciplinary management of the older adult with cancer. In A. S. Luggen & S. E. Miener (Eds.), *Handbook for the care of the older adult with cancer* (pp. 25-34). Pittsburgh: Oncology Nursing Press.

Travis, S. S., Loving, G., McClanahan, L., & Bernard, M. (2001). Hospitalization patterns and palliation in the last year of life among residents in long-term care. *The Gerontologist, 41,* 153-160.

Tuchman, L. I. (1996). The team and models of teaming. In P. Rosin, A. Whitehead, L. I. Tuchman, G. S. Jesien, A. L. Begun, & L. Irwin (Eds.), *Partnerships in family-centered care* (pp. 119-143). Baltimore: Paul Brookes Publishing.

U.S. General Accounting Office. (2000, September). *Medicare: More beneficiaries use hospice, yet many factors contribute to shorter stays* (GAO/T-HEHS-00-201). Washington, DC: U.S. General Accounting Office, Health, Education and Human Services Division.

vonGuten, C. F., Ferris, F. D., & Emanuel, L. (2000). Ensuring competency in end-of-life care: communication and relational skills. *Journal of the American Medical Association, 284*(23), 3051-3057.

Wachter, R. M., & Goldman, L. (1996). The emerging role of "hospitalists" in the American health care system. *New England Journal of Medicine, 335,* 514-517.

Wiener, R. L., Eton, D., Gibbons, V. P., Goldner, J. A., & Johnson, S. H. (1998). A preliminary analysis of medical futility decision making: Law and professional attitudes. *Behavioral Sciences and the Law, 16,* 497-508.

Zerzan, J., Stearns, S., & Hanson, L. (2000). Access to palliative care and hospice care in nursing homes. *Journal of the American Medical Association, 284,* 2489-2494.

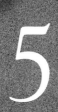

5

ETHICAL AND LEGAL ASPECTS OF DYING AND HEALTH CARE RESOURCE ALLOCATION

Anita J. Tarzian and Judith K. Schwarz

INTRODUCTION

Ethics refers to a framework or guideline for determining what is morally good (right) or bad (wrong). This process has become increasingly difficult when making health care decisions at the end of life, particularly for older individuals residing in the United States. There are many reasons for this increased difficulty. Medical research and technology have extended life spans, which, together with the aging of the "baby boomer" generation, has shifted population age demographics toward the older adult. Indeed, the fastest growing age demographic in the United States is persons 85 years and older. While on the one hand this is a marker of success, on the other hand, it forces more complex decisions to be made about when, if ever, to place limits on the use of medical interventions for the older adult. Should the focus be on life prolongation regardless of quality of life? How should decisions be made about allocating limited medical resources to older adults, who have less time to reap the benefits of expensive and potentially risky medical therapies?

In discussing "ethics at the end of life," *end of life* usually serves as a euphemism for the process of dying and death. The term is generally reserved for those who are expected to die within a given time frame (e.g., less than 6 months) from an incurable, progressive disease. By this definition, the "end of life" is not restricted to the older adult. Yet, as one ages and surpasses his or her estimated life expectancy, mortality looms closer regardless of health status, causing most to include the older adult in discussions of ethics at the end of life. This is likely what prompted one healthy 90-year-old woman to tell her health care providers (HCPs) that she was 10 years younger

than she was to ensure that they would not "give up too easily" in providing her medical care.

Should age be considered in a discussion of health care ethics at the end of life? If so, how? How do the answers to these questions differ depending on whether one is considering an individual elder patient or society at large? What framework might guide the discussion of these issues to promote ethical decision making and practice among HCPs? Consider the following approach, which is actually a combination of many theoretical approaches.

PROMOTING ETHICAL PRACTICE–DOING AND BEING

Various ethical frameworks exist to guide HCPs in sorting through ethical issues in policy making and clinical practice. Generally speaking, they can be categorized according to whether they provide guidelines of what to *do* in a given situation (*doing*) or whether they address *how* an ethical agent should act (*being*). Maximizing benefits over harms (i.e., application of the combined principles of *beneficence* and *nonmaleficence*) is an example of *doing*, and is relevant for both clinical decision making and public policy making. At the extreme, ethically right or wrong actions are based solely on identifiable (and typically measurable) outcomes—this is known as *consequentialism*. The maxim "seek the greatest benefit for the greatest number" is one form of consequentialism, that of *utilitarianism*. The principle of autonomy is often considered under the broader principle of *respect for persons*, and guides HCPs to respect mentally competent patients' health care wishes and protect mentally incompetent or decisionally incapacitated patients from being harmed. The principle of *justice* addresses what should be done to ensure equal health care access and fair resource allocation.

Many also acknowledge the importance of ethical frameworks that focus on character traits of the ethical agent (*being*). Nurses who cultivate positive virtues and caring behaviors are thought to be oriented toward ethical actions from an "inside out" approach. For example, nurses who cultivate the virtue of *benevolence* are oriented toward implementing *beneficent* actions. The problem with an approach that is focused solely on virtues or character traits is that it does not give specific direction about what to do when faced with an ethical dilemma. It assumes that nurses who cultivate the virtue of benevolence will naturally act beneficently. Many ethicists acknowledge that virtue and care ethics must be coupled with guidelines for good action, such as *principalism*. Principalism teaches that we must identify potential harms and goods and try to minimize the former (nonmaleficence) and maximize the latter (beneficence). Advocating for a patient to be able to continue living independently as he or she wishes (or, alternatively, seeking other living arrangements if independent living would put the patient at undue risk) is informed by the principle of respect for persons. Yet, using principles alone as decision-making guides can reduce the moral encounter to one of superficially applying rules in a "cookbook"-like fashion. The authors feel that ethical decision making should be informed by an *orientation toward good action*, which we call a framework of "being"—caring is one way of being that orients the nurse toward good action. Virtues such as compassion and loyalty are other examples. In this chapter, when we refer to ethical principles, we do so with the implicit recognition that applying principles to ethical decision making at the bedside (i.e., "doing") is best achieved when virtues that promote caring and reflective thought are fostered throughout the health care professional's education, training, and practice (i.e., "being").

ETHICS AND THE LAW

It is often the case when ethical dilemmas arise in health care institutions that staff ask the question, "What does the law say?" Although this is an understandable question, it is important to realize that *ethical* and *legal* are not synonymous.

There are some who think that Dr. Jack Kevorkian's actions to assist individuals in committing suicide were ethically right, although Michigan state law prohibits assisted suicide. Likewise, others feel that the assisted suicide that Oregon physicians have legally been permitted to provide since 1997 is ethically wrong. City, county, state, and federal laws are created through legislative processes, and typically serve to protect individual rights and liberties, such as those granted in the U.S. Constitution. The legal system generally has a higher threshold for deeming an act as "wrong" and punishable because its purpose is to protect citizens and promote their well-being, but not to legislate morality.

Most laws that influence ethical decision making in health care are grounded in the concept of *respect for individual autonomy* and the right of citizens to retain control over their own persons. As long as individuals are not in danger of harming themselves or others, laws generally allow them to make their own health care choices. Distinctions can be made between liberty and welfare rights. *Liberty rights*, such as the right of privacy, are entitlements ensuring that an individual is left free from unwanted and unwarranted interference—they entail no obligation other than noninterference. In contrast, *welfare rights* are those that another party, such as the government, has an obligation to provide, such as basic education and protection from violent crime. Currently, basic (i.e., nonemergency) health care is not viewed as a positive right for all U.S. citizens, a topic we will revisit at the end of this chapter.

The relationship between ethics and the law is more easily understood when considering specific examples, such as the difference between mental competency and decisional capacity. Both are rooted in the ethical principle of respect for persons. However, *mental competency* is strictly a legal determination made by a judge as to whether an individual has the cognitive ability to make rational choices that do not put him or her or others in danger of undue harm. For example, a hospital may petition a court to appoint a legal guardian for an elder hospitalized patient who needs surgery but has no identified family members or legal surrogate who can consent to the surgery. The judge, based on psychiatric evaluations of the patient, will determine globally whether this patient has the mental capacity to make health care decisions for him- or herself. If a judge determines that the patient does not, a guardian will be appointed to make health care decisions for him or her. The guardian will then make a decision about whether or not to consent to the surgery. Whether or not a judge determines that such a patient is mentally incompetent and appoints a legal guardian, an evaluation of the patient's *decisional capacity* to consent to the surgery should also take place. Decisional capacity is evidenced if an individual states a consistent preference among available options, if that preference is based on sound reasoning (i.e., is consistent with the individual's values and beliefs), and if the individual demonstrates an understanding of the likely risks and benefits of his or her choice. In summary, *mental competence* is a legal term referring to a *global* assessment of a person's ability to make rational decisions, and *decisional capacity* is a clinical term that refers to a patient's ability to make a rational *individual* decision.

An elder person who has mild to moderate dementia may be deemed *mentally incompetent* by the legal system, but a health care professional or legal guardian may determine that the individual has the decisional capacity to make *certain* choices about his or her health care or living situation. Often elder persons demonstrate capacity that "waxes and wanes." Clinicians who know the patient well are often able to suggest the most opportune time of day to discuss treatment options with him or her. Typically, the threshold for determining decisional capacity is higher if the anticipated outcome carries a riskier potential harm, such as death. That is, it is ethically justifiable that a person who consents to a leg amputation to save his or her life does not undergo the same level of scrutiny of decisional capacity as the person who refuses the amputation, but the person refusing the amputation may be allowed to do so if he or she demonstrates the criteria for decisional capacity.

Recent evidence has highlighted the importance of assessing decisional capacity among ill older adults. Cassell, Leon, and Kaufman (2001) found signs of cognitive impairment affecting judgment in sicker, hospitalized patients who were otherwise competent adults. They found

that sick individuals had the same decision-making ability as preadolescent children, thus questioning the assumed decisional capacity of ill adults. Along similar lines, Dr. Marie Nolan, a nurse researcher, and her colleagues at Johns Hopkins University have been interviewing individuals at different time points who have four different types of terminal diseases with different trajectories to death, ranging from an average of 6 to 9 months (metastatic lung cancer) to 2 to 4 years (amyotrophic lateral sclerosis or "Lou Gehrig's disease"). These researchers have found that, as patients experience increased dependence as a result of disease progression and symptom exacerbation, they tend to prefer that decisions be made for them by physicians who have consulted them about their preferences. If their symptoms abate and they regain independence, they tend to prefer taking a more active role in medical decision making (Nolan, 2001).

Thus, just as mental incompetence may coexist with the decisional capacity to consent to or refuse certain medical interventions, mental competence may coexist with evidence of decisional incapacity, particularly during health crises or illness exacerbations. The ethical principles of respect for persons, nonmaleficence, and beneficence require that an ill patient's decision-making capacity be assessed and that assistance with health care decisions be provided as needed by trusted surrogates, with HCPs providing necessary information, support, and advocacy.

ISSUES AT THE END OF LIFE
Identifying Benefits and Harms

Generally speaking, the goal of ethical action and decision making involves avoiding or minimizing harms and, if possible, maximizing benefits. This may sound simple—in theory. Yet, as most nurses know, it can be much harder in practice. One person may find the side effects of chemotherapy for advanced cancer (i.e., "harm") not worth the benefit of a few months of extended life, particularly if those extra months are spent enduring various chemotherapy-induced side effects. Another person may take the opposite view. Such differences in what one considers beneficial and harmful are grounded in a person's core beliefs and values. One person's values or beliefs, for example, may obligate him to extend life as long as possible. Another person's beliefs may lead her to seek assisted suicide to avoid anticipated suffering or being a burden to others. HCPs involved in caring for patients who make such choices may experience conflict when their own values diverge from those of the patient.

In a country as ethnically diverse as the United States, exploring an individual's core beliefs and values in order to identify what he or she considers harmful and beneficial is anything but simple. The tendency to project our own values and beliefs onto others puts us at risk for making unwarranted assumptions about what others consider helpful and harmful. Consider the case of Mrs. W., an elder African American nursing home resident who has severe dementia. Mrs. W. is contracted in a fetal position, cannot eat or drink by mouth, and receives nutrition through a gastrostomy tube. She makes moaning sounds and sucks her thumb, but cannot speak or interact with others. The day shift nurse caring for Mrs. W. thinks to herself, "This is no life! She should never have had this G-tube inserted. I can't believe she has a full code status. What a tragedy this is!" In contrast, the evening shift nurse cannot imagine depriving nutrition to a patient like Mrs. W., who is not able to maintain her caloric needs through oral intake. Mrs. W.'s daughter, a devout Pentecostal Christian, believes that her mother's soul still communicates with God, and this gives the daughter great comfort. She can't understand why the doctor brought up the issue of code status, because it is clearly God who will decide when it is her mother's time to "return to God's kingdom."

It is not hard for most nurses to recognize that the day shift nurse's perceptions about quality of life and suffering are different from those of Mrs. W.'s daughter and the evening shift nurse, but this still leaves a few questions unanswered, such as, "Yes, but is this what *Mrs. W.* truly wanted?" and "Does it make sense to pay exorbitant sums to keep people like Mrs. W. alive when so many others in this country don't even have access to basic health care?" These are two different questions. The first asks what is ethically justifiable for an individual patient—Mrs. W. The latter asks a bigger question—one about how we as a society should best allocate health care resources. Let's first consider the question about individual patients.

Advocating for What Patients Want

When older adult individuals can no longer make decisions for themselves, the first standard that surrogates (i.e., legally recognized decision makers, usually family members) should employ in making health care decisions for such individuals is the "substituted judgment" decision. The surrogate should make decisions based on what the elder individual would have wanted, based on available evidence in the form of stated or written wishes. Since the Patient Self-Determination Act of 1990, written advance directives (also known as "living wills") have been looked upon as the "gold standard" for substituted judgments in medical decision making. However, except for certain populations of individuals, completion rates for advance directives still run only 4% to 25% (Perkins, 2000). Furthermore, when individuals do complete advance directives, physicians often do not use them to guide medical care. This may be due to differing interpretations of the written stipulations of the document, such as it becoming effective only when the individual is "terminally ill" or "imminently dying." Even when those conditions are met, specific information about the decisionally incapable patient's wishes may not be evident, such as whether, by refusing "all medical interventions that prolong life," an individual meant to exclude administration of antibiotics to treat pneumonia or a trial of mechanical ventilation to reverse potentially treatable respiratory distress (Perkins, 2000). Confusion may also arise if an individual has written health care instructions in the form of an advance directive *and* has appointed a health care agent. Which is the better standard for judging what the patient would have wanted?

A recent Maryland case gives one example of placing the priority on an individual's stated wishes. A Maryland nursing home resident had completed a written advance directive and had also appointed her son as her health care agent. She explicitly rejected tube feedings in the instructional portion of her written directive. Subsequently, she was hospitalized and became decisionally incapacitated. During her hospitalization, the son urged the physicians to insert a feeding tube, which they did. When the woman returned to the nursing home, staff tried to comply with her written advance directive by using the feeding tube only to administer medications, but soon after being threatened with a lawsuit by the son, they started administering tube feedings. In turn, the state Office of Health Care Quality (OHCQ) assessed a $10,000 civil penalty against the nursing home for violating the resident's right to compliance with her written end-of-life wishes. An administrative law judge upheld the monetary penalty after the facility challenged the OHCQ action (Schwartz, 2002). The judge's decision was based on the clear refusal of tube feedings in the woman's written advance directives. Even though the woman also appointed her son as her health care agent, his obligation in that role is to try to make decisions based on what his mother would have wanted, if those wishes are known (surrogate decision making). The judge showed a preference for honoring the written advance directives over the directives of an appointed health care agent that run contrary to the patient's written wishes. In other states, the health care agent's judgments might be given more priority. The ethical imperative, though, is to attempt to identify what the patient would have wanted and honor those wishes.

Consider another case, that of Mr. B., a 65-year-old retired fisherman who has suffered a severe hemorrhagic stroke. Neurologists hold out the possibility that, with aggressive medical interventions, he might survive and regain some functional and cognitive abilities, although the latter would require extensive rehabilitation. Mr. B. has not appointed anyone as his health care agent or completed a written advance directive. Close family members describe him as a fiercely independent man who avoided doctors and hated having to depend on others for anything. The family requests that life-sustaining therapies be withdrawn and that he be allowed to die. This is where substituted judgment decisions become difficult. Family members believe that Mr. B. would rather die than survive in a highly or even moderately compromised state. Although the latter is probable, it is not a certainty—that is, Mr. B. may have less impairment than anticipated. Moreover, family members cannot know for sure whether Mr. B., if he survives with moderate impairment, might be satisfied with that outcome. In this case, it might be ethically justifiable for life-sustaining interventions to be

withheld or withdrawn based on a substituted judgment standard, but, because the outcome of death is irreversible, such a decision must not be taken lightly. A family conference should be held in which all key decision makers and HCPs are present to discuss the medical facts and pros and cons of treatment options. Ideally, an ethics consultation would be requested and such a meeting and discussion would be the focus of the ethics consultation process. What is *legally* allowed is different from what is *ethically* allowed. State laws differ on such matters. Typically, the law prioritizes individual autonomy (i.e., honoring patients' wishes) and, when evidence of this is lacking, errs on the side of life rather than death. The differences lie, in part, on what counts as "evidence" for a patient's wishes.

In addition to lack of evidence of an individual's wishes, substituted judgment decisions can be problematic in other ways. Research has shown less than ideal correlation between patients' wishes and family members' perceptions of patients' wishes (Fagerlin, Ditto, Danks, Houts, & Smucker, 2001; Hare, Pratt, & Nelson, 1992; Sulmasy et al., 1998). Although other research suggests that elders who are very ill prefer family members to make health care decisions for them (Puchalski et al., 2000), these elder individuals may erroneously assume that family members know what they (the patients) want. Another factor to consider is the stability, or lack thereof, of stated end-of-life preferences, which have been shown to change over time (Lockhardt, Ditto, Danks, Coppola, & Smucker, 2001; Nahm & Resnick, 2001). Moreover, some have pondered what has been referred to as the "someone else problem" (DeGrazia, 1999; Kuhse, 1999). If an individual undergoes immense psychological change as a result of progression of a disease such as Alzheimer's, is he or she the same person as his or her prior self? Should prior stated wishes apply to this "new" self, particularly when following the previous directions do not *currently* seem to be in the patient's best interests (e.g., a demented elder nursing home resident who seems happy, enjoying "I Love Lucy" reruns on television and other simple pleasures, develops treatable pneumonia, but her previous wishes stipulate that she would not want any life-prolonging treatments, including antibiotics, if she lost her cognitive capacity). For a more in-depth discussion of these issues, the reader is referred to Dresser (1995), Callahan (1995), and Newton (1999). These cases present examples of true ethical dilemmas, when all available options entail a compromise of ethical values or principles. The best that HCPs can do in these situations is to gather all the key decision makers together in a safe environment and discuss the available options, with input from any sources that might provide insight, such as a chaplain, ethics consultant or consult team, and any involved health care staff. The focus of such discussion should be to advocate for the patient by identifying what he or she would have wanted, and, if that is not possible, to have a discussion in which all the available facts can be considered to determine what would be in the patient's best interests.

Questions about honoring a decisionally incapable patient's prior stated wishes are particularly vexing when HCPs encounter advance directives that place atypical limits on end-of-life care options. For example, some advance directives have precluded tube feeding *and spoon feeding* in the event that the patient stops eating on his or her own. If an individual with such an advance directive resides in a nursing home, staff will likely find it difficult to resist spoon feeding the resident if he or she accepts food that is offered. Kapp (2001) reported cases of individuals executing advance directives with provisions such as, "When I only have [x] dollars remaining in my bank account, stop all medical treatment keeping me alive, because I don't want excessive health care expenses to erode the estate I wish to leave to my family" (p. 255). Although HCPs can take comfort in knowing that these kinds of directives are not the norm, situations similar to these and those mentioned above will inevitably be encountered by surrogates and HCPs. Again, an ethics consult is recommended for cases in which the "right thing to do" is not apparent. HCPs should not assume that their facility has no ethics consult service, because many facilities (e.g., long-term care facilities) have partnerships with local hospitals or belong to a network of facilities through which an ethics consult can be requested. Again, in the absence of ethics consult availability, a patient care conference to assist with the decision-making process should be arranged.

Advocating for What Is in the Patient's Best Interest

When it is not known what a decisionally incapable older adult would have wanted regarding medical interventions, the next standard for surrogate decision making is the "best interests" standard. The surrogate decision maker is expected to select the intervention that will most benefit the patient; decisions are based on what is in the individual's best interests, all things considered. That is, the surrogate objectively weighs the expected benefits and burdens of the medical intervention and chooses the option that maximizes benefits and minimizes burdens. As we saw earlier, this is easier said than done. By whose standard is "best interest" judged? Some research provides insight into what most individuals would want for themselves or a loved one. For example, Lockhart et al. (2001) found that most people think about their health status more in terms of their functional ability than their disease. These researchers interviewed adults over the age of 65, and found that these elders assessed the states of coma, chronic severe pain that cannot be controlled, inability to communicate through any means, and inability to reason or remember as representing very poor quality of life. When asked to rate their preference for life or death in these states, most evidenced a preference for death. However, from 10% to 33% of 50 individuals who were followed up for a second interview conducted, on average, 10.7 months after the first, changed their preferences upon follow-up interviews. For example, 33% of those rating inability to reason and remember as a "fate worse than death" at the initial interview changed their rating to a "fate better than death" at follow-up interview. Gjerdingen, Neff, Wang, and Chaloner (1999) surveyed 84 cognitively intact men and women 65 years and older and found that approximately three fourths said they would not want cardiopulmonary resuscitation (CPR), use of a ventilator, or artificial feedings with milder forms of dementia, and 95% would not want these procedures with severe dementia. Schneiderman, Kronick, Kaplan, Anderson, and Langer (1994) found that "most seriously ill patients consider the costs and burdens they might place on others in weighing decisions about their own medical treatment" (p. 111).

EVIDENCE-BASED PRACTICE

Reference: Nahm, E. S. & Resnick, B. (2001). End-of-life treatment preferences among older adults. *Nursing Ethics*, 8, 533–543.

Research Problem: To identify older adults' end-of-life treatment preferences (ELTPs) and compare after 1 year.

Design: Descriptive study using structured interviews.

Sample and Setting: 140 out of 207 residents in a continuing care retirement community were interviewed twice, 1 year apart. All scored 24 or above on a Mini-Mental State Examination and had at least a high school education. Seventy-seven percent were female and 79% unmarried, with a mean age of 85 years.

Methods: As part of a yearly health check, participants were interviewed by graduate nursing students to elicit their ELTPs, including their desire for cardiopulmonary resuscitation (CPR), major surgery, ventilator placement, dialysis, blood transfusions, artificial nutrition and hydration, diagnostic tests, antibiotics, or pain medications.

Results: Most participants did want the following treatments if medically necessary: antibiotics (95%),

diagnostic testing (94%), pain medications (84%), blood transfusions (71%), and major surgery (55%). About half of the participants did not want CPR (53%), to be put on a ventilator (49%), or dialysis. Regarding artificial nutrition and hydration, 36% wanted it, 15% wanted it started but stopped if there was no improvement, and 40% did not want it. After 1 year, there was a slight increase in the percentage of residents who wanted CPR and blood transfusions and a slight decrease in the percentage that wanted to be put on a ventilator.

Implications for Nursing Practice: In providing information about advance directives, nurses should discuss specific pros and cons of each end-of-life treatment option with patients while they remain cognitively competent. ELTPs need to be reassessed at least yearly because they may change over time.

Conclusion: Elder persons generally wish to receive medical treatments that could restore their health, such as antibiotics, diagnostic testing, blood transfusions, or surgery. Preferences for more invasive treatments such as CPR, dialysis, ventilator placement, and artificial nutrition and hydration were more variable. The nurse has an obligation to inform elder patients about treatment pros and cons as they relate to advance directive options, and to reassess preferences regularly.

In addition to research about what end-of-life care elder individuals perceive that they would want, research on outcomes of medical interventions has provided insight into best interest considerations. For example, evidence has shown that tube feedings in patients with advanced dementia in general do not prevent aspiration pneumonia, prolong survival, reduce the risk of pressure sores or infections, improve function, or provide palliation (Finucane, Christmas, & Travis, 1999). Counseling the surrogate of a patient with advanced dementia that withholding or withdrawing his or her loved one's tube feedings is likely to be in the patient's best interests provides a good example of how

evidence-based research can inform ethical decision making.

Autonomy: A Family Affair?

Many in the bioethics field have begun to realize that the overemphasis on individual autonomy belies the reality that people live in a community and are often more willing to sacrifice some of their autonomy for the well-being or peace of mind of those they love. Moreno (1992) referred to the belief that autonomous individuals are not embedded in a social context as the "myth of the asocial being" (p. 53). Likewise, Jecker (1990) described the many ways that family members and "intimate others" contribute to medical decision making. Puchalski and colleagues (2000) found that 71% of older inpatients and 78% of seriously ill adult inpatients would prefer to have their family and physician make resuscitation decisions for them.

In many other cultures, the centrality of the family in medical decision making does not come as a surprise, because the family (i.e., nuclear *and* extended family) plays a much more central role in daily life and decision making. This might lead to clashes between HCPs in the United States and members of other cultural groups, who may, for example, request that a HCP withhold the truth of an elder family member's medical diagnosis or prognosis from him or her. Freedman (1993) pointed out that patients have a right, but not a duty, to know the truth about their medical condition. That is, they are entitled to receive medical information that is relevant to their condition and any medical treatments they might undergo, and HCPs are obligated to explain such information in a way that patients can understand. However, patients are not *obligated* to have all medically relevant information divulged to them by the HCP. Some elders may prefer to exert their autonomy by delegating decision making to another family member. In these cases, informed consent for procedures or therapies is obtained through the designated family member, with HCPs checking in with the patient at regular intervals to ascertain whether more medical information is desired. Regardless of how decision making might be shared among family members, it is important for HCPs to include involved family members of elder patients in the patient's plan of care, particularly at the end of life. When death is expected, the goals of care can reasonably be extended to include minimizing future regrets of the patient's loved ones.

DIFFICULT END-OF-LIFE DECISIONS
Withholding Versus Withdrawing Medical Treatments

When continued use of life-sustaining treatment serves only to prolong the dying process, HCPs may recommend that those treatments be withdrawn. Decisionally capable individuals have both a legal and moral right to refuse to accept or continue unwanted treatments, whether life sustaining or not. With just one exception—the

1988 New York Court of Appeals decision in *In re Westchester County Medical Center* (1988)—virtually all courts agree that an incompetent person's right to refuse medical treatments (i.e., via their prior stated wishes) should be equal to a competent person's right to do so (Ahronheim, Moreno, & Zuckerman, 1994). Courts have also rejected the idea that withdrawal of life-sustaining treatment constitutes suicide or homicide, finding instead that the actual cause of death is the patient's underlying disease or injury. There is a clear consensus among ethicists and legal experts that there is no relevant distinction between a decision not to begin treatment and a decision to withdraw treatment already begun. Specifically, whatever legal or moral justifications support a decision to withhold medical treatments (e.g., their use is not expected to benefit the patient) should be equally applicable to support the decision to withdraw life-sustaining treatments (e.g., benefits of their continued use do not outweigh the burdens). The following criteria could be used to justify *either* withdrawing or withholding life-sustaining treatments: the wishes of a decisionally capable patient, instructions in an advance directive or an appointed surrogate's decision on behalf of an incompetent patient, evaluation of the patient's best interests, or a clinician's determination that the treatment is "medically ineffective" (i.e., of no medical benefit to the patient in light of his or her current condition) (Ahronheim et al., 1994). Despite this consensus among ethical and legal experts, some HCPs may decide not to initiate a particular life-sustaining treatment for fear that, once begun, it could not be stopped or withdrawn. Yet this deprives the patient of the opportunity to try a potentially useful treatment.

Decisions about the benefits and burdens of artificial nutrition and hydration are often particularly difficult. In a study of 1446 physicians and nurses, Solomon and colleagues (1993) reported that 34% of medical attending physicians and 45% of surgical attending physicians indicated that, even when all other forms of life support, including mechanical ventilation and dialysis, were stopped, nutrition and hydration should always be continued. Although a majority of the Supreme Court justices concluded that artificial nutrition and hydration constitute medical treatment that can be withheld or withdrawn like other treatments that no longer benefit the patient, decisions about their use can cause much heartache for family members and clinicians.

Despite extensive geriatric and bioethics literature supporting the conclusion that use of feeding tubes is neither mandatory nor likely to prolong survival (Finucane et al., 1999; Lynn & Childress, 1986), family members often fear that their loved one will otherwise "starve to death." Families or other surrogates may also be led to believe that they have no alternative but to agree to the placement of a feeding tube in order to prevent suffering, excessive weight loss, or aspiration pneumonia. The need for nurses to function as educators and advocates in these situations is clear. Decisions about use of feeding tubes should reflect the preferences and values of the patient, and should also reflect a clear determination of the goals of care when patients enter the terminal phase of dementia, which is often signaled by abnormal swallowing and difficulty with eating. Because of the growing body of research that concludes that tube feeding seldom achieves the intended goal of extending life, preventing aspiration pneumonia, or preventing suffering, geriatricians are increasingly recommending to patients and their families that nutrition be provided orally, not through a feeding tube, during the final stage of dementia (Gillick, 2000). When family members do not know their loved one's wishes regarding use of feeding tubes, Gillick argues that clinicians should not assume, as a default position, that a person with advanced dementia would want a gastrostomy tube and subsequent tube feedings.

When patients are terminally ill and death is expected, nurses who embrace palliative goals of care and strive to keep dying patients comfortable may nonetheless experience difficulty distinguishing among interventions that allow, hasten, or cause death. When life-sustaining treatments are withheld or withdrawn at the informed request of a decisionally capable person or the surrogate for an incompetent patient, the patient is "allowed" to die of his or her underlying disease, an action previously known as "passive euthanasia." Most bioethicists and palliative care clinicians reject this label as inappropriate and confusing because such acts are neither passive nor acts of killing the patient. Allowing death to occur by removing interventions that are disproportionately burdensome to a patient demonstrates respect for that patient's right of self-determination and autonomy, and is recognized as a professionally sanctioned end-of-life nursing intervention. As previously noted, although a consensus supports the absence of any moral or legal distinction between withholding and withdrawing life-sustaining treatments, clinicians who are expected to participate in the withdrawal of such treatments may *feel* that these two acts are quite different. Withdrawing feels "worse" than withholding because it may cause clinicians to believe that they are directly involved in *causing* that patient's death.

Nurses may find guidance in their profession's written position statements and the newly revised American Nurses Association (ANA) Code of Ethics for nurses (ANA, 2001). In its statement opposing nurse participation in assisted suicide, the ANA (1994) acknowledged the difficulty of finding a balance between "the preservation of life and the facilitation of a dignified death" (p. 1), and advised nurses to recognize how their own feelings could influence their end-of-life clinical decisions. Finding that balance may be particularly difficult for nurses who provide palliative care to elder patients who may be experiencing pain or other symptoms of suffering that they are incapable of verbally describing. Nurses and other clinicians describe conflicting emotions that result from interventions that allow, hasten, or indirectly cause death. Although legally and ethically supported as good end-of-life care, doing the "right thing" for patients does not always feel right.

Edwards and Tolle (1992), two physician-ethicists, eloquently described the emotional anguish that accompanied their participation in withdrawing a ventilator from a patient who knew that he would die as a consequence. They detailed the steps they took to ensure that he was decisionally capable; that his wish was informed, durable, and uncoerced; and that he would receive adequate sedation to prevent suffering any feelings of suffocation or pain during the withdrawal. They also acknowledged the difficulty of titrating sedation when the intended goal is relief of suffering without deliberately causing a respiratory arrest. Their description of the conflict they experienced between their intellectual judgment and their affective response is instructive:

A venous line was placed. We looked into the face of an alert man who we knew would soon die. Our more rational intellects told us that his disease, not us, would be the cause of his death. Deep feelings, on the other hand, were accusing us of causing death. From deep within us, feelings were speaking to us, making accusations, "You're really killing him, practicing active euthanasia, deceptively rationalizing with your intellects that there is a difference." (Edwards & Tolle, 1992, pp. 255-256)

Nurses describe similar feelings of conflict when providing opiate analgesia to symptomatic dying patients in doses that they fear may hasten dying. Most experienced palliative care clinicians agree that providing dying patients with effective relief of pain and suffering is a moral imperative, and freeing patients from pain may facilitate peaceful dying. Although, in theory, most nurses would endorse the truism that the correct dose of analgesia is whatever dose is necessary to relieve the patient's suffering, in practice, many nurses fear being morally or legally responsible for hastening a patient's death (Solomon et al., 1993). In a study by Volker (2001), an experienced oncology nurse wrote about her feelings of conflict and uncertainty when a symptomatic and desperately ill patient died immediately after she administered a bolus dose of morphine:

"I felt guilty. The question was, of course, did that dose of morphine cause further respiratory compromise and hasten her death? Intellectually I knew better—that it [her death] would probably have happened anyway that day. I kept trying to reassure myself that I was an experienced professional with expertise in caring for patients in pain . . . surely this had happened to every physician and nurse at least once. Maybe I had overstepped my bounds? Maybe I was treating the family member (and myself?) instead of the patient?" (p. 45)

This nurse wondered about the possibility that she had killed her patient, despite her intellectual "certainty" that the patient was dying from very advanced disease.

The ANA position statements on assisted suicide (ANA, 1994) and the promotion of comfort and relief of pain in dying patients (ANA, 1991), together with the newly revised Code of Ethics (ANA, 2001), unequivocally call for nurses to provide interventions to relieve pain and other symptoms of suffering in the dying patient, "even when those interventions entail risks of hastening death." However, the following stipulation is added: "[N]urses may not act with the sole intent of ending a patient's life even though such action may be motivated by compassion, respect for patient autonomy and quality of life considerations" (ANA, 2001, p. 8). The ANA position statement on pain relief is even more specific about hastening death: "[T]he increasing titration of medication to achieve adequate symptom control, even at the expense of life, thus hastening death secondarily, is ethically justified" (ANA, 1991, p. 1). The content of these professional guides raises two issues. The first is the question of whether appropriate use of opiate analgesia has an associated risk of hastening death. The second involves the nature of clinicians' intentions in end-of-life care.

Experts in pain management and palliative care maintain that, when opioids are used appropriately, clinically significant respiratory depression is a rarely occurring side effect because tolerance to the sedating and respiratory depressant effects of opioid use develops relatively quickly when compared with tolerance to its analgesic effects (Foley, 1991; Quill, 1998). Others note that, "the clinical impression of those treating pain in the terminally ill with opioids is that the patient's death is related to the progression of the disease, not to the use of opioids" (Manfredi, Morrison, & Meier, 1998, p. 1390). Several small studies have provided additional empirical support that use of opioids in dying patients does not increase the likelihood of a hastened death and may, under some circumstances, prolong life (Campbell, Bezek, & Thill, 1999; Wilson et al., 1992).

That having been said, many experienced hospice and oncology nurses describe a different clinical reality—instances of opiate-related hastening of death are not uncommon and generally not associated with feelings of conflict. As a participant in a study of nurses' experiences of requests for assistance in dying noted in caring for symptomatic dying patients, "if a hastened death occurs secondarily as a result of giving opiates for pain—that's not a problem" (Schwarz, 2002, p. 239). Participants in this study did not feel moral conflict because they believed their intentions were "good"—to relieve the patient's suffering, not to cause death. Other studies of nurses' end-of-life experiences report similar findings about hastening death (Ferrell, Virani, Grant, Coyne, & Uman, 2000; Matzo & Schwarz, 2001).

When evaluating the moral permissibility of particular end-of-life interventions, many clinicians and ethicists use the *principle of double effect* to distinguish currently permissible acts that may hasten death (e.g., foregoing or withdrawing life-sustaining treatments and use of high-dose opiates) and those that are deemed impermissible (e.g., assisted suicide and active euthanasia). The principle of double effect was first developed by Roman Catholic moral theologians in the Middle Ages and is currently used as a guide to clinical decision making in situations when it is impossible for an agent to avoid all harmful consequences of a single action (Quill, Dresser, & Brock, 1997). The traditional formulation stipulates that four conditions must be met before an act with both good and bad outcomes may be justified: (1) the act itself must not be intrinsically wrong and not be in a category that is absolutely prohibited, such as the killing of innocent persons; (2) the agent must intend only the good and not the bad effect, although the bad effect, such as respiratory depression following administration of opiates, may be foreseen; (3) the bad effect, such as death, must not be the means used to bring about the good effect, such as the relief of suffering; and (4) the good results must outweigh the bad effect—the bad effect can be permitted only when there is a proportionally grave reason for it (Beauchamp & Childress, 1989; Quill et al., 1997).

The principle of double effect, properly applied, requires that the agent intend only the good effect and not the bad, but does not answer the question of what is a good or bad outcome when dying patients are suffering and may wish for death. Some clinicians and philosophers question the usefulness of applying this principle to clinical cases because they believe that, when clinicians face "real" cases that involve conflicts in values, their intentions are often multiple, complex, and conflicted (Quill et al., 1997).

Gauthier (2001), a philosopher, noted that the principle of double effect is often represented as a kind of "mathematical formula for determining the moral permissibility of an action . . . if one simply plugs in the action, its effects, and the intentions of the agent, the answer will be obvious and consistent for anyone who applies the formula correctly" (p. 45). Gauthier argued that, instead, clinical application of the principle

always involves questions that are either impossible to answer with any confidence (i.e., the agent's intentions) or based entirely on personal values (such as whether the good effect outweighs the bad). This, she concludes, explains why people differ in their moral evaluation of the same action despite appropriately applying this principle. Other philosophers agree that there is often serious difficulty in the identification of one's actual intentions, as well as the determination of what counts as an intended effect (Beauchamp & Childress, 1989).

Questions about Intentions

Sulmasy (1998) stated that a thorough understanding of the principle of double effect was essential so that clinicians could maintain their opposition to euthanasia and assisted suicide while still providing adequate pain relief to dying patients. He argued that, in clinical situations where high doses of opioids were necessary for relief of a dying patient's suffering, although the clinician might *hope* for his or her patient's death, expect it, or even pray for it, that was not the same as being committed to bringing about the patient's death "as the condition that fulfills her intention. Desire and belief are not intentions . . . Intention seems to involve something over and above belief and desire. It involves commitment" (Sulmasy, 1998, p. 59).

Some palliative care clinicians question the need to appeal to the principle of double effect as moral justification for providing good pain management. They argue that patients have an absolute moral right to receive effective pain management; the clinician's duty to treat pain is thus a moral imperative that requires no additional justification. Cherny and Coyle (1999) stated that, "to leave a person in avoidable pain is a fundamental breach of [his or her] human rights" (p. 644). One of the increasingly recognized reasons for this unfortunate reality is clinicians' fear of causing an opiate-related hastened death by providing the "last dose" before death (Ferrell et al., 2000; Solomon et al., 1993; Volker, 2001).

Support for appeal to the principle of double effect persists, despite questions raised about its application to clinical cases and confusion about specifying the nature of the agent's "intent." Application of the principle of double effect is recognized as an effective means to encourage nurses to appropriately administer opiates to symptomatic dying patients despite the possibility of secondarily hastening death. Nurse experts in palliative care maintain that

[t]he principle of double effect is an essential ethical construct for nurses to understand if they are going to adequately control complex symptoms at the end of life . . . Giving a patient who is dying, hypotensive, and in pain sufficient opioid dosages to control the pain is good palliative care and not euthanasia (Coyle & Layman-Goldstein, 2001, p. 413).

Ultimately, then, the ethical justification of unintentionally hastening death through withholding or withdrawing medical therapies or administering palliative interventions lies in the judgment that the benefits outweigh the burdens (when a comprehensive definition of each of the latter is understood). HCPs must avoid the language of "withholding care" at the end of life—the correct term is *withholding medical interventions. Care* should never be withheld or withdrawn, particularly at the end of life. Furthermore, HCPs should eliminate references to "doing nothing" versus "doing everything"—the euphemisms often used to refer to how to treat patients at the end of life when a do-not-resuscitate order is or is not in place. "Doing everything" must be redefined to encompass the full panoply of palliative options, and patients and family members should be assured that the palliative approach involves a different vision of "doing everything."

Assisted Suicide and the Older Adult

Suicide is an act of intentional self-inflicted death, and "parasuicide" occurs when a person attempts suicide but does not succeed in dying. Older adults (over age 65) commit suicide at a higher rate than other groups in the population, two to three times even the rate for teenagers. Elders made up 12.6% of the 2000 population but committed 18.1% of suicides, whereas the young (ages 15 to 24) made up 13.9% of the population and committed 13.6% of all suicides (American Association of Suicidology, 2002). At all ages, men have higher successful suicide rates than women, and the rate of suicide increases with age. Seventy percent of older men who commit suicide do so with firearms, and elder white men are at greatest risk for suicide as a result of

feelings of hopelessness, depression, poor quality of life, and ready access to such lethal means as guns (Bangar et al., 1998). Women have a higher parasuicide rate than do men: three women attempt suicide for each attempt by a man. Some speculate that reported rates actually underestimate the true incidence of suicide among elders because incidents of treatment refusal and accidents may mask actual suicides (Francis, 1998).

The question of what to make of these findings is unclear. Some might believe these data illustrate the independence of last acts chosen by autonomous elder persons, while others would find support for fears that elders are at heightened risk for untimely deaths because they have, as a group, an increased likelihood of being depressed, incompetent, and vulnerable. Is it appropriate to consider elder persons less able to make reasoned choices because of the multiple losses—physical, social, and cognitive—that are associated with advanced age? To be capable of making a reasoned choice, an individual must be able to identify and articulate her or his values, understand and employ relevant information about the consequences of available alternatives to achieve those values, and choose among alternatives based on some connection between those values and consequences. Although most experts agree that there are no grounds for assuming that age alone compromises reasoning ability, there are special concerns about the presence of undiagnosed and untreated depression among elders.

There is a well-recognized link between the presence of untreated depression and suicide, and some consider depression to be the strongest risk factor for suicide. Because suicide rates increase with age, depression among older adults is a significant risk factor for suicide (Moscicki, 1997). Lynn, Schuster, and Kabcenell (2000) noted that, whereas depression is overlooked in most adults, it is unrecognized in those who are terminally ill and is "virtually ignored in elderly patients" (p. 247). There are a number of reasons for this: clinicians do not screen patients for depression, and older depressed patients may believe that there is no hope to treat their depression, or blame themselves for their feelings, or feel reluctant or ashamed to discuss their unhappiness. Depression can also be caused by medical conditions and medications, and antidepressant medications have been found to reduce depressive symptoms for 80% of older adult suicidal patients (Bangar et al., 1998). Among elders, physical debility, the death of loved ones, reduced independence, and economic instability all contribute to the incidence of depression.

Screening for depression should become a routine part of a nursing assessment, just as pain is. Chochinov, a psychiatrist, recommended that clinicians simply ask patients, "Are you feeling depressed?" In studies conducted with patients receiving palliative care for advanced cancer, he and his colleagues found that this single-item interview question was as valid as other screening tools, such as the Beck Depression Inventory Short Form (Chochinov, Wilson, Enns, & Lander, 1997). Experts agree that depression is a highly treatable condition, even among the terminally ill; psychostimulants have been found effective for patients in severe distress who need a rapidly acting intervention with few side effects (Block & Billings, 1994).

Patient Requests for a Hastened Death

Some elder patients may express distress about the diminished quality of their lives, and "wonder" out loud whether anything can be done to hasten a prolonged dying process. At other times, patients may explicitly ask their nurse for assistance in dying. We are beginning to learn about reasons some patients request an assisted death, in part because of the results of the ongoing social experiment in assisted suicide in Oregon, the only state that legally permits physician-assisted suicide. The Oregon Death with Dignity Act was approved twice by voters in 1994 and 1997, and allows terminally ill citizens of that state to request a lethal dose of drugs if two physicians confirm that the individual has less than 6 months to live, is mentally competent to make that choice, and is acting voluntarily. The individual must also be able to self-administer the lethal medication. If it is determined that the applicant is suffering from a psychological disorder, including depression, that causes impaired judgment, no lethal medication can be prescribed until or unless the disorder is treated.

As of 2001, a total of 91 Oregon citizens, most of whom (77%) were suffering from cancer, have committed suicide using the law, and their median age was 69 years (range 25 to 94). The most frequently presented reasons for the request for lethal drugs were "fear of decreasing ability to do enjoyable activities" and "fear of losing autonomy," followed by "fear of losing control of bodily function" and "fear of being a burden." Inadequate control of pain was not a significant reason for these requests (International Task Force, 2003).

Many more persons received lethal prescriptions (140) than used them, suggesting that individuals who wished to control the circumstances of their dying were concerned that their suffering might become intolerable and they wanted a safeguard against that possibility. Ganzini and colleagues (2000) reported that, when the attending physician implemented a substantive palliative intervention, such as better pain management or referral to a hospice program, 46% of those patients changed their minds about assisted suicide, as compared with 15% of those for whom no such interventions were made. Similar findings were reported in a qualitative study of nurses who were asked by patients to provide assistance in dying. When good palliative end-of-life care was provided, most patients withdrew their requests, and unmanaged pain was not the primary reason for such requests (Schwarz, 2002). Nurses in this study also found that the meaning of the request for assistance in dying was not always what it seemed, and a careful assessment was always required.

One clear implication of these findings is that nurses must remain open to hear their patients' stories, and be committed to remaining present to their patients, because many dying patients fear abandonment above all things. Patients with advanced terminal disease often have thoughts about suicide, and it is important for clinicians to encourage patients to express such feelings and to explore with the patient the meaning of these thoughts or wishes (Block & Billings, 1994; Coyle, 1992).

When older adults and/or dying patients or their surrogates request that all life-sustaining treatments be withdrawn so that the patient can die, nurses might wonder whether respecting such requests would morally involve them in helping a patient to die. Although, as we previously noted, there is no question about the existing legal right that competent persons have to refuse unwanted treatments, regardless of the reason or their medical condition, that may not always answer the moral question for nurses. Thomasma (1999), who argues for the need to coordinate practical ethical judgments with theory and public policy issues in the complex world of caring for the aged, noted that,

Often in the clinical setting, older patients, say those over 80, request that nothing further be done to prolong their life. They do not want to die anymore than any of the rest of us. But they seem to have passed beyond the stage of clinging to life the way younger people do. (p. 157)

He cited Fletcher, who observed that, "physicians often ignore, compromise, or even deny a patient's right to die . . . Physicians are less prone than some patients and ethicists to acknowledge that the patient has a moral right to choose to die" (Thomasma, 1999, p. 157).

In 2000, there were 4 million people over 85 years of age in the United States, up from 3 million in 1994 (*http://www.againgstats.gov/chart book2000/population.html*); these "oldest old" are the most rapidly growing age group. About half of this age group require placement in long-term care settings or home health care; providing hospitalized care to persons over age 85 costs three times as much as care for those under age 65 for the same illness (Thomasma, 1999). In the next section we explore several approaches to how care and costs of care can be compassionately and justly managed.

EVIDENCE-BASED PRACTICE

Reference: Marwit, S. J., & Datson, S. I. (2002). Disclosure preferences about terminal illness: An examination of decision-related factors. *Death Studies, 26,* 1–20.

Research Problem: To determine patient preferences for the context within which they would prefer to receive news of a terminal prognosis.

Design: Mailed questionnaire.

Sample and Setting: 112 of 130 members of cancer support groups in Missouri, Illinois, and Kansas (26 men and 86 women ages 29 to 85, mostly white).

Methods: In addition to other measures, the questionnaire assessed preferences for level of disclosure (full, partial, or nondisclosure) and for pathway of disclosure (from physician to patient only, from physician to patient in the presence of a loved one, or from physician to loved one only).

Results: Participants chose full disclosure significantly more often than nondisclosure, with men preferring it more than women did. No one endorsed nondisclosure when a partial disclosure option was made available. Participants whose previous experience with death had resulted in a reduced fear of death were significantly more likely to express a preference for full disclosure than participants whose previous experiences resulted in an increased fear of death. Younger participants and those who had attended college were slightly more likely to prefer full disclosure. About two thirds of participants preferred disclosure in the presence of a loved one. Those whose previous experience resulted in a reduced fear of death, along with patients having 12 years or less of education, were more likely to prefer having a loved one present when receiving negative prognostic information.

Implications for Nursing Practice: Preferences for level and pathway of disclosure should be assessed and accommodated. Individuals belonging to groups known to prefer nondisclosure of negative medical information may actually prefer less than immediate full disclosure rather than total nondisclosure.

Conclusion: Most individuals prefer full disclosure of negative medical information from the health care provider in the presence of a loved one. Variables affecting preferences for level and pathway of disclosure include age, level of education, and previous experience with death.

ALLOCATING HEALTH CARE RESOURCES—AND JUSTICE FOR ALL

Earlier we discussed the case of Mrs. W., the nursing home resident with end-stage dementia who was receiving tube feedings and had a "full code" status. We considered the question of what to do for Mrs. W. as an individual patient. Now we will consider the question of what to do for the population of elder individuals in this country with end-of-life medical needs. Because the ability of the nurse to advocate for individual patients is dependent on the greater context of how health care is provided at the societal level, it is imperative that nurses, both as health care professionals and as citizens, concern themselves with issues of health care allocation and just distribution of resources. The ethical principle of *justice* is more likely to enter into such discussions.

The United States has adopted an approach toward providing health care to its citizens that reflects its struggle with opposing political ideologies, which place differing values on government subsidies, government regulation, the free market, and the role of the private sector. Most U.S. citizens are medically insured through employer-based coverage. The next biggest insurer is the government, which has two forms of *socialized insurance:* Medicare and Medicaid (i.e., the government is the payer, but the actual health care services are provided by private not-for-profit and for-profit HCPs or health care institutions). In addition, there are two forms of *socialized medicine* in the United States: the Department of Veterans Affairs and the bulk of the armed forces health care system (i.e., the government finances *and administers* health care services) (Reinhardt, 1993). Those individuals receiving health care services who do not have health care insurance may rely on indigent funds or charity, or they may pay out of pocket. Emergent health care treatment may be obtained by anyone residing in the United States through the Emergency Medical Treatment and Active Labor Act (EMTALA), a statute passed as part of the Comprehensive Omnibus Budget Reconciliation Act of 1986. EMTALA mandates that a patient presenting to a hospital must be provided with "an appropriate medical screening examination" to determine if he or she is suffering from an "emergency medical condition," in which case the hospital is obligated to either provide treatment to stabilize the patient or transfer the patient to another hospital, in accordance with the statute's directives (*http://www.emtala.com*). However, a third-party payer, or the patient, will be billed for the treatment provided through EMTALA.

In the year 2000, 72.4% of people in the United States were covered by private insurance (64.1% employment based), 13.4% by Medicare, 10.3% by Medicaid, and 3% by the military. Fourteen percent (38,683,000) of Americans were uninsured. The percentage of uninsured individuals is higher among ethnic minorities (32.7% for Hispanics, 19.5% for blacks, and 10.1% for non-Hispanic whites over the 3-year period from 1998 to 2000) (U.S. Census Bureau, 2000). Even among the insured, rising out-of-pocket health care expenses threaten to exceed what individuals can reasonably afford. The escalating cost of prescription drugs is a cause for concern among older adults, most of whom do not have prescription coverage. A study by the Harvard School of Public Health revealed that 32% of U.S. older adults reported having no drug coverage, with 20% paying $50 to $100 per month out of pocket for drugs and 16% paying more than $100 per month. Of U.S. older adults who reported 1999 out-of-pocket drug expenses over $100 per month, 15% reported not filling a prescription because they could not afford it, 18% reported having problems paying medical bills, and 29% reported having problems meeting daily living expenses (Harvard School of Public Health, 2000).

Lack of access to health care is also a problem for many older adults, who may have difficulty getting to a clinic or may not have health care facilities available where they live (particularly emergency rooms, through which EMTALA is invoked). One particular access issue of concern to U.S. elders and their family members is nursing home placement, which may be covered by the state Medicaid program if an elder individual qualifies. However, the federal government and a majority of states let nursing homes restrict the number of people they serve who are eligible for Medicaid, so individuals might have difficulty finding a Medicaid-funded nursing home placement (AARP, 2003). Furthermore, long-term care costs are placing a tremendous strain on state

Medicaid budgets, something that does not bode well for the long-term stability of state Medicaid programs.

Another access issue of concern for older adults is the underutilization of hospice services. Although the Medicare hospice benefit has been available since 1986, a substantial portion of terminally ill elders are not offered the option of electing hospice coverage, or are referred too late in the illness trajectory to benefit from the services hospice provides (Frantz, Lawrence, Somov, & Somova, 1999). Elder nursing home residents are included among those underserved by hospice (Keay & Schonwetter, 2000). There are many reasons for the underutilization of less invasive, more holistic approaches to end-of-life care, such as those provided by hospice. Kapp (2001) identified several, including the practice of defensive medicine to avoid lawsuits, effects of media coverage that feed public expectations of medical miracles, education and socialization of health care professionals that instill an ethos that "death is the ultimate failure, to be avoided as long as possible by any means available," and "a powerful bias in favor of maximizing the aggressive use of advanced technological intervention whenever possible" (p. 253).

Indeed, the United States is recognized as the global leader in developing and refining cutting-edge medical technology, which fosters dependence on that technology for a variety of reasons. Partly because of this preference for and dependence on high-tech diagnostics and medical interventions, the United States is also recognized as the industrialized nation that least effectively and efficiently allocates health care resources to its citizens. Compared to other industrialized nations, the United States commits a higher percentage of its gross national product (14%) and spends more per capita ($5,035 in 2001) on health care, but cannot boast better outcomes, as indicated by the high number of under- and uninsured, particularly among vulnerable and disadvantaged populations such as children, the poor, and ethnic minorities (Levit, Smith, Cowan, & Lazenby et al, 2003). Most agree that reform is in order. Attempts to curb health care spending, such as the Medicare Diagnosis-Related Group program, and other forms of capitated payment schemes, such as those provided by managed care organizations, have slowed the rate of increase of

spending, but have not accomplished the goal of promoting *just allocation* of health care resources. So what, exactly, would the latter entail?

Theories of *distributive justice* include giving all persons of equal status an equal share, or allocating resources according to need, effort, contribution, merit, or free market exchanges. The language of "rights" is sometimes invoked but can be ambiguous. What does it mean to have a "right to health care"? Sometimes rights are tied to basic human needs (e.g., something necessary to sustain biologic existence, such as air, food, water, and shelter). The assumption is that, in order to have the opportunity to flourish, humans must be assured of having their basic biologic needs met. Yet, in modern industrialized societies, human flourishing is dependent on much more than the mere provision of basic biologic needs—for example, one needs education and the support of a community of others (Loewy, 1996).

In the authors' opinion, a "just society" is one whose privileged citizens stand in solidarity with those in the society who are vulnerable (such as children and older adults) and disadvantaged (such as the poor and those who face discrimination). The privileged, then, have an obligation to "level the playing field" and lessen the burdens of the disadvantaged. However, debates continue as to whether and how various needs of the citizenry should be provided by the government. One thing is certain: With more of our population aging and fewer young people in the workforce to provide a tax base, spending limits cannot be ignored for long. It is projected that, by 2040, older adults will comprise one fifth of the population, and almost half the health care expenditures will be made in their behalf (Rice, 1990). Is there a limit to how much we will spend on health care, and, if so, how should decisions be made about how much to spend, and how to allocate those health care dollars?

Options for Health Care Reform

Full treatment of the subject of health care reform is beyond the scope of this chapter, but the subject is one with which nurses should familiarize themselves. For a more comprehensive discussion of this topic, the reader is referred to Reinhardt (1993, 1996). *Health care reform* refers to strategies to reduce the number of individuals in this country with no health care insurance, ensure access to health care for all who need it, and provide a more just distribution of health care resources. Different approaches have been suggested to work toward these goals. The ANA endorses a plan for health care reform that involves providing government-subsidized universal health insurance coverage. By eliminating the large number of uninsured, this would relieve HCPs from sharing the cost of covering them. Other suggested strategies include cost control through spending limitations, quality assurance initiatives that track outcomes and promote evidence-based medicine, case management oversight, malpractice tort reform (limiting amounts that can be awarded for medical malpractice lawsuits), and simplification of paperwork and administrative bureaucracy (which some have shown is responsible for up to one fourth of health care costs).

An important component of health care reform would involve creating a more efficient system in which maximal health care outcomes are achieved for the dollars spent. HCPs and citizens alike have to consider both what is good for the individual *and* what is good for society at large—we all share obligations to minimize waste and maximize efficiency in the provision of health care. This is different from rationing, which is discussed in the next section. Decisions about efficiency are based on outcomes and cost, whereas rationing decisions are based purely on availability or cost. Refraining from ordering a magnetic resonance imaging scan for a patient if the same information can be gained from a radiograph or even a thorough physical exam and medical history is an example of good stewardship of health care resources, whereas not offering kidney dialysis to individuals over a certain age is an example of rationing.

The obligation to maximize efficiency does not trump the nurse's role as advocate for the whole patient—body, mind, and spirit. "Efficiency" does not exclude caring. Perhaps a useful framework to refer to is that of Erich Loewy's (1997) *rational compassion*, which requires that HCPs' compassion in caring for individual patients be informed by rationality or reason, such as a consideration of evidence-based research outcomes and distributive justice issues. Likewise, when considering populations of individuals, to counter the distance one has

from actual patients, *compassionate rationality* is required—the act of informing rational decisions with compassion, remembering that decisions made at the aggregate level will ultimately affect individuals who live in a community of others. As Loewy (1997) stated:

> Reason without compassion can easily be cold, analytic, and basically not only inhumane but . . . unhuman . . . If, however, compassion unleavened by reason were my only motivating force, I might well act impulsively, foolishly, and ultimately destructively or perhaps even unethically . . . Our actions must steer between the Scylla of callousness and the Charybdis of sentimentality." (pp. 122–123)

Having acknowledged the need to couple compassion with reasoned judgments, it is important to recognize the limitations and dangers inherent in applying efficacy data about groups of people to patients at the bedside. For example, evidence that a large percentage of Medicare dollars are spent in an elder person's last month of life may imply that aggressive end-of-life medical treatment is not achieving the goal of extending life among these elders, who might be better served by a palliative care/hospice approach. However, physicians claim that they cannot predict with enough accuracy who among the elders receiving aggressive medical treatment will die and who will live. Moreover, research has not demonstrated definitively that cost savings will be incurred by limiting aggressive end-of-life interventions (Emanuel, 1996; Scitovsky, 1994).

Making efficacy judgments in health care should be approached with caution. There is a real danger that vulnerable patients, particularly ill elders, will fall victim to some HCP's erroneous assumptions about what counts as "worthwhile" treatment. For example, it has been shown that HCPs tend to underrate chronically ill patients' quality of life (Sprangers & Aaronson, 1992; Woodend, Nair, & Tang, 1997). The same concerns discussed earlier about the slippery slope in legalizing assisted suicide are relevant here. The public trusts HCPs to protect the patients entrusted to their care—particularly the very ill, elders, and disabled individuals. If the role of the HCP shifts too far away from that of patient advocate to that of health care resource manager, HCPs may lose that public trust. Furthermore, if it becomes the expected norm that only health care interventions that have measurable benefits need be administered, there is a risk that biased definitions of "benefit" will unjustly disadvantage the disabled, chronically ill, or cognitively impaired, who may stand less chance of evidencing "measurable" improvements. Again, the concept of compassionate rationality is important here—outcomes research should inform health care decisions both in policy making and at the bedside, but a perspective grounded in compassionate, humane care and advocacy for the most vulnerable should be the compost in which just resource allocation decisions are planted.

With those caveats acknowledged, a reasonable place to focus attention in the responsible allocation of health care resources is the limitation of medical interventions that elder patients do not want, and those that do not produce a worthwhile benefit. Regarding the former, aggressive life-sustaining therapy (e.g., CPR attempts, use of mechanical ventilation, and tube feedings) is most often mentioned. Generally, it is preferable to discuss goals of care with patients and family members in advance of a health care crisis. Effective communication and proactive planning is likely a more efficacious, as well as compassionate, approach to avoid wasting health care dollars on medically ineffective and invasive end-of-life interventions. However, the luxury of pre-hospital health care planning conversations is not available to intensive care unit (ICU) staff, who must make life-and-death decisions about patients who are usually not known to them. Although communication upon admission to an ICU is the cornerstone of providing good end-of-life care, sometimes the "choices" that are offered to family members for the patient's plan of care are not really choices at all. Offering CPR to the patient who is not expected to benefit from it is one example. Yet, in other cases, HCPs must be careful not to project their own judgments about what they consider to be acceptable outcomes onto patients and families.

Some health care institutions are implementing medical futility or "medically ineffective treatment" policies, which provide a mechanism that allows two physicians to certify that a given medical intervention, such as CPR, would be "medically ineffective" for a given patient and thus would not be attempted, even if the patient's surrogate requested that it be attempted. One

definition of medically ineffective treatment is "treatment that, as certified by the attending and consulting physicians to a reasonable degree of medical certainty, will neither prevent or reduce deterioration of the health of an individual nor prevent the impending death of an individual" (Schwartz, p. 4, 2000).

The term *medically ineffective* is favored over *medical futility* because the former emphasizes that the goal being sought is a medical outcome that can be evaluated objectively, rather than subjectively. That is, there is objective evidence that CPR will, at best, only prolong the inevitable death of a patient with multisystem organ failure or end-stage metastatic cancer who is imminently dying. The term *objective evidence* is not meant to imply medical certainty, but, rather, that the treatment would not produce its intended goal "to a reasonable degree of medical certainty," which is the standard most often applied when asking patients to consent to most medical interventions. The more general "futility" term, by comparison, is less clear. An intervention can only be deemed futile in relation to an identified goal. If a patient's family has a qualitative goal in mind, such as extending life (or even attempting to do so) regardless of medical outcome, CPR may not be futile in that it may achieve the desired goal.

Critics charge that decisions to withhold or withdraw treatments based on medical ineffectiveness criteria are disguised forms of health care rationing. Others support the use of policies to limit certain treatments based on medical ineffectiveness criteria, and point out that no HCP is obligated to provide a treatment that will not benefit the patient. For a more in-depth discussion of these issues, the reader is referred to Schneiderman (1992) and Schneiderman, Jecker, and Jonsen (1996).

Problems arise when medical interventions in end-of-life care do not meet the criteria for medical ineffectiveness—for example, the use of renal dialysis in persons in a persistent vegetative state. In addition, as mentioned above, difficulties with "futility" judgments are encountered when family members of imminently dying, unconscious patients have other goals in mind for continuing or implementing life-sustaining medical interventions. These may include extending their loved one's life for religious reasons, or to reach an important date such as a wedding anniversary, or because of feelings of guilt. Bringing up the exorbitant cost of the medical care being provided at such a time hardly evokes the spirit of compassionate rationality. Indeed, although financial cost often influences decisions made at the bedside, typically because of the reimbursement limitations by third-party payers, cost alone should not guide such decisions. Good health care provision involves seeking positive outcomes for patients based on their personal wishes and medical needs by using the least burdensome and least wasteful methods to achieve those outcomes, ideally through a holistic approach to care. Thus, if a dying patient who would have preferred a less invasive approach ends up in an ICU receiving aggressive life-sustaining therapy, *good care* has not been provided.

In cases where patients and/or family members consistently choose to implement aggressive life-sustaining interventions, even though death is the inevitable outcome, resorting to implementation of a medically ineffective treatment policy should be the last resort (Wear & Logue, 1995). Consistent and open communication between family members and the health care team is the key to avoiding such confrontations—communication in which the goals of treatment are explained, criteria are identified to determine if goals are being met, and new goals are set if previously identified goals are not met within a predetermined time frame (Curtis et al., 2001; Mularski, Bascom, & Osborne, 2001).

HCPs may be justified in withholding truly medically ineffective treatment such as CPR attempts for the dying elder patient with multisystem organ failure. Hopefully, this will be approached with compassion and in such a way that the family members are supported through the process. In some cases, family members may feel relieved that the decision was "taken away from them," although this should not be assumed. When medical ineffectiveness cannot be established for a treatment that family members request be continued (e.g., kidney dialysis for the patient in a persistent vegetative state), decisions to withdraw or withhold such treatments should be acknowledged as rationing decisions, and should be made at the population level through an explicit (ideally, a democratic) process. Health care rationing is discussed in the next section.

Health Care Rationing: Implicit, Explicit, and Age-Based

Rationing refers to deciding who gets what amount of a limited resource. The complex system by which donor organs are allocated is an example of *explicit* rationing of a limited resource. In the United States, we tend to reject explicit rationing while denying that *implicit* rationing is pervasive. Churchill (1988, p. 645), wrote:

"Our market-driven health care system is a de facto rationing scheme. Current scatter-shot health policies are a mish-mash of reactive programs designed to patch and plug a price-rationing system. The result is a secondary system that rations, among other ways, by age (Medicare), by disease (end-state renal disease), by media appeal (parents pleading for livers for their children), and by provider philanthropy. Meanwhile, a powerful set of mythic beliefs keeps the acknowledgment of rationing in the background, through the use of utopian assessments of our abilities and myopia about our needs. The hard choices of scarcity, we tell ourselves, can be avoided by efficiency, technological innovation, cutting the defense budget, or outproducing needs. In fact, no society has been able to avoid rationing its health services. The only question is how to do it justly."

Most ethicists agree that health care rationing is inevitable. Therefore, explicit rationing, which should be informed by a theoretical framework and subject to public discourse and decision/policy-making due process, is ethically superior to implicit rationing, which tends to be uninformed by theory, reactive instead of proactive, and nondemocratic. The most common form of implicit rationing in the United States is price rationing. The problem with explicit rationing in the United States is that it would be difficult, if not impossible, to create just rationing schemes before rectifying the current health care access and delivery injustices that exist in this country. For example, Hispanics and African Americans are over-represented among the uninsured, and African Americans have been shown to receive less aggressive medical interventions than European Americans (Kressin & Petersen, 2001). Serious initiatives to rectify these injustices would have to be made before disadvantaged individuals would be expected to participate in rationing schemes. Universal health care insurance would be a necessary start. Deciding what would be included in a minimal insurance coverage plan, if done through a democratic process, could be one form of explicit rationing. The Oregon Medicaid program, although not without flaws, provides an example of this approach (Blumstein, 1997; Fleck, 1994; Glass, 1998).

It has been pointed out that age-based rationing already occurs in the United States through the Medicare program. That is, elders are *favored* in that they, unlike children in this country and the nonworking people who do not qualify for Medicaid, are assured of health care coverage. Some suggest that age-based rationing that would limit certain medical interventions (e.g., no renal dialysis or organ transplants, and certain other life-extending therapies, to those over a certain age) would be justified based on egalitarian and utilitarian arguments. The egalitarian argument is that individuals should receive a greater investment of resources when they are young to allow them to be well-functioning citizens, with the understanding that, as they get older, they will receive fewer resources to ensure that the next generation is able to enjoy the same investment of resources in their youth (Daniels, 1985). The problem with that argument is the same as the caveat mentioned above—not all citizens enjoy the same access to resources before they reach their senior years. Furthermore, Jecker (1991) argued that age-based rationing would unjustly disadvantage women, whose life opportunities may have been limited as a result of sex discrimination, who provide the bulk of child and family member caregiving, and who, comprising a greater percentage of older adults, would be subjected to age-based rationing more often than their male counterparts. Finally, there is evidence that age-based rationing already exists implicitly (Fishman, 1989; Ward, 2000), and would only further disadvantage elder persons and erode their trust in the health care system (and further diminish the respect owed to them) if it were formalized through explicit rationing schemes.

A utilitarian argument for age-based rationing is based on poorer outcomes in older adults for certain medical interventions, based on available evidence such as "quality-adjusted life years" (Dolan, 2001). Yet critics of this approach argue that age alone is an insufficient predictor of health care outcomes, and that, if rationing of medical interventions were to be based on outcomes, such decisions should be made based on overall health indicators rather than age alone. (Dean [1999] presented a more in-depth discussion of the challenges inherent in using quality of life as an outcome measure, particularly for rationing purposes.) Many have observed that the U.S. culture is youth oriented and does not afford the older adult the respect that other cultures bestow upon their elders. We are a death-denying culture that seeks to defy individual mortality, and thus defy the aging process. Some argue that elders have a duty to accept the limits of their natural life span and avoid requests beyond that point for expensive life-extending medical technology (Callahan, 1987). However, most agree that the health care reforms needed in this country cannot be achieved through strict age-based rationing (what some refer to as "hard rationing"). Rather, instead of placing no limits on aggressive, life-extending medical technology while price-rationing the more effective, efficient, and humanistic primary care, we should re-envision our health care priorities to focus on quality, justice, and caring rather than life extension alone. As Churchill wrote:

"Most patients would not bankrupt their family and deny their children a fair start in life by striving for a last, expensive extension of their own lives. Neither should we extend our lives at the margins if by so doing we deprive nameless and faceless others a decent provision of care. And such a gesture should not appear to us as a sacrifice, but as the ordinary virtue entailed by a just, social conscience." (1988, p. 647)

Clearly, decisions about withholding or withdrawing life-sustaining therapy at the end of life can weigh heavily on HCPs. However, the more seemingly mundane decisions about resource allocation for elder patients in the HCP's office or clinic may be the more difficult ones on which to reach consensus about what is just. A step in the right direction would be to put health care decisions in the hands of health care professionals and the inevitable rationing decisions in public forums where they can be debated and approached rationally, and compassionately.

CONCLUSION

In this chapter we have briefly touched on legal and ethical issues that influence the care of the elder patient. At the beginning of the chapter, we discussed a framework for ethical decision making that couples *doing* with *being*. This orients the nurse to focus on making a particular decision for a particular patient, while also being centered and fully present to the patient as well as focused on "the big picture." Health care decision making for individual patients is complex, but that complexity is manageable by systematically exploring benefits and burdens for an individual patient and exhausting multiple perspectives to identify those benefits and burdens. This is best accomplished through a holistic, team approach. Concerns about hastening death, although common among HCPs, should not impede access of the dying older adult to palliative interventions that can minimize his or her suffering. Indeed, more timely and universal access to good palliative end-of-life care for elders is a necessary response to higher suicide rates and increased demand for legalized assisted suicide. It should be recognized as another vision of "doing everything" at the end of life.

On par with the framework of *doing* and *being* to guide individual ethical decision making, Loewy's description of *rational compassion* and *compassionate rationality* expands the level of focus beyond the individual patient to the community at large. It is clear that our present system of health care resource allocation in the United States is unjust. Minimizing waste and maximizing beneficial outcomes for individual patients is the first step toward reform, yet often excludes those who are uninsured or without adequate access to health care. Although redressing the injustices will not likely be accomplished by resorting to strict age-based rationing, it is inevitable that rationing needs to be a component of health care reform. Such rationing should be explicit rather than implicit, should take place not at the bedside but at the community level within a democratic process, and must be preceded by access to health care for all individuals in this country. Nurses as health care professionals have a responsibility to advocate for their patients. Nurses as citizens have a responsibility to advocate for the health of their society and the justice of its approach to allocating health care resources.

REFERENCES

Ahronheim, J., Moreno, J., & Zuckerman, C. (1994). *Ethics in clinical practice.* Boston: Little, Brown.

AARP. (2003). *Medicaid: Paying for nursing home care.* Retrieved from http://www.aarp.org/confacts/health/medicaidnurse.html

American Association of Suicidology. (2002). Year 2000 official final data on suicide in the United States. In *United States suicide statistics.* Retrieved from http://www.suicidology.org/displaycommon.cfm?an=1&subarticlenbr=21

American Nurses Association. (1991). *Position statement on the promotion of comfort and relief of pain in dying patients.* Washington, DC: Author.

American Nurses Association. (1994). *Position statements: Assisted suicide.* Retrieved from http://nursingworld.org/readroom/position/ethics/etsuic.htm

American Nurses Association. (2001). *Code of ethics for nurses with interpretive statements.* Washington, DC: Author.

Bangar, B., Berman, A. L., Maris, R. W., Silverman, M. M., Harris, E. A., & Packman, W. L. (1998). *Risk management with suicidal patients.* New York: Guilford Press.

Beauchamp, T. L., & Childress, J. F. (1989). *Principles of biomedical ethics* (3rd ed.). New York: Oxford University Press.

Block, S. D., & Billings, A. J. (1994). Patient requests to hasten death: Evaluation and management in terminal care. *Archives of Internal Medicine, 154,* 2039-2047.

Blumstein, J. F. (1997). The Oregon experiment: The role of cost-benefit analysis in the allocation of Medicaid funds. *Social Science and Medicine, 45,* 545-554.

Callahan, D. (1987). *Setting limits.* New York: Simon and Schuster.

Callahan, D. (1995). Terminating life-sustaining treatment of the demented. *Hastings Center Report, 25,* 26.

Campbell, M. L., Bizek, K. S., & Thill, M. (1999). Patient responses during rapid terminal weaning from mechanical ventilation: A prospective study. *Critical Care Medicine, 27,* 73-77.

Cassell, E. J., Leon, A. C., & Kaufman, S. G. (2001). Preliminary evidence of impaired thinking in sick patients. *Annals of Internal Medicine, 134,* 1120-1123.

Cherny, N., & Coyle, N. (1999). The application of ethical principles in the management of cancer pain. In G. Aronoff (Ed.), *Evaluation and treatment of chronic pain* (3rd ed., pp. 643-654). Baltimore: Williams & Wilkins.

Chochinov, H. M., Wilson, K. G., Enns, M., & Lander, S. (1997). "Are you depressed?": Screening for depression in the terminally ill. *American Journal of Psychiatry, 154,* 674-676.

Churchill, L. R. (1988). Should we ration health care by age? *Journal of the American Geriatrics Society, 36,* 644-647.

Coyle, N. (1992). The euthanasia and physician-assisted suicide debate: Issues for nursing. *Oncology Nursing Forum, 19*(Suppl. 7), 41-46.

Coyle, N., & Layman-Goldstein, M. (2001). Pain assessment and management in palliative care. In M. L. Matzo & D. W. Sherman (Eds.), *Palliative care nursing: Quality care to the end of life* (pp. 363-486). New York: Springer.

Curtis, J. R., Patrick, D. L., Shannon, S. E., Treece, P. D., Engelberg, R. A., & Rubenfeld, G. D. (2001). The family conference as a focus to improve communication about end-of-life care in the intensive care unit: Opportunities for improvement. *Critical Care Medicine, 29*(2 Suppl.), N26-N33.

Dean, H. E. (1990). Political and ethical implications of using quality of life as an outcome measure. *Seminars in Oncology Nursing, 6,* 303-308.

Daniels, N. (1985). *Just health care.* Cambridge, UK: Cambridge University Press.

DeGrazia, D. (1999). Advance directives, dementia, and 'the someone else problem.' *Bioethics, 13,* 373-391.

Dolan, P. (2001). Utilitarianism and the measurement and aggregation of quality-adjusted life years. *Health Care Analysis, 9*(1), 65-76.

Dresser, R. (1995). Dworkin on dementia: Elegant theory, questionable practice. *Hastings Center Report, 25,* 35.

Edwards, M. J., & Tolle, S. W. (1992). Disconnecting a ventilator at the request of a patient who knows he will then die: The doctor's anguish. *Annals of Internal Medicine, 117,* 254-256.

Emanuel, E. J. (1996). Cost savings at the end of life. What do the data show? *Journal of the American Medical Association, 275,* 1907-1914.

Fagerlin, A., Ditto, P. H., Danks, J. H., Houts, R. M., & Smucker, W. D. (2001). Projection in surrogate decisions about life-sustaining medical treatments. *Health Psychology, 20*(3), 166-175.

Ferrell, B., Virani, R., Grant, M., Coyne, P., & Uman, G. (2000). Beyond the Supreme Court decision: Nursing perspectives on end-of-life care. *Oncology Nursing Forum, 27,* 445-455.

Finucane, T. E., Christmas, C., & Travis, K. (1999). Tube feeding in patients with advanced dementia: A review of the evidence. *Journal of the American Medical Association, 282,* 1365-1370.

Fishman, S. K. (1989). Health professionals' attitudes toward older people. *Dental Clinics of North America, 33,* 7-10.

Fleck, L. M. (1994). Just caring: Oregon, health care rationing, and informed democratic deliberation. *Journal of Medicine and Philosophy, 19,* 367-388.

Foley, K. M. (1991). The relationship of pain and symptom management to patient requests for physician-assisted suicide. *The Journal of Pain and Symptom Management, 6,* 289-297.

Frantz, T. T., Lawrence, J. C., Somov, P. G., & Somova, M. J. (1999). Factors in hospice patients' length of stay. *American Journal of Hospice & Palliative Care, 16,* 449-454.

Freedman, B. (1993). Offering truth: One ethical approach to the uniformed cancer patient. *Archives of Internal Medicine, 153,* 572-576.

Ganzini, L., Nelson, H. D., Schmidt, T. A., Kraemer, D. F., Delorit, M. A., & Lee, M. A. (2000). Physician's experience with the Oregon Death with Dignity Act. *New England Journal of Medicine, 342*(8), 557-563.

Gauthier, C. C. (2001). Active voluntary euthanasia, terminal sedation, and assisted suicide. *The Journal of Clinical Ethics, 12,* 43-50.

Gillick, M. R. (2000). Rethinking the role of tube feeding in patients with advanced dementia. *New England Journal of Medicine, 342,* 206-210.

Gjerdingen, D. K., Neff, J. A., Wang, M., & Chaloner, K. (1999). Older persons' opinions about life-sustaining procedures in the face of dementia. *Archives of Family Medicine, 8,* 421-425.

Glass, A. (1998). The Oregon Health Plan: Development and implementation of an innovative method of delivery of health care services to the medically indigent. *Cancer, 82*(10 Suppl.), 1995-1999.

Hare, J., Pratt, C., & Nelson, C. (1992). Agreement between patients and their self-selected surrogates on difficult medical decisions. *Archives of Internal Medicine, 152,* 1049-1054.

Harvard School of Public Health. (2000). *US seniors bear drug cost hardship compared to similar nations* Retrieved from http://www.hsph.harvard.edu/press/releases/press05082000.html

In re Westchester County Medical Center, 72 N.Y.2d. 517, 534 N.Y.S.2d 886 (1988).

International Task Force on Euthanasia and Assisted Suicide. (2003). *5 Years under Oregon's assisted suicide law.* Retrieved from http://www.internationaltaskforce.org/orstats.htm

Jecker, N. S. (1990). The role of intimate others in medical decision making. *The Gerontologist, 30,* 65-71.

Jecker, N. S. (1991). Age-based rationing and women. *Journal of the American Medical Association, 266,* 3012-3015.

Kapp, M. B. (2001). Economic influences on end-of-life care: empirical evidence and ethical speculation. *Death Studies, 25,* 251-263.

Keay, T. J., & Schonwetter, R. S. (2000). The case for hospice care in long-term care environments. *Clinics in Geriatric Medicine, 16,* 211-223.

Kressin, N. R., & Petersen, L. A. (2001). Racial differences in the use of invasive cardiovascular procedures: Review of the literature and prescription for future research. *Annals of Internal Medicine, 135,* 352-366.

Kuhse, H. (1999). Some reflections on the problem of advance directives, personhood, and personal identity. *Kennedy Institute of Ethics Journal, 9,* 347-364.

Levit, K., Smith, C., Cowan, C., Lazenby, H., Sensenig, A., & Catlin, A. (2003). Trends in health care spending, 2001. *Health Affairs, 22*(1).

Lockhart, L. K., Ditto, P. H., Danks, J. H., Coppola, K. M., & Smucker, W. D. (2001). The stability of older adults' judgments of fates better and worse than death. *Death Studies, 25,* 299-317.

Loewy, E. H. (1997). *Moral strangers, moral acquaintances, and moral friends: Connectedness and its conditions.* Albany: State University of New York.

Loewy, E. H. (1996). *Textbook of healthcare ethics.* New York: Plenum Press.

Lynn, J., & Childress, J. (1986). Must patients always be given food and water? In J. Lynn (Ed.), *By no extraordinary means* (pp. 47-60). Bloomington: Indiana University Press.

Lynn, J., Schuster, J. L., & Kabcenell, A. (2000). *Improving care for the end of life: A sourcebook for health care managers and clinicians*. New York: Oxford University Press.

Manfredi, P. L., Morrison, R. S., & Meier, D. E. (1998). The rule of double effect [Letter]. *Journal of the American Medical Association, 338,* 1390.

Matzo, M. L., & Schwarz Kennedy, J. (2001). In their own words: Oncology nurses respond to patient requests for assisted suicide and euthanasia. *Applied Nursing Research, 14,* 64-71.

Moreno, J. D. (1992). The social individual in clinical ethics. *The Journal of Clinical Ethics, 3*(1), 53-55.

Moscicki, E. K. (1997). Identification of suicide risk factors using epidemiologic studies. *Suicide, 20,* 506.

Mularski, R. A., Bascom, P., & Osborne, M. L. (2001). Educational agendas for interdisciplinary end-of-life curricula. *Critical Care Medicine, 29*(2 Suppl.), N16-N23.

Nahm, E., & Resnick, B. (2001). End-of-life treatment preferences among older adults. *Nursing Ethics, 8,* 533-543.

Newton, M. J. (1999). Precedent autonomy: Life-sustaining intervention and the demented patient. *Cambridge Quarterly of Healthcare Ethics, 8,* 189-199.

Nolan, M. (2001, October 4). Panel discussion on the ethics of allocation. Presented at a meeting on "The Ethics of Health Care: An Assessment in Germany and the United States." The Catholic University of America, Washington, DC.

Perkins, H. S. (2000). Time to move advance care planning beyond advance directives. *Chest, 117,* 1228-1231.

Puchalski, C. M., Zhong, Z., Jacobs, M. M., Fox, E., Lynn, J., Harrold, J., et al. (2000). Patients who want their family and physician to make resuscitation decisions for them: Observations from SUPPORT and HELP. Study to Understand Prognoses and Preferences for Outcomes and Risks of Treatment and Hospitalized Elderly Longitudinal Project. *Journal of the American Geriatrics Society, 48*(5 Suppl.), S84-S90.

Quill, T. E. (1998). Principle of double effect and end-of-life pain management: Additional myths and a limited rule. *Journal of Palliative Medicine, 1,* 333-336.

Quill, T. E., Dresser, R., & Brock, D. (1997). The rule of double effect—a critique of its role in end-of-life decision making. *New England Journal of Medicine, 337,* 1768-1771.

Reinhardt, U. E. (1993). Reforming the health care system: The universal dilemma. *American Journal of Law and Medicine, 19*(1-2), 21-36.

Reinhardt, U. E. (1996). Rationing health care: What it is, what it is not, and why we cannot avoid it. *Baxter Health Policy Review, 2,* 63-99.

Rice, D. P. (1990). The medical care system: Past trends and future projections. In P. R. Lee & C. L. Estes (Eds.), *The Nation's Health* (3rd ed.). Boston: Jones and Bartlett.

Schneiderman, L. J. (1992). Futility and rationing. *American Journal of Medicine, 92,* 189-196.

Schneiderman, L. J., Jecker, N. S., & Jonsen, A. R. (1996). Medical futility: Response to critiques. *Annals of Internal Medicine, 125,* 669-674.

Schneiderman, L. J., Kronick, R., Kaplan, R. M., Anderson, J. P., & Langer, R. D. (1994). Attitudes of seriously ill patients toward treatment that involves high costs and burdens on others. *The Journal of Clinical Ethics, 5,* 109-112.

Schwartz, J. (2000, May 1). *Summary of the Health Care Decisions Act.* Retrieved from http://www.oag.state.md.us/Healthpol/HCDAsummary.pdf

Schwartz, J. (2002, Spring). Legal update on advance directives in Maryland. *Mid-Atlantic Ethics Committee Newsletter,* p. 8.

Schwarz, J. K. (2002). *Assistance in dying: The nurse's experience.* Unpublished doctoral dissertation, New York University.

Scitovsky, A. A. (1994). "The high cost of dying" revisited. *Milbank Quarterly, 72,* 561-591.

Solomon, M., O'Donnell, L., Jennings, B., Guilfoy, J. B., Wolf, S., Nolan, K., et al. (1993). Decisions near the end of life: Professional views on life-sustaining treatments. *The American Journal of Public Health, 83,* 14-22.

Sprangers, M. A., & Aaronson, N. K. (1992). The role of health care providers and significant others in evaluating the quality of life of patients with chronic disease: A review. *Journal of Clinical Epidemiology, 45,* 743-760.

Sulmasy, D. P. (1998). Killing and allowing to die: Another look. *The Journal of Law, Medicine & Ethics, 26,* 55-64.

Sulmasy, D. P., Terry, P. B., Weisman, C. S., Miller, D. J., Stallings, R. Y., Vettese, M. A., et al. (1998). The accuracy of substituted judgments in patients with terminal diagnoses. *Annals of Internal Medicine, 128,* 621-629.

Thomasma, D. C. (1999). Stewardship of the aged: Meeting the ethical challenge of ageism. In honor of Joseph Fletcher. *Cambridge Quarterly of Healthcare Ethics, 8,* 148-159.

U.S. Census Bureau. (2002). Table A: People without health insurance for the entire year by selected characteristics: 1999 and 2000. In *Health insurance coverage 2000.* Retrieved from http://www.census.gov/hhes/hlthins/hlthin00/hlthtables00.html

Volker, D. L. (2001). Perspectives on assisted dying: Oncology nurses' experiences with requests for assisted dying from terminally ill patients with cancer. *Oncology Nursing Forum, 28,* 39-49.

Ward, D. (2000). Ageism and the abuse of older people in health and social care. *British Journal of Nursing, 9,* 560-563.

Wear, S., & Logue, G. (1995). The problem of medically futile treatment: Falling back on a preventive ethics approach. *The Journal of Clinical Ethics, 6,* 138-148.

Wilson, W. C., Smedira, N. G., & Fink, C. (1992). Ordering and administration of sedatives and analgesics during the withholding and withdrawing of life support from critically ill patients. *Journal of the American Medical Association, 267,* 949-953.

Woodend, A. K., Nair, R. C., & Tang, A. S. (1997). Definition of life quality from a patient versus health care professional perspective. *International Journal of Rehabilitation Research, 20*(1), 71–80.

COMMUNICATION ISSUES IN ADVANCE CARE PLANNING

Kathleen Ouimet Perrin

INTRODUCTION

"I'd like to speak with you about the type of care you would like to receive if you were very ill, probably dying. Have you ever thought about that before? What do you think would be important to you at the end of your life? What type of care would help you obtain that? Whom would you like to make a decision about your care if you couldn't? Have you talked with anyone about what you would want or have you completed an advance directive? Would you want to have medical interventions tried at the end of your life that might offer a slim possibility of prolonging your life?" Although such a barrage of questions at one time would be inappropriate, it is important to talk about these issues with older adults, whether they are patients, family members, or significant others.

People over the age of 65 account for nearly 75% of the deaths in this country (Haynor, 1998). Yet, because it is difficult for health care providers and family members to initiate conversations about the end of life, many older adults die without their preferences for end-of-life care being known or respected (Bedell & Delbanco, 1984; Cotton, 1993; SUPPORT Principal Investigators, 1995). Although most elders desire to participate in discussions about end-of-life care with their families (High, 1994; O'Brien, Grisso, & Maislin, 1995) and/or with health care providers (O'Brien et al., 1995; Wetle, Levkoff, Cwikel, & Rosen, 1988), they are unwilling to initiate the discussion (Silverman & Vinicky, 1991). If a health care provider or family member does not ask the types of questions listed previously, the wishes of the elder for end-of-life care may go unspoken and unfulfilled.

END-OF-LIFE CARE PLANNING

Martin, Emanuel, and Singer (2000) stated that one of the most important elements of end-of-life care is communication among patients, health care providers, and families about goals and treatments at the end of life. They suggested that, although written advance directive forms may be used, they are seldom completed and have little impact on such specific end-of-life interventions as cardiopulmonary resuscitation (CPR). They urged that the goal of advance planning at the end of life be seen not as controlling each treatment decision but rather as helping the patient and family achieve a sense of control of the dying process. They believe advance care planning should be used to determine settings for care and limits for life-sustaining treatments that may inappropriately prolong dying.

Martin et al. (2000) recommended that the process of advance planning involve a reflective discussion of the patient's values, goals, and preferences in a noncrisis setting. They see a completed advance directive form not as a central feature of end-of-life planning but as a worksheet for assisting the planning process. Martin et al. suggested that an appropriate advance planning form or discussion would allow a patient, the family, and health care providers to think about and articulate values, goals, and preferences relevant to health care decisions. Silverman and Vinicky (1991) recommended including questions such as the following in a values history:

What do you think will be important to you when you are dying?

What is your attitude toward death?

How do you feel about technology that might prolong your life?

Although they advocated asking a patient about his or her values, Martin et al. (2000) cautioned that there has been only a weak correlation between the statement of a person's values and his or her specific preferences. In contrast to a values approach, a goals-based discussion would help the person to articulate an overall goal for end-of-life care, such as "Keep me comfortable at all costs" or "Keep me alive until my grandchild is born." Decisions about specific interventions are made in line with the person's overall goal. Finally, the person may have preferences about specific treatments at the end of life, such as "Whatever happens to me, I don't want to have that breathing tube in again." When a patient has a specific disease with a known course and an anticipated series of treatments, Martin et al. (2000) recommended that any discussion of patient preferences be tailored to the patient's specific disease and anticipated treatments. Patients are thus urged to consider the options they are most likely to confront.

When there is an open process of communication and discussion among patient, family, and health care providers, appropriate advance planning may occur and directives may be developed. If a written directive is to result from the process, Martin et al. (2000) recommended that it include a statement of patient values or goals, some indication of patient preferences in specific circumstances, and an identification of a durable power of attorney for health care purposes or a health care proxy. However, not all patients are able to complete all three components. Some patients, even though competent, are unable to decide what specific treatments they would want at the end of life; others are unable to identify a person they trust to serve as a proxy decision maker.

ADVANCE DIRECTIVES

The two most common types of advance directives recognized in the United States are instructional directives, such as living wills or medical directives, and proxy designates, such as health care proxies or durable powers of attorney for health care purposes. Instructional directives identify the amount and type of care that a patient would wish to receive if certain conditions are met. In the case of the living will, the patient affirms that, if he or she is terminally ill, he or she does not wish to be treated with any life-sustaining treatments. There are two major problems with the living will. First, it is not always clear when a person is dying. In the Study to Understand Prognoses and Preferences for Outcomes and Risks of Treatments (SUPPORT) (SUPPORT Principal Investigators, 1995), comprising seriously ill patients, many of the patients were still predicted to have a 50% chance of surviving at least 2 months as recently as 2 days before they died. Also, health care providers are reluctant to recognize that patients with some diagnoses, particularly heart failure, are dying (Forbes, 2001). Furthermore, the patient does not usually have an opportunity to refuse specific treatments.

Medical directives are more specific; they allow patients to specify their desires for or refusals of specific treatments under certain circumstances should they become incapacitated. For example, patients might indicate that they did not wish to be resuscitated (using a do-not-resuscitate [DNR] order) or would not want to be intubated, be ventilated, receive nasogastric feedings, or be dialyzed under specific circumstances, such as becoming comatose. The major problem with medical directives that are not specific to a patient's illness is that the patient's situation may not be similar enough to the circumstance described in the advanced directive for anyone to determine how the patient would wish to be treated. Teno, Licks, and Lynn (1997) found that directives were specific enough in only 3% of actual circumstances to guide decision making. Other problems with medical directives are that they do not allow for advances in medical treatment or for the patient to change his or her mind about one of the interventions or situations without changing the directive. The medical directive may only represent the patient's desires for treatment at the time the directive was completed, not at the time treatment is being planned.

Proxy designates were developed to alleviate such situations. They permit a person to appoint an agent to make health care decisions for the person should he or she become incapacitated. These directives allow for greater flexibility and more relevance to the patient's specific situation. Molloy et al. (1996) noted that the capacity required to designate a proxy is considerably less than that needed to envision scenarios and complete a medical directive. Thus proxy designations may be more appropriate for people who, although competent, are having difficulty understanding options and making decisions about end-of-life care. However, there are disadvantages. The proxy designate may not realize the level of responsibility that being a health care proxy entails and may have difficulty making a decision. The proxy may also confound his or her interests with those of the patient and fail to act in the patient's best interests (Perrin, 1997).

ELDERS' PREFERENCES FOR END-OF-LIFE CARE

In the United States, only about 20% to 30% of older adults have completed any type of advance directive, although three fourths or more of the residents in long-term care facilities may have a DNR order (Molloy et al., 2000). DNR orders represent the most common type of advanced planning done for older adults in this country (Eun-Shim & Resnick, 2001; Ghusn, Teasdale, & Jordan, 1997; Nolan & Bruder, 1997). They are also often viewed as a "practical place to start" (Smith et al., 1997) and are often the first step in considering treatment limitation at the end of life. When a DNR order is written, the patient or proxy designate and health care providers concur that, if the patient is dying, the health care team will not make any attempt to stop the process or bring the patient back to life.

Most health care providers believe that it is quite reasonable for older adults to forgo CPR because CPR is rarely successful when attempted on older adults. Buchanan (1998) estimated that 2 long-term care residents out of every 100 who receive CPR survive to hospital discharge, and both would most likely have significant neurologic impairments. Murphy, Murray, Robinson, and Campton (1989), in a study of older adults receiving CPR in hospital, rehabilitation, and long-term care settings, found that 22% of patients survived the initial resuscitation attempt, but only 3.8% of the patients survived to hospital discharge. In a study by Banja and Bilsky (1993), no patients survived to hospital discharge after resuscitation in a rehabilitation hospital. Survival rates after CPR for all age groups have stayed consistent for three decades at about 13% (Schneider, Nelson, & Brown, 1993). Marik and Craft (1997) found that patients who

survived to hospital discharge following CPR had one reversible condition, were otherwise healthy, and had suffered a sudden, unexpected dysrhythmia. Thus it seems very reasonable for an older adult with multiple chronic illnesses to forgo CPR.

The majority of clearly competent elders living in community or long-term care facilities would prefer not to be resuscitated if they were gravely ill and probably dying (Diamond, Jernigan, Moseley, Messina, & McKeown, 1989; Eun-Shim & Resnick, 2001; Kellogg et al., 1992; Wagner, 1984). However, elders who have moderate to severe impairment in daily decision-making skills but are still alert and conversant may prefer CPR (O'Brien et al., 1995). Molloy et al. (1996) stated that there was no "gold standard" for determining when an older adult has the capacity to make decisions about end-of-life care, and there is a lack of consensus about what tool ought to be used to measure capacity and who ought to administer the assessment. Eun-Shim and Resnick (2001) stated that capacity must be clinically determined because the person must be shown to be able to understand and appreciate the consequences of his or her end-of-life treatment plan. Bradley, Walker, Blechner, and Wetle (1997) found that 48% of decisionally competent nursing home residents did not receive information about end-of-life treatment choices and advance directives, while 34% of partially or totally confused patients did. In Chapter 7, Mitty and Mezey discuss competency testing and end-of-life care decision making for people who are not competent or lack capacity to make a decision.

Practitioners have wondered if age and changes in health status affect the stability of patient preferences about end-of-life care. Eun-Shim and Resnick (2001) explored the preferences for end-of-life care of competent elders living in a continuing care retirement community. Their study found that slightly more than half the participants did not want to receive CPR, to be put on dialysis, to be put on a ventilator, or to receive tube feedings. Nearly all would want to receive antibiotics (95%), diagnostic testing (94%), and pain medication as needed (84%). When the same individuals were followed up 2 years later, there was a slight increase in the number of people who wanted CPR and a slight

EVIDENCE-BASED PRACTICE

Reference: Eun-shim, N., & Resnick, B. (2001). End of life treatment preferences among older adults. *Nursing Ethics*, 8, 533-544.

Research Problem: This study explored the end-of-life treatment preferences (ELTPs) among older adults and compared those preferences to preferences expressed by the same people a year earlier to identify characteristics and continuity of preferences.

Design: This was a descriptive study.

Sample and Setting: 191 of 207 residents living in a continuing care retirement community participated in the study.

Methods: As part of a yearly health check, residents were interviewed by graduate nursing students and asked if, in the event of medical necessity, they would be willing to accept any of the following medical interventions: cardiopulmonary resuscitation (CPR), major surgery, ventilator therapy, dialysis, blood transfusion, artificial nutrition and hydration, diagnostic tests, antibiotics, or pain medications.

Results: The findings of this study indicate that about half of participants did not want CPR, ventilator therapy, or dialysis. There was no relationship between ELTPs and chronic illness. There was a statistically significant difference between the older adults' preferences for some of the interventions (CPR, blood transfusions, and ventilator therapy) between the two interviews.

Implications for Nursing Practice: Discussions with older adults about the pros and cons of each therapy should begin in the community while people are still physically healthy and cognitively intact. Factors influencing ELTPs need to be examined further.

Conclusion: The findings from this study suggest that many older adults do not want aggressive interventions at the end of life but choose interventions that may keep them comfortable. However, treatment decisions may change over time.

reduction in the number of people who wanted to be put on a ventilator. Their findings were comparable to those of Kohut et al. (1997), who noted that, although most preferences about end-of-life treatment do not change, most people change one of their preferences. However, these findings are in contrast to earlier findings by Schonwetter, Teasdale, Taffet, Robinson, and Luchi (1991) and Everhart and Pearlman (1990), who concluded that, despite changes in health care status and education, patient's preferences were stable over time.

How informed are health care providers about their patients' preferences for or against CPR or other possible medical interventions? In 1984, Bedell and Delbanco noted that only 19% of patients had discussed their preferences about CPR with their physician. The SUPPORT study demonstrated that the majority of patients who died in intensive care units had never communicated their thoughts about resuscit-

ation to their physicians (SUPPORT Principal Investigators, 1995). Ghusn et al. (1997) could find documentation of discussion of DNR decisions in the records of only 27% of residents of a long-term care facility. O'Brien et al. (1995) found that only 12% of residents of long-term care facilities had discussed their preferences with their health care providers. Puopolo (1997) studied critical care nurses, only 13% of whom had had direct discussion of their patients' CPR preference with the patients. Yet the nurses could accurately predict a patient's preference 76% of the time. How do health care providers learn what might be affecting their patients' wishes?

There are personal and ethnic factors that account for some of the differences among elders in preferences for or against CPR and other life-sustaining technologies. Mezey, Leitman, Mitty, Bottrell, and Ramsey (2000) found that white, college-educated patients were more likely to know about advance directives and be willing to forgo CPR. Eun-shim and Resnick (2001) noted that their sample included a large proportion of college-educated people and postulated that this factor might explain why a majority of elders did not want CPR. O'Brien et al. (1995) and Blackhall et al. (1999) noted that African American patients were more likely to request CPR and ask to be kept alive on life-sustaining technologies. Romero, Lindeman, Koehler, and Allen (1997) stated that Hispanics were more likely to choose CPR, intubation, antibiotics, and tube feedings and were also unlikely to have heard of living wills or advance directives.

Several reasons for the difference in preferences between white and minority individuals have been postulated. African American and Hispanic patients demonstrated a deep distrust of the health care system in ethnographic interviews (Blackhall et al., 1999). They may fear signing an advance directive, believing that it will merely provide the health care system with another opportunity to deny them care, and they would rather err on the side of overtreatment than undertreatment (O'Brien et al., 1995). Ethnographic interviews of Mexican Americans by Blackhall et al. (1999) revealed that they did not believe the interventions would have been suggested if the patient were going to die and the case were truly hopeless. Vaughn, Kiyasu, and McCormick (2001) noted that health care providers are uncomfortable discussing end-of-life issues with minorities, such as Japanese American patients, and that the patients were more likely to entrust such decisions to their families, as were Korean Americans (Blackhall et al., 1999).

Preference of Elders for Family Decision Makers

Elders of all ethnic groups are more likely to speak with a family member about end-of-life care than with a health care provider. This does not mean that they have completed a health care proxy or durable power of attorney for health care purposes. Rather, most elders have simply discussed their preferences for end-of-life care with at least one family member (High, 1993). When asked whom they believe knows them well enough and whom they would trust to make a health care decision for them, elders overwhelmingly (94%) choose family members, primarily spouses or adult children. Confidence and trust in family members to make any necessary decision for them may be a major reason older adults do not complete advance directives (High, 1994).

High (1994) believes that elders prefer family decision makers for a variety of significant and appropriate reasons. The family member has an inherent knowledge of the culture, values, and expectations of the patient and is usually concerned with the patient's welfare. In most instances, High believes family members choose appropriately based on the patient's values, and best interests. High suggested that too much emphasis has been placed on disagreement and abuse within families and not enough on family empowerment and good-faith decision making. He suggested that elders' preferences for family decision makers ought to be recognized and advance directives should be encouraged only for those who "have very specific or unusual preferences, do not want family to serve as substitute decision makers or have disagreements with family or have no family" (High, 1994, p. S17).

Elders say they have thought at least a "moderate amount" about whom they would want to make health care decisions for them if they become incapacitated (Lo, McLeod, & Saika, 1986). Overwhelmingly, they would choose to have their families make such decisions without the benefit of a written directive (High, 1994; Lo et al., 1986; Nolan, 2000). Although the elders in one study realized that having a written advance directive would help their families to know their wishes and possibly prevent guilt among family members over the decision, most elders still did not complete advance directives (Nolan, 2000). These elders wanted their families to decide about end-of-life care based on their families' best judgments in the specific situation. Perhaps this is because these elders put their trust in their families and not in a piece of paper (High, 1993). Or it might be because elders believe that the family is the center of their lives (Blustein, 1993) and no individual can be completely autonomous; any decision made for one individual affects the entire family. In High's (1993) study, none of the elders stated that they always expected to make their own decisions. Most elders realize that their families will be profoundly affected by providing or paying for their health care. Thus elders may believe their families ought to have a significant role in determining what is the most appropriate end-of-life care.

Martin et al. (2000) emphasized that making a decision about end-of-life care ought to be done in a family context. They believe that having discussions with patients about end-of-life care "helps patients prepare for death, is influenced by personal relationships, is a social process and occurs within the context of family and loved ones" (p. 1672). They asserted that the primary value of end-of-life care planning is to allow the patient and family to prepare for death and dying and to find ways to cope with the impending death. Thus they believe one reason patients may communicate about end-of-life issues with families more often than health care providers is that the discussion may help the family to resolve any outstanding issues and become ready for the patient's death.

PHYSICIAN INVOLVEMENT IN END-OF-LIFE DECISION MAKING

Although most elders have had discussions about end-of-life care preferences with at least one family member, few patients have had such discussions with their physicians (Emanuel, Barry, Stoeckle, Ettelson, & Emanuel, 1991; O'Brien et al., 1995). Although patients are willing and eager to engage in such a discussion, they believe it is not their role to initiate the discussion (Emanuel et al., 1991). Thus they wait for their physicians to start the conversation. Unfortunately, the physician usually does not. Reasons physicians may be reluctant to initiate such conversations are found in Box 6-1.

Although they do not tend to initiate end-of-life conversations with patients, most physicians (82%) believe it is their responsibility to begin the discussion (Markson et al., 1997) and to

---

Box 6-1 Physician Reluctance Regarding Patient Preferences

1. Personal discomfort with discussing death and dying (Ventres, Nichter, Reed, & Frankel, 1992). If the physician believes that the patient is dying because the physician has failed and there is no more that he or she can do, the physician is less likely to discuss CPR preference with the patient.

2. Lack of physician education and experience in conducting such a conversation (Tulsky, Chesney, & Lo, 1995). Resident physicians learn early in the course of their education that various attending and older residents have differing views on how and when end-of-life discussions should occur. Unfortunately, according to Tulsky and colleagues, resident physicians receive very little education in how to conduct a discussion about end-of-life preferences, and consequently they "often did not provide essential information" (p. 436).

3. Fear that the patient will believe the physician has "given up on and is abandoning the patient" (Cotton, 1993). Some doctors say they have difficulty discussing end-of-life care without conveying a sense of hopelessness to the patient. Kohn and Menon (1988) stated that physicians may be unwilling to bring up the issue until a crisis develops because they are afraid of unnecessarily alarming the patient.

4. The physician may feel legally or morally bound to treat until death is proximate (Hanson, Tulsky, & Danis, 1997). About 10% of physicians believe they must treat all patients with maximal interventions and that to limit treatment is morally and ethically unacceptable. Another larger group of physicians believes that it is inappropriate to discuss treatment limitation until the patient is certainly going to die. Unfortunately, if discussion waits until the patient is definitely dying, the patient frequently no longer has the capacity to participate in decision making about her or his end-of-life care.

5. Concern about the amount of time such a conversation will require (Emanuel et al., 1991). Some physicians fear that having discussions about end-of-life care planning, which are not reimbursable, may be very time consuming. Studies indicate that, although it takes only approximately 10 to 16 minutes of physician time in discussion with a patient and/or family for a DNR decision to be reached, this is often just the first in a series of end-of-life decisions (Smith et al., 1997; Tulsky et al., 1995).

write the appropriate orders. Some physicians (Reckling, 1997) report that they prefer that nurses and other health care providers not discuss these issues with patients. The result is that each group—health care providers, patients, and families—talks among itself about appropriate end-of-life care, but the groups do not talk with each other (Kohn & Menon, 1988). Less than a tenth of patients have spoken with their physicians when planning an advance directive, and the majority of patients with advance directives have never been asked by or told their physicians whether they have advance directives (Teno et al., 1997). Thus, unfortunately, conversations about end-of-life care among physicians, patients, and families usually do not occur until a crisis develops.

Researchers have documented concerns with how physicians engage in end-of-life care discussions in crisis situations. In Tulsky et al.'s (1995) study, conversations about resuscitation lasted about 10 minutes and the resident physicians dominated the speaking time. Tulsky et al. did not believe that the information the residents provided to patients/families was adequate for them to make decisions about CPR. For example, only 13% of physicians mentioned the futility of CPR and the chance of the patient surviving. Additionally, residents did not allow patients or families many opportunities to ask questions, and elicited information about the patient's values and goals in end-of-life care less than 10% of the time.

Hanson et al. (1997) reported similar findings. They noted that, because physicians tended to focus on treatment descriptions rather than listening to patient concerns, their understandings of patient preferences remained poor even after face-to-face discussions. They stated that physicians tended to be coercive in forcing their opinions. Markson et al. (1997) surveyed physicians who admitted that they would attempt to persuade patients to change decisions that they believed were not well informed (91%), medically reasonable (88%), or in the patient's best interest (88%). Ventres et al. (1992) concluded that "Physicians' presentation of opinions to patients are not neutral. Options are often presented in such a way as to influence DNR decision-making" (p. 163), and that communication strategies "may work to distance physicians from their patients at times when it is imperative for them to explore the values and wishes of the patient" (p. 165).

According to Ventres et al. (1992), physicians use three common prototypes to approach the discussion of DNR orders with patients and families. The first might be described as legalistic or technical. In this situation, the physician might ask, once the patient has become incapacitated, whether the patient has an advance directive or has a health care proxy and if someone can produce the appropriate papers. In the second approach, the physician might admit there were no further medical treatments that might lead to a cure and ask the patient or family what the patient would want for end-of-life care. In the third approach, the physician might mention that there were legal requirements that CPR be attempted at the end of life unless a DNR order was written. The physician would next ask the patient's and/or family's opinion about the appropriateness of administering a painful and probably useless treatment.

ROLE OF THE NURSE IN ADVANCE CARE PLANNING AND END-OF-LIFE DECISION MAKING

According to the American Nurses Association (ANA, 1996), in a position statement revised in 1995, nurses have a responsibility to facilitate informed decision making about end-of-life care, including but not limited to the discussion of advance directives. The ANA also recognizes that nurses have roles as educators about end-of-life care and as patient advocates to assure that appropriate end-of-life care is provided. Thus nursing responsibilities in advance planning may predominate at two times, when a plan for end-of-life care is being developed and when a plan for end-of-life care is being implemented.

The nurse may be involved in assisting a patient or resident to consider or plan for end-of-life care when the elder is admitted to a hospital or long-term care facility. Or, in their roles as educators, nurses may encounter elders in the community who wish to discuss end-of-life care planning. For example, some critical care nurses are actively promoting end-of-life planning through television programming, group discussions, and community meetings. Most patients agree that it is when they are relatively well, which most believe they are even on hospital admission, that they ought to be considering end-of-life care planning (Nolan & Bruder, 1997).

The ANA concurs that nurses need not focus on completion of an advance directive during such discussions but instead ought to provide education about possibilities at the end of life and explore patients' values, wishes, and preferences. Davison and Degner (1998) suggested that a logical place to begin the discussion is determining how much control the person wishes to exert over his or her end-of-life care. They utilized a card sort that establishes three categories of patient decision making: active, collaborative, and passive (Box 6-2). Davison and Degner suggested that, once it has been determined what role the patient wishes to assume in decision making and whom the patient wishes to include in the decision-making process, then it is the nurse's role to initiate appropriate discussion and education among decision makers.

Because most patients desire that they and their families have at least some input into end-of-life decisions, Davison and Degner (1998)

Box 6-2 Patient Decision-Making Categories

Active: The person might select "I prefer to make the final selection about which treatment I will receive." The patient might also choose to have the family make the final decision; a definitive choice for the family to decide is also seen as an active decision by the patient. (p. 134)

Collaborative: The person would choose from the card sort: "I prefer that my doctor and I (or my family and my physician) share the responsibility for deciding which treatment is best for me."

Passive: The person would select a choice such as: "I prefer to leave all decisions concerning my treatment to my physicians." The person might suggest that the physician consult with the person or family for an opinion, but in this selection, the final decision is the physician's alone.

Adapted from Davison, J., & Degner, L. F. (1998). Promoting patient decision making in life-and-death situations. *Seminars in Oncology Nursing, 14*(2), 129-136.

---

recommended that the nurse next focus on identifying the patient's and families' goals and values, as well as their understanding of the possibilities and results of the use of life-sustaining technologies at the end of life. The nurse might begin such a discussion by saying:

"I want you to imagine that you were diagnosed as having a terminal illness. By that I mean you were dying from the illness and would not be likely to get better no matter what treatment your doctor prescribed. What would matter to you? How would you like to be cared for at that time?"

This is the step that most physicians avoid. It is difficult because it is imperative that the health care provider listen actively to the patient's and family's concerns, questioning and clarifying what they desire without imposing his or her own values and goals. What the nurse is attempting to learn is what this person and his or her family believe they will value as the end of life approaches. Most elders have a strong tendency to favor limitation of treatment when they are unlikely to return to their baseline functioning or are probably dying (Gillick & Mendes, 1996), but this is not always true, and some elders wish to continue to live until specific events occur or goals are reached. This is the nurse's opportunity to learn what the elder and family believe will probably be important as the end of life approaches.

After the patient's and family's goals and values have been explored, the nurse should assess what they understand about the use of life-sustaining treatment. According to Silveira, DiPiero, Gerrity, and Freudener (2000), a significant proportion of outpatients misunderstand options at the end of life. This is not particularly surprising because many Americans obtain their information about life-sustaining technology and end-of-life care from television. Diem, Lantos, and Tulsky (1996) documented that, in reality-based television medical shows, nearly all patients survive CPR, while in fictional shows such as "ER," approximately 75% of patients survive CPR. This serious misinformation often needs to be dispelled before patients and families consider what types of life-sustaining interventions they would desire at the end of life.

According to the ANA, nurses have an important role in educating patients and their families about their options at the end of life. This includes a discussion of the experience and outcomes of such treatments as CPR and ventilation. The description of CPR should be accurate and include all of the elements of resuscitation (aeration with intubation, chest compressions, defibrillation, etc.). However, it is important that the nurse allow the patient and family to develop their own opinions and come to their own conclusions. Just as physicians can color their discussions to patients and families with their perspectives on life-sustaining interventions, so can nurses. Many nurses have very negative remembrances of CPR (Page & Meerabeau, 1996), and it is quite possible for nurses to convey these impressions to their patients and the families. Nurses might begin discussion of specific preferences for life-sustaining treatments in a way similar to that with which they began discussion of the patient's values and goals for end-of-life care, such as

"I want you to imagine that you are very close to dying and would not be likely to get better no matter what treatment your doctor prescribed. What type of medical interventions would you want us to try in an attempt to prolong your life and delay your death?"

The final step in the development of an end-of-life care plan should involve an interdisciplinary meeting for development of the plan. The meeting should involve at least the patient and physician but also family and other health care providers if appropriate and the patient so desires. At this meeting, the patient and family can clarify any questions they might have about end-of-life care options and develop a plan, possibly a written directive. Hopefully, the final plan would include the extent to which the patient desires to be involved in the decision making, the role he or she wishes his or her family or physician to play, the patient's goals or values for end-of-life care, any specific desires the patient has for specific interventions to be utilized or withheld at the end of life, and a choice of health care proxy, if appropriate. The more physicians and other health care providers are involved in developing a plan for end-of-life care for a patient, the more likely the plan is to be followed when the patient becomes ill and a decision needs to be made.

Once the person becomes ill and enters the health care system, the ANA recommends that the nurse assume the role of advocate for the patient's end-of-life care preferences. On the person's admission to a health care institution, the patient and family must be asked whether the patient has an advance directive and, if a directive exists, whether they can produce a copy. Before assuming that the directive should come into effect, the nurse or another health care provider needs to inquire whether the patient still wants the directive to take effect. As previously noted, many patients change their minds about portions of their advance directive as they age and their health status changes. However, only one member of the health care team needs to inquire of the patient about the patient's current thoughts and feelings. The spouse of one patient who had declined all life-sustaining technologies recalled his wife being asked by 13 health care providers in 24 hours if she had changed her mind. Communication among health care providers about advance directives is essential.

Communication between health care institutions is also essential. One major problem with existing advance directives is that they are lost when the patient is transferred from one institution to another. If, as health care providers, we are asking people to complete advance directives prior to the development of an illness, we ought to be able to arrange for communication regarding the directive between facilities.

When directives exist, the nurse may use the directive to help families to understand and follow the choices laid out in the directive for a family member who has become gravely ill and is incapacitated. When a patient has stated in a directive that he or she wishes to have life-sustaining interventions such as CPR or intubation withheld, the family often feels relieved to know that they are not making the choice. Some families experience guilt over making a decision that could deprive a family member of even the smallest possibility of continued survival.

However, when a patient becomes suddenly, gravely ill, it is much more likely that, if a directive exists, the patient's choices will not be clearly related to the specific circumstances the patient is experiencing. Or, most likely of all, no advance directive will exist. When the patient is

EVIDENCE-BASED PRACTICE

Reference: Mezey, M. D., Leitman, R., Mitty, E. L., Bottrell, M. M., & Ramsey, G. C. (2000). Why hospital patients do and do not execute an advance directive. *Nursing Outlook*, 48(4), 165-171.

Research Problem: This study examined the extent to which race, education, language, and income are associated with reasons for executing or not executing an advance directive.

Design: This was a descriptive study.

Sample and Setting: A sample of 1016 patients was randomly drawn from lists of patients discharged from four tertiary care hospitals in New York City.

Methods: A survey developed for the study, consisting of 75 items, was administered by telephone interview to patients who had been discharged within the previous 3 months from the four New York City hospitals.

Results: Twenty percent of participants had an advance directive at the time of the survey. White respondents, respondents with higher income, and respondents with some college education were significantly more likely to have an advance directive. The most frequently cited reasons for having an advance directive were "wanting to make up own mind," "felt it would help my family or give peace of mind," and "don't want to be kept alive with tubes in a coma."

Implications for Nursing Practice: Of the patients who did not have an advance directive, less than 50% cited any of the reasons used in the study as their reasons for not executing a directive. Reasons why patients may choose not to execute an advance directive are insufficiently understood.

Conclusion: Findings from this study suggest that level of education is the most important factor in differentiating among patients who do and do not have advance directives.

---

gravely ill, it is often the nurse who notices first that death is approaching. Clear communication to the family and physician is essential at this time because the family frequently has not considered death as an alternative (Caswell & Omery, 1990). Families need adequate, consistent information in terms that they can understand. Woods, Beaver, and Luker (2002) described this as having the family get the whole story. Norton and Talerico (2000) cautioned that families need health care providers to use words such as "death" and "dying"; that vague language makes families become confused. It is especially important, according to Norton and Talerico, that health care providers not use terms like "better" when a patient's condition has temporarily stabilized but the overall prognosis is unchanged, because this leads to conflicting impressions among family members and family disagreement about treatment. Another word that confuses family members is "hope." Health care providers often use the term when there is

hope for a good death or pain control, whereas for family members, hope primarily means survival. Norton and Talerico (2000) recommended that nurses be specific in identifying that they are hoping for a good death or pain control for the patient, not continued life.

When death appears imminent, nurses may introduce the discussion of withholding or withdrawing of life-sustaining interventions, such as CPR, intubation, and ventilation. There are two common ways that nurses begin a discussion of these interventions (Norton & Talerico, 2000). One of them is to tell the family that there are legal requirements that all people receive CPR (even when it is unlikely to be of any benefit to the person) unless a DNR order is written. This is often an easier way to begin the discussion if the family has not completely acknowledged that the patient is probably dying. However, it may prevent the family from acknowledging and discussing the nearness of the patient's death. Another common approach is to acknowledge

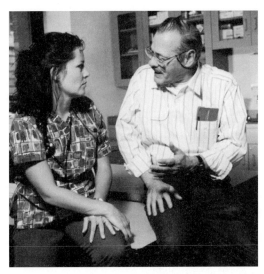

The importance of discussing health issues. (Courtesy Mathy Mezey.)

that the patient is gravely ill, probably dying, and ask the family which vision of the patient's death would be in the patient's best interests: one in which he or she was surrounded by family with the lights lowered and was receiving medication for pain and symptom relief, or one in which he or she was surrounded by health care personnel who were providing CPR. A discussion of the likelihood of survival following CPR should also be included.

Most patients and families want to discuss end-of-life care with their nurse, but they need to hear the same message from the elder's physician. Thus the nurse must be in communication with the physician about the elder patient's prognosis and the patient and family's preferences about end-of-life care. Hanson et al. (1997) noted that one reason for delays in the withdrawal of patient treatments is that, although patient preferences are documented, they are not communicated to physicians so that the physicians actually appreciate the patient's wishes. When there are differences in expectations of patient outcome or confusion over the appropriateness of various therapies, interdisciplinary patient care conferences are very appropriate.

Discussion about CPR with families or patients in crisis cannot come as a barrage of

questions all at once from multiple health care providers. Just as the questions at the beginning of the chapter are best asked of well elders a few at a time to help them to plan for end-of-life care, it is best if the seriously ill patient and/or family have some time to consider end-of-life care. Thus withholding CPR is often discussed first, and gradually questions concerning withholding or withdrawal of other life-sustaining interventions are introduced.

CONCLUSION

As the ANA has noted in its position statement, it is the responsibility of nurses to facilitate informed decision making for patients at the end of life. This responsibility begins when the nurse encourages an elder to consider what would be important to him or her at the end of life, continues with the nurse educating the elder about end-of-life care options, and is completed when the nurse advocates for and delivers the type of care the older adult desires at the end of his or her life. However, this process of communication about end-of-life care is not solely the responsibility of the patient and the nurse; it is an interdisciplinary process that includes at least the physician and family in addition to the older adult and nurse.

REFERENCES

American Nurses Association. (1996). American Nurses Association position statement on nursing and the Patient Self-Determination Act. In *Compendium of ANA position statements* (pp. 106-108). Washington, DC: Author.

Banja, J. D., & Bilsky, G. S. (1993). Discussing cardiopulmonary resuscitation with elderly rehabilitation patients. *American Journal of Physical Medicine and Rehabilitation, 72,* 168-171.

Bedell, S. E., & Delbanco, T. L. (1984). Choices about cardiopulmonary resuscitation in the hospital: When do physicians talk with patients? *New England Journal of Medicine, 310,* 1089-1092.

Blackhall, L. J., Frank, G., Murphy, S. T., Michel, V., Palmer, J. M., & Azen, S. P. (1999). Ethnicity and attitudes towards life sustaining technology. *Social Science and Medicine, 48,* 1779-1789.

Blustein, J. (1993). The family in medical decision making. *Hastings Center Report, 23*(3), 6-13.

Bradley, E., Walker, L., Blechner, J. D., & Wetle, T. (1997). Assessing capacity to participate in discussions of advance directives in nursing homes: Findings from a study of the

Patient Self-Determination Act. *Journal of the American Geriatrics Society, 45,* 79-83.

Buchanan, S. F. (1998). Guardians of care: Geriatrics and the law. *Clinical Geriatrics, 6*(12), 79-81.

Caswell, D., & Omery, A. (1990). The dying patient in the critical care setting: Making the critical difference. *AACN Clinical Issues in Critical Care Nursing, 1*(1), 178-186.

Cotton, P. (1993). Talk to people about dying—they can handle it, say geriatricians and patients. *Journal of the American Medical Association, 269,* 321-323.

Davison, J., & Degner, L. F. (1998). Promoting patient decision making in life-and-death situations. *Seminars in Oncology Nursing, 14*(2), 129-136.

Diamond, E. L., Jernigan, J. A., Moseley, R. A., Messina, V., & McKeown, R. A. (1989). Decision making ability and advance care directive preferences in nursing home patients and proxies. *The Gerontologist, 29,* 622-626.

Diem, S. J., Lantos, J. D., & Tulsky, J. A. (1996). Cardiopulmonary resuscitation on television: Miracles and misinformation. *New England Journal of Medicine, 334,* 1578-1582.

Emanuel, L. L., Barry, M. J., Stoeckle, J. D., Ettelson, L. M., & Emanuel, E. J. (1991). Advance directives for medical care—a case for greater use. *New England Journal of Medicine, 324,* 889-895.

Eun-shim, N., & Resnick, B. (2001). End of life treatment preferences among older adults. *Nursing Ethics, 8,* 533-544.

Everhart, M. A., & Pearlman, R. A. (1990). Stability of patient preferences regarding life sustaining treatments. *Chest, 97,* 160-164.

Forbes, S. (2001). This is heaven's waiting room: End of life in one nursing home. *Journal of Gerontological Nursing, 27*(11), 37-45.

Ghusn, H. F., Teasdale, T. A., & Jordan, D. (1997). Continuity of do-not-resuscitate orders between hospital and nursing home settings. *Journal of the American Geriatrics Society, 45,* 465-469.

Gillick, M. R., & Mendes, M. L. (1996). Medical care in old age: what do nurses in long-term care consider appropriate? *Journal of the American Geriatrics Society, 44*(11), 1322-1325.

Hanson, L. C., Tulsky, J. A., & Danis, M. (1997). Can clinical interventions change care at the end of life? *Annals of Internal Medicine, 126,* 381-388.

Haynor, P. M. (1998). Meeting the challenge of advance directives. *American Journal of Nursing, 98*(3), 16-29.

High, D. M. (1993). Advance directives in the elderly: A study of intervention strategies to increase use. *The Gerontologist, 33,* 344-349.

High, D. M. (1994, November-December). Families roles in advance directives. *Hastings Center Report, Special Supplement,* pp. S16-S18.

Kellogg, F. R., & Ramos, A. (1995). Code status decision making in a nursing home population: processes and outcomes. *Journal of the American Geriatrics Society, 43*(2), 113-121.

Kohn, M., & Menon, G. (1988). Life prolongation: Views of elderly outpatients and health care professionals. *Journal of the American Geriatrics Society, 36,* 840-844.

Kohut, N., Sam, M., O'Rourke, K., MacFadden, D. K., Salit, I., & Singer, P. A. (1997). Stability of treatment preferences: Although most preferences do not change, most people change some of their preferences. *The Journal of Clinical Ethics, 8*(2), 124-135.

Lo, B., McLeod, G., & Saika, G. (1986). Patient attitudes to discussing life-sustaining treatments. *Archives of Internal Medicine, 146,* 1613-1315.

Marik, P. E., & Craft, M. (1997). An outcomes analysis of in-hospital cardiopulmonary resuscitation: The futility rationale for do not resuscitate orders. *Journal of Critical Care, 12*(3), 142-146.

Markson, L., Clark, J., Glantz, L., Lamberton, V., Kern, D., & Stollermna, G. (1997). The doctor's role in discussing advance preferences for end-of-life care: perceptions of physicians practicing in the VA. *Journal of the American Geriatric Society, 45*(4), 399-406.

Martin, D. K., Emanuel, L. L., & Singer, P. A. (2000). Planning for the end of life. *The Lancet, 356,* 1672-1677.

Mezey, M. D., Leitman, R., Mitty, E. L., Bottrell, M. M., & Ramsey, G. C. (2000). Why hospital patients do and do not execute an advance directive. *Nursing Outlook, 48*(4), 165-171.

Molloy, D. W., Guyatt, G. H., Russo, R., Goeree, R., O'Brien, B., Dedard, M., et al. (2000). Systematic implementation of an advance directive program in nursing homes. *Journal of the American Medical Association, 283,* 1437-1443.

Molloy, D. W., Silberfield, M., Darzins, P., Guyatt, G. H., Singer, P. A., Rush, B., et al. (1996). Measuring capacity to complete an advance directive. *Journal of the American Geriatrics Society, 44,* 660-664.

Murphy, D. J., Murray, A. M., Robinson, B. E., & Campton, E. W. (1989). Outcomes of cardiopulmonary resuscitation in the elderly. *Annals of Internal Medicine, 111,* 199-205.

Nolan, M. T., & Bruder, M. (1997). Patients' attitudes toward advance directives and end-of-life treatment decisions. *Nursing Outlook, 45*(5), 204-208.

Norton, S. A., & Talerico, K. A. (2000). Facilitating end-of-life decision-making: strategies for communicating and assessing. *Journal of the American Geriatrics Society, 44*(11), 1322-1325.

O'Brien, L. A., Grisso, J. A., & Maislin, G. (1995). Nursing home residents preferences for life sustaining treatments. *Journal of the American Medical Association, 274,* 1775-1779.

Page, S., & Meerabeau, L. (1996). Nurses' accounts of cardiopulmonary resuscitation. *Journal of Advanced Nursing, 24,* 317-325.

Perrin, K. O. (1997). Giving voice to the wishes of elders for end of life care. *Journal of Gerontological Nursing, 23*(3), 18-27.

Puopolo, A. L., Kennard, M. J., Mallatratt, L., Follen, M. A., Desbiens, N. A., Conners, Jr., A. F., Califf, R., Walzer, J.,

Soukup, J., Davis, R. B., & Phillips, R. S. (1997). Preferences for cardiopulmonary resuscitation. *Image—the Journal of Nursing Scholarship, 29*(3), 229-235.

Reckling, J. B. (1997). Who plays what role in decisions about withholding and withdrawing life-sustaining treatment? *Journal of Clinical Ethics, 8*(1), 39-45.

Romero, L. J., Lindeman, R. D., Koehler, K. M., & Allen, A. (1997). Influence of ethnicity on advance directives and end of life decisions. *Journal of the American Medical Association, 277*, 298.

Rosenfeld, K. E., Wenger, N. S., & Kagawa-Singer, M. (2000). End-of-life decision making: a qualitative study of elderly individuals. *Journal of General Internal Medicine, 15*(9), 620-625.

Schneider, A. P., Nelson, D. J., & Brown, D. D. (1993). In-hospital cardiopulmonary resuscitation: A 30-year review. *Journal of the American Board of Family Practice, 6*, 91-101.

Schonwetter, R. S., Teasdale, T. A., Taffet, G., Robinson, B. E., & Luchi, R. J. (1991). Educating the elderly: Cardiopulmonary resuscitation decisions before and after intervention. *Journal of the American Geriatrics Society, 39*, 372-377.

Silveira, M. J., DiPiero, A., Gerrity, M. S., & Freudener, C. (2000). Patients' knowledge of options in end-of-life care: Ignorance in the face of death. *JAMA, 284*, 2483-2488.

Silverman, H. J., & Vinicky, J. K. (1991, June). Advance directives: The patients values history. *Clinician Reviews*, pp. 73-87.

Smith, T. J., Desch, E. E., Hackney, M. E., & Shaw, J. E. (1997). How long does it take to get a "do not resuscitate" order? *Journal of Palliative Care, 13*(1), 5-8.

SUPPORT Principal Investigators. (1995). A controlled trial to improve care for seriously ill hospitalized patients: The Study to Understand Prognoses and Preferences for Outcomes and Risks of Treatments (SUPPORT). *Journal of the American Medical Association, 274*, 1591-1598.

Teno, J., Licks, S., & Lynn, J. (1997). Do advance directives provide instructions that direct care? *Journal of the American Geriatrics Society, 45*, 500-507.

Tulsky, J. A., Chesney, M. A., & Lo, B. (1995). How do medical residents discuss resuscitation with patients? *Journal of General Internal Medicine, 10*, 436-442.

Vaughn, G., Kiyasu, E., & McCormick, W. C. (2000). Advance directive preferences among subpopulations of Asian nursing home residents in the Pacific Northwest. *Journal of the American Geriatrics Society, 48*, 554-557.

Ventres, W., Nichter, M., Reed, R., & Frankel, R. (1992). Do-not-resuscitate discussions: A qualitative analysis. *Family Practice Research Journal, 12*, 157-169.

Wagner, A. (1984). Cardiopulmonary resuscitation in the aged: A prospective study. *New England Journal of Medicine, 310*, 1129-1130.

Wetle, T., Levkoff, S., Cwikel, J., & Rosen, A. (1988). Nursing home resident participation in medical decisions: Perceptions and preferences. *The Gerontologist, 28*(Suppl.), 32-37.

Woods, S., Beaver, K., & Luker, K. (2000). Users' view of palliative care services: ethical implications. *Nursing Ethics: an International Journal for Health Care Professionals, 7*(4), 314-326.

7

ADVANCE DIRECTIVES: OLDER ADULTS WITH DEMENTIA

Ethel L. Mitty and Mathy D. Mezey

INTRODUCTION

Advance directives allow individuals to direct the health care they want or do not want in the event that they lack decision-making capacity at the time a medical decision needs to be made. Thus an advance directive is an attempt by an individual to exercise control over his or her person, provide guidance to those who will make health care decisions for him or her, and reduce conflict among those with a sincere and vital interest in his or her well-being, including health care professionals. Decision making by and for a cognitively impaired individual raises ethical and legal concerns. Typically, the question is posed as, "At what point in a dementing illness is the personal right of self-determination relinquished or lost, and relegated by design or default to another decision maker?" Given that the diagnosis of dementia is generally made after the disease has progressed to the point where there are noticeable signs of memory loss and impaired judgment, we suggest that the first question to be asked is, "How can we determine if the individual has the requisite capacity to understand and create an advance directive?" Advance care planning can serve the best interests of the demented person, and should be addressed early in the course of the disease. Yet advance planning is not without barriers, not the least of which is that many physicians and nurses believe that cognitively impaired individuals are unable to state their treatment preferences; therefore, the person so affected is unlikely even to be approached to talk about advance planning.

This chapter briefly reviews the demographics and trajectory of dementia, describes advance directives, and then addresses advance care planning from the perspective of decision-making capacity assessment, ethical issues, and surrogate decision making.* Aspects of proxy education and mediation for treatment decision disharmony are then discussed in order to enrich the knowledge and skills associated with the nurse's competency to respect the patient's views and wishes during end-of-life care.

DEMENTIA

Knowledge of the course of dementia is important because, by describing the disease trajectory, the person's right to self-determination (i.e., to create an advance directive) might still be honored after the diagnosis is made. It is estimated that 1% of persons age 60 years and older evidence some, if not all, symptoms characteristic of dementia. Dementia is a category of cognitive dysfunction that includes Alzheimer's disease and related dementias (44%), vascular dementia (47%), and other etiologies (9%) (American Psychological Association, 1997). Prevalence increases exponentially with each age group, from 10% of 65-year-olds to 47% of those 85 years old and older (Evans et al., 1989). Approximately 43% of nursing home residents (Harrington, Carillo, & Wellin, 2001) have moderate to severe dementia, generally of the Alzheimer's type. Of the 1.5 million older adults in assisted living residences, 40% have mild to moderate dementia and 15% have severe dementia (National Center for Assisted Living, 2001). At this time in the United States, approximately 1.8 million people are in the final stage of dementia (Morrison & Sui, 2000); more than 7 million

---

Competency is a legal determination of decision-making ability; *capacity* is a clinical determination of this ability and is the term that is used in this chapter.

EVIDENCE-BASED PRACTICE

Reference: Fazel, S., Hope, T., & Jacoby, R. (2000). Effect of cognitive impairment and premorbid intelligence on treatment preferences for life-sustaining medical therapy. *American Journal of Psychiatry, 157,* 1009-1011.

Research Problem: The influence of cognitive impairment, premorbid intelligence, and decision-making capacity regarding life-sustaining treatments (LSTs).

Design: Descriptive; correlational.

Sample and Setting: 100 community dwelling elders, 60 years of age or older, with a diagnosis of moderate dementia (n = 50) or not cognitively impaired (n = 50).

Methods: Three clinical vignettes, each describing a realistic situation in which an advance directive would influence treatments to be provided or withheld, were written. After administration of the Mini-Mental Status Examination (MMSE) and the National Adult Reading Test, each subject was asked his or her treatment preference using a semistructured interview that reflected the legal standards of competence (i.e., capacity).

Results: No significant difference was found between the subjects with and without dementia with regard to treatment preference. Those subjects opting for LSTs had lower MMSE scores and less decision-making capacity than those subjects who refused such interventions. Premorbid intelligence did not influence treatment choices. Cognitively impaired subjects (MMSE score of 20) and those who did poorly on a previously validated instrument to assess legal competence were judged incapable of executing an advance directive.

Implications for Nursing Practice: Cognitive impairment influences LST preferences; the greater the impairment, the greater the likelihood that the elder will want LSTs. Nurses should talk with patients who have mild to moderate cognitive impairment, and their families, about end-of-life treatment preferences before significant cognitive deterioration presents. It is important that patients and their families understand the benefit, burdens, and risks of LSTs and consider the value of these interventions for the quality of the elder's life when he or she is profoundly incapacitated.

Conclusion: Advance care planning with patients and their families, prior to the onset of cognitive impairment, can better reflect the genuine treatment preferences of patients at the end of their lives, and avoid the heartache and costs that attend futile LST interventions.

people are projected to be afflicted by the year 2040 (Office of Technology Assessment, 1990).

A variety of scales and measures are used to test for the presence and severity of cognitive impairment and Alzheimer's disease. Progression is inexorable and, to some degree, predictable. The Global Deterioration Scale (GDS) (Reisberg, Ferris, deLeon, & Crook, 1982) uses a clinical continuum from normal age-related changes to severe Alzheimer's disease. The Mini-Mental Status Examination (MMSE) (Folstein, Folstein, & McHugh, 1975), a widely used screening instrument for dementia, is strongly correlated with the global stages of

Alzheimer's disease described in the GDS. The Functional Assessment Staging Technique (Reisberg, 1988) identifies the progress and prognosis of Alzheimer's disease and details progressive functional losses.

Life span after diagnosis can be 3 to 15 years, characterized by an at-first insidious but always relentless impairment of memory and reasoning (Damasio, 1996). Characteristically, short-term memory loss is followed by lapse of recognition of known faces and places, decrease in affective tone, unwise financial or property decisions, deteriorated social relationships, impairment in abstract thinking, and growing evidence of poor judgment. Variations in onset include paranoid behavior, nighttime disorientation, problems with word-finding, alteration in the ability to visualize more than one object at a time, and inability to recognize previously known routes. Typically, the functional losses that accompany deterioration of memory and intellect appear later in the course of the disease. Indeed, some patients are able to learn new motor skills while experiencing devastating loss of information-processing ability. The natural history of Alzheimer's disease is that most patients die from other diseases of old age, not Alzheimer's disease. Special care units for patients with dementia, provided in 22% of nursing homes (Teresi, Grant, Holmes, & Ory, 1998), can increase survival in comparison to standard care (Volicer, 1994).

Severity of dementia is characterized as mild, moderate, or severe. In its mildest form or early stages, most individuals are able to live independently, attend to their personal hygiene and self-care needs, and exercise a reasonable degree of judgment about routine matters. As the disease progresses, there are growing risks to safety and well-being. Independent living may no longer be possible, and some degree of supervision and oversight of self-care and decision making is warranted. The severely demented person is so compromised that self-care ability and decision-making and language skills are largely absent. It is clear, then, that advance care planning and decision making by the individual in the early or mild stage of Alzheimer's disease provides the most opportune if not best, or last, chance to honor self-determination. Research indicates that individuals with mild to moderate Alzheimer's disease have the ability to make some, but not all, treatment choices (Marson, Chatterjee, Ingram, & Harrell, 1996; Sansone & Nichols, 1997) and are able to respond consistently to questions about their treatment preferences and choices (Feinberg & Whitlatch, 2002).

ADVANCE DIRECTIVES

It is extremely likely that decisions about life-sustaining treatments will occur at some point in the future of the patient with Alzheimer's disease, and, given the long course of the disease, those decisions could lie a considerable time ahead. Imagining such a future scenario, by the patient as well as family members or a significant other, can be difficult because it seems so far into the

future and can be emotionally laden; therefore, these very important discussions and decisions might not be made or are hurriedly gone over. A small pilot study of patients with mild to moderate dementia found that planning for hypothetical future illness did not precipitate any adverse consequences, such as agitation or depression; their decisions were consistent and rational (Finucane, Brock, Roca, & Kawas, 1993). It is important to keep in mind, however, that advance planning decisions by a person afflicted with dementia will deny them access to new knowledge and relevant information that may surface between the time the directive is created and when it is activated (Dresser, 1995). It follows, then, that autonomous decision making is not honored if the person's wishes and preferences were based on erroneous or missing information.

Values histories are documents that can guide decision makers for the incapacitated person and have been upheld by the courts. A values history contains open-ended statements that help an individual think about dependency on others, family burden, pain and suffering, and quality of life (compared to life at any cost) (Center for Health Law and Ethics, 2003; Gibson, 1990; Schirm & Stachel, 1996). The person's thoughts and feelings about trust and confidence in their caregivers and physician to make health care decisions for them are also elicited. The last section of the values history addresses the person's attitudes toward dying and death, preferred location of death, and the use of life-sustaining treatments in the face of terminal or irreversible chronic illness, such as Alzheimer's disease. There is evidence that individuals with mild cognitive impairment (MMSE score of 17 to 24) are able to express values more easily by stating "yes" or "no" than by responding to open-ended questions (Karel, Moye, & Oville, 1996).

The two most commonly used advance directives are the living will (LW) and the durable power of attorney for health care, or health care proxy (HCP) as it is more commonly known (state-specific versions of both of these documents are accessible at *http://www.partnershipforcaring.org*). Although do-not-resuscitate (DNR) orders are often construed as an advance directive, DNR orders in most states fall under a different set of statutes than do LWs and HCPs (Patient Self-Determination Act, 1990).

Generally used to declare wishes to refuse, limit, or withhold life-sustaining treatments under certain circumstances, LWs are recognized by statute in all states except New York, Massachusetts, and Michigan. Case law in New York allows the court to recognize the LW as satisfying the state's evidentiary requirement of "clear and convincing evidence." The HCP permits health care decision making by a designated other for an individual who lacks decisional capacity for the specific health care decision that needs to be made. Whereas a LW requires treatment decisions to be made in advance, the HCP requires that the individual designate another person, presumably known and trusted, to make health care decisions should the individual lose the capacity to do so. Unlike the LW, the HCP can apply to all health care decisions, including those regarding withholding or withdrawing life-sustaining treatment. In some states, however, the proxy may not make decisions about the use of artificial nutrition or hydration unless the individual stated such preference in writing in an HCP or LW document. Recently, several states have added a section on organ donation (i.e., "anatomical gift") to the standard HCP document that allows individuals to indicate if they wish to donate their organ(s). However, the agent cannot effect this wish unless he or she is also the identified decision maker for organ donation, a distinct statutory authority separate from health care agency.

The Physician Orders for Life-Sustaining Treatment (POLST) program, initiated in Oregon in 1995, is a state-endorsed protocol to honor an individual's wish to die in a familiar setting (such as the home) without unwanted, aggressive life-supporting interventions by emergency medical services personnel (Center for Ethics in Health Care, 2003; Dunn et al., 1997). Four separate categories of physician's orders address cardiopulmonary resuscitation (CPR) versus DNR orders; an order to transfer only if comfort measures fail versus aggressive life-sustaining treatments; antibiotics for comfort only versus intramuscular antibiotics for curative purposes; and parenteral feeding (including intravenous) for the short term versus the long term, or not at all. These treatment options go beyond the typical HCP and LW and carry the full weight of physician authority. Ongoing re-evaluation indicates that Oregon nursing home residents

with POLSTs received significantly higher levels of comfort care and fewer aggressive life-sustaining interventions than those without POLSTs (Tolle, Tilden, Nelson, & Dunn, 1998). In addition, more deaths occurred outside hospitals, and there was less use of CPR and more orders for narcotic analgesics at the time of death for nursing home residents with POLSTs. The Kaiser Permanente managed care system has adopted the protocol for its members in long-term care facilities (Spann & Christopher, 1999).

The "Five Wishes" document bears many similarities to the values history, POLST, LW, and HCP; it is legally valid in all but 15 states (Aging with Dignity, 2003). Using open-ended statements, the individual completing the Five Wishes document expresses wishes about the person to make health care decisions for him or her, the medical treatment wanted and not wanted, the degree of comfort wanted, how he or she wants to be physically and emotionally supported, and what he or she wants loved ones to know. The document also provides space for persons to state what they would like said about them at their funeral and what burial arrangements they would like. Although there are no published reports about use of this document by persons with dementia, there is no reason to presume that a person with mild cognitive impairment would be unable to express his or her wishes through this document.

Given that only 20% to 25% of the adult population of the United States has executed an advance directive of any kind, it is estimated that only 15% of community-dwelling elders have an advance directive (Bradley, Wetle, & Horwitz, 1998). Of the slightly under 1.6 million nursing home residents, approximately 50% have some kind of directive; however, there are extreme regional variations in advance directive completion within and between states. More residents have DNR orders than a LW or HCP (Castle & Mor, 1998). The number of nursing home residents with Alzheimer's disease or other dementias who have a LW or HCP is not known. Among those with an advance directive, it is also not known when the directive was created.

DECISION-MAKING CAPACITY ASSESSMENT

Decisional capacity is an issue with every consent to treatment, agreement to be a research subject, or creation of an advance directive. The standard

EVIDENCE-BASED PRACTICE

Reference: Carney, M. T., Neugroschl, J., Morrison, R. S., Marin, D., & Siu, A. L. (2001). The development and piloting of a capacity assessment tool. *The Journal of Clinical Ethics, 12,* 17-23.

Research Problem: Development of a capacity assessment tool (CAT) to determine capacity for a specific decision.

Design: Comparison of CAT score with psychiatrist determination of capacity; correlational.

Sample and Setting: 20 English-speaking patients, 65 years of age or older, in geriatric inpatient unit.

Methods: Participants were randomly assigned to a physician bedside interview using the CAT or psychiatric "gold standard" assessment; both were based on the four standards for determining cognitive capacity: ability to communicate, describe a choice, understand risks and benefits, and reason. Overall capacity assessment for the specific decision was also measured.

Results: The psychiatrist determination and CAT interview scores agreed at least 95% of the time on all measures except Describing Choices (80% agree-

ment). Regarding the components of capacity, communication was easily achieved, followed by ability to describe a choice, and ability of the participant to state his or her reasons. Only about 50% of subjects were able to describe risks and benefits, whether by psychiatric or CAT assessment.

Implications for Nursing Practice: Investigators felt that house staff had a possible advantage in conducting the capacity evaluation because they had known the patient over a period of time, knew when moments of maximum lucidity were likely to occur, and could draw on the patient's resources, including family. By virtue of the greater time nurses spend with patients in comparison even to house staff, the CAT administered by a professional nurse might better reflect patients' decision-making capacity, thereby affording more patients the right to make their own health care decisions, given the level of risk of the decision.

Conclusion: The CAT requires further testing, possibly comparing physician and nurse scores as well. The CAT has the potential to expand the window of opportunity for decision making for many individuals labeled incapacitated (or, erroneously, "incompetent").

---

for determining whether an individual has sufficient decisional capacity to make a health care decision is raised in relationship to the complexity and risk associated with the decision (Midwest Bioethics Center, 1996). Evidence of decision-making capacity requires the ability to communicate a choice; understand relevant information; comprehend the risks, benefits, options, and consequences; and rationally manipulate information. The capacity to complete an advance directive requires that the individual demonstrate understanding and appreciation that the choices expressed in an advance directive will be acted upon in the future, when the person no longer has decision-making capacity; that some of the choices will involve medical interventions, some of which could lead to the person's death or

a permanent comatose state; and that another person can be selected to make these decisions (Silberfeld, Nash, & Singer, 1993). Most elder patients understand that the purpose of an advance directive is to make their health care choices known and subsequently honored when they no longer have decisional capacity.

Not surprisingly, the capacity to engage in advance health planning after being diagnosed with Alzheimer's disease is often questioned. Although the diagnosis of dementia does not establish lack of capacity to make a decision about current or future treatments, the observed cognitive deficits that support the diagnosis raise questions about the person's ability to understand and process information about his or her medical condition(s), probable course, and treatment

Box 7-1 **Standard Script to Inform an Individual about the Right to Create a Health Care Proxy**

Paraphrased recall: the individual is asked to state in his or her own words what he or she just heard; synonyms are acceptable for the key words (IN CAPITAL LETTERS).

Step 1. HEALTH CARE DECISIONS
You have the RIGHT to make CHOICES about your HEALTH CARE as long as you are able. You have the FREEDOM to SELECT TREATMENTS you want. As long as you are able, you are ENTITLED to make DECISIONS about your HEALTH CARE.

Step 2. APPOINTMENT
You have the right to ASK someone to make HEALTH CARE DECISIONS for you if you get so sick that you cannot make them yourself. You can CHOOSE someone to make your HEALTH CARE DECISIONS for you. If you get so sick that you cannot make your own HEALTH CARE DECISIONS, the person you SELECT will make them for you.

Step 3. TREATMENT
(Name of person chosen) could choose a treatment for you that might involve LIFE AND DEATH. If you were critically ill, (name of person chosen) would make treatment decisions about your care. Some of the treatments could affect whether you LIVE OR DIE.

Step 4. HEALTH CARE PROXY
You can SIGN A PAPER, called a HEALTH CARE PROXY, that allows (name of person chosen) to make health care choices for you. If you SIGN this paper, (name of person chosen) will be allowed to make treatment decisions for you. (Name of person chosen) is allowed to make health care choices for you once you SIGN a HEALTH CARE PROXY.

From Mezey, M., Teresi, J., Ramsey, G., Mitty, E., & Bobrowitz, T. (2000). Decision-making capacity to execute a health care proxy: Development and testing of guidelines. *Journal of the American Geriatrics Society, 48*, 179-187.

preferences (Lynn et al., 1999). This is compounded by the fact that physicians are not always knowledgeable about the components of decision-making capacity, fail to differentiate between competence and capacity, and are prone to question a patient's capacity when the decision is not in line with the physician's recommendation (Carney, Neugroschl, Morrison, Martin, & Siu, 2001).

It is erroneous to assume that capacity is either present or absent. Capacity is a complex of specific abilities, not a single, global ability. Cognitive impairment or a diagnosis of dementia/Alzheimer's disease does not constitute incapacity. The concept of "decision-specific capacity" holds that individuals with impaired, fluctuating, or questionable cognitive ability may have the capacity to make some but not all health care decisions. In this view, capacity is a threshold requirement to make an autonomous decision (Applebaum & Gutheil, 1991). The capacity to create an advance directive is different from the capacity to give informed consent for treatment (Marson et al., 1996; Mezey, Teresi, Ramsey, Mitty, & Bobrowitz, 2000; Silberfeld et al., 1993). The decisional complexity associated with creating a HCP is less than that with a LW, for which the ability to contemplate and reason about treatment options that might be needed in the future must be contemplated by the individual. The risk associated with creation of a LW is greater; therefore, the threshold capacity to create a HCP is lower and less stringent than for a LW (Miller, 1995). Thus a person may lack the decisional capacity to make a decision about artificial feeding but may have sufficient capacity to appoint a proxy or agent to make decisions for him or her (Mezey, Mitty, Bottrell, Ramsey, & Fisher, 2000; Mezey, Teresi, et al., 2000).

There are no professionally agreed upon clinical guidelines, no single instrument or "gold standard," for capacity determination. A substantial body of research indicates that physicians, including psychiatrists, lack the skill and experience to determine a demented person's ability to participate in advance planning; standard tests of mental status are used incorrectly to judge this ability (Kapp & Mossman, 1996; Marson et al., 1996). The informed consent process used to determine a person's understanding regarding information about a HCP can be based on the process used to obtain consent for treatment but is considerably simplified for the person with questionable or fluctuating decisional capacity (Silberfeld et al., 1993). Given that the person diagnosed with dementia may experience depression and despair, the "windows of lucidity" associated with fluctuating capacity are an opportunity to hold a structured yet sensitive discussion about treatment choices and care at the end of life.

Guidelines that lower the threshold necessary to execute a HCP define capacity in relationship to a specific health care decision rather than construing it as an "all-or-none" ability that a person has or does not have (Kapp & Mossman, 1996; Mezey, Teresi, et al., 2000). In this view, the threshold need be no higher than that needed to make a decision about something relevant to everyday life, such as choosing a physician. As suggested by Silberfeld et al. (1993), capacity determination guidelines should ask two basic questions: "Is the person willing at this time to make choices about the future use of life-sustaining treatments?" and "Does the person want to appoint someone to make these decisions for him or her?" A series of follow-up questions to confirm understanding should then be asked if the person answers affirmatively.

Capacity is operationalized as "understanding" in guidelines developed by Mezey, Teresi, et al. (2000; see also Pruchno, Smyer, Rose, Hartman-Stein, & Henderson-Laribee, 1995), drawing on the work of Applebaum and Grisso (1987). Using "paraphrased recall" and "recognition" to determine the person's understanding of the HCP information presented, the four-step guidelines include informing the individual by using a *standard script*, determining understanding using *standard questions*, evaluating response to the questions using *standard scoring*, and establishing consistency of the decision using a *safeguard measure* (Box 7-1). Among 200 nursing home residents, almost three fourths of whom had MMSE scores of less than 20, 77% demonstrated sufficient understanding (capacity) to name someone to make health care decisions for them.

Approximately 30% of residents with severe dementia (MMSE score of 0 to 10) demonstrated sufficient understanding to name/choose an agent. In a follow-up interview 24 hours later, 92% of all residents named the same person, establishing the consistency or stability of a decision necessary to meet informed consent standards (Dubler, 1985). The data suggest that the guidelines were more efficient and accurate than the MMSE in identifying nursing home residents with the requisite understanding (capacity) to create a HCP.

ADVANCE DIRECTIVES AND DEMENTIA RESEARCH

There are differences between an advance directive for health care (therapeutic) decision making and a research advance directive. Several bioethicists suggest that a primary motivation to create a health care advance directive is to avoid medical overtreatment, whereas the motivation to create a research advance directive must arise not from self-interest, but from altruism (Berghmans, 1998; Sachs, 1994). An advance directive for nontherapeutic research must address the probability of greater than minimal risk or burden to the demented person, yet it is virtually impossible to give advance consent for a future experiment about which the nature and methods of the research are, as yet, unformulated and unknown. Hence, the responsibility of a proxy decision maker for research consent and participation should require that the proxy has substantive awareness of the person's wishes, feelings, and preferences about participation in research and that the proxy should also "monitor" the research process with regard to adverse effects on the demented person. As Berghmans (1998) rightly suggested, an agent's duty to act and decide in the person's best interest is challenged by research participation involving more than minimal risk or burden, and "undermines the moral authority of the proxy to give consent for an incompetent demented subject in this type of research" (p. 36). (The role of a proxy decision maker, overall, is briefly discussed in the last portion of this chapter.)

Several states and the National Bioethics Advisory Commission (NBAC) have recommended and moved toward policy formulation that permits capacitated individuals to give "advance consent" to research participation after decision-making capacity is lost (NBAC, 1999). The individual would select someone to act as his or her decision maker with regard to all issues involving his or her research participation. Although this chapter does not permit extensive discussion of the issues surrounding the formidable research dilemma of research on or with demented persons, concerns include the adequacy of information and discussion conducted with the capacitated individual prior to creating an advance research directive, the potential for substantial physical and/or psychological risk without the probability of a direct health benefit, the degree and methods of assessing the participant's research experience given his or her impaired communication and means of expression, and the safeguards embedded in the research design to promote and protect the welfare of the research subject (Dresser, 2001).

ETHICAL ISSUES IN ADVANCE PLANNING BY PATIENTS WITH DEMENTIA

Capacity for health care decision making is a critical ethical issue. Based on the autonomy principle, an individual determined to have decisional capacity should be encouraged to make his or her own health care decisions. However, those without such capacity need to be protected from making poor and/or risk-laden decisions, based on the principles of beneficence and nonmaleficence. Whereas a low-level or limited ability to make health care decisions is acceptable if the chosen treatment has a high likelihood of benefit and a low risk of burden (losses, pain, etc.), a higher standard of capacity must be demonstrated if the choice carries high risk and/or limited probability of benefit and/or the individual refuses an intervention that not only would appear to be in his or her best interest but represents sound clinical advice.

The representativeness of an advance directive created when an individual had full or even somewhat diminished capacity is a major ethical issue and speaks to an individual's continuing "personhood." Representativeness also addresses the notion of "precedent autonomy," which holds that the currently incapacitated person was, at one time, fully competent to weigh choices and make decisions and that the protection of that

freedom and right is exercised by honoring advance directive instructions. Yet others argue that slavish adherence to advance directive instructions leaves no room for changes of mind, if the person still has that capacity, nor does it recognize that the incapacitated person is not at all the same person who created the advance directive several years earlier (Parfit, 1984). Indeed, it is further suggested that individuals with moderate to severe dementia are unlikely to be in as much subjective distress, or have such a miserable quality of life, as those who see and care for them presume (Dresser, 1995).

Several arguments are marshaled to set limits on the treatment preferences expressed by the formerly competent but now demented individual. It is important to note that treatment wishes that may be in dispute could be either to refuse or to demand certain treatments. The first argument proposes the notion that personal identity arises from a person's history: thoughts, emotions, and memories (Parfit, 1984). In the event of drastic change to these cognitive and psychological features, as in Alzheimer's disease, the person who now exists is a different person than the one who existed prior to the profound mental changes. The second position refutes the "different person" notion and takes the position that the now-incapacitated person is the same person who expressed treatment preferences, but that there may be valid reasons to disregard those wishes. In this view, a previously capacitated person's refusal of life-sustaining treatment should not override the person's autonomy rights if it appears that the now-incapacitated person is deriving some enjoyment from life, is not in physical pain, and does not appear unhappy (Kadish, 1992). The "take-away" message of this line of reasoning is that we should not be in such a terrible rush to honor wishes to refuse certain treatment interventions. In this view, also, a request for aggressive life-sustaining treatment expressed prior to the onset of dementia that would impose significant pain or burden without any benefit does not have to be honored. Given both contexts, compassion for the person has equal merit as autonomy; the decision to be made derives from caring and beneficence (to do good; to do no harm). A third argument in line with the positions noted above holds that the now-incapacitated person may have substantially different interests than those that existed when he or she was capacitated.

Some ethicists caution against not honoring a previously expressed treatment preference by a now-demented individual because this could signify "undervaluing the lives of. . . . vulnerable individuals" (Dresser & Whitehouse, 1994, p. 6). Concerns are raised that life-sustaining treatments such as antibiotics, fluid and nutritional support, surgery, and CPR might be prematurely withheld from a person who is not in the last stage of Alzheimer's disease. It is argued that most dementia patients, until the terminal phase, have an "experiential world" that consists of emotions, thoughts, and perceptions and that they deserve an approach that considers "what it is like" to be the person whose treatment decisions must be made by others (Dresser & Whitehouse, 1994). Put simply, but not simplistically, it means "crawling into their skin." Yet the exceedingly complex concept of "quality of life" is an aspect of making treatment decisions for others, *and* in respect of their advance stated wishes, that confounds most professional and family caregivers. In the absence of any communication and expressive power, or any windows of lucidity, facial expressions and other behaviors usually occurring in the more advanced stages of dementia can provide clues to what the person is experiencing and feeling.

It has been suggested that advance care planning is more than preparation for incapacity and death. It is not simply an expression of autonomy and self-determination. If the creation of a HCP is construed as a "social process" that is embedded in interpersonal relationships (Singer et al., 1998), then the notion of health care agency—making health care decisions for another—is a "covenant" of trust and understanding between two individuals (Fins, 1999). As such, any deviation from a duly created advance directive should be based on context, facts, and the benefits and burdens predicted to occur with and without the intervention. Each patient is case specific; there are no explicit standards and scales to guide this assessment. This applies, as well, to the incapacitated person about whom we know nothing, who never created an advance directive, and whose treatment wishes are not known. It is also suggested that decision maker(s) need to recognize the tension between societal and culturally laden views on respect for life versus the allocation of (scarce) resources, and the external and internal influence this might have on their treatment decisions. In addition, there is some concern that undertreatment of incapacitated patients without surrogates could happen in a managed care environment (Meier, 1997). Finally, the family role in treatment decision making is no small consideration, especially in the presence of a duly executed HCP and appointed proxy/agent. Health care professionals need to find ways to include the family in health care decision making that simultaneously do not diminish the authority of the agent and recognize family interest in the patient's care.

PROXY (SURROGATE) DECISION MAKING

A health care agent (proxy or surrogate) is authorized and required by law to make decisions for the now-incapacitated person that the person would make for him- or herself if able to do so. Decision making occurs in two ways: the first, *substituted judgment*, calls on the surrogate's knowledge of the person's wishes, preferences, values, and principles, and, if possible, his or her past decision making. This standard asks the decision maker to infer how the patient would evaluate the benefits and burdens of a treatment him- or herself. Ways to assist the surrogate decision maker in exploring the options and consequences can include questions such as, "If the patient could join the discussion, what would he say?" and "When faced with similar situations in the past, how did she decide?" The second type of decision making, the *best interest* standard, asks the surrogate decision maker to evaluate benefits and burdens based on an objective assessment of what is in the patient's best interest, relying on the notion of what an average person in the patient's particular situation would consider beneficial or burdensome (Kopelman, 1997). Sometimes called the "reasonable person" standard, the proxy must consider more than what is in the patient's medical best interest (Bosek, Savage, Shaw, & Renella, 2001). To facilitate a best interest determination, one can ask "What does this patient have to gain or lose as a result of this decision? In what ways will he or she be better or worse off as a result of this decision?" It is important to keep in mind that the substituted judgment and best interest standards do not often work as discrete entities. A study of spouses'

EVIDENCE-BASED PRACTICE

Reference: Volicer, L., Cantor, M. D., Derse, A. R., Edwards, D. M., Prudhomme, A. M., Gregory, D. C. R., et al. (2002). Advance care planning by proxy for residents of long-term care facilities who lack decision-making capacity. *Journal of the American Geriatrics Society, 50,* 761-767.

Research Problem: Advance care planning (ACP) by proxies of decisionally incapacitated long-term care (LTC) residents.

Design: Descriptive.

Sample and Setting: Oregon LTC facilities ($n = 8$); Veterans Health Administration (VHA) LTC facilities ($n = 10$).

Methods: The study included a review of VHA policies regarding proxy authorization to limit care absent a written formal advance directive; a survey of state statutes and recent case law regarding ACP by proxies; an evaluation of the Physician Orders for Life-Sustaining Treatment (POLST) form; and the outcome of discussions of focus groups composed of LTC/VHA clinicians.

Results: There are no uniform guidelines for process or documentation when proxies of incapacitated

VHA residents authorize a do-not-resuscitate order even in the absence of an advance directive. Some states do not permit proxy decision making regarding life-sustaining treatment decisions. The POLST form was found to be effective; resuscitation and life-sustaining treatment preferences of LTC residents in Oregon tended to be universally followed. VHA clinicians felt that the absence of documented advance care decisions often led to unwanted or ineffective aggressive medical care and were unaware of two VHA facilities with policies for ACP by proxies for incapacitated residents.

Implications for Nursing Practice: Nurses should communicate regularly with a proxy to keep him or her informed about the patient's current status. An oral directive is acceptable in most courts as a genuine expression of a person's wishes. Given the few moments of lucidity for many demented patients, nurses need to be literally tuned in to hear those verbal expressions—and document them.

Conclusion: Proxies and clinicians need to work together to develop appropriate advance care plans; the best time to do this is when the patient is relatively stable, prior to an acute event or disease exacerbation when decisions are often made under stress.

decision making for patients with Alzheimer's disease found that fewer than half used substituted judgment decision making (Mezey, Kluger, Maislin, & Mittelman, 1996).

Surrogate decision making needs to be prepared for and is best done over time. Persons in the early or mild stages of Alzheimer's disease are most likely able to talk about what they like, what they value, and what kinds of intensive medical care they might want at the end of life, such as ventilator support, artificial nutrition, and invasive diagnostic tests. The accuracy of substituted judgments in comparison to what patients would select for themselves is approximately 65%; however, prior discussion with a patient increases concordance between the patient and the proxy decision (Sulmasy et al.,

1998). Close family members are slightly better surrogate decision makers than an elder patient's physician and, in the absence of a living will or evidence that the family is acting contrary to a patient's best interest, a family's substituted judgment is "the best available evidence of the elder patient's wishes" (Tomlinson, Howe, Notman, & Rossmiller, 1990). Research results indicate that substituted judgment decisions tend to favor treatment rather than non- or undertreatment. In a sense, these latter findings are troubling because, in the absence of a more explicit indication of a patient's refusal of certain treatments, the elder patient's rights may have been violated. The Department of Veterans Affairs has initiated and provided recommendations for advance care planning by the proxy (surrogate decision maker) of a now-incapacitated resident who may or may not have created an advance directive. In the absence of a written directive, the proxy uses substituted judgment and the best interest standard to guide decisions (Volicer et al., 2002).

Professional Responsibility for Proxy Education and Decision Making

Decision making for another is not an easy responsibility. It is emotionally laden, almost always culturally infused, and fertile ground for new or resurgent interfamily conflict. Among the barriers to effective and reasonably comfortable health care decision making for another are the need to differentiate the agent's needs from those of the patient, scant or no guidance from the patient, inadequate communication with and marginalization by professional health care providers, making decisions about treatments that did not exist when the patient had the capacity to talk about his or her treatment preferences, insufficient time to consider the options and consequences of a treatment choice, lack of understanding of the proxy's legally authorized role by the health care team as well as the proxy him- or herself, and the proxy's willingness to make decisions (Bosek et al., 2001; Post, Blustein, & Dubler, 1999).

The capacitated patient who chooses to forego further life-sustaining interventions (or death-prolonging ones) has most likely thought deeply about his or her own future pain and suffering and that of his or her significant others, and has weighed the benefits and burdens of a medical intervention on the expected trajectory of his or her illness. Personal, religious, spiritual, and philosophical values are part of this decision making. For the proxy, a decision to refuse or withdraw a life-sustaining treatment is no doubt embedded in the proxy's grief surrounding the death of a loved one. End-of-life decision making for another is a formidable task indeed. Unfortunately, the faithfulness and loyalty with which physicians (should) relate to their patients is not extended to the proxy (Dubler, 1995). The same full extent of truth-telling, disclosure, and informed consent inherent in the doctor–patient relationship should adhere to the doctor-proxy relationship; very often, it does not (Loewy, 1998). The relationship of nurses and physicians to proxy decision makers is often unidirectional:

The proxy is someone of whom demands are made but is rarely treated as someone to whom obligations and accountability are due (Dubler, 1995). Nurses can influence and change the relationship between the health care team and the proxy such that the proxy is accorded respect, compassionately informed, and guided with appropriate information in a timely way.

Mediating Differences of Opinion

Differences of opinion about health care needs, interests, and choices are likely to occur among proxies, families, and health care providers. Mediation can "level the playing field" by improving communication so that all parties can voice their concerns for the patient and reduce if not avoid power struggles between the proxy and concerned family, friends, and others. The person acting as mediator is generally trained to use "problem-solving tools," but, even in the absence of formal training, the neutral person who convenes the parties has to be mindful that different cultures, ethnic groups, and professional groups have different ways of communicating and making decisions. Most of the health care decisions to be made by a proxy are ones that require immediate action. Therefore, mediation is sensitive to the time constraints and the needs of the situation. The first "rule" of mediation is to avoid describing the disagreement as a "conflict"; the parties themselves do often not view it that way, and labeling it as such is not helpful.

The hallmarks of mediations are to identify the concerned parties, determine their needs and interests, provide relevant information, identify options, and promote agreement about the "best" decision. Once there is agreement about the clinical information, the goals of care should be identified and discussed. It is important that the non-health care parties understand the medical facts. A reasonable next step is to establish how decisions by or for the patient were made in the past. Were they patient or family driven? It is extremely important to identify, also, if there is one person to whom the patient and/or family deferred or whom they sought for his or her opinion prior to a major decision; this individual may or may not be the current proxy decision maker. The next step explores the presence or applicability of any ethical principle or legal issue that is relevant to reaching a decision. The

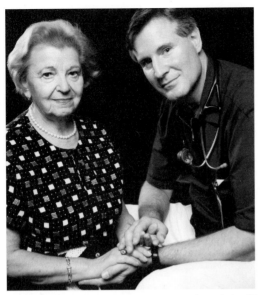

Promoting quality of life through the nurse-patient relationship. (Courtesy Mathy Mezey.)

"principled solution" that emerges from mediation is one that reflects "fairness of process" (Dubler & Marcus, 1994).

CONCLUSION

The cognitively impaired older adult must be afforded every protection, support, and opportunity to profess his or her health care wishes. The HCP advance directive is best suited for this purpose; the elder is choosing someone he or she presumably knows and trusts to make decisions for the elder when he or she is no longer capable of doing so. To optimize the elder's ability to create a HCP advance directive, the health care professional should identify the best time of day and environment for advance planning discussions; use the person's strengths; ameliorate the perverse effect of medication, pain, and stress; and provide adequate time. Specific end-of-life treatment measures can be difficult to discuss because of the need to predict and imagine possible future scenarios with a cognitively impaired person; also, among some cultures these kinds of discussions, planning for death, are taboo (Mitty, 2001). Nevertheless, health care measures that are desired as well as those that are not wanted

can be addressed broadly as comfort measures, rather than as specific interventions. Selection of the hospice benefit for elders with Alzheimer's disease and end-of-life care that provides options that favor aggressive comfort measures and bereavement support for families is vital. Additionally, this support should be extended to the proxy, who might not be a family member.

Life is a narrative story. To disregard an elder's choices is not only "unjustified paternalism," but it dishonors the person's life (Dresser, 1995). To the extent that an advance directive expresses a patient's wishes—explicitly in a LW or through the person standing in for him or her, the chosen proxy decision maker—autonomy is preserved and the person's life story is honored. Those who love and care for the patient can be assisted to make the best possible decision by thinking about what he or she would have chosen if given the opportunity. It is an honor to be asked to be a surrogate decision maker, and is a unique responsibility that is almost existential in nature. Nurses are best placed to assist the patient and proxy partnership to continue and complete the narrative.

REFERENCES

Aging with Dignity. (2003). *Five wishes*. Retrieved from http://www.agingwithdignity.org/5wishes.html

American Psychiatric Association. (1997). Practice guidelines for the treatment of patients with Alzheimer's disease and other dementias of late life. *American Journal of Psychiatry, 154*(5 Suppl.), 1-39.

Applebaum, P. S., & Grisso, T. (1987). The MacArthur Treatment and Competence Study: I. Mental illness and competence to consent to treatment. *Journal of Law and Human Behavior, 19*, 105-174.

Applebaum, P. S., & Gutheil, T. (1991). *Clinical handbook of psychiatry and law*. Baltimore: Williams & Wilkins.

Berghmans, R. L. P. (1998). Advance directives for non-therapeutic dementia research: Some ethical and policy considerations. *Journal of Medical Ethics, 24*, 32-37.

Bosek, M. S. DeW., Savage, T. A., Shaw, L. A., & Renella, C. (2001). When surrogate decision-making is not straightforward: Guidelines for nurse administrators. *JONAs Healthcare Law, Ethics, and Regulation, 3*(2), 47-57.

Bradley, C. H., Wetle, T., & Horwitz, S. M. (1998). The Patient Self-Determination Act and advance directive completion in nursing homes. *Archives of Family Medicine, 7*, 417-423

Carney, M. T., Neugroschl, J., Morrison, R. S., Martin, D., & Siu, A. L. (2001). The development and piloting of a capacity assessment tool. *The Journal of Clinical Ethics, 12,* 17-23.

Castle, N. G., & Mor, V. (1998). Advance care planning in nursing homes: Pre- and post the Patient Self-Determination Act. *Health Services Research, 33,* 101-124.

Center for Ethics in Health Care. (2003). *The Physician Orders for Life-Sustaining Treatment program (POLST).* Retrieved from http://www.ohsu.edu/ethics/polst.htm

Center for Health Law and Ethics. (2003). *The institute and health law and ethics.* Retrieved from http://ipl.unm.edu/chle

Damasio, A. R. (1996). Alzheimer's disease and related dementias. In J. C. Bennett & F. Plum (Eds.), *Cecil textbook of medicine* (20th ed., pp. 1992-1994). Philadelphia: Saunders.

Dresser, R. (1995). Dworkin on dementia: Elegant theory, questionable policy. *Hastings Center Report, 25*(6), 32-38.

Dresser, R. (2001). Advance directives in dementia research: Promoting autonomy and protecting subjects. *IRB: Ethics & Human Research, 23*(1), 1-6.

Dresser, R., & Whitehouse, P. (1994). The incompetent patient on the slippery slope. *Hastings Center Report, 24*(4), 6-12.

Dubler, N. N. (1985). Some legal and moral issues surrounding informed consent for treatment and research involving the cognitively impaired elderly. In M. Kapp, N. E. Pies, & A. E. Doudera (Eds.), *Legal and ethical aspects of health care for the elderly* (pp. 247-257). Ann Arbor, MI: Health Administration Press.

Dubler, N. N. (1995). The doctor-proxy relationship: The neglected connection. *Kennedy Institute of Ethics Journal, 5*(4), 289-306.

Dubler, N. N., & Marcus, L. J. (1994). *Mediating bioethical dispute: A practical guide.* New York: United Hospital Fund.

Dunn, P. M., Schmidt, T. A., Carley, M. M., Donius, M., Weinstein, M. A., & Dull, V. T. (1997). A method to communicate patient preferences about medically indicated life-sustaining treatment in the out-of-hospital setting. *Journal of the American Geriatrics Society, 44,* 785-791.

Evans, D. A., Funkenstein, H., Albert, M. S., Scherr, P. A., Cook, N. R., Chown, M. J., et al. (1989). Prevalence of advance directives in a community-based population of older persons. *Journal of the American Medical Association, 262,* 551-556.

Feinberg, L. F., & Whitlatch, C. J. (2002). Are persons with cognitive impairment able to state consistent choices? *Gerontologist, 41*(3), 374-382.

Fins, J. J. (1999). From contract to covenant in advance care planning. *Journal of Law, Medicine & Ethics, 27*(1), 46-51.

Finucane, T. E., Brock, B. A., Roca, R. P., & Kawas, C. H. (1993). Establishing advance medical directives with demented patients: A pilot study. *The Journal of Clinical Ethics, 4,* 51-54.

Folstein, M. F., Folstein, S. E., & McHugh, P. (1975). Mini-mental state: A practical method for grading the cognitive state of patients for the clinician. *Journal of Psychiatric Research, 12,* 189-198.

Gibson, J. McI. (1990). National Values History Project. *Generations, 14*(Suppl.), 51-53.

Harrington, C., Carillo, H., & Wellin, V. (2001). *Nursing facilities, staffing, residents and facility deficiencies, 1994-2000.* San Francisco: University of California, School of Nursing, Department of Social and Behavioral Sciences.

Kadish, A. (1992). Letting patients die: Legal and moral reflections. *California Law Review, 80,* 857-858.

Kapp, M., & Mossman, D. (1996). Measuring decisional capacity: Cautions on the construction of a "capacimeter." *Psychology, Public Policy and Law, 2,* 73-95.

Karel, M., Moye, J., & Oville, A. (1996, November 19). *Assessing values and competency for health care planning in cognitively impaired older adults.* Presented at the Annual Meeting of the Gerontological Society of America, Boston.

Kopelman, L. M. (1997). The best-interests standard as threshold, ideal, and standard of reasonableness. *Journal of Medical Philosophy, 22,* 271-289.

Loewy, W. H. (1998). Ethical considerations in executing and implementing advance directives. *Archives of Internal Medicine, 126,* 1227-1232.

Lynn, J., Teno, J., Dresser, R., Brock, D., Nelson, H. L., Nelson, J., et al. (1999). Dementia and advance-care planning: Perspectives from three countries on ethics and epidemiology. *The Journal of Clinical Ethics, 10,* 271-285.

Marson, D. C., Chatterjee, A., Ingram, K. K., & Harrell, L. E. (1996). Toward a neurological model of competency: Cognitive predictors of capacity to consent in Alzheimer's disease using three different legal standards. *Neurology, 46,* 666-672.

Meier, D. E. (1997). Voiceless and vulnerable: Dementia patients without surrogates in an era of capitation. *Journal of the American Geriatrics Society, 45,* 357-377.

Mezey, M., Kluger, M., Maislin, G., & Mittelman, M. (1996). Life-sustaining treatment decisions by spouses of patients with Alzheimer's disease. *Journal of the American Geriatrics Society, 44,* 144-150.

Mezey, M. D., Mitty, E. L., Bottrell, M. M., Ramsey, G. C., & Fisher, T. (2000). Advance directives: Older adults with dementia. *Clinics in Geriatric Medicine, 16,* 255-268.

Mezey, M., Teresi, J., Ramsey, G., Mitty, E., & Bobrowitz, T. (2000). Decision-making capacity to execute a health care proxy: Development and testing of guidelines. *Journal of the American Geriatrics Society, 48,* 179-187.

Midwest Bioethics Center. (1996). *Ethics Committee Consortium: Guidelines for the determination of decisional incapacity.* Kansas City, MO: Author.

Miller, T. (1995). Advance directives: Moving from theory to practice. In P. Katz, R. I. Kane, & M. Mezey (Eds.), *Quality care in geriatric settings.* New York: Springer.

Mitty, E. (2001). Ethnicity and end-of-life decision making. *Reflections on Nursing Leadership, 27*(1), 28-31.

Morrison, S. E., & Siu, A. L. (2000). Survival in end-stage dementia following acute illness. *Journal of the American Medical Association, 284,* 47-52.

National Bioethics Advisory Commission. (1999). Research involving persons with mental disorders that may affect decision making. Vol. 2: Commissioned papers (pp. 5-28). Rockville, MD: Author.

National Center for Assisted Living. (2001). *Facts and trends, 2001: The assisted living sourcebook.* Washington, DC: Author.

Office of Technology Assessment. (1990). *Confused minds, burdened families: Finding help for people with Alzheimer's disease and other dementias* (OTA-BA-403). Washington, DC: Author.

Parfit, D. (1984). *Reasons and persons.* Oxford, UK: Oxford University Press.

Patient Self-Determination Act of 1990, 42 U.S.C. §§ 1395c, 1396a (West Supp. 1991).

Post, L. F., Blustein, J., & Dubler, N. N. (1999). Introduction: The doctor-proxy relationship. *Journal of Law, Medicine & Ethics, 27,* 5-12.

Pruchno, R. A., Smyer, M. A., Rose, M. S., Hartman-Stein, P. E., & Henderson-Laribee, D. L. (1995). Competence of long-term care residents to participate in decisions about their medical care: A brief objective assessment. *The Gerontologist, 35,* 622-629.

Reisberg, B. (1988). Functional Assessment Staging (FAST). *Psychopharmacological Bulletin, 24,* 653-655.

Reisberg, B., Ferris, S., de Leon, M., & Crook, T. (1982). The Global Deterioration Scale for assessment of primary degenerative dementia. *American Journal of Psychiatry, 139,* 1136-1139.

Sachs, G. A. (1994). Advance consent for dementia research. *Alzheimer Disease and Associated Disorders, 8*(Suppl. 4), 19-27.

Sachs, M., & Siegler, M. (1991). Guidelines for decision making when the patient is incompetent. *Journal of Critical Illness, 1,* 348-359.

Sansone, P., & Nichols, J. (1997, Fall). *The right to choose capacity study.* Paper presented at the New York Ethics Network, New York.

Schirm, V., & Stachel, L. (1996). The values history as a nursing intervention to encourage use of advance directives. *Applied Nursing Research, 9*(2), 93-96.

Silberfeld, M., Nash, C., & Singer, P. (1993). Capacity to complete an advance directive. *Journal of the American Geriatrics Society, 41,* 1141-1143.

Singer, P. A., Martin, D. K., Lavery, J. V., Thiel, E. C., Kelner, M. K., & Mendelssohn, D. C. (1998). Reconceptualizing advance care planning from the patient's perspective. *Archives of Internal Medicine, 158,* 879-884.

Spann, J., & Christopher, M. (1999). *Implementing end-of-life treatment preferences across clinical settings* (Community-State Partnerships to Improve End-of-Life Care, No. 3). Kansas City, MO: Midwest Bioethics Center.

Sulmasy, D., Terry, P., Weisman, C. S., Miller, D. J., Stallings, R. Y., Vettese, M. A., et al. (1998). The accuracy of substituted judgments in patients with terminal diagnoses. *Annals of Internal Medicine, 128,* 621-629.

Teresi, J. A., Grant, L. A., Holmes, D., & Ory, M. G. (1998). Staffing in traditional and special dementia care units: Preliminary findings from the NIA Collaborative Studies. *Journal of Gerontological Nursing, 24*(1), 49-53.

Tolle, S. W., Tilden, V. P., Nelson, C. A., & Dunn, P. M. (1998). A prospective study of the efficacy of the Physician Order for Life Sustaining Treatment (1995-1997). *Journal of the American Geriatrics Society, 46,* 1097-1102.

Tomlinson, T., Howe, K., Notman, M., & Rossmiller, D. (1990). An empirical study of proxy consent for elderly persons. *The Gerontologist, 30,* 54-64.

Volicer, L. (1994). Impact of special care units for patients with advanced Alzheimer's disease on patient discomfort and cost. *Journal of the American Geriatrics Society, 42,* 597-603.

Volicer, L., Cantor, M. D., Derse, A. R., Edwards, D. M., Prudhomme, A. M., Gregory, D. C. R., et al. (2002). Advance care planning by proxy for residents of long-term care facilities who lack decision-making capacity. *Journal of the American Geriatrics Society, 50,* 761-767.

8

FAMILY CAREGIVERS OF DYING ELDERS: BURDENS AND OPPORTUNITIES

Valerie Swigart

Mr. J., an 84-year-old with a history of diabetes mellitus, hypertension, coronary heart disease, heart surgery (saphenous vein bypass grafting), stroke, peripheral vascular disease, and a non-healing wound on the right lower extremity, died 2 weeks ago. His daughter, a 61-year-old school teacher, offers the following narrative:

I took care of Dad for the last 8 years. My husband and I have a home about 20 miles from where Dad lived. I'm an only child, so there was no one else to help. My husband retired early because of poor health, our kids live out of state, and I am still teaching third graders. My mom died 25 years ago, and Dad remarried. He retired at 60 from a good job as personnel director for a steel company. He was a "take charge" kind of guy. He and my stepmom, Lydia, traveled a lot while they were well. We are a small family, and we had a lot of good times, until her emphysema incapacitated Lydia. She was on oxygen for a year. Dad took good care of her, but his health suffered. He had a mild stroke right after she died. He had been on some medicines for his blood pressure and diabetes for years. He had circulation problems in his feet. The stroke made him weak in his left arm, and he couldn't think quite as clearly. I was driving the 30 miles to his place three times a week, paying his bills, trying to see that he took his medication, and getting him to appointments with his doctors.

On a regular checkup, his internist thought he needed his heart checked more closely. They found blockages. The way they explained it, surgery was a matter of life or death. Dad decided to have the surgery. It was very tough; his lungs

filled up twice. We thought he was going to die, but he made it through. The place on his leg where they took the graft never healed right. Then he fell one evening in his apartment and opened up the area on his leg. At that point, I was driving up to his apartment every other day to change the dressings and check on him. He refused to let me hire help. I was exhausted. I have blood pressure problems and macular degeneration, so I don't see that well. Then he got an infection and had to go to the hospital. Again, we almost lost him, but he pulled through. He was too weak to go back to his place, so I found a nursing home closer to me.

Well, they really tried to get him better in the nursing home, but the leg just got all black. One doctor said it needed to be amputated. Dad adamantly refused. He said, "I don't want to be a ragtag old man. I want to die in one piece." He was in a lot of pain. Then when he got medication for the pain, he became irrational. I don't think he ever slept an entire night in that nursing home. The staff really didn't like him.

One night they called me at 2:00 AM. They said he was toxic and sent him to the hospital. He had to go to the ICU. He was not able to talk coherently. I knew that he did not want an amputation. Apparently he was too sick for that anyhow. By the next day he was in a coma. He was just lying there, unable to talk, unable to eat. They had to put a tube in his bladder. They kept using the needles, pushing and prodding him. I winced every time they came to do something else to him. He had made it through so much. He had left the hospital so many times. We are not religious people, but I did ask God, "What should I do?" Dad had a living will, but it sure didn't cover this situation.

Then, after 3 days of that, I looked at him and knew that his poor old body had taken all it could. He would not want to go on in that state of deterioration. I wanted him to have every chance to live; you just don't take life away from someone. I talked to a friend who knew Dad. We talked about what a good life Dad had. He was really quite a dapper guy. He just would not want his body mistreated like that. She advised using hospice. I went back into the ICU and told them to stop taking blood from him. The young ICU doctor would not listen to me. So I said, "Maybe we should have an ethics committee consult." His eyes widened. He said, "Oh, OK, what is it you want to do?" We called hospice. That day they shifted Dad to the regular unit, then out to the hospice. He never woke up.

It was quiet there in the hospice. My husband and I talked a lot about what an exciting life my Dad had had. The nurses encouraged me to talk to my Dad, even though he couldn't respond. I told him good-bye, and he squeezed my hand. A day later, I was right there holding his hand when he took his last breath. It was not easy, but I knew I was doing what I needed to do. He was a tough one, but I know he loved me. I did my best to take care of him. It took years off of my life. I'm sorry he had so much suffering near the end. I still wonder if, morally, I did the right thing.

INTRODUCTION

The family is central to care of the dying elder. Advanced illness is an experience shared by the elder and the family. Death, particularly of an elder, may be expected, yet dying and death are a family crisis, and, as in all crises, the situation has inherent burdens and opportunities for those involved. For family members, the shared experience of dying can be a time of great stress or burden and, at the same time, can be an opportunity for unexpected growth and reaching new potential.

The family or intimate network has always been considered the focus of palliative care (Davies, Reimer, & Martens, 1994; Rando, 2000). This contrasts with the more common patient-centered approach, wherein the patient is seen as the focus of care and viewed as a member of the family. The family has been conceptualized as a part of the palliative care team or as the hub of a wheel around which the interdisciplinary team are arrayed like spokes (Gunten, 2002). Family members, defined here as those with committed familial or emotional bonds with the dying elder, have participatory and decision-making roles in the care of the dying person. Thus the term *family* includes not only biologically related persons but also those persons who constitute the dying person's circle or intimate network (Doka, 1993; Rando, 2000).

In this chapter, using a family systems approach, the family is viewed as complex, interactive, and dynamic. The family is the client (Gilliss, 1991), and information exchange is a primary operative concept. The inputs to the family are information from outside and from inside the system. Outputs are communications to others outside of the family and to those within the system. The family system can be best understood by developing knowledge of its structural features, such as the flow of the information exchange and the beliefs, attitudes, and culture(s) of those involved (Buckley, 1967). The beliefs, attitudes, and culture of the family give meaning to the information received and create patterns of communication networking made up of loops, paths, and feedback mechanisms.

Communication processes directly impact the quality of family life (Faulkner, 1998), the process of caregiving for the dying elder (Krause, 1991), and the ongoing health of the family (Larson & Tobin, 2000). Palliative care, whether in the home, hospital, or nursing home, must be family centered (Teno, Casey, & Edgeman-Leviton, 2001). Saunders (1982) defined four domains of palliative care: the physical, psychological, social, and spiritual. Ideally, the nurse enters the intimate circle of caregivers as a "surrogate friend" to the family (Kissane, Spruyt, & Aranda, 2000, p. 382). The nurse assesses and implements the physical aspects of care, such as symptom relief; attends to practical and financial issues; and uses communication to assist with psychosocial-spiritual aspects, such as loss, suffering, and finding meaning in the experience. The nurse assists the patient–family system to work through the dying and death of their family member, while minimizing burdens and maximizing opportunities.

This chapter describes the burdens and opportunities inherent in or evolving out of caregiver work during the dying process of an elder family member. A brief discussion of the impact of modern medicine and technology on the family unit of the elder is followed by a more detailed exploration of how the changing trajectories of illness and the site of dying have impacted the burdens and opportunities inherent in the role of family caregiver. Burdens and opportunities are discussed separately for the convenience of explanation. In reality, the two aspects may be experienced simultaneously. The associations between burdens, suffering, finding meaning, self-transcendence, opportunities, and sociohistorical-cultural issues are explored.

The importance of considering the historical, social, and cultural factors that impact the receptivity of families to palliative care interventions are also highlighted. Dying and death are culturally laden, and the determination of what are or are not burdens and opportunities may be influenced by the culture of the family; therefore, some general points about consideration of cultural differences are discussed. The literature base for this chapter reflects Anglo-American health care theory and practice. The following description of trajectories of illness and dying is applicable only to those countries with health care systems similar to that of United States.

ILLNESS AND DYING TRAJECTORIES

The illness, dying, and death trajectories of older adults and their families in the United States have been profoundly affected by changes in biomedical science occurring in the last 60 years. Advances in public health, knowledge of the human body, use of technology, and control of some diseases has increased the average American life span to about 80 years (Brock & Foley, 1998). Until the mid-20th century, most persons died from infection or injury. The trajectory of dying was a sharp decline over a short period of time (Teno, Weitzen, Fennel, & Mor, 2001). It was common for persons with severe chronic illness (such as emphysema) to die in middle age; they are now living to old age (Lynn, 2000). Only about one third of American elders will die having had limited and manageable chronic illness, such as osteoarthritis or hearing deficit. Over two thirds of elders will die having had serious, complex, progressively worsening chronic illness. Lynn and Forlini (2001) suggested that the term *serious and complex (and*

eventually fatal) be used to describe these conditions (p. 316).

According to Lynn and Forlini (2001), the trajectory of illness experienced by the elder with serious and complex chronic illness and his or her caregiving family falls into one of three categories: (1) a short period of decline at the end of life, typical of cancer; (2) a slow downward illness trajectory, marked by periods of relative stability and exacerbations with unpredictable timing of death, which characterizes dying with chronic organ system failures; or (3) progressive self-care deficits and a slow deterioration to death, such as that resulting from frailty of old age, stroke, or dementia.

The trajectory of illness and dying impacts the length of caregiving and the degree and pattern of uncertainty burdening the family. For example, an older adult may be well except for manageable chronic illness, but then receives an abrupt life-threatening diagnosis, such as pancreatic cancer. The individual loses weight and has a precipitous functional decline signaling approaching death (Teno et al., 2001). In this illness trajectory, the family has time to develop an understanding of the illness and adapt to the situation. The fairly predictable terminal phase allows for final good-byes and resolutions. This is the classic hospice care situation, and considerable attention has been given to ways health care providers can provide support. In actuality, only 23% of elders die from cancer (Brock & Foley, 1998).

The situation for families of persons with long-term, complex, chronic illness is especially problematic. The sharply varying but downward-sloping trajectory of illness of the individual with serious and complex chronic health problems creates a lengthy caregiving experience with repeated episodes of acute illness. Teno et al. (2001) have documented that more than 40% of persons dying of diabetes, congestive heart failure, and chronic obstructive heart disease had significant impairments in activities of living 1 year prior to death. The elder and the family caregivers experience a prolonged, varying course of ups, when daily life and relationships continue, and downs, when survival is often in question (Lynn & Forlini, 2001). The repeated cycles of uncertainty and recovery can create an enduring sense of hope for cure; that hope for cure, in the face of futility, may interfere with the realization that death is imminent and may obstruct the transition to hope for a peaceful death (Lynn, 2001). Thus the long history of multiple periods of threat and uncertainty regarding the survival of the family member, and the short period of terminal illness, usually occurring in the hospital setting, make preparation of the family for dying and death particularly difficult (Rando, 2000).

Family caregiving, for an elder member who experiences the trajectory of illness involving progressive loss of cognitive function, is lengthy, and the dying process can often be complicated by the patient's inability to communicate. A study using interviews of family members of 6748 decedents over age 65 revealed that behavioral problems were evident in 20% of the elders during the last year of life, and 68% of those with behavioral problems lived the majority of their last year in their homes (Bedford, Melzer, & Guralnick, 2001). The psychological impact of caring for an individual who is unable to provide reciprocity, may have behavioral problems, or has lost the personality characteristics of the loved one may interfere with caregivers' abilities to affirm the ill person's dignity (Yang & Kirshling, 1992), and may dramatically impact the family's adjustment to dying and death (Jones & Martinson, 1992).

LOCATION OF DYING AND DEATH

As the cause of death has changed in the last 60 years, so has the place. Viewing health care providers as agents of cure and the hospital as the preferred place for medical care are relatively new phenomena. Prior to the 1930s, death occurred at home, and young family members were included in the experience and supported. Nurses visited or were employed for "private duty" with the family. In the middle of the 20th century, with the biomedical revolution, the hospital became the preferred site for illness, dying, and death. Dying became a medicalized, isolated process, hidden especially from young family members (Gunten, 2002). Privacy disappeared; family interaction occurred in waiting rooms in hospitals rather than in living rooms at home. Modern technologies increased the uncertainty, drama, and ethical ambiguity of dying (Callahan, 1993).

A Gallup poll in 1997 found that 90% of the U.S. population would prefer to die at home (Center for Gerontology and Health Care Research, 2000); however, Fried, van Doorn, O'Leary, Tinetti, and Drickamer (1999) and Steinhauser et al. (2000) found elder Americans less interested in dying at home, citing family burden and dislike of having a dead body in the home. Although a shift from hospital- to home-based care of dying persons is taking place (Grady, 1999), about 52% of Americans still die in the hospital (Center for Gerontology and Health Care Research, 2000), and more elders are dying in nursing homes. In some states, one third of older adults die in nursing homes, and it is estimated that, within the next 40 years, 40% to 50% of Americans will die in nursing homes (Teno, 2002). Hospice care is available in hospital, home, and nursing home settings, and serves about one fourth of dying Americans; patients with a diagnosis of cancer comprise 57% of hospice admissions. Hospice use by persons with chronic, life-threatening illnesses, such as end-stage lung or heart disease, is growing (National Hospice and Palliative Care Organization, 2002). The high incidence of multiple and serious chronic illnesses and the associated uncertainty about when death will occur are reasons why many elder–family units do not consider hospice care (Lynn & Forlini, 2001). Palliative care programs are being developed to better provide for the end-of-life needs of hospitalized patients and their families. A survey in 1998 revealed that only 28% of hospitals provide hospice care and only 15% have any formalized protocols for end-of-life care (Quill, 2002).

The expanding numbers of elder persons, the changing trajectory of illness of dying elders, limitations placed on the length of hospitalization, and the persistent scarcity of in-hospice care have profoundly impacted the caregiving burdens of family members of aging Americans. Approximately 45% of elder Americans will have been seriously and chronically ill with noncancer disease or will have suffered from cognitive deficits before death. Therefore, the classic time frame of the cancer-patient-in-hospice care model does not apply for a large number of elder patient–family units. Most family caregivers of elders will have been caring for the chronically ill individual for many years prior to the advanced stages of illness. The effects of long-term in-home provision of care on the health of caregivers must be taken into consideration.

BURDENS OF LONG-TERM CAREGIVING IN THE HOME

Long-term caregiving, whether required because of a complex chronic illness or dementia or during the prolonged terminal phase of an illness, may endanger the physical and psychological health of the caregiver. Although the impact of caregiving varies with the length and complexity of caregiving, race, advanced age, employment status, and social support, overall, home-based caregivers have been found to be at risk for poor health outcomes (Aranda, 1997; Hileman, Lackey, & Hassanein, 1992; Scharlach, Midanik, Runkle, & Soghikian, 1997) and higher mortality (Schultz et al., 1999).

Although there is some evidence that older caregivers may be more accepting of the caregiver role (Oberst, Thomas, Gass, & Ward, 1989), the increased frequency of chronic illness and the average lower income of older persons may result in increased vulnerability for poor outcomes (Clipp & George, 1993). Elder spouses are especially vulnerable (Navaie-Waliser et al., 2002). The tasks of caring for a chronically ill or dying elder, such as assistance with washing, feeding, toileting, getting out of bed, walking, or positioning in bed, all require time and considerable strength. Problems such as incontinence significantly increase the workload for home cleanliness and laundry (Krause, 1991). Home-based caregivers are called on to manage multiple medical regimens. These may include managing drug delivery systems, such as pumps and spinal ports; monitoring symptom relief and ongoing treatment of disease problems; changing dressings; and providing treatments such as rectal suppositories or range-of-motion exercises.

Home-based family caregivers have reported increased stress, anxiety, depression, and reduced self-esteem (Kissane, Bloch, Burns, McKenzie, & Posterino, 1994; Kissane et al., 2000) and perceived decline in health (Stetz, 1989). The family must transition from a time of regular schedules and usual events to schedules focused on the ill or dying family member. Care at home may require changes in the location of furniture or sleeping quarters. Hours are spent waiting in doctor's offices, performing the activities of caring, or simply being at home because the ill person cannot be left alone (Rose, 1998; Roy, 1998). Caregivers have reported foregoing established social interaction and personal pleasures, lack of sleep, and decreased participation in health maintenance activities (Hileman et al., 1992). Rando (1993) found that caring for a member with long-term illness predisposed family members to depletion of resources and complicated mourning.

Burdens of Caregivers of Elders with Dementia

The burdens of caregiving for the dying elder who has dementia can be particularly complicated and painful. Elder spouses providing long-term care to cognitively impaired elders are especially vulnerable. Caring for a loved one with dementia and experiencing the death of that person can result in severe psychosocial stressors and be a source of continuing depression (Blasi, Hurley, & Volicer, 2002; Robinson-Whelen, Yuri, MacCallum, McGuire, & Kiecolt-Glaser, 2001). Davies (2001) pointed out that it is important to the caregiver that the recipient acknowledge the many acts and sacrifices of caregiving. Caregivers whose efforts were unacknowledged or minimized felt unappreciated and exhausted; some confessed that they were "waiting" for the patient to die (p. 356).

Jones and Martinson (1992) identified the acute grief experienced by caregivers of patients with Alzheimer's disease while the individual was alive; it was theorized that this was related to the "immediate and permanent loss of the relative's human abilities and personhood" (p. 175). Grieving occurred and intensified during the caregiving experience and created agonizing emotional distancing. Distancing or detachment was less when the recipient was able to continue some meaningful communication and to show affection. The bereavement response to the actual death of the relative was accompanied by increased grief, feelings of relief, and often guilt. How these emotions of family caregivers are expressed when the elder is in pain or is dying has not been explored.

Burdens of Family Caregivers in the Nursing Home and Hospital

Family members caring for ill or dying elders in the nursing home or hospital setting also experience the burdens of caregiving. Although having less responsibility for the day-to-day physical needs of the elder, the burdens of "being there," protecting and advocating for the elder, and participating in critical decisions are substantial (Dunne & Sullivan, 2000; Swigart, 1995; Tilden, Tolle, Nelson, & Fields, 2001). Family members attending to relatives in the hospital or nursing home experience role conflict, guilt, depressive symptoms, anxiety, stress, and fatigue (Bull, Jervis, & Her, 1995; Forbes, Bern-Klug, & Gessert, 2000).

Recent studies have documented poor control of pain in nursing home residents (Teno, Weitzen, Wetle, & Mor, 2001); low use (16%) of hospice care; delay of hospice referral until, on average, 1 week before death; and lack of attention to family members' desires to attend the death of their family member (Forbes, 2001; Happ et al., 2002). All of these factors negatively impact the experience of family members.

Fifty-five to 60% of older adults die in the hospital (Field & Cassel, 1997). In-hospital care

---

EVIDENCE-BASED PRACTICE

Reference: Tolle, S. W., Tilden, V. P., Rosenfeld, A. B., & Hickman, S. E. (2000). Family reports of barriers to optimal care of the dying. *Nursing Research, 49*, 310-317.

Research Problem: In order to improve care of the dying, researchers need to identify barriers to optimal care.

Design: Descriptive, survey.

Sample and Setting: A systematic random sampling technique was used to select 475 family caregivers in Oregon who were interviewed by telephone in their homes 2 to 5 months after the death of a family member.

Methods: Family members were interviewed using a 58-item questionnaire developed by the investigators. The first 55 items were forced choice and the last three were open-ended. Numerical data were analyzed using SPSS 8.0 and narrative data were reduced using thematic analysis.

Results: The average age of the decedents was 77 years, and 98% were white. The average age of the caregivers was 60 years; most were either spouses or adult offspring. Twenty-eight percent of the decedents died in the hospital, 38% in nursing homes, and 28% in private homes. Sixty-eight percent of the caregivers reported that the decedent had a living will. Ninety-seven percent believed that the decedent's preference for treatment had been respected; this did not vary across settings. Twenty percent of the sample were dissatisfied with physician availabil-

ity, and 8% were dissatisfied with nurse availability. Thirty-four percent of caregivers indicated that their relative was in moderate to severe pain during the last week of life. Although the level of pain was highest in hospitalized patients, families reported more difficulty with management of pain in the home setting. Communication problems, uncaring attitudes on the part of physicians, and medical treatment problems were reported as most problematic.

Implications for Nursing Practice: The finding that one third of the sample reported that their relative was in moderate to severe pain during the last week of life is unsettling. Oregon has one of the highest rates of morphine prescriptions per capita in the United States. Nurses must continue to be concerned about pain and consider new ways for management. Nurses need to attend to family members' preparation for and education regarding pain control. Family members' interpretations of and reaction to pain in their dying relative need to be explored. Because the debate about end-of-life care in Oregon has raised most citizens' awareness of these issues, generalizability of the findings of this study to other states is in question. The authors suggest that the study may be a bellwether for changes emerging in end-of-life care throughout the United States.

Conclusion: Despite a generally positive profile in a state where the conversation about the quality of dying and death has been ongoing, persistent barriers to optimal care of the dying were clearly evident. Primary problems were level of pain, management of pain, and dissatisfaction with physician availability.

at the end of life has been reported as failing to serve the needs of elder patients and their family members. Nearly half of the seriously ill patients who are in intensive care units (ICUs) spend their last 8 to 10 days comatose and on mechanical ventilation. Twenty-two percent of those who are conscious experience moderate to severe pain (SUPPORT Principle Investigators, 1995). Elders whose illness trajectories reach finality with a sudden life-threatening illness or at the end of one of multiple hospitalizations for complex, serious chronic illness die in a hospital bed. In hospitals, particularly in critical care settings, opportunities for the family to integrate awareness of dying, to begin to develop a new self-identity through the dying process, and to become socially and psychologically prepared for the death of their relative are markedly absent (Seymour, 1999).

Caregiving family members in hospitals and nursing homes may be additionally burdened by participation in end-of-life decision making for an incapacitated elder. Much has been written about advance care planning and the need for patient and/or family discussions about preferences at the end of life (Azoulay et al., 2000; Lilly et al., 2000; Rier, 2000; Wros, 1994). Advance directives and living wills, although certainly still advised, are completed by less that one fourth of Americans (Emanuel, Barry, Stoeckle, & Emanuel, 1991). Interpretation of these documents in actual clinical situations is difficult, and some reports (Forbes, 2001; Reilly, Teasdale, & McCullough, 1994; Teno, 1997) have indicated that they are underused by clinicians. Family members continue to have an active role in decisions to implement, continue, or discontinue life-supporting treatments.

Forbes et al. (2000) studied family caregiver end-of-life decision making for nursing home residents with dementia. Caregivers described making end-of-life decisions in the context of overwhelming burden and underlying guilt related to placing the relative in the nursing home. Forbes noted that the family members received no counsel regarding the expected trajectory of physical and cognitive losses. Additionally, family members were not able to recognize recurring pneumonia, dysphagia, or decreased mentation as heralding the end of life; rather, these are seen as emergent problems to be fixed.

The extreme stress experienced by family members assisting with end-of-life decisions for a critically ill relative in the hospital has received considerable attention (Tilden, Tolle, Nelson, Thompson, & Eggman, 1999; Tolle, Tilden, Rosenfield, & Hickman, 2000). Swigart, Lidz, Butterworth, and Arnold (1996) described the burdensome and stressful experience of family members as they attempted to seek out information about the course of the illness and treatment. Inconsistencies and lack of physician time were frustrating. Family members carried out cognitive, emotional, and social work in order to be able to "reframe" from a hope for recovery to hope for a peaceful death (Swigart et al., 1996, p. 486). Not all families were able to make this transition. In the intensive care setting, not being able to have the opportunity to say good-bye or to feel a sense of interpersonal closure with the dying relative was common, and traumatic reactions (recurring thoughts about mistreating or causing the death of the relative, and nightmares) have been reported by family members (Swigart, Lidz, Butterworth, & Arnold, 1998). Long-term high levels of stress in family members involved in life support decisions have been documented (Tilden et al., 2001).

Little has been written specifically about the unique situation of the seriously chronically ill elder and his or her family. The frequency of serious illnesses, hospitalizations, and "close calls" with death may create a delay in the ability to recognize the closeness of death, exemplified by the following family member's statement, "Yeah, well, dad was a fighter. The way I look at it, if there is any chance at all for him to recover, I wanted him to have that chance. He would have wanted it, and I wanted it that way. He got better before. I thought he could do it again." (Swigart et al., 1998). Often in such situations, despite long-term serious illness, when the end of life does come, family members perceive the death as sudden and unexpected. Too often, the patient has been too ill to participate in resolutions and good-byes, never having considered him- or herself to be dying. Family members continue to suffer, having had no opportunity to find meaning or comfort in the dying process (Tilden et al., 2001).

Burden of Reciprocal Suffering

Whether in the home, nursing home, or hospital, the psychosocial-spiritual impact of dealing with illness and dying, of witnessing deterioration, dependency, pain, and suffering, and of anticipating separation and loss can be very burdensome to the family (Rando, 2000). Sherman (1998) described the combined physical, emotional, social, and spiritual distress of the family during the terminal illness as "reciprocal suffering." The patient suffers as he or she considers the loss of his or her life and all of the connections of life. The family, facing the approaching death of a valued family member, attempts to deal with the loss of that family member. The impending death of a loved one disrupts the basic sense of security of being in the world (Seale, 1998). At the end of life, the family members feel and share the dying member's physical and existential distress. They feel the threat and fear of death, the grief associated with sharing life's ending, the loss of control, and the shame as the body weakens and deteriorates (Kissane et al., 2000). Family members suffer as they face the impending loss of the dying member and the other multiple burdens of caregiving (Sherman, 1998).

Suffering, to some extent, universally accompanies dying and death, even when physical pain is not experienced or is skillfully controlled (Byock, 1996). Use of the biomedical model and existing technology to relieve suffering related to pain or other symptoms is an important aspect of palliative care. However, understanding emotional or existential suffering requires moving beyond the biomedical model. "Suffering" is defined as feeling pain, distress, or loss; or as undergoing or passing through (Abate & Jewell, 2001). Suffering is distress brought on by the actual or perceived impending threat to the integrity or continued existence of the intact or whole person (Cassel, 1982) or family unit. "Reciprocal" refers to two concepts so related that, if the first determines the second, then the second determines the first (Abate & Jewell, 2001). Thus the reciprocal suffering of the family is, at least in part, an existential crisis, created by a threat to self-identity as a family. Reciprocal suffering includes mutually experienced pain, distress, and loss felt as family members realize the impermanence of their experienced relationships and family structure.

In Western culture, the pursuit of individuality is highly regarded; the notion that a "deeply felt" state such as suffering is reciprocal may seem foreign. Reciprocal suffering can be understood by considering the "self" as a social construct; we cannot conceive of who we are without reference to others. We grow and live within the context of others and of a shared language, which we use to explain to ourselves, and to others, who we are. Cassel (1991) referred to this as the "inescapable intimacy in which we are all bound" (p. 31). The idea of social bonds is important to understanding the interdependence and reciprocity of family life. The person exists inescapably in linkage with others. Loss of that linkage is, in part, a loss of self. Just as self-identity is rooted in the past, self-identity is perceived as continuing into the future. Suffering begins with awareness of a future wherein some elements of identity that provide purpose and meaning to ongoing life are about to be lost (Cassel, 1991).

For the family, the impending loss represents a loss of the identity of the family inclusive of the dying member—that is, the "whole family" will no longer exist. The family as it exists in the present will not go on. Cassel (1991) suggested that relief of suffering for the dying person includes giving up the "myself of tomorrow" (p. 25). For family members, too, the relief of existential suffering may be the intrapsychic reformation of the family; that is, the family members

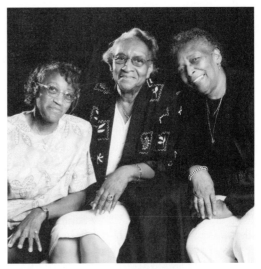

Achieving quality of life in older women. (Courtesy Mathy Mezey.)

and family as a unit are able to give up the existing "family of tomorrow" and envision a new such family without the loved one.

The multiple physical, psychological, social, and existential burdens of family caregiving for an elder dying family member have been described, and the relatively new concept of reciprocal suffering has been discussed. Cassel (1982) noted that suffering associated with loss of part of the "self" is ameliorated by finding meaning and transcendence, and that "the sufferer is not isolated by pain but is brought closer to a transpersonal source of meaning and to the human community" (p. 644). Suffering has been associated with "finding personal meaning in circumstances of loss, illness, limitation, dependency, and death" (Kenny, 1997, p. 30). If pain is controlled and suffering is not overwhelming, facing and coping with hardship creates a search for meaning (Steeves & Kahn, 1987). These statements may apply to the family as well.

OPPORTUNITIES FOR CAREGIVERS OF THE DYING OLDER ADULT

Although much has been published about the dying person finding hope and experiencing meaning in the dying process, little has been written about the positive aspects or opportunities for the family caregivers of a dying person. Gribich (2001) noted that caregivers of family members with terminal cancer who were able to explore issues and spend quality time with their dying relative during the terminal phase of illness felt valued and happy. Time with the dying member was considered a gift. Gribich stated, "When the patient was able to respond and to appreciate this love, much of the negative emotion experienced was alleviated and the caregiver's self-worth was heightened" (2001, p. 35). Yang and Kirshling (1992), studying caregivers of elders dying in hospice, found that caregivers' positive experiences included learning about aging and the caregiving process and "finding meaning" for themselves (p. 180).

Enyert and Burman (1999) interviewed seven in-home caregivers 6 to 12 months following the death of a family member. These family members, all of whom had had time to reflect on their caregiving experience, recognized the hardship of their caregiving, but they attributed meaning to their caregiving because it was important to the

then-dying family member. Meaning was related to the ability to "do for," to "be with," and to fulfill self-defined roles. Enyert and Burman noted a "common thread of commitment" running through the interviews (1999, p. 460). The family members indicated that the caregiving experience had created a new appreciation of "little things" and "down to life things." After the caregiving experience, these elements of life seemed to matter more. Several of the caregivers discussed a clearer sense of the relationship of human life to a higher power or God. Interviewees reported feelings of satisfaction about the caring experience that made them want to go on to help others. These positive aspects of caregiving are identified as self-transcendence.

Self-Transcendence and Finding Meaning

Self-transcendence is considered a positive developmental outcome of "going through" life-threatening experiences, such as breast cancer (Coward, 1989, 1991). Self-transcendence was first discussed by Frankl, a psychiatrist, as he described the life-affirming psychological state and behaviors that followed the experience of having been in and survived life in a Nazi concentration camp. Frankl (1963, 1966) proposed that people make meaning of their lives and events in their lives in three ways: (1) by contributing to the world, (2) by being receptive to others, and (3) by accepting inevitable life events. Thus caregivers may make meaning out of the hardships of caregiving by contributing time, energy, patience, and love; by being receptive to the needs of the ill relative; and by accepting rather than resisting and questioning the dying process.

Self-transcendence has been further described as "the expansion of one's conceptual boundaries inwardly through introspective activities, outwardly through concern about others' welfare, and temporally by integrating perceptions of one's past and future to enhance the present" (Reed, 1991, p. 5). Life events that increase awareness of personal mortality are associated with achieving this advanced level of developmental maturity. Facing and journeying through the death of a loved one is certainly an experience of mortality, an experience that provokes questions regarding the meanings in one's life as well as the meaning of one's life (O'Connor, Wicker, & Germino, 1990).

Borneman and Brown-Saltzman (2001) stated that "[t]he ability to transcend truly is a gift of the human spirit and frequently occurs after a long struggle and out of suffering. It is often unclear which comes first—does meaning open the door for transcendence, or quite the opposite, does the act of transcendence bring the meaning?" (p. 421). It is likely that, for the family caregivers of dying older adults, transcendence and finding meaning are dynamic, interrelated processes. The everyday tasks and thoughts that make up the caregiving experience come together in such a way that they are personally rewarding. Palliative care providers can maximize the rewarding aspects of caregiving by addressing the symptom management and comfort needs of the patient, by mobilizing resources to help with caregiving tasks, and by providing emotional support and education that take into consideration the socio-historical-cultural factors that impact the family's burdens and opportunities.

Culturally Sensitive Support for the Caregiver Family

Palliative care is a philosophy that provides comfort and support to patients and families while being sensitive to and respectful of their values, traditions, religious beliefs, and culture (Matzo & Sherman, 2001). Care of the dying individual and family includes supporting family members as they carry out essential end-of-life tasks. According to Cohen and Cohen (1981) and Corr (1992), these tasks include (1) physical tasks focused on bodily needs and minimizing physical distress; (2) psychological tasks including moving from denial to acceptance of the approaching death, maintaining a functional equilibrium, providing security, meeting needs for the patient's autonomy, regulating affect, and providing some richness in living; (3) social tasks involving interpersonal attachments and establishment of relationships with health care providers; and (4) spiritual tasks centered on identification, development, or reaffirmation of sources of spiritual energy and hope.

Not all families are able to complete these tasks. Some families "negotiate the bumps on the road as they encounter them," recognizing each other's gifts, respecting each other's autonomy,

dealing with differences in a positive manner, and communicating clearly and directly. Others get "stuck in the rut of conflicts," unable to find common ground (Mulder & Gregory, 2000, p. 27). Chapter 6 provides more information about family function, communication, and interaction.

Whether the family is able to carry out all the tasks or just some of them, family members face the end-of-life situation with their own particular sets of values and cultural orientation. Those values and cultural orientation impact how family members perceive the tasks to be carried out for their relative. Family members develop their own perception of what "should" be done for the dying family member according to what they have learned through experience, family stories, experts within the culture, reading, and education. Many areas of palliative care, such as pain control, feeding, informing the patient of terminal diagnosis, and mourning practices, are culturally mediated (Crawley, Marshall, Lo, & Koenig, 2002). Providing culturally sensitive palliative care can enhance caregivers' opportunities for finding meaning in the dying and death of their relative.

ENHANCEMENT OF PALLIATIVE CARE BY CONSIDERING SOCIOHISTORICAL-CULTURAL FACTORS

Consideration of sociohistorical-cultural factors is essential to palliative care. Health care providers are challenged to examine the family's and their own social, generational, and cultural differences. Palliative care providers have expertise in providing quality of life even as death approaches. Current Anglo-American theory suggests that the following components are necessary to a peaceful death: effective control of pain and other symptoms, the patient and family fully informed of the terminal illness, making time and space for intimacy, opportunities to review relationships, reconciliation of enmities, conflict resolution among family members, and saying final good-byes (Cassel & Foley, 1999; Field & Cassel, 1997; Oberst et al., 1989; Seale, 1998). However, applying any one of these components without consideration of the family's cultural needs can create dissonance and increase the burdens of caregiving.

According to Berger (1998), "Assessments of good and harm are culturally mediated" (p.

2085). How family members reflect upon and eventually come to feel about their part in the dying and death of their spouse or relative is largely impacted by whether they have fulfilled their own interpretation of their personal, social, and cultural roles. Nuland (1993) summarized this sentiment in the statement, "Death belongs to the dying and to those who love them" (p. 265).

Western society has promoted vigorous attention to individual determination, disclosure, and informed consent. Such cultural bias needs some scrutiny. For example, in Italy disclosing the diagnosis of cancer is believed to disrupt the serenity of the terminally ill, while in the Navajo culture, explicit discussion of a terminal diagnosis is thought, in some way, to cause the death (Berger, 1998; Carrese, 2000). Thus what is accepted and thought best in Anglo-American culture is viewed as rude or failing to protect the patient in other cultures.

In order to provide palliative care that will maximize family members' opportunities for growth, providers must develop both cultural sensitivity and cultural competence. Cultural sensitivity has two components: (1) the awareness of how the family culture shapes values, beliefs, and worldviews; and (2) how one's own values, beliefs, and worldview may differ from that of the family. The next step is then cultural competence, or learning about the specific cultural needs. Knowledge of specific cultural needs can be obtained from family members by displaying interest and listening, by investigating the literature, and through a cultural "insider" who understands the family's culture (Crawley et al., 2002).

CONSIDERATION OF VARIABILITY OF TRANSITIONS FROM LIFE TO DEATH

Attention to the variability in the trajectory of illness and in values held concerning the use of medical treatment near the end of life is essential. Variability in end-of-life transitions influences communications and the use of established components of palliative care practice. The communication models for end-of-life care developed over the last 30 years have focused on the cancer patient. These models may have limited application for the approximately 45% of elders who experience trajectories of disease that are charac-

terized by progressive loss of cognitive function or long-term, complex, serious chronic illness.

Elders with severe cognitive dysfunction may be unable to understand that their lives are ending, and may be unable to participate with family members in resolutions and good-byes. Although research such as that by Forbes et al. (2000) greatly enhances our understanding of the experience of these family members, new models for assisting family members to understanding the natural trajectory of severe cognitive impairment are sorely needed.

The values held by hospitalized dying elders and their families who have battled serious, complex chronic illness for years and enter the hospital expecting that medicine will once again "fix" the situation are problematic even when palliative care is provided. Arnold (2000), a hospital-based palliative care physician, pointed out that the sociohistorical-cultural association of the hospital with cure, use of technology, and control of disease (even in advanced age) interferes with dialogue about death. According to Arnold, hospitalized patients and their family members do not want to talk about death, either because they are in the hospital to get better or because they find the subject too difficult. This is consistent with what Byock (2002) referred to as secular society's symbolization of hospitals as "temples of death denial" (p. 284). Thus discussions are often put off or not accepted, and the end arrives unexpectedly, absent of resolutions and good-byes. Citing Kaufman (1998), Arnold called for a broad reconsideration of medicine's dominant role in social life, a reshaping of institutional practices and values, and a reacknowledgment of the highly variable transition process from life to death. Examining the association of the trajectory of illness with factors such as uncertainty, death anxiety, and willingness to participate in advance care planning could be fruitful. Research focused on ways to help elders and their family members with the uncertainty created by the interface of technology and health care is needed.

Case Study Conclusion

When caring for the family of the dying elder, health care providers must assess the limitations and assets of the family members involved and

EVIDENCE-BASED PRACTICE

Reference: Forbes, S., Bern-Klug, M., & Gessert, C. (2000). End-of-life decision making for nursing home residents with dementia. *Journal of Nursing Scholarship, 32*, 251-258.

Research Problem: Little is known about family surrogate decision making about end-of-life treatment by family members of nursing home residents with dementia.

Design: Descriptive, qualitative, naturalistic inquiry.

Sample and Setting: Twenty-eight family members of nursing home residents with severe dementia participated in four 2-hour focus group discussions held in four nursing home facilities.

Methods: An experienced focus group leader asked research-driven questions such as: "What is the most difficult decision you have made for your family member?" and "With regard to your family member, what does quality at the end of life mean to you?" Focus group sessions were tape-recorded, transcribed, coded, and analyzed using processes of decontextualization and recontextualization.

Results: The researchers elicited descriptions of significant emotional burdens, unrelenting guilt, an acute sense of responsibility, and the emotional turmoil of death as a tragedy versus death as a blessing. The family members discussed the pain of loss of

the relationship with the loved one and of the relative's loss of personhood. The family members were unable to conceptualize the trajectory of the dementing disease. None was able to identify that pneumonia, dysphagia, and deteriorating cognition were evidence that the end of life was approaching. Participants were unprepared to make end-of-life treatment decisions. No family member had talked with a trusted, consistent health care provider about what to expect during the last years or months of the trajectory of dementing illness.

Implications for Nursing Practice: Family members need assistance in processing difficult and painful emotions, understanding the trajectory of severe cognitive loss, and identifying what decisions might impede a natural death. They need to be aware of comfort or palliative care options. Methods to initiate advance care planning prior to the onset of dementia or with family surrogate decision makers in the nursing home setting are needed.

Conclusion: Family members of nursing home residents in this study received no education regarding the illness trajectory or expected dying process of their elderly family member with dementia. The absence of that information and carrying the guilt of being unable to care for the elder themselves, resulted in an inability to perform optimally as surrogate desision makers at the end of the life of their incapacitated relative.

---

consider the historical, social, and cultural factors that impact the burdens and opportunities of family members providing care. The prevalence of long-term serious, chronic illness and its impact on the elder and the family must be considered. The case presented at the beginning of this chapter, of the 61-year-old daughter caring for her father during the last 8 years of his life, is typical of the elder living to old age with multiple serious, chronic health problems. In the case, the father also was a long-term care provider, having taken care of his wife who was disabled by emphysema for many years. Both the father and

the daughter neglected their own health while caregiving. Additionally, both strongly valued personal independence. The need for reconciling the desire to maintain independence with the need for assistance and support from the formal health care system and from the community is dramatized in this case. Innovative ways of informing in-community needy elders and their family members of available resources, and approaches that facilitate acceptance of resources, are needed.

The sociohistorical-cultural factors in this case are not overtly dramatic. Yet consider the strong historical themes of family cohesiveness, hard work, and pursuit of "the good life." The social factors of loyalty, respect of the daughter for her father's wishes, and self-sacrifice characterized the years of caregiving. This daughter certainly was committed to her father, and she was able to "do for" and "be with." In the years of caregiving preceding his death, she carried out self-defined cultural roles. Near the end of her father's life, in the ICU, she was distressed and confused. She persisted in "doing for" and "being with" her father, and, because he could no longer speak for himself, she recognized the need to speak for him. Yet the control of caregiving had shifted to ICU health care providers and basic palliative care was absent. A team approach, advance care planning from the time of admission (or preferably years before), support concerning prognosis from physicians, attention to pain and discomfort from the nursing staff, and a visit from the chaplaincy would have benefited this daughter and her father.

The daughter's reciprocal suffering near the end of her father's life is depicted in part by the expression, "I winced every time they came to do something else to him." However, it was not her physical sense of his suffering that brought her to decide to abandon hopes for recovery and, instead, seek a peaceful death; rather, it was a shared existential suffering. She understood her father's regard for the integrity of his body and control over his body. This case demonstrates some resolution, precipitated initially by a knowledgeable friend who helped her to recognize that her father had had a good life and that hospice services were appropriate at that time. Then, in hospice, the coaching of hospice nurses facilitated her sense of closure and saying good-bye. However, it was too late for exchange of words of appreciation or for developing more clarity about the father's specific preferences. In the case presented, the daughter continued, just 2 weeks after her father's death, to have ambivalence about whether she did the right thing. She could benefit from bereavement follow-up and counseling. There is the hope that, with time, the uneasiness will be outweighed by the sense of having done all that could be done. The burdens of the daughter in this case are clearly evident; the opportunities of caregiving remain more obscure.

What meaning did the dying and death of her father hold for this daughter? She indicated that she had done "the best" that she could under the circumstances and that she did what she "needed to do." These statements suggest some fulfillment of self-defined roles. How could health care providers have better served this family? If ICU care of this elder had included just one nurse or physician who could have interpreted the father's advanced stage of serious chronic illness, and helped this daughter to realize that "death is real and there are real human limits to preventing it" (Benner, 2001, p. 358), perhaps less suffering would have occurred. In this case, despite the uncertainty often escalated by many "close calls" with death, the daughter was gradually able to face the inevitable. She reviewed the positive aspects of her father's life with a friend. If the curative agenda of the ICU had given way to a "carative" agenda, with "social space for dying" (Benner, 2001, p. 358), such as inclusion of the time-honored rituals of reminiscing and narrative reflection on the life of the dying loved one, then perhaps her decisions would be less painful and less regretted. Leaders in the critical care field have recently begun to pursue provision of palliative care in hospital and intensive care settings. ICU palliative care, using interdisciplinary teams to improve pain and symptom management, patient and family communication, and shared decision making is one of the newest types of palliative care (Curtis & Rubenfeld, 2001; Robert Wood Johnson Foundation, 2002). Palliative care has the potential to significantly decrease the burdens and to increase the possible opportunities for personal growth of patients and family members experiencing dying and death in the ICU setting.

CONCLUSION

In all settings, a careful examination of what satisfaction, psychological comfort, feeling in control, and being supported mean to the dying patient and family members must be considered (Chochinov, 2002). Each family will have its own way of dealing with dying and death; care should be consistent with the historical, social, and cultural values of the dying elder and the family members. For elders and their families, a significant part of the history is linked to the trajectory of illness. Attention to historical, social, and cultural values enhances the possibility that the family's experience of the dying and death of their loved one will be meaningful to them.

Opportunities are embedded in the process of finding meaning and transcendence. Each family ascribes their own unique meaning or importance to the notion of dying with dignity, including practical matters such as basic comfort, the tone or quality of care, and consideration of the "soul" or spirit" (Chochinov, 2002, p. 2254).

Providing comfort and support to the dying elder patient has a reciprocal and often lasting effect on the family. Dying and death are times of crisis, and, as such, they are remembered vividly by the family. Thus the palliative care provided to the patient and family, whether in the home, hospital, or nursing home, is important in the present and in the future of the family unit. Family members' experiences associated with the dying and death of a close relative can produce negative and lasting disturbances in health; or, in contrast, the experiences can become part of personal growth and contribute to the family legacy.

REFERENCES

Abate, F., & Jewell, E. (2001). *The new Oxford American dictionary*. New York: Oxford University Press.

Andershed, B., & Ternestedt, B. (2001). Development of a theoretical framework describing relatives in palliative care. *Journal of Advanced Nursing, 34*, 554-562.

Aranda, M. P. (1997). The influence of ethnicity and culture on the caregiver stress and coping process: Sociocultural review and analysis. *The Gerontologist, 37*, 342-354.

Arnold, R. M. (2000). Ambivalence and ambiguity in hospitalized critically ill patients and its relevance for palliative care. *Journal of Palliative Medicine, 3*, 23-28.

Azoulay, E., Chevret, S., Lelue, G., Pochard, F., Adrie, C., & Canoui, P. (2000). Half of intensive care unit patients experience inadequate communication with physicians. *Critical Care Medicine, 28*, 3044-3049.

Bedford, S., Melzer, D., & Guralnick, J. (2001). Problem behavior in the last year of life: Prevalence, risks, and care receipt in older Americans. *Journal of the American Geriatrics Society, 49(5)*, 590-595.

Benner, P. (2001). Death as human passage: Compassionate care for persons dying in critical care units. *American Journal of Critical Care, 10*, 355-359.

Berger, J. T. (1998). Culture and ethnicity in clinical care. *Archives of Internal Medicine, 158*, 2085-2090.

Blasi, Z., Hurley, A., & Volicer, L. (2002). End of life care in dementia: A review of problems, prospects, and solutions in practice. *Journal of the American Medical Directors Association, 3(2)*, 57-65.

Borneman, T., & Brown-Saltzman, K. (2001). Meaning in illness. In B. R. Ferrell & N. Coyle (Eds.), *Textbook of palliative nursing* (pp. 415-424). New York: Oxford University Press.

Brock, D. B., & Foley, D. J. (1998). Demography and epidemiology of dying in the U.S. with emphasis on deaths of older persons. *The Hospice Journal, 13(1-2)*, 49-60.

Buckley, W. (1967). *Sociology and modern systems theory.* Englewood Cliffs, NJ: Prentice Hall.

Bull, M., Jervis, L., & Her, M. (1995). Hospitalized elders: The difficulties families encounter. *Journal of Gerontological Nursing, 21(6)*, 19-23.

Byock, I. (1996). The nature of suffering and the nature of opportunity at the end of life. *Clinical Geriatric Medicine, 12*, 237-252.

Byock, I. (2002). The meaning and value of death. *Journal of Palliative Care, 5(2)*, 279-288.

Callahan, D. (1993). Pursuing a peaceful death. *Hastings Center Report, 4*, 33-38.

Carrese, J. (2000). Bridging cultural differences in medical practice: The case of discussing negative information with Navajo patients. *Journal of General Internal Medicine, 15*, 92-96.

Cassel, C. K., & Foley, K. M. (1999). *Principles for care of patients at the end of life: An emerging consensus among the specialties of medicine.* New York: Milbank Memorial Fund.

Cassel, E. J. (1982). The nature of suffering and the goals of medicine. *New England Journal of Medicine, 306*, 640-645.

Cassel, E. J. (1991). Recognizing suffering. *Hastings Center Report, 15(2)*, 24-31.

Center for Gerontology and Health Care Research. (2000, August 31). *Brown atlas of dying–site of death: 1989-1997. Retrieved June 6, 2002, from the Brown Medical School Web site: http://www.chcr.brown.edu/dying/brownatlas.htm*

Chochinov, H. M. (2002). Dignity-conserving care—a new model for palliative care: Helping the patient feel valued. *Journal of the American Medical Association, 287*, 2253-2260.

Clipp, E. C., & George, L. K. (1993). Dementia and cancer: A comparison of spouse and caregivers. *The Gerontologist, 33*, 534-541.

Cohen, M., & Cohen, E. (1981). Behavioral family systems intervention in terminal care. In H. Sobel (Ed.), *Behavior therapy in terminal care: A humanistic approach.* Cambridge, MA: Ballinger.

Corr, C. A. (1992). A task-based approach to coping with dying. *Omega–Journal of Death and Dying, 24*, 81-94.

Coward, D. D. (1989). The lived experience of self-transcendence in women with advanced breast cancer. *Nursing Science Quarterly, 3*, 162-169.

Coward, D. D. (1991). Self-transcendence and emotional well-being in women with advanced breast cancer. *Oncology Nursing Forum, 18*, 857-863.

Crawley , L., Marshall, P., Lo, B., & Koenig, B. (2002). Strategies for culturally effective end-of-life care. *Annals of Internal Medicine, 136(9) supplement*, 673-679.

Curtis, J. R., & Rubenfeld, G. D. (2001). *Managing death in the intensive care unit: The transition from care to comfort.* New York: Oxford University Press.

Davies, B. (2001). Supporting families in palliative care. In B. R. Ferrell & N. Coyle (Eds.), *Textbook of palliative nursing* (pp. 363-373). New York: Oxford Press.

Davies, B., Reimer, J. C., & Martens, N. (1994). Family functioning and its implications for palliative care. *Journal of Palliative Care, 10*(3), 29-36.

Doka, K. J. (1993). *Living with life-threatening illness: A guide for patients, their family and caregivers.* Lexington, MA: Lexington Books.

Dunne, K., & Sullivan, K. (2000). Family experiences of palliative care in the acute hospital setting. *International Journal of Palliative Nursing, 6*(4), 170-178.

Emanuel, L., Barry M., Stoeckle, L., & Emanuel, E. (1991). Advance directives for medical care: A case for greater use. *New England Journal of Medicine, 324,* 889-895.

Enyert, G., & Burman, M. (1999). A qualitative study of self-transcendence in caregivers of terminally ill patients. *American Journal of Hospice & Palliative Care, 16,* 455-462.

Faulkner, A. (1998). ABC of palliative care: Communication with patients, families, and other professionals. *British Medical Journal, 316,* 130-132.

Field, M. J., & Cassel, C. K. (Eds.). (1997). *Approaching death: Improving care at the end of life* (Committee on Care at the End of Life, Division of Health Care Services, Institute of Medicine). Washington DC: National Academy Press.

Forbes, S. (2001). This is heaven's waiting room: End of life in one nursing home. *Journal of Gerontological Nursing,* 37-45.

Forbes, S., Bern-Klug, M., & Bessert, C. (2000). End-of-life decision making for nursing home residents with dementia. *Journal of Nursing Scholarship, 32,* 251-258.

Frankl, V. (1959). *Man's search for meaning: An introduction to logotherapy* (3rd ed.). New York: Simon & Schuster.

Frankl, V. (1966). Self-transcendence as a human phenomenon. *Journal of Humanistic Psychology, 6,* 97-106.

Fried, T. R., van Doorn, C., O'Leary, J. R., Tinetti, M. E., & Drickamer, M. A. (1999). Older persons' preferences for site of terminal care. *Annals of Internal Medicine, 132,* 419.

Gillis, C. L. (1991). Family nursing research, theory and practice. *Image: Journal of Nursing Scholarship, 23,* 19-22.

Grady, P. (1999) Improving care at the end of life: Research issues. *Journal of Hospice and Palliative Nursing , 1*(4), 151-155.

Grbich, C. (2001). The emotional and coping strategies of caregivers of family members with a terminal cancer. *Journal of Palliative Care, 17*(1), 30-36.

Gunten, C. F. von (2002). Secondary and tertiary palliative care in US hospitals. *Journal of the American Medical Association, 28,* 875-881.

Happ, M. B., Capezuti, E., Strumpf, N., Wagner, L., Cunningham, S., Evans, L., et al. (2002). Advance care planning and end-of-life care for hospitalized nursing home residents. *Journal of the American Geriatrics Society, 50,* 829-835.

Hileman, K., Lackey, N., & Hassanein, R. (1992). Identifying the needs of home caregivers of patients with cancer. *Oncology Nursing Forum, 19,* 771-777.

Jones, P., & Martinson, I. (1992). The experience of bereavement in caregivers of family members with Alzheimer's disease. *Image: Journal of Nursing Scholarship, 24,* 172-176.

Kaufman, S. R. (1998). Intensive care, old age, and the problem of death in America. *The Gerontologist, 38,* 715-725.

Kenny, N. P. (1997). Ethical implications of human suffering. *Humane Health Care, 13*(2), 27-30.

Kissane, D. W., Bloch, S., Burns, W. I., Mckenzie, D. P., & Posterino, M. (1994). Psychological morbidity in families of care recipients with cancer. *Psycho-oncology, 3,* 47-56.

Kissane, D., Spruyt, O., & Aranda, S. (2000). Palliative care: New approaches to the problem of suffering. *Australian and New Zealand Journal of Medicine, 30,* 377-384.

Kruse, A. (1991). Caregivers coping with chronic disease, dying and death of an aged family member. *Reviews in Clinical Gerontology, 1,* 411-415.

Larson, D. G., & Tobin, D. R. (2000). End-of-life conversations: Evolving practice and theory. *Journal of the American Medical Association, 284,* 1573-1578.

Lilly, C. M., DeMeo, D. L., Sonna, L. A., Haley, K. J., Massaro, A. F., Wallace, R. F., et al. (2000). An intensive communication intervention for the critically ill. *American Journal of Medicine, 109,* 469-475.

Lynn, J. (2000). Learning to care for people with chronic illness facing the end of life. *Journal of the American Medical Association, 284,* 2508-2511.

Lynn, J. (2001). Serving patients who may die soon and their families: The role of hospice and other services. *Journal of the American Medical Association, 285,* 925-932.

Lynn, J., & Forlini, J. H. (2001). "Serious and complex illness" in quality improvement and policy reform for end-of-life care. *Journal of General Internal Medicine, 16,* 315-319.

Matzo, M. L., & Sherman, D. W. (2001). Palliative care nursing: Ensuring competent care at the end of life. *Geriatric Nursing, 22,* 288-293.

Mulder, J., & Gregory, D. (2000). Transforming experience into wisdom: Healing amidst suffering. *Journal of Palliative Care, 16*(2), 25-29.

National Hospice and Palliative Care Organization. (2002, August). *Facts and figures on hospice care in America.* Retrieved September 2, 2002 from http://www.nhpco.org/public/articles/coo1.doc

Navaie-Waliser, M., Feldman, P., Gould, D., Levine, C., Kuerbis, A., & Donelan, K. (2002). When the caregiver needs care: Plight of vulnerable caregivers. *American Journal of Public Health, 92,* 409-413.

Nuland, S. B. (1993). *How we die: Reflections on life's final chapter.* New York: Knopf.

Oberst, M. T., Thomas, S. I., Gass, K. A., & Ward, S. E. (1989). Caregiving demands and appraisal of stress among family caregivers. *Cancer Nursing, 12,* 209-215.

O'Connor, K. A., Wicker, C., & Germino, B. (1990). Understanding the cancer patient's search for meaning. *Cancer Nursing, 13,* 167-175.

Quill, T. (2002). In-hospital end of life services: Is the cup 2/3 empty or 1/3 full. *Medical Care, 40*(1), 4-6.

Rando, T. A. (1993). *Treatment of complicated mourning.* Champaign, IL: Research Press.

Rando, T. (2000). *Clinical dimensions of anticipatory mourning.* Champaign, IL: Research Press.

Reed, P. (1991). Self-transcendence and mental health in oldest-old adults. *Nursing Research, 40,* 5-11.

Reilly, R. V., Teasdale, T. M., & McCullough, L. B. (1994). Projecting patients' preferences from living wills: An invalid strategy for management of dementia with life-threatening illness. *Journal of the American Geriatrics Society, 42,* 997-1003.

Rier, D. A. (2000). The missing voice of the critically ill: A medical sociologist's first-hand account. *Social Health, 22,* 251-259.

Robert Wood Johnson Foundation. (2002, September). Retrieved September 2, 2002 from the Promoting Excellence in End-of-Life Care Web site: http://www.promotingexcellence.org/content/critical_care.html

Robinson-Whelen, S., Yuri, T., MacCallum, R., McGuire, L., & Kiecolt-Glaser, J. K. (2001). Long-term caregiving: What happens when it ends. *Journal of Abnormal Psychology, 110,* 573-584.

Rose, K. (1998). Perceptions related to time in a qualitative study of informal carers of terminally ill cancer patients. *Journal of Clinical Nursing, 7,* 343-350.

Roy, D. J. (1998). Waiting for the unexpected. *Journal of Palliative Care, 14*(4), 3-4.

Saunders, D. C. (1982). Principles of symptom control in terminal care. *Medical Clinics of North America, 66,* 1169-1183.

Scharlach, A. E., Midanik, L. T, Runkle, M. C., & Soghikian, K. (1997). Health practices of adults with elder care responsibilities. *Preventative Medicine, 26,* 342-354.

Schulz, R., Beach, S., Lind, B., Martire, L., Zdaniuk, V., Hirsch, C., et al. (2001). Involvement in caregiving and adjustment to death of a spouse: Findings from the Caregiver Health Effects Study. *Journal of the American Medical Association, 285,* 3123-3129.

Seale, C. (1998). Theories in health care and research: Theories and studying the care of dying people. *British Medical Journal, 317,* 1518-1520.

Semour, J. (1999). Revisiting medicalization and natural death. *Social Science and Medicine, 49,* 691-704.

Sherman, D. W. (1998). Reciprocal suffering: The need to improve family caregivers' quality of life through palliative care. *Journal of Palliative Medicine, 1,* 357-366.

Steeves, E., & Kahn, D. (1987). Experience of meaning in suffering. *Image: Journal of Nursing Scholarship, 19,* 114-116.

Steinhauser, K. E., Christakis, N. A., Clipp, E. D., McNeilly, M., McIntyre, L., & Tulsky, J. (2000). Factors considered important at the end of life by patients, family, physicians, and other care providers. *Journal of the American Medical Association, 284,* 2476-2482.

Stets, K. M. (1989). The relationship among background characteristics, purpose in life and caregiving demands on perceived health of spouse caregivers. *Scholarly Inquiry in Nursing Practice, 3,* 133-153.

SUPPORT Principal Investigators. (1995). A controlled trial to improve care for seriously ill hospitalized patients: The Study to Understand Prognoses and Preferences for Outcomes and Risks of Treatment. *Journal of the American Medical Association, 274,* 1591-1598.

Swigart, V. A. (1995). Recognizing and respecting family judgment. *The Journal of Clinical Ethics, 6,* 85-87.

Swigart, V., Lidz, C., Butterworth, V., & Arnold, R. (1996). Letting go: Family decisions to forgo life support. *Heart and Lung: The Journal of Critical Care, 25,* 483-494.

Swigart, V., Lidz, C., Butterworth, V., & Arnold, R. (1998). [Family member interviews]. Unpublished raw data.

Teno, J. M. (1997). Do advance directives provide instructions that direct care? *Journal of American Geriatrics Society, 45,* 508-512.

Teno, J. M. (2002). Now is the time to embrace nursing homes as a place of care for dying persons. *Innovations in End of Life Care, 4*(2), 1-3.

Teno, J., Casey, V. A., & Edgeman-Leviton, S. (2001). Patient-focused, family-centered end-of-life medical care. *Journal of Pain and Symptom Management, 22,* 738-751.

Teno, J. M., Weitzen, S., Fennell, M., & Mor, V. (2001). Dying trajectory in the last year of life: Does cancer trajectory fit other diseases. *Journal of Palliative Medicine, 4,* 457-464.

Teno, J. M., Weitzen, S., Wetle, T., & Mor, V. (2001). Persistent pain in nursing home residents. *Journal of the American Medical Association, 285,* 2081.

Tilden, V. P., Tolle, S. W., Nelson, C. A., & Fields, J. (2001). Family decision-making to withdraw life-sustaining treatments from hospitalized patients. *Nursing Research, 50,* 105-115.

Tilden, V. P., Tolle, S. W., Nelson, C. A., Thompson, M., & Eggman, S. C. (1999). Family decision making in foregoing life extending treatments. *Journal of Family Nursing, 4,* 426-442.

Tolle, S. W., Tilden, V. P., Rosenfeld, A. G., & Hickman, S. E. (2000). Family reports of barriers to optimal care of the dying. *Nursing Research, 49,* 310-317.

Wros, P. (1994). The ethical context of nursing care of the dying patients in critical care. In P. Benner (Ed.), *Interpretive phenomenology: Embodiment, caring and ethics in health and illness* (pp. 255-277). Thousand Oaks, CA: Sage.

Yang, C., & Kirschling, J. (1992). Exploration of factors related to direct care and outcomes of caregiving: Caregivers of terminally ill older persons. *Cancer Nursing, 15,* 173-181.

9

SUFFERING, LOSS, GRIEF, AND BEREAVEMENT

Robert L. Arnold and Kathleen Egan

INTRODUCTION

Change and loss as a result of illness and death are a part of our experience as humans. A person's ability to adapt to these changes often underscores how he or she has lived. Is the end of life perceived as a natural part of one's life, or is it viewed as unnatural or abnormal? Is it viewed as a time of growth and transition, or as dysfunctional and depressing? The manner in which one approaches end-of-life issues will determine one's experience with this transition. This is true of all persons involved, including patients, families, health care professionals, and nurses.

Older adults bring exciting challenges and wonderful opportunities to nurses providing end-of-life care. A lifetime of experiences shape a patient's thoughts, feelings, attitudes, and perceptions. Sensitivity to these factors in concert with content knowledge and skill development provide nurses with a unique opportunity to provide care that is patient and family directed and meets the physical, psychosocial, and spiritual needs of older adults and their families at the end of life.

SUFFERING, LOSS, GRIEF, AND BEREAVEMENT: EFFECTS ON PATIENTS, FAMILIES, AND NURSES

Grief is a process. Each survivor and professional caregiver experiences grief in his or her own way. Coping skills are developed and used in accordance with one's own cultural norms, belief systems, faith systems, and life experiences. Grief begins before the death for the patient, family, and significant others as they anticipate and experience a variety of losses. Grief continues for the survivors with the death of the patient. The grief process is not always orderly and predictable,

and it usually includes a series of stages and/or tasks that a person moves through to help resolve grief (Table 9-1). This is sometimes referred to as "grief work" (Lindemann, 1994). No one really "gets over" a loss, but we can heal and learn to live with a loss and/or live without the deceased.

Early definitions of grief suggested that it is primarily an emotional response to a loss, is individualized, and includes the personalized feelings and responses that are experienced regarding real or anticipated loss (Despelder & Strickland, 1987; Doka, 1989). New thought posits that grief is an "interdimensional experience" that involves a person's mind, heart, body, and spirit (Arnold & Eagan, 2002). When change and loss as a result of illness and death are experienced, one's thought processes (intrapersonal) and affective (emotional), interpersonal (social), physical (body), and functional (activities of daily living) aspects are all influenced.

Suffering is defined as "the condition of tolerating or enduring evil, injury, pain or death or the source of pain or distress." Cassell (1991) defined suffering as "the state of severe distress associated with events that threaten the intactness of a person" (p. 33). Suffering impacts the person's mind and spirit, as well as his or her body; much suffering occurs in the absence of physical pain. Suffering may be acute or chronic. Acute suffering may emerge from a sudden critical event that is being experienced. Chronic suffering may be experienced as a result of a life-changing event that has long-term consequences for an individual.

Loss is defined as the absence of a possession or future possession (Corless, 2001). The value of the possession is determined by, and unique to, the person experiencing the loss. Losses are expe-

Table 9-1 **Stages and Tasks of Grief**		
Stage of Grief	Tasks	Characteristics
Stage 1: Notification and shock	Share acknowledgment of the reality of the loss by assessing the loss, recognizing the loss	• Assists the survivor in coping with the initial impact of the death • Survivor may have feelings of numbness, difficulties with decision making, poor daily functioning, emotional outbursts, denial, isolation, avoidance • Feelings should eventually decrease and subside as the survivor moves onto the next stage
Stage 2: Experience the loss emotionally and cognitively	Share in the process of working through the pain by reacting to, expressing, and experiencing the pain of separation/grief	• Confrontation, anger, bargaining, depression • Survivor may be angry at loved one who has died, "abandoned them," "left them behind"; anger may be directed at physician, nurse, other health care professionals, family members, friends • Survivor may feel guilt based on perceptions that he or she, or others, did not do enough to prevent the death, he or she did not take good enough care of the deceased • Survivor may ask questions: "What if . . ."; "If only . . ." • Survivor may experience sadness, loneliness, emptiness, lack of interest in daily life, insomnia, loss of or increase in appetite, apathy, disorganization
Stage 3: Reintegration	Reorganize and restructure family systems and relationships and reinvest in other relationships and life pursuits by adjusting to an environment without the deceased, relinquishing old attachments, forming new identity without deceased, adapting to new role while retaining memories	• Survivor may begin to reorganize his or her life, find hope in the future, feel more energetic, participate in social events, read acceptance

Sources: Corless, I. B. (2001). Bereavement. In B. R. Ferrell, & N. Coyle. (Eds.). *Textbook of palliative nursing care.* New York: Oxford University Press; Kübler-Ross, R. (1969). *On death and dying.* New York: MacMillan; Rando, T. A. (1984). *Grief, dying and death: clinical interventions for caregivers.* Champaign, Ill: Research Press; Worden, J. W. (1991). *Grief counseling and grief therapy: a handbook for the mental health practitioner* (2nd ed.). New York: Springer Press.

rienced in daily life, such as through divorce or children leaving home. Feelings of loss may also occur before a death. These feelings may be present for the patient, family, and significant others as they anticipate future losses. These losses may include declining health, changes in or loss of autonomy, role changes, and the loss of life. Most losses will trigger mourning and grief and accompanying feelings, behaviors, and reactions to the loss.

Mourning is the outward social expression of a loss (Corless, 2001). How a person outwardly expresses a loss may be dictated by cultural norms, customs, and practices, including rituals and traditions. Some cultures may be very emotional and verbal in their expression of loss, wailing or crying loudly, whereas others may show little reaction to loss, appearing stoic and business-like. Religious and cultural beliefs may also dictate how long one mourns and how the survivor "should" act during the bereavement period. In addition, outward expression of loss may be influenced by the individual's personality and life experiences.

Bereavement involves grief and mourning and includes the inner feelings and outward reactions of a person. It is often said that a person surviving a death has a "bereavement period." This may be the time it takes for a person to feel the pain of loss, mourn, grieve, and adjust to a world without the physical, psychological, and social presence of the deceased.

It is the nurse's responsibility to be aware of the cultural characteristics of grief and mourning for patients, family members, and significant others for whom they care. Many resources, including books, Internet sites, local churches, cultural associations, and clubs, can assist in cultural education. Asking the patient, family, and significant others directly about their culture and customs can create an understanding regarding cultural behaviors, reactions, rites, rituals, and traditions surrounding loss, grief, mourning, death, and the afterlife (Geissler, 1994; Lipson, Dibble, & Minarik, 1996).

TYPES OF GRIEF

The nurse should identify the type of grief experienced by the patient and family members, based on characteristics and signs/symptoms of grief, to be able to implement appropriate bereavement interventions (Table 9-2). Types of grief include anticipatory grief, normal grief, and complicated grief. Complicated grief has identified subtypes: chronic grief, delayed grief, exaggerated grief, and masked grief. In addition, there are special considerations for children (children's grief) (Wolfelt, 1990) and for persons faced with social sanction and stigma surrounding illness and death.

Anticipatory Grief

Anticipatory grief occurs before a loss in association with the diagnosis, acute and chronic illness, and terminal illness as experienced by the patient, family, and caregivers. These feelings and perceptions include fear regarding the actual or potential loss of health, loss of independence, loss of a body part, loss of financial stability, loss of choice, and loss of mental function.

Experiencing anticipatory grief may be helpful and provides time for preparation for loss, acceptance of loss, finishing unfinished business, life review, and conflict resolution. For survivors, anticipatory grief provides time for preparing for life without the deceased, including preparation for role change and mastering life skills.

For older adults, it is clear that these feelings and perceptions may be a part of everyday life as a consequence of the aging process. The natural changes in a person's physical, cognitive, and social status as he or she ages may trigger increased fear and anxiety about the future. Add to this the rendering of a life-limiting diagnosis, and the potential for triggering anticipatory grief reactions increases exponentially.

Normal Grief

Normal grief is present when feelings, behaviors, and reactions to a loss are consistent with expectations of a person's experience, culture, social role, and relationship with the deceased. Normal grief reactions to a loss can be physical, emotional, cognitive, and behavioral (Box 9-1).

In older adults, the assessment of normal grief reactions must be placed in an interdimensional context (Arnold & Egan, 2002; Egan, 2000). Assessment must evaluate the individual along physical, functional, intra- and interpersonal, and spiritual dimensions. Paramount is the assessment of the older adult's loss history, current support systems, and long-term coping strategies. When assisting older adults with change and loss as a result of illness and death, understanding what is "normal" for them is paramount. Respecting their wishes and their ways of coping is a gentle and respectful method of care (Table 9-3).

Complicated Grief

Risk factors for complicated grief include sudden or traumatic death, suicide, homicide, a

Table 9-2 **Types of Grief**

Type of Grief	Definition	Characteristics
Anticipatory Grief (Rando, 2000; Evans, 2001)	Anticipated and real losses associated with diagnosis, acute and chronic illnesses, and terminal illness. Experiencing anticipatory grief may provide time for preparation for loss, acceptance of loss, finishing unfinished business, life review, and resolving conflicts. For survivor, anticipatory grief provides time for preparing for life without deceased, including preparation for role change, mastering life skills such as paying bills and learning how to manage a checkbook.	With acute illness, chronic illness, accidents, and other changes in health, a patient may experience loss of general health, loss of functionality, loss of independence, loss of role in the family (breadwinner, caregiver), and loss of lifestyle as a result of dietary or activity restrictions. Loss of a limb or body part (breast, uterus) may cause loss of self-confidence, changes in perception about body image. Family members, significant others will also experience losses when patient is ill, including loss of role in the family, loss of relationship, loss of finances, loss of security, loss of companionship, loss of relationship. AIDS can cause multiple losses over short periods of time, such as loss of a job, material possessions, body image as a result of changes in physical appearance, functionality, privacy (the secret is out), friends, partners, and social acceptance. With diagnosis of terminal illness, additional losses may include loss of control (choice), loss of physical and/or mental function, loss of relationships, loss of body image, loss of future, loss of dignity, loss of life.
Normal Grief (Doka, 1989; Parkes, 1999; Worden, 1991)	Also known as uncomplicated grief. Normal feelings, reactions and behaviors to a loss; grief reactions can be physical, psychological, cognitive, behavioral.	Reactions to loss can be physical, psychological, and cognitive.
Complicated Grief		Those at risk for any of the four types of complicated grief may have experienced loss associated with
Chronic Grief	Normal grief reactions that do not subside and continue over very long periods of time.	• traumatic death • sudden, unexpected death such as heart attacks, accidents • suicide
Delayed Grief	Normal grief reactions that are suppressed or postponed. The survivor consciously or unconsciously avoids the pain of the loss.	• homicide • dependent relationship with deceased • old-old person or those with chronic illnesses (survivor may have difficulty believing death actually occurred after years of remissions and exacerbations)
Exaggerated Grief	Survivor resorts to self-destructive behaviors such as suicide.	• death of a child • multiple losses • unresolved grief from prior losses
Masked Grief (Brown-Saltzman, 1998; Corless, 2001; Loney,	The survivor is not aware that behaviors that interfere with normal functioning are a result of the loss.	• concurrent stressor (the loss plus other stresses in life, such as divorce, a move, children leaving home, other ill family members, financial issues)

Table 9-2 **Types of Grief—cont'd**

Type of Grief	Definition	Characteristics
Masked Grief—cont'd 1998; Parkes, 1999; Worden, 1991)		• history of mental illness or substance abuse • patient's dying process was difficult, including poor pain and symptom management, psychosocial and/or spiritual suffering • poor or few support systems • no faith system, cultural traditions, religious beliefs Complicated grief reactions can include any of the normal grief reactions, but the reactions may be intensified, prolonged, last more than a year, and/or interfere with the person's psychological, social, and physiologic functioning. Other complicated grief reactions may include: • severe isolation • violent behavior • suicidal ideation • workaholic behavior • severe deterioration of functional status • symptoms of post-traumatic stress disorder • denial beyond normal expectation • severe or prolonged depression • loss of interest in health and/or personal care • severe impairment in communication, thought, or motor skills • ongoing inability to eat or sleep • replacing loss and relationship quickly • social withdrawal • searching and calling out for deceased • avoidance of reminders of the deceased • imitating the deceased Survivors experiencing complicated grief should be referred to a grief and bereavement specialist/counselor.
Disenfranchised Grief (Doka, 1989)	The grief encountered when a loss is experienced and cannot be openly acknowledged, socially sanctioned, or publicly shared. Usually employers do not recognize survivor experiencing disenfranchised grief for time off for funeral/memorial service, grief. May not be recognized by biologic family members and may be excluded from rites, rituals, and traditions for loss.	Those at risk for experiencing disenfranchised grief include partners of HIV/AIDS patients, ex-spouses, ex-partners, fiancé(e)s, friends, lovers, mistresses, co-workers, children experiencing the death of a step-parent, and others persons close to the patient but not biologic family members. The mother of a stillborn infant may also experience disenfranchised grief because society may not acknowledge a relationship between the mother and a child who experienced death prior to birth.

AIDS, acquired immunodeficiency syndrome; *HIV*, human immunodeficiency virus.

Sources: Doka, K. (1989). Grief. In R. Kastenbaum & B. Kastenbaum. (Eds.) *Encyclopedia of death* (p. 127). Phoenix: The Oryx Press; Parkes, C. M. (1999). *Bereavement: studies of grief in adult life*. London: Tavistock; Worden, J. W. (1991). *Grief counseling and grief therapy: A handbook for the mental health practitioner* (2nd ed.). New York: Springer Press; Corless, I. B. (2001). Bereavement. In B. R. Ferrell & N. Coyle. (Eds.). *Textbook of palliative nursing care*. New York: Oxford University Press; Brown-Saltzman, K. (1998). Transforming the grief process. In R. Carroll-Johnson, L. Gorman, & N. J. Bush. *Psychosocial nursing care: along the cancer continuum*. Pittsburgh: Oncology Nursing Press, Inc.

Box 9-1 **Normal Grief Reactions**

Physical	Emotional	Cognitive	Behavioral
• Hollowness in stomach	• Numbness	• Disbelief state of	• Impaired work
• Tightness in chest	• Relief	depersonalization	performance
• Heart palpitations	• Emancipation	• Confusion	• Crying
• Sensitivity to noise	• Sadness	• Inability to	• Withdrawal
• Breathlessness	• Yearning	concentrate	• Avoiding reminders of
• Weakness	• Anxiety	• Idealization of the	the deceased
• Tension	• Fear	deceased	• Seeking or carrying
• Lack of energy	• Anger	• Preoccupation with	reminders of the deceased
• Dry mouth	• Guilt and	thoughts or image	• Overreactivity
• Gastrointestinal	self-reproach	of the deceased	• Changed relationships
disturbances	• Shame	• Dreams of the deceased	
• Loss of libido	• Loneliness	• Sense of presence	
• Increase or loss of	• Helplessness	of deceased	
appetite	• Hopelessness	• Fleeting tactile, olfactory,	
• Weight gain or loss	• Abandonment	visual, and auditory	
• Exhaustion	• Loss of control	hallucinatory experiences	
• Tight throat	• Emptiness	• Search for meaning in	
• Vulnerable to illness	• Despair	life and death	
• Restlessness	• Ambivalence		
• Headaches	• Loss of ability		
• Dizziness	for pleasure		
• Muscle aches	• Shock		
• Sexual impotency			
• Insomnia			
• Tremors, shakes			

Sources: Doka, K. (1989). Grief. In R. Kastenbaum & B. Kastenbaum. (Eds.). *Encyclopedia of death* (p. 127). Phoenix: The Oryx Press; Parkes, C. M. (1999). *Bereavement: studies of grief in adult life*. London: Tavistock; Worden, J. W. (1991). *Grief counseling and grief therapy: a handbook for the mental health practitioner* (2nd ed.). New York: Springer Press.

dependent relationship with the deceased, chronic illness, the death of a child, experiencing multiple losses, unresolved grief from prior losses, concurrent stressors, experiencing a difficult dying process (e.g., one marked by pain and suffering), lack of support systems, and crises of faith. Complicated grief reactions may include severe isolation, violent behavior, suicidal ideation, workaholic behavior, severe or prolonged depression, replacing the loss and relationships quickly, searching and calling out for the deceased, avoidance of reminders of the deceased, or imitating the deceased. Four types of complicated grief have been identified: chronic grief, delayed grief, exaggerated grief, and masked grief.

Chronic grief is characterized by normal grief reactions that do not subside and continue over very long periods of time (Worden, 1991). For older adults, this may be assessed through listening to their stories of past losses and how they have adjusted to the loss. If their expressions of grief have become part of an everyday pattern for months or even years, intervention may be required. Often older adults identify or define themselves by their losses. Their identities may be based on being a victim instead of a survivor. Titles such as "widow" are often embraced and support chronic grief in older adults.

Delayed grief is characterized by normal grief reactions that are suppressed or postponed as the

Table 9-3 **Interdimensional Assessment of Grief**				
Physical	Functional	Interpersonal	Intrapersonal	Spiritual
Appetite	Activities of daily	Relationships	Mood	Beliefs
Sleeping patterns	living	Family roles	Stress level	Hope
Energy level	Personal hygiene	Social status	Concentration	Search for
Sexual function	Mobility/	Social skills	Thoughts on	understanding
Blood pressure	transportaion	Communication	dying, death,	Search for purpose
Digestive	Economic status	skills	life, living	and meaning
processes	Productivity at		Focus on health	Need to ask "the
General health	work or school		Sense of self,	big" questions
			identity	

survivor consciously or unconsciously avoids the pain of the loss (Worden, 1991). Often delayed grief is supported by one's real or perceived role in a family system. For older adults, being perceived as the person who is wise, philosophical, strong, or comforting to others may place that person in a role that focuses on others and not him- or herself. Similarly, in situations where older adults may need to adapt to a new financial plan, home, or role, and/or learn new tasks as a part of everyday living, the introduction of these changes may put their grief on hold. Often older persons experiencing delayed grief will begin to process their feelings when their life begins to settle into a new pattern.

Exaggerated grief is present when a person resorts to self-destructive behavior (Worden, 1991). In these cases, unhealthy coping strategies are adopted to ease emotional and spiritual pain. The abuse of drugs and alcohol, engaging in unsafe sex, and the expression of suicidal ideation and suicide attempts are all examples of exaggerated grief. In older adults, it is important to assess for these psychological and behavioral symptoms. Often they are brought about by great stress and anxiety relative to a diagnosis, decline, or death. It is also important to understand the history of the older adult. If there is a history of depression, substance abuse, and/or suicide attempts, it is important to create an environment of safety by including the resources and support of an interdisciplinary team. Bringing resources together can help to ensure safety.

Masked grief is present when a person is not aware that the behaviors in which he or she is engaging interfere with normal functioning and are a result of a loss (Worden, 1991). In older adults, masked grief may present itself in the form of overcommitment to work or volunteer activities. These create distractions, and the elder may work intensely beyond expected parameters; often this creates tension in his or her personal life. Stable relationships begin to fail, and this unintentionally compounds the sense of loss. In contrast, some elders become overly dependent. This condition is driven by a fear of isolation, feelings of helplessness, and a fear of separation from loved ones. Such dependent behavior can strain existing relationships as well, spawning rejection or enabling behavior within a person's social support system. Nurses can help the elder recognize the symptoms of masked grief and offer options that create balance and support empowerment.

Disenfranchised Grief

Disenfranchised grief is encountered when a loss is experienced and cannot be openly acknowledged, socially sanctioned, or publicly shared (Doka, 1989). Those at risk include partners of patients with ex-spouses, ex-partners, fiancé(e)s, friends, lovers, mistresses, and co-workers.

For older adults, systems supporting disenfranchisement may have been present for years and may be compounded by present life events.

For older adults who become separated from family, friends, and community as a result of placement in an assisted living facility or nursing home, participation in the rites and rituals that honor the life, and acknowledge the death, of significant others may be restricted. Similarly, in our mobile society, distance and travel expenses may inhibit participation in funerals and memorials services.

Many older adults also form deep, loving relationships later in life and choose not marry because of the economic constraints related to retirement benefits. Often participation of the partner in end-of-life decisions is restricted because of this lack of legal relationship. He or she may be left out of health care decisions, funeral planning, and ongoing participation in the deceased's family system. Feelings of anger, sadness, and isolation are common in persons experiencing this type of disenfranchised grief. Nurses can assist by validating the person's loss, acknowledging the relationship, and providing opportunities to honor the memory of the loved one.

THEORIES OF GRIEF

Many theorists have developed models of grief, most of which include a series of stages that describe the cognitive, emotional, and spiritual status of the grieving person. Included in each stage is a series of identified tasks (Table 9-4). Successful completion of these tasks assists in adaptation to life without the deceased (Corless, 2001; Kübler-Ross, 1969; Rando, 1984). Competing theories use different language to describe the stages and tasks of grief. However, most models include some shared concepts, generally comprising three stages: (1) notification

Table 9-4 Theoretical Stages and Tasks of Grief

Kübler-Ross' (1969)	Parkes' Stages (1987)	Bowlby's Stages (1980)	Wordon's Tasks (1991)	Rando's Process of Bereavement (1993)
1. Denial	1. Alarm	1. Numbing	1. Accept reality of the loss	1. Recognize the loss and death
2. Anger	2. Searching	2. Searching & longing	2. Experience the pain of grief	2. React to, experience, and express the separation and pain
3. Bargaining	3. Mitigation	3. Disorganization & despair	3. Adjust to an environment without the deceased	3. Reminisce
4. Depression	4. Anger & guilt	4. Reorganization	4. Withdraw emotional energy and reinvest in another relationship	4. Relinquish old attachments
5. Acceptance	5. Gaining a new identity			5. Readjust and adapt to the new role while maintaining memories, and form a new identity.
				6. Reinvest

Source: Rando, T. A. (1999). *Clinical dimensions of anticipatory mourning: Theory and practice in working with the dying, their loved ones, and caregivers.* Champaign, IL: Research Press.

and shock, (2) experiencing the loss emotionally and cognitively, and (3) reintegration into life without the deceased.

The tasks of stage 1 (*shock and notification*) include sharing and acknowledging of the reality of the loss and recognizing the loss. A person may experience feelings of numbness, shock, poor daily functioning, isolation, and avoidance of the topic. This may occur at the time of diagnosis, during a major decline, or at the time of death.

In older adults, it is important to provide support based on their reactions to the loss. Providing too much information or using complex language may exacerbate the feelings of being shocked and overwhelmed; much of the detailed information may be ignored or forgotten. Nurses can assist by being honest, gentle, and patient. Important information may need to be written down in print large enough for the elder to see, repeated, or presented at a time of decreased emotion. It is also important to assess for patient and family support persons during this time of loss and change. The nurse should identify support that will focus on the health and safety of the older adult during this period of shock.

The tasks of stage 2 (*experiencing the loss emotionally and cognitively*) include sharing in the process of working through the pain of the loss. Dying patients must adjust to the reality of their illness and death. Family members and significant others may feel anger at the elder who is ill or has died. They may express feelings of isolation and abandonment. Anger may be directed at physicians, nurses, family, friends, God, and oneself. Feelings of guilt are often based on perceptions and personal choices that may have influenced the present state of affairs—for example, a person who smoked cigarettes may be dying of cancer or lung disease, or a substance abuser may now have liver disease; or a person who did not take time to call or visit may experience feelings of guilt and regret for his or her past actions.

Other feelings typical of this stage include, but are not limited to, sadness, loneliness, emptiness, and reduced interest in daily life and pleasurable activities. Behavioral changes may include insomnia, changes in appetite, being distracted, and a general sense of disorganization. This may also be a time when issues of a religious or spiritual nature may emerge. Questions of faith, purpose, and transcendence may be examined at this time.

In older adults, this stage is important; it is a time to sort out thoughts and feelings. Support and assistance during this stage can promote healing and growth at the end of life. Nurses can facilitate this process by listening, validating feelings, and providing realistic and positive guidance.

The tasks of stage 3 (*reintegration*) include the reorganization and restructure of family systems and relationships and reinvestment in other or new relationships. Successful negotiation of this phase results in survivors who hope in the future, feel more energetic, participate in social events, and experience an acceptance of death. Challenges and opportunities abound for older adults at this stage. Older adults are often retired or working part time; therefore, their time is their own. Opportunities to make new friends, develop new skills, and engage in pleasurable activities are limited only by access, motivation, and health.

THE NURSE'S ROLE

Western culture is influenced by a value of youth, beauty, health, and fitness. Simultaneously, it is avoidant of illness and disability and is death denying. In denying death, Western culture denies the need to express grief and feel the pain that accompanies a loss. These feelings are normal, natural, and necessary for growth and healing. The nurse's role in facilitating the grief process includes assessing grief and assisting the survivor to feel the loss, express the loss, and complete the tasks of the grief process. Grief affects patients, families, and significant others physically, psychologically, socially, and spiritually. Nurses should utilize an interdisciplinary team (e.g., nurses, social workers, volunteers, grief and bereavement counselors, chaplain, and physician) to facilitate a healthy transition through the grief process. Each discipline can contribute its expertise to the bereavement plan of care.

Assessing Grief in Older Adults

The grief assessment includes the patient, family members, and significant others and should begin at the time the patient is admitted to a hospital, nursing facility, or assisted living facility, or at the time of diagnosis of acute, chronic, or terminal illness. Grief assessment continues throughout the course of an illness for the patient, family members, and significant others and for the bereavement period after the death. Grief should be assessed frequently during the bereavement period to alert the nurse to possible signs/symptoms/reactions of complicated grief (see Table 9-2) (Corless, 2001; Brown-Saltzman, 1998). When assessing grief in older adults, the nurse should assess for the type of grief, the presenting reactions, the stage and/or tasks of grief presented by the patient and family, and factors that support or inhibit a safe and healthy transition through the grief process.

Many elder caregivers do not care for themselves when caring for their loved ones living with a life-limiting disease. Therefore, assessment of the caregiver should also include a general health checkup, an assessment of somatic symptoms, dental and eye exams as appropriate, a nutritional evaluation, a sleep assessment, an examination of the ability to maintain work and family roles, a determination of whether there are major changes in the presentation of self, an assessment of changes resulting from the death

EVIDENCE-BASED PRACTICE

Reference: Schulz, R., Beach, S. R., Lind, B., Martire, L. M., Zdaniuk, B., Hirsch, C., et al. (2001). Involvement in caregiving and adjustment to the death of a spouse: Findings from the Caregiver Health Effects Study. *Journal of the American Medical Association, 285*, 3123-3129.

Research Problem: The bereavement experience(s) among three groups of elder caregivers varies according to their degree of involvement in the care of loved ones.

Design: Prospective, population-based cohort study, self-report.

Sample and Setting: The study was conducted in four U.S. communities between 1993 and 1998. A total of 129 caregivers ages 66 to 96 participated. The three groups studied were defined as noncaregivers ($n = 40$), caregivers reporting no strain (stress) ($n = 37$), and strained caregivers ($n = 52$). Objective self-report measures were used to assess health outcomes for each group.

Methods: Outcome measures included the Center for Epidemiological Studies–Depression Scale (CES-D); use of depression medication; weight change; and the presence, absence, degree, and frequency of unhealthy coping strategies. These measures were used pre- and postdeath over a 4-year period to assess change over time.

Results: The noncaregivers experienced the most difficulty in bereavement. Nonstrained caregivers demonstrated little change, and strained caregivers indicated an improvement in health and well-being.

Implications for Nursing Practice: The findings of this study suggest that caregiver involvement, stressful or not, correlated with healthy bereavement. Caregivers (spouses) with limited involvement in the care of their loved ones were at greater risk for complicated bereavement. Facilitating communication and participation of caregivers in the care process may act as a preventive measure and support healthy grief and bereavement. Nurses working with patients in long-term, custodial, and acute inpatient settings should be especially sensitive to this dynamic. In addition, sensitivity to elder caregivers who are uninvolved and isolated may require greater advocacy and health care team involvement. The assessment of supportive resources and referral for bereavement support services may be warranted.

Conclusion: Therefore it is important for nurses to understand the influence caregiving may have on the bereaved and to invite family participation in the care of dying patients.

and the difficulties with these life changes, and an assessment of social networks (Corless, 2001). For persons experiencing signs and symptoms of complicated grief, the nurse should make a referral to a bereavement specialist (Glass, Cluxton, & Rancour, 2001).

Nursing Interventions for Grief and Bereavement

Patient- and Family-Directed Plan of Care

After the initial assessment, the nurse, in collaboration with the older adult, family, and members of their health care team, may create a bereavement plan of care. This plan of care focuses on the goals identified by the older adult. When implementing bereavement interventions, the nurse should maintain an accepting, nonjudgmental attitude and an awareness of each survivor's individual needs, strengths, challenges, and traditions. Sensitivity to the practices of specific cultures in mourning and grief reactions

should be respected and honored and may be helpful in providing support (Egan, 2000).

What Do I Say?

Nurses may fear "saying the wrong thing" to an older adult or his or her family when death is present, or they may fear not knowing what to say to a survivor. The listing of unhelpful and helpful comments provided in Table 9-5 may assist the nurse in guiding dialogue with older adults who are grieving and bereaved.

Interventions for Anticipatory Grief

Often older adults and/or their family members experiencing anticipatory grief require the same grief interventions as a survivor of a deceased patient. Anticipatory grief interventions may include emotional support, encouragement of discussion regarding the anticipated loss, assistance with role changes, presentation of educational resources to teach new life skills, engagement in life review, education regarding the signs and

Table 9-5 Unhelpful and Helpful Comments in Speaking with the Bereaved

Unhelpful Comments	Helpful Comments
I know exactly how you're feeling.	I am sorry that you are going through this painful process.
I can imagine how you are feeling.	It must be hard to accept that this has happened.
I understand how you are feeling.	It's OK to grieve and be really angry with God and anyone else.
I'm always here for you, call me if you need anything.	I can bring dinner over either Tuesday or Friday Which will be better for you?
You should be over it by now. It's time you moved on.	Grieving takes time. Don't feel pushed to hurry through it.
You had so many years together. You are so lucky.	I did not know _____, will you tell me about him? What was your relationship like?
At least you have your children.	It's not your fault. You did everything you could do.
You're young, you'll meet someone else.	What's the scariest part about facing the future alone without _____?
At least her suffering is over. She is in a better place now.	You will never forget _____, will you?
He lived a really long and full life.	It's not easy for you, is it? What about your relationship will you miss the most?
How old was he?	He meant a lot to you.

Adapted from Klein, S. (1998). *Heavenly hurts: Surviving AIDS-related deaths and losses*. New York: Baywood Publishing Company.

symptoms of disease progression and the dying process, and encouragement of the elder patient and family members to complete unfinished business. The nurse should work to be truly present, listening actively and providing gentle touch and reassurance.

Opportunities to decrease feelings of loss may also include reassurance that adaptive equipment (e.g., wheelchairs to minimize loss of mobility) will be available should it ever be required. Generation of advance directives should be encouraged to minimize an elder patient's and/or family's feelings of fear and loss of control in decision making.

Grief Interventions

There are a number of interventions to support healthy and safe grieving for older adults. Being present, active listening, gentle touch, and appropriate silence are also very supportive to a grieving elder. Normalizing the grief process and the unique as well as common aspects of grief is also helpful in reducing anxiety and feelings of isolation. Validating the loss and encouraging the expression of feelings may reduce feelings of anger, sadness, and guilt and help to promote emotional balance. Helping to identify support systems that currently exist in the older adult's life may affirm that he or she is cared for and will not be alone in grief.

In some cases, the use of bereavement specialists and referral to bereavement resources can promote healing. It is always important to be mindful of complications or barriers to healthy grieving. For persons experiencing disenfranchised grief, the nurse and health care team may be the only persons who may be willing to acknowledge and validate the survivor's relationship with the deceased, his or her feelings and grief reactions, and the need for ritual in saying goodbye.

A comprehensive assessment may determine the need for additional assistance. Identifying resources and making referrals is an essential intervention strategy, and an interdisciplinary approach to care is strongly recommended. For example, the survivor may have spiritual issues that would best be addressed by the pastoral care worker. A financial counselor might best assist the survivor with financial concerns and/or life skills in paying bills. In addition, the nurse should assess for signs/symptoms of complicated grief and make referrals to bereavement specialists, psychologists, or physicians as needed.

Completion of the Grieving Process

No one can predict when a person's grief work will be complete, and some experts argue that this work is never completely finished. There will always be times when a memory or an object, an anniversary of the death, or feelings of loss occur and the accompanying sadness and guilt are experienced. In addition, change and loss as a result of illness and death occur and reoccur across the life span; therefore, the adaptation may fluctuate in intensity but is often ongoing. Grief can diminish and healing occur as the pain of the loss decreases, and as survivors adapt to life without the deceased and physically, psychologically, and socially reinvest in other relationships and commitments.

DEATH ANXIETY, CUMULATIVE LOSS, AND GRIEF: THE NURSE'S JOURNEY
Death Anxiety

In most health care settings, the nurse will care for older adults with life-threatening illnesses and experience their death. Working with dying patients can trigger the nurse's awareness of personal loss and fears about his or her own death and mortality. The nurse may also fear expressing emotion in a medical setting that promotes "control." Death anxiety occurs when the nurse is confronted with fears about death and has few resources or support systems to explore and express thoughts and emotions about dying and death (Buckman, 1998; Vachon, 2001).

When overwhelmed by death anxieties, nurses may use various defenses to allay fears, including focusing only on physical care needs, evading emotionally sensitive conversations with older adults and their families, speaking only when spoken to by patients, and talking only about topics that are comfortable for the nurse. These behaviors result in emotional distancing, avoidance, and withdrawal from dying elder patients and their families at a time when they need intensive, compassionate interpersonal care and active involvement by the nurse. Nurses should be aware of their own feelings, responses, and reactions to death so they can convey caring, acceptance, and respect for elder patients and their families and communicate effectively.

One's comfort with death is affected by personality; cultural, social, and spiritual belief systems; life experiences; and experiences with death. Adapting to caring for the dying may require the nurse to explore, experience, and express his or her personal feelings regarding death. Personal death awareness activities/exercises, as well as discussion of belief systems about death and the afterlife with friends, peers, and pastoral care workers, can be helpful. Self-exploration and reflection may promote an understanding and acceptance of death (Vachon, 2001).

Adapting to Cumulative Loss: Survival Skills for Nurses

Cumulative loss is a succession of losses experienced by nurses who work with patients with life-threatening illnesses and their families (Table 9-6). Nurses can experience anticipatory and normal grief before and after the death of a patient. Not only is loss painful, but, when a nurse is exposed to death frequently, he or she may not have time to resolve the grief issues associated with one patient before another patient dies (Vachon, 2001).

Nurses new to working with dying patients may need to adapt emotionally and spiritually to caring for the terminally ill. The five stages of adaptation for nurses caring for dying patients and their families are intellectualization, emotional survival, depression, emotional arrival, and deep compassion (Harper, 1994). Working through these stages is crucial to assist the nurse in relieving anxiety about dying and death, attaining personal and professional growth, and adapting to comfortably caring for patients at the end of life and their families (Harper, 1994; Vachon, 2001).

A host of factors influence the nurse's adaptation process, including professional training, personal death history, life changes, and available support systems. Professional training has a strong influence on a nurse's professional behavior and personal approach to care. In the past, health care professionals were often told to control emotions and to emotionally distance themselves from patients and families. However, patients and families require intense interpersonal involve-

ment and compassionate care at the end of life. Nurses may benefit by verbalizing their feelings and expressing their emotions. This helps nurses to process loss and grief and provide quality care at the end of life.

Similarly, one's personal death history influences adaptation and resiliency in dealing with cumulative loss. Past experiences with death on a personal and/or professional level and possible unresolved grief issues can influence the professional's ability to cope with caring for dying patients and their families.

Stressful life changes will also influence the ability of a nurse to cope with the stress present in providing end-of-life care. Stressful life changes may include a death in the family, caring for elder parents, separation from loved ones, children leaving home, divorce, and illness. These changes may signify losses, trigger grief responses, and make it difficult for the nurse to cope.

The presence or absence of support systems can influence the nurse's ability to move through the stages of adaptation. Emotional support provided by peers, family, co-workers, and instructors increases the capacity to adapt to and cope with the care of those who are dying (Vachon, 2001). Finding balance and assessing and utilizing a wide range of support systems is as important for nurses as it is for patients and families.

Balance is the ability to provide compassionate, quality care to dying patients and their families and find personal satisfaction in the work of professional nursing. The purpose of a system of support is to balance the effects of death anxiety and cumulative loss by assisting the nurse in exploring and expressing feelings associated with anxiety, loss, and grief, and in adapting to caring for the dying patient and family.

When assessing support systems, two questions should be considered, First, does the setting support or inhibit the nurse's professional adaptation, growth, and development in caring for dying patients and families? Second, does the setting provide a supportive environment where the nurse feels safe to express death anxiety, emotions, loss, and grief?

Creating a Supportive Environment

Creating and maintaining a supportive environment is essential for personal and professional

Table 9-6 Coping with Professional Anxiety in Terminal Illness

Stage I (0-3 mo) Intellectualization	Stage II (3-6 mo) Emotional Survival	Stage III (6-9 mo) Depression	Stage IV (9-12 mo) Emotional Arrival	Stage V (12-24 mo) Deep Compassion
Professional knowledge	Increasing professional knowledge	Deepening of professional knowledge	Acceptance of professional knowledge	Refining of professional knowledge
Intellectualization	Less intellectualization	Decreasing intellectualization	Normal intellectualization	Refining intellectual base
Anxiety	Emotional survival	Depression	Emotional arrival	Deep compassion
Some uncomfortableness	Increasing uncomfortableness	Decreasing uncomfortableness	Increasing comfortableness	Increased comfortableness
Agreeableness	Guilt	Pain	Moderation	Self-realization
Withdrawal	Frustration	Mourning	Mitigation	Self-awareness
Superficial acceptance	Sadness	Grieving	Accommodation	Self-actualization
Providing tangible services	Initial emotional involvement	More emotional involvement	Ego mastery	Professional satisfaction
Utilization of emotional energy on understanding the setting	Increasing emotional involvement	Overidentification with the resident	Coping with loss of relationship	Acceptance of death and loss
Familiarizing self with policies and procedures	Initial understanding of the magnitude of the area of practice	Exploration of own feelings about death	Freedom from concern about own death	Rewarding professional growth and development
Working with families rather than residents	Overidentification with the resident's situation	Facing own death	Developing strong ties with dying residents and families	Development of ability to give of one's self
		Coming to grips with feelings about death	Development of ability to work with, on behalf of and for the dying resident	Human and professional assessment
			Development of professional competence	Constructive and appropriate activities
			Productivity and accomplishments	Development of feelings of dignity and self-respect
			Healthy interaction	Ability to give dignity and self-respect to dying resident
				Comfortableness

Source: Harper, B. C. (1994). *Death: The coping mechanism of the health professional.* Greenville, SC: Southeastern University Press.

health. The presence and combination of formal and informal support systems can do much to support nurses providing end-of-life care. Formal support may include preplanned gatherings where nurses can express feelings in a safe environment and postclinical debriefings after stressful clinical experiences. These opportunities can help relieve anxieties by allowing nurses to relate the emotion to the experience and explore and express feelings related to dying and death. Events that acknowledge loss provide an opportunity to express grief. Planned memorial services assist in honoring the lives of patients and the value of the work of the nurse.

Informal support in the work setting may include one-to-one sharing of experiences with co-workers, peers, an instructor, a pastoral care worker, and/or a physician. Finding persons who are trusted and caring can create a milieu of emotional safety and support when needed most. Health care settings, where help may be requested as needed, can be very supportive. Supervisors, mentors, and instructors can provide moral support to nurses providing end-of-life

---

EVIDENCE-BASED PRACTICE

Reference: Evans, W. M., Bilbeau, D. L., & Mullen-Conley, K. (2001). Coping strategies used in residential hospice settings: Findings from a national study. *American Journal of Hospice & Palliative Care*, 18(2), 102-110.

Research Problem: Professional caregivers utilize a number of strategies for coping with the deaths of patients in residential hospices in the United States.

Sample and Setting: Using the *Guide to National Hospices, 1996-1997*, 10 residential hospices employing a total of 199 professional caregivers were identified for inclusion in the study. Seven of the 10 sites responded; in all, 69 questionnaires were returned. The respondents were one-third certified nurse assistants, one-third registered nurses, and one-third other professional caregivers.

Methods: Subjects were asked to think about a patient death that had occurred within the past 6 months that was particularly stressful to them. They were asked to describe the patient, their own coping strategies, and their satisfaction with the experience. Participants at each site were asked to complete the Ways of Coping Questionnaire (WCQ) (Folkman & Lazarus, 1988). The WCQ is a 66-item tool that describes a person's coping process relative to a specific event.

Results: Findings indicated that "positive reappraisal" was the most frequently used coping strategy. Eighty-five percent of the respondents indicated that they used "prayer" in coping with loss.

Implications for Nursing Practice: This study suggests that many residential hospice employees experience death as an opportunity for personal and spiritual growth. Employees who were dissatisfied with their end-of-life experience(s) reported confrontational coping styles, had a higher need for control by accepting greater responsibility for patient outcomes, and used escape-avoidance strategies in dealing with the stress of caring for the dying. These strategies that attempt to "control" or "fix" the patient are incongruent with best practices in patient and family value-directed care and lead to greater stress. The implications of nurses experiencing chronic stress include, but are not limited to, burnout, poor health, and poor patient care outcomes. The results of this study suggest that professional caregivers (nurses) may benefit from intentional support in the form of in-service training and environmental interventions. Education supporting personal and professional growth in the midst of loss and change and creating and maintaining a healthy balance are suggested.

Conclusion: Therefore, it is important for nurses to develop an awareness of their own personal coping style and connect to resources that support professional health and well-being.

care. This is especially true when a grieving family member visits, and/or at the time of the patient's death. The presence of an experienced peer can greatly decrease anxiety and provide immense support to the nurse. Nurses will often find comfort in knowing they are not alone. In addition, spiritual care providers can assist the nurse in spiritual reflection, exploration, and spiritual replenishment as he or she experiences the loss of patients and examines issues of transcendence and transformation.

Knowledge is power. Education and skill development in end-of-life care promote competence and self-confidence. This has the potential to decrease anxiety in caring for patients and their families at the end of life and promote a sense of professional health. Health care settings that promote professional development can also promote professional health and quality care.

Nurses have a personal and professional responsibility to seek out support systems to cope with death anxiety, loss, and grief. They should learn to acknowledge their limitations; be willing to ask for help from co-workers and other professionals (e.g., social workers, pastoral care workers, supervisors, and instructors); engage in personal reflection, physical exercise, and relaxation techniques; and take the time to socialize and play.

CONCLUSION

Nursing care of and responsibilities to the older adult do not end with the death of the patient. When working with older adults, the experience of loss, grief, and bereavement should be assessed at each encounter with elders, and bereavement care should continue after the death of the patient. End-of-life care is at its best when an interdisciplinary approach is used. Care plans that are directed by the older adult with his or her family are best suited to meeting the unique aspects of care when dealing with change and loss as a result of illness and death. Suffering, loss, grief, and bereavement are all important issues to address in providing quality end-of-life and palliative care to older adults. Similarly, nurses are human too; nurses should work to recognize and respond to their own grief in order to provide quality palliative care.

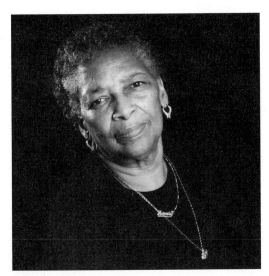

Reflecting on the meaning of life in older age. (Courtesy Mathy Mezey.)

REFERENCES

Arnold, R., & Egan, K. (2002). *Growth and opportunity at the end-of-life: The experience model of care.* Largo, FL: The Hospice Institute of the Florida Suncoast.

Brown-Saltzman, K. (1998). Transforming the grief process. In R. Carroll-Johnson, L. Gorman, & N. J. Bush (Eds.), *Psychosocial nursing care: Along the cancer continuum.* Pittsburgh: Oncology Nursing Press.

Buckman, R. (1998). Communication in palliative care: A practical guide. In D. Doyle, G. W. C. Hanks, & N. MacDonald (Eds.), *Oxford textbook of palliative medicine* (2nd ed., pp. 141-156). New York: Oxford University Press.

Cassell, E. J. (1991). *The nature of suffering and the goals of medicine.* (p. 33). New York: Oxford University Press.

Corless, I. B. (2001). Bereavement. In B.R. Ferrell & N. Coyle (Eds.), *Textbook of palliative nursing care.* (pp. 647-662). New York: Oxford University Press.

Corr, C., Nabe, C. & Corr, D. (2000). *Death and dying, life and living.* (3rd ed., pp. 209-243). Belmont, CA: Wadsworth.

Despelder, L. A., & Strickland, A. L. (1987). *The last dance* (2nd ed., p. 207). Mountain View, CA: Mayfield Publishing Company.

Doka, K. (1989). Grief. In R. Kastenbaum & B. Kastenbaum (Eds.), *Encyclopedia of death* (p. 127). Phoenix, AZ: The Oryx Press.

Egan, K. (2000). Patient and family directed care. In *Initial hospice training orientation manual.* Largo, FL: The Hospice Institute of the Florida Suncoast.

Evans, W. M., Bilbeau, D. L., & Mullen-Conley, K. (2001). Coping strategies used in residential hospice settings: findings from a national study. *American Journal of Hospice and Palliative Care, 18*(2), 102-110.

Folkman, S., & Lazarus, R. (1988). *Ways of coping Questionnaire review set*. Manual, test booklet, scoring key. Redwood City, CA: MindSpring.

Geissler, E. (1994). *Pocket guide to cultural assessment*. St. Louis: Mosby.

Glass, E., Cluxton, D., & Rancour, P. (2001). Principles of patient and family assessment. In B. R. Ferrell & N. Coyle (Eds.), *Textbook of palliative nursing*. (pp. 37-52). New York: Oxford University Press.

Harper, B. (1994). *Death: The coping mechanism of the health professional*. Greenville, SC: Southeastern University Press.

Kübler-Ross, E. (1969). *On death and dying*. New York: Macmillan.

Lindemann, E. (1994). Symptomatology and management of acute grief. *American Journal of Psychiatry, Sesquicentennial Suppl, 151*(6), 155-160.

Lipson, J., Dibble, S., & Minarik, P. (1996). *Culture and nursing care: A pocket guide*. San Francisco: The Regents, University of California.

Loney, M. (1998). Death, dying and grief in the face of cancer. In C.C. Burke (Ed.). *Psychosocial dimensions of oncology care*. Pittsburgh, PA: Oncology Nursing Press Inc.

Parkes, C. M. (1999). *Bereavement: Studies of grief in adult life*. London: Tavistock.

Rando, T. A. (1984). *Grief, dying and death: Clinical interventions for caregivers*. Champaign, IL: Research Press.

Rando, T. A. (1999). *Clinical dimensions of anticipatory mourning: Theory and practice in working with the dying, their loved ones, and caregivers*. Champaign, IL: Research Press.

Vachon, M. (2001). The nurse's role: The world of palliative care nursing. In B. R. Ferrell & N. Coyle (Eds.), *Textbook of palliative nursing*. (pp. 647-662). New York: Oxford University Press.

Wolfelt, A. (1990, March/April). Bereavement and children: Adolescent mourning, a naturally complicated experience. Part II. *Bereavement Magazine*, pp. 34-37.

Worden, J. W. (1991). *Grief counseling and grief therapy: A handbook for the mental health practitioner* (2nd ed.). New York: Springer.

DISEASE-RELATED PALLIATIVE CARE NURSING

Janet L. Abrahm

Older adults tend to have many chronic diseases that lend themselves more to medical management than to cure. The challenge for nurses in maximizing quality of life is to help patients and families optimize treatment of the disease and the relief of symptoms. For nurses to accomplish this, they must have an understanding of the incidence and prevalence of diseases that commonly afflict older adults, the elements of comprehensive assessment, co-morbiditys and complications, emergency situations, and the typical monitoring and treatment regimens that are effective. It is important to understand family concerns and caregiver fears. Finally, nurses must understand each disease's trajectory, and how to promote health and well-being for the older adult population dying from these diseases. This section of the book, therefore, is devoted to a review of the common disease processes that afflict older adults: heart disease; cancer; stroke, coma, brain death; dementia and neuro-degenerative disease; end-stage renal disease; chronic lung disease, and end-stage liver disease.

Congestive heart failure is a condition in which comprehensive monitoring and care significantly improve patient functioning. Case managers working with patients with class III and IV heart failure help them avoid hospitalization, minimize dyspnea and edema, and maximize independent functioning. Communication and education have been the key. Simple measures are very effective: asking patients to call when weight increases by 2 pounds, educating about diet, and paying careful attention to medication regimens. What can be most difficult for families is the "saw tooth" shape of the dying trajectory in patients with congestive heart failure. It may be very hard to determine which exacerbation is likely to be the fatal one, and, consequently, how much life-sustaining technology is reasonable.

Cancer in older adults usually has a more straightforward trajectory, once the disease becomes refractory to first or second line therapy. Goals of care can therefore be easier to establish, but it is equally important to deliver accurate prognoses. Patients who think they have a >10% chance of living 6 months often chose aggressive life-prolonging measures; only those who think they have <10% chance may chose comfort care. Cancer in older adults offers significant opportunities, but also significant challenges to delivering palliative care. Pain, for example, is poorly treated in older adults. Patients are reluctant to complain: they want to be good patients, they feel pain is part of getting old, and they want to use their pain to monitor their response to cancer treatment. Physicians, in turn, under-medicate older adults, and may not take the time needed to find the right combination of medications that minimize sedation, confusion, and constipation. Delirium, too, either from the tumor or medications used for palliation, can go unrecognized and be a serious source of distress.

As with cancer, dementia and neurodegenerative diseases have well-defined landmarks that indicate that the patient is dying. Imparting an understanding of these to caregivers and other family members can help them cope with the demands of care, make decisions about the most appropriate setting of care, and define advance care plans.

The older adult patient who develops end-stage renal disease may elect to stop dialyses. Renal failure may be caused by a variety of disease processes. Therefore, while the metabolic implications may be similar, the needs of the diabetic patient, the patient with heart failure, the patient with obstructive disease, or with atherosclerotic vascular problems are quite different. Their co-morbidity's, experiences with the health care system, and outcomes of dialysis also differ. One of the major challenges, then, is to be of assistance as they and their families consider discontinuing dialysis. Understanding and sharing the potential burdens and benefits, the physical manifestations of renal failure, and the techniques by which suffering can be ameliorated all help families and patients make this final choice an informed one.

Patients with chronic lung disease have a similarly difficult choice: that of intubation. Many of them have experienced intubation once or many times. As painful as those memories may be, the recollection of the symptoms that preceded the intubation may lead patients to feel that they have no other choice. Careful discussions of all that can be done to alleviate those symptoms will help reassure patients who would prefer not to have to be maintained on ventilators. The older adult patients can also be reassured that much can be done to alleviate the day-to-day symptoms experienced. The anxiety that exacerbates their sensation of breathlessness can be treated effectively both by educated family members and professional caregivers using non-pharmacologic, as well as pharmacologic methods. Dyspnea arising from deconditioning can be improved even in patients with significant disease. Educating family members can decrease their sense of helplessness and panic and they can become valued allies in the care of these patients.

Palliative care and hospice teams are experienced in caring for patients with all the diseases discussed in this section. Unfortunately, the criteria to determine eligibility for hospice and palliative care and the availability of health care resources have been barriers to quality end of life care for older adults. Current criteria for enrollment of patients with dementia or chronic lung disease allow only the very sickest to be enrolled, late enough in the course that the family is able to benefit only minimally from the services provided. The expense of palliative medications needed by patients with stage IV congestive heart failure, with advanced pulmonary hypertension, or with bowel obstruction from cancer often means that hospice programs with limited resources cannot afford to enroll them. Until the situation changes, nurses from other care settings will continue to provide the majority of palliative and end-of-life care for older adults. The section that follows will assist nurses in providing quality care to the older adult experiencing a variety of advanced illnesses.

Judith B. Dyne

Mrs. C., 82, is brought into the doctor's office today by her daughter for a follow-up appointment. Mrs. C. was recently discharged from the hospital after treatment of an episode of congestive heart failure (CHF). She has been a client for the past 10 years. Mrs. C. was diagnosed with CHF 3 years ago, and has been hospitalized numerous times with exacerbation of symptoms.

Her daughter tells the nurse that her mom has been very depressed and despondent since her discharge, and keeps talking about "giving up," and not wanting to go to the hospital again. In the discussion with Mrs. C., she restates her desire to stay at home with her family, and not be rehospitalized if she has another episode of shortness of breath. She wants to discuss how she can manage her symptoms at home, and what other medications can be used to give her some relief. The nurse reviews her medication profile and sees that she has been on a loop diuretic and an angiotensin-converting enzyme inhibitor for the past 2 years. A previous note refers to the fact that Mrs. C. alluded to the idea of remaining at home at her last visit, but wanted to discuss her options with her family. She tells the nurse that the discussion with her family did not go well, and that they want her to continue with all therapy, including going to the hospital again if needed.

The nurse, as her health care provider, must address these issues with Mrs. C. and her daughter. Questions that the nurse should consider include

Are there any other treatments that could provide symptomatic relief?

What is the nurse's role relative to other members of the health care team (e.g., collaborating physician, cardiologist) in the communication of the wishes of Mrs. C?

What referrals would need to be made if Mrs. C. elects to receive palliative care?

INTRODUCTION

Coronary artery disease, which ultimately develops into end-stage congestive heart failure, is a major problem for older adults in the United States today. End-stage heart disease affects elders not only as an unrelenting disease state, but also as a condition that daily affects their quality of life. Unremitting dyspnea, orthopnea, dobutamine therapy, intravenous diuretics, and hospital admissions are the norm in end-stage heart disease, rather than the exception. Despite the aggressive medical interventions available, clients continue to suffer. What care can nurses offer these elder individuals, and what options should be addressed with both the patient and his or her family? This chapter explores these issues utilizing the most current evidence regarding end-of-life care options related to end-stage heart disease in the older adult population.

EPIDEMIOLOGY AND ETIOLOGY OF END-STAGE HEART DISEASE

Heart disease is a problem of epidemic proportions. Heart failure is the end stage of heart disease. As the population ages, this disease and its sequelae raise issues regarding quality of life, treatment options, and the impact on society and health care economics. It is primarily a disease of older adults and the number one cause of death in this country. The Framingham Study (Ho, Pinsky, Kannel, & Levy, 1993), which began in

1948 with a cohort of over 5000 male and female subjects, was the first large-scale study that looked at heart disease and heart failure in the United States. On routine examinations of the subjects in this study, it was found that the rate of CHF increased in men from 8 per 1000 at ages 50 to 59 years to 66 per 1000 at ages 80 to 89 years. In women, the prevalence estimates increase from 8 per 1000 to 79 per 1000 in the same age categories (Ho et al., 1993). In part, these estimates differ because women live longer than men do, even with heart disease. One in three women over the age of 65 has some form of cardiovascular disease, which accounts for the greater proportion of deaths from heart disease in this age group ("Neither Prevention nor Cure," 1999).

Considered the hallmark study in modern cardiology, the Framingham study provided the data on which many worldwide clinical trials on heart disease and heart failure have been based. Over the years of observing these patients and their offspring, this study found no decrease in the incidence of heart failure despite the improved detection and treatment of coronary artery disease. In fact, the incidence of CHF has been found to increase sharply with age in both sexes, and doubles with each decade (Kannel, 2000). According to the American Heart Association's (AHA's) 2002 *Heart and Stroke Statistical Update*, there are 4,790,000 Americans alive with CHF today, with 550,000 new cases diagnosed each year. Of these, 2,360,000 are men and 2,440,000 are women, and 10 per 1000 are older than 65 years of age.

After the diagnosis of CHF, the median survival is 1.7 years in men and 3.2 years in women (National Heart, Lung and Blood Institute, 1996). After a myocardial infarction (MI), death will occur within 6 years (in 22% of men and 46% of women) (AHA, 2002). Deaths from CHF have been exponentially increasing as much as 145% in the period from 1979 to 1999, with an overall death rate of 18.8% (19.4% for white males, 21.9% for black males, 18.2% for white females, and 19.4% for black females) (AHA, 2002). Those with CHF have a five times greater likelihood of sudden death as compared to the general population.

Disability from heart failure is also an issue today, in terms of both quality of life and health care costs. The diagnosis of CHF is overwhelm-

ing the health care system. In the last 10 years, it is reported that there were 15 million office visits and 7 million hospital days attributed to the treatment of heart failure, costing approximately $38.1 billion in outpatient dollars alone (Goldstein, 2001). Hospitalizations of older adults with CHF are on the rise, and CHF is the number one diagnosis for admission (Kannel, 2000). Among nursing home residents (National Center for Health Statistics, 1997), 25.8% of elder residents had a primary diagnosis of cardiovascular disease on admission (highest disease category). The latest statistical report by the AHA (2002) estimated direct and indirect costs of cardiovascular disease and stroke in the United States to be in the billions of dollars (Table 10-1).

PATHOPHYSIOLOGY OF HEART FAILURE

In order to lay a foundation for understanding heart failure in the elder population, it is important to review the structural changes that occur in the senescent heart. In elder patients who are free of heart disease or hypertension, there is an increase in the left ventricular wall thickness, septal hypertrophy, and a reduction of diastolic compliance, which are physiologic changes that naturally occur (Taylor, 2001). The hypertrophy results from an increased afterload on the left ventricle, which is caused by increased pressure in the aorta that leads to decreased compliance of the ventricles. As one ages, there is also an increase in collagen accumulation in the left ventricle, which adds to the diastolic rigidity (Taylor, 2001).

The aging process also affects valvular structure. The leaflets of the aortic and mitral valves become calcified (aortic/mitral stenosis), and there is a consistent increase in the circumference of all four heart valves. There is also an increased incidence of atrial fibrillation in patients who have calcium deposition in the mitral valve. Idiopathic bundle branch fibrosis may also occur with increasing age, and may be a cause of increased risk of heart block in elders. The arterial walls also become less elastic and distensible, and systolic hypertension can occur (Taylor, 2001).

CHF can be described as a clinical syndrome characterized by pulmonary or systemic congestion, or both, with diminished or limited cardiac output. This decrease in cardiac output

Table 10-1 Estimated Direct and Indirect Costs (in Billions of Dollars) of Cardiovascular Diseases and Stroke United States: 2002

	Heart Disease*	CAD	Stroke	Hypertensive Disease	Congestive Heart Failure	Total Cardiovascular Disease†
Hospital/nursing home	$81.0	$41.8	$24.5	$8.6	$15.4	$126.1
Physicians/other professionals	15.3	8.6	2.4	8.6	1.6	29.9
Drugs/medical durables	5.2	1.6	3.1	1.7	2.4	11.7
Home Health Care	13.5	6.2	0.8	15.5	2.0	31.8
Total Expenditures†	$115.0	$58.2	$30.8	$34.4	$21.4	$199.5

*This category includes coronary heart disease, congestive heart failure, part of hypertensive disease, cardiac dysrhythmias, rheumatic heart disease, cardiomyopathy, pulmonary heart disease, and other or ill-defined "heart" diseases.
†Totals do not represent sums of data in rows or columns because of rounding and overlap of categories.
Adapted from American Heart Association. (2002). *Heart and stroke statistical update*. Dallas: Author.

causes the associated symptoms of dyspnea, fatigue, and peripheral edema. The heart is unable to pump sufficient amounts of blood to meet the metabolic demands of the body (Michaels & Frances, 2001). It is the decreased myocardial contractile state that leads to a decreased stroke volume (volume of blood ejected by the ventricle with each heartbeat), which triggers acute compensatory neurohormonal mechanisms. These neurohormonal responses include sympathetic nervous system changes (increased heart rate), increased inotropy (increased contractile state in viable myocardium), arteriolar constriction (to maintain organ perfusion), and activation of the renin–angiotensin system (which mediates arteriolar vasoconstriction and retention of sodium). These compensatory mechanisms in the acute phase attempt to maintain adequate cardiac output and vital organ perfusion. However, when heart failure occurs on a chronic basis, ventricular remodeling develops in response to these neurohormonal influences (Woods, Froelicher, & Motzer, 2000). The ventricle takes on a spherical instead of an oval shape in order to make the most of Starling's law. This law states that, if the myocardial fibers can be stretched by increased volume of blood within the ventricle, the force of contraction will be greater and the ventricle will more completely empty (Lamb, 1984).

When this adaptation occurs, the combination of the neurohormonal response and the ventricular remodeling cause myopathy, which is a response to the increased afterload and fluid retention. Ventricular filling pressures (preload) increase further, the myocardial fibers overstretch, the mechanism of Starling's law fails, cardiac output is compromised, and the increased pressure in the left ventricle backs up into the pulmonary vasculature. The heart can no longer meet the metabolic needs of the body for oxygen delivery to the tissues, and systolic hypoperfusion, severe vasoconstriction (increased afterload), and poor pump performance occur.

The effect of the inflammatory mediators on cardiac dysfunction has also been investigated. Mann (2001) believes that inflammatory mediators, such as tumor necrosis factor, interleukin-1, interleukin-6, and nitric oxide, negatively affect cardiac tissues in the same way that other substances or mechanisms cause heart dysfunction. Mediator modulation may become the goal of emerging classes of therapeutic agents.

Heart failure can be due to heart muscle abnormalities, ventricular systolic dysfunction, dysrhythmias, valve malfunction, and myocardial rupture (rare) (Hudak, Gallo, & Morton, 1998). Muscle abnormalities include MI, ventricular aneurysm, cardiomyopathy (excessive hypertrophy from pulmonary hypertension), aortic stenosis, and systemic hypertension (Hudak et al., 1998).

Ventricular dysfunction can be due to either systolic dysfunction or diastolic dysfunction.

Systolic dysfunction occurs when the contractility of the heart is compromised, which is measured by the left ventricular ejection fraction (LVEF). The normal LVEF is approximately 60%, but, with systolic heart failure, the LVEF is below normal, usually less than 40%. In end-stage heart failure resulting from systolic dysfunction, the LVEF can be as low as 15% to 20%. Common causes of systolic dysfunction are ischemic heart disease, cardiomyopathy, volume overload (valvular insufficiency), and pressure overload (hypertension or valvular stenosis).

In diastolic dysfunction, the LVEF is normal or hyperdynamic (>60%), but the ability of the ventricle to relax and fill is compromised (poor compliance). This type of dysfunction accounts for approximately 50% of all cases of heart failure (Michaels & Frances, 2001). Causes may include ischemic heart disease with aging, myocardial hypertrophy, and restrictive cardiomyopathy. It is important to note that, as a result of the aging process, the relaxation of the heart in diastole is sometimes delayed, which causes a decrease in the filling time (Michaels & Frances, 2001).

Disorders of the cardiac rhythm—bradycardia, tachycardia, and ventricular and atrial dysrhythmias—can also contribute to heart failure. If loss of filling pressure or filling time occurs as a result of these dysrhythmias, stroke volume is affected and cardiac output decreases.

Valvular malfunction, which contributes to both systolic and diastolic heart failure, also plays a part in CHF. Valvular malfunction results from either pressure overload or volume overload. With age, the heart valves become calcified, leading to stenosis or narrowing of the valve diameter. The resulting pressure overload, which most often exists in the aortic valve, slowly progresses over time. Volume overload, which is present in valvular insufficiency or regurgitation, most often occurs in the mitral and aortic valves. This condition also progresses insidiously, unless there is an associated acute cause, such as endocarditis, papillary muscle or chordae tendineae rupture, or interventricular rupture following a MI (Laurent-Bopp, 2001).

Heart failure is classified using the New York Heart Association (NYHA) Functional Classification (Box 10-1). The severity of symptoms in the older adult with end-stage heart

disease places him or her in NYHA class III or IV, with associated radical clinical dysfunction affecting the quality of life of the individual (Criteria Committee of the NYHA, 1964).

CHF is also classified according to the side of the heart that is affected. The right ventricle and left ventricle are independent of each other, but are serially connected. To function effectively, both ventricles must maintain equal outputs. Unless the patient has a history of chronic lung disease, the left ventricle is usually the first to become dysfunctional. This is typically because the left ventricle must generate higher pressures than the right ventricle in order to maintain adequate cardiac output. The left ventricle must generate a great deal of force to eject its contents in systole (which in turn requires adequate oxygen). If the systemic vascular resistance is high (high blood pressure), it increases afterload, which ultimately decreases stroke volume. If the left ventricle fails, there is backward flow of blood into the pulmonary capillaries, which eventually transudates into the alveoli. The clinical symptoms are related to the elevated pulmonary pressures and decreased cardiac output. High blood pressure, myocardial ischemia, aortic stenosis or insufficiency, and mitral stenosis or insufficiency can also cause left ventricular failure.

Box 10-1 The New York Heart Association Functional Classification

Class I	Cardiac disease without resulting limitations of physical activity
Class II	Slight limitation of physical activity—comfortable at rest, but ordinary physical activity results in fatigue, palpitation, dyspnea, or anginal pain
Class III	Marked limitation in physical activity—comfortable at rest, but less ordinary physical activity causes fatigue, palpitation, dyspnea, or anginal pain
Class IV	Inability to carry on any physical activity without discomfort or symptoms at rest

Criteria committee the New York Heart Association. (1964). *Diseases of the heart and blood vessels: Nomenclature and criteria for diagnosis* (6th ed.). Boston: New York Heart Association.

Right ventricular failure is caused by increased pulmonary pressure. This increased pressure is usually due to chronic lung disease, pulmonary emboli, or left-sided heart failure. The clinical signs are those associated with increased systemic venous pressure, which gives rise to the signs of dependent peripheral edema. Although initial heart failure may be either right or left sided, in end-stage heart failure it is both, or biventricular.

HEART FAILURE AND DEPRESSION

Clinical studies have reported that depression following a MI can be associated with poorer outcomes (Barefoot, Helms, & Mark, 1996). A study by Frasure-Smith, Lesperance, and Talajic (1995) documented an increase in morbidity and mortality of four- to fivefold in the first 18 months after an MI in those patients who were also clinically depressed. Jaarsveld, Sanderman, Miedema, Ranchor, and Kempen (2001), using the HR-QL tool, measured health-related quality of life in patients with acute MI or CHF. The authors found more depression and poorer social and role functioning in the CHF group compared to the reference group, with decline in the first year after diagnosis. In patients with MI, there was no significant difference in role functioning on the HR-QL as compared to the reference group.

What is the link? It is known that cortisol levels are persistently high in patients with depression, which in turn leads over time to hypertension (increased afterload), increase in heart rate (decreased ventricular filling time), immunodepression, increased gluconeogenesis, inhibition of growth and reproduction systems, shunting of blood to the central nervous system, and the development of maladaptive neural and hormonal pathways (Rossen & Buschmann, 1995). It has also been found that proinflammatory cytokines, which are activated in the stress response, have major effects on the serotonergic system by reducing the available serotonin, which leads to not only depression, but also to increased platelet aggregation and, ultimately, coronary artery occlusion (Kubzansky & Ichiro, 2000).

The largest U.S. study documenting a link between depression and heart disease was done by the National Health and Nutrition Examination Survey (NHANES), which began in 1960 with 6672 subjects. More than 14,000 people were subsequently followed. One of the subsets of this study included measures of anxiety and depression and their relationship to hypertension (Jonas, Franks, & Ingram, 1997). A secondary analysis of these data by Ferketich, Schwartzbaum, Frid, and Moeschberger (2000) followed over 5000 women and 2800 men for 10 years and found that depression increased the risk of heart disease by approximately 75%.

In addition, depression may be common in the elder population with chronic heart failure, which can contribute to the loss of functional ability. Symptoms of physical aches and pains, difficulty sleeping, fatigue, or diminished capacity to do day-to-day activities often occurs. There is loss of the ability to live independently, which exacerbates the depression even further. For mild depression psychotherapy alone may be sufficient, however in those with chronic illnesses, like CHF, combination therapy to include counseling and antidepressant medications may be indicated. Follow up to assess treatment effects is imperative especially in the first three months of treatment as nonadherence is a problem (Barefoot, Helms, & Mark, 1996).

CLINICAL SIGNS AND SYMPTOMS OF CHF

In evaluating the clinical signs of CHF, it is important for nurses to understand the symptoms of both right and left heart failure. An elder may have typical right or left heart failure symptoms, but patients with end-stage heart disease often have biventricular heart failure, in which combined symptoms occur. The symptoms of both right ventricular and left ventricular failure are outlined in Box 10-2. The severity and progression of the symptoms is dependent on the extent of the failure and the type of dysfunction. Early in the disease process, when cardiac output decreases as a result of heart failure, compensatory mechanisms come into play to keep tissue perfusion intact. The sympathetic nervous system releases catecholamines, which cause increases in the heart rate, systemic vascular resistance, preload, afterload, and contractility. These same compensatory mechanisms eventually cause the symptoms of CHF as the ventricles begin to fail and LVEF declines.

RIGHT HEART FAILURE	**LEFT HEART FAILURE**
• Jugular vein distention	• Dyspnea, orthopnea, paroxysmal nocturnal dyspnea
• Dependent edema	• Pulmonary edema
• Hepatojugular reflex	• Irritating dry cough
• Splenomegaly	• S_3, S_4 heart sounds
• Decreased breath sounds	• Crackles, wheezing
• Weight gain of >2 lb/day	• Pulsus alternans (every other QRS complex on the ECG is lower voltage)
• Liver engorgement	• Hypoxemia, low Sao_2
• Nausea + vomiting	• Low hemoglobin (shunting)

ECG, electrocardiogram; Sao_2, arterial oxygen saturation.

Dyspnea is the initial manifestation of CHF in most patients. Fatigue, weakness, cachexia, malnutrition, and low urinary output then develop. When left untreated, cardiogenic shock, marked hypoperfusion of poorly oxygenated blood to the tissues, and death will eventually result. Heart failure should always be ruled out in patients who present with recurrent pulmonary infections, those with frequent exacerbations of chronic obstructive pulmonary disease, and elders who experience acute confusion.

PHYSICAL ASSESSMENT OF CHF
The goal of physical assessment is to assess the type of heart failure (right, left, or biventricular) and the severity of the condition. Assessment of the older adult with heart failure would include cardiac, pulmonary, integumentary, gastrointestinal, and functional assessments.

Cardiac Assessment
Knowledge of the heart rate and rhythm is essential to determine the presence of dysrhythmias that are compromising the function of the heart. Change in the pulse is usually the initial response to decreased cardiac output. Pulsus alternans, or alternating pulse, may be present as a result of the altered function of the left ventricle. This is manifested by strong beats alternating with weak beats on palpation and low-voltage QRS complexes on the electrocardiogram (ECG).

On palpation of the chest wall, the point of maximum impulse, which normally is at the fifth intercostal space in the midclavicular line, will be displaced laterally to the left toward the axilla. This displacement is due to the enlarged, hypertrophied left ventricle. In patients with heart failure, a third heart sound (S_3) is often the first clinical sign of CHF and is highly specific. This is a result of overfilling of the ventricle and reduced cardiac output. A fourth heart sound may also be heard, indicating chronic ischemic disease and lack of ventricular compliance. It is also important to be alert for murmurs.

Jugular vein pulses can estimate the venous pressure, and should be assessed while the patient is positioned at a 45-degree angle. Jugular vein distention (JVD) indicates right ventricular failure. The hepatojugular reflex should also be elicited, which is done by pressing on the right upper quadrant of the abdomen. When there is increased peripheral venous pressure, the compression of the abdomen causes increased blood flow to the right atrium, which causes the right atrial pressure to rise, in turn engorging the jugular vein and causing JVD. Increase in the JVD by at least 3 cm is considered a positive sign (Ducas, Madger, & McGregor, 1983).

Pulmonary Assessment
When pulmonary pressures are elevated, the hydrostatic pressure within the pulmonary capillaries surrounding the alveoli is elevated. This occurs as the left ventricle fails and causes backward flow. This increased pressure causes transudation of the fluid within the capillaries into the alveoli. This accumulated fluid is heard as "crackles" when the patient inspires. These crackles do not clear with coughing and are initially heard in the dependent portions of the lung. As pulmonary pressures continue to rise with left heart failure, these breath sounds can be heard throughout both lung fields. Sometimes crackles cannot be heard because of the increased lymphatic drainage in the lungs, and the only manifestation of pulmonary congestion may be wheezing (Shamsham, 2000).

Pleural effusions can also be present. Dyspnea increases as fluid accumulates in the alveoli, oxygen saturation decreases, and the patient feels as if he or she is drowning.

Integumentary Assessment

Dependent edema is a hallmark sign of right heart failure and biventricular failure. Edema should be assessed by palpation in the ankles and the feet, and in the sacral area in those patients who are bedridden. This edema may lead to stasis dermatitis, hyperpigmentation, and ulceration. The temperature of the skin is also very helpful in assessing cardiac output. Cool, clammy, diaphoretic skin is an indicator of peripheral vasoconstriction, which is a sign of increased sympathetic nervous system response, a compensation for decreased cardiac output.

Gastrointestinal Assessment

As mentioned in Box 10-2, liver enlargement occurs with heart failure (right ventricular or biventricular) as a result of venous congestion. The liver, when engorged, can be felt below the right costal margin of the ribs. In advanced heart failure, the spleen can also be palpated below the left costal margin.

Functional Status

In end-stage heart disease, symptoms of biventricular failure such as dyspnea, weakness, and fatigue are present in the physical assessment. It is important for health care providers to evaluate the impact of these symptoms on daily functioning by completing patient interviews or questionnaires at every visit. For the home care, hospice, long-term care, and advanced practice nurse, this assessment often helps to determine the plan of care and expectations regarding level of future functioning. This assessment is completed using various methods, depending on the setting. In addition to the NYHA Functional Classification system, the Dartmouth COOP charting system and the Short Form 36 (SF-36) are appropriate in primary care, skilled nursing home, and home care functional assessment.

The Dartmouth COOP chart system (Fig. 10-1) was developed by the Dartmouth Primary Care Cooperative Information Project a decade ago, and offers the practitioner a brief, practical method to assess functional status in both adults and adolescents (Nelson, Wasson, Johnson, & Hays, 1996). The COOP/WONCA version is a self-scoring system that can be used with adult patients, and is composed of charts encompassing different areas of functional status. Physical factors, emotional factors, daily activities, social

activities, social support, pain, and overall health are represented, each depicted by a drawing illustrating the level of functioning. High scores indicate an *unfavorable* self-assessment of that function, or a limitation. These charts are simple to administer and take very little time for the patient to complete. Elder patients can easily follow the directions, pictures can be enlarged if necessary, and the questionnaire can be interpreted easily. In some practices these charts are bar-coded so that a health report can be generated and elders can immediately see what health problems should be addressed. The system has been tested by practitioners in many different specialties, including those treating patients with CHF (Jenkinson, Jenkinson, Shepperd, Layte, & Petersen, 1997). When used longitudinally, changes that are made in the patient's plan of care can be assessed before and after intervention to ascertain whether they are effective. This system can also be used to guide management decisions, provide feedback on patient satisfaction, and predict outcomes regarding mortality.

Another functional assessment tool developed by the Measures Outcome Study is the SF-36 (Ware & Sherbourne, 1992). This 36-item questionnaire measures eight dimensions of health—physical functioning, bodily pain, general health, vitality, social functioning, role emotional, mental health, and health transition—covering three areas of general concern to individuals: functional status, well-being, and overall evaluation of health. This tool asks the patient to evaluate his or her status on each of the dimensions over the past year. The eight dimensions are scored on a scale of 0 to 100, with 0 being the worst possible health status and 100 being the best possible status (O'Mahoney, 1998). O'Mahoney (1998) found that this tool was suitable for interview administration, but found it was not useful in administration by mail in the elder population. When Jenkinson et al. (1997) evaluated both this scale and the Dartmouth COOP system for use in CHF patients, the SF-36 was found to be useful in assessing health status, but only modest expectation of improvement was reported by these patients. This was thought to be due to the significant compromise of functional capacity that is associated with CHF. The researchers also found that elders' physical activity was limited. Patients reported that treatment with angiotensin-converting

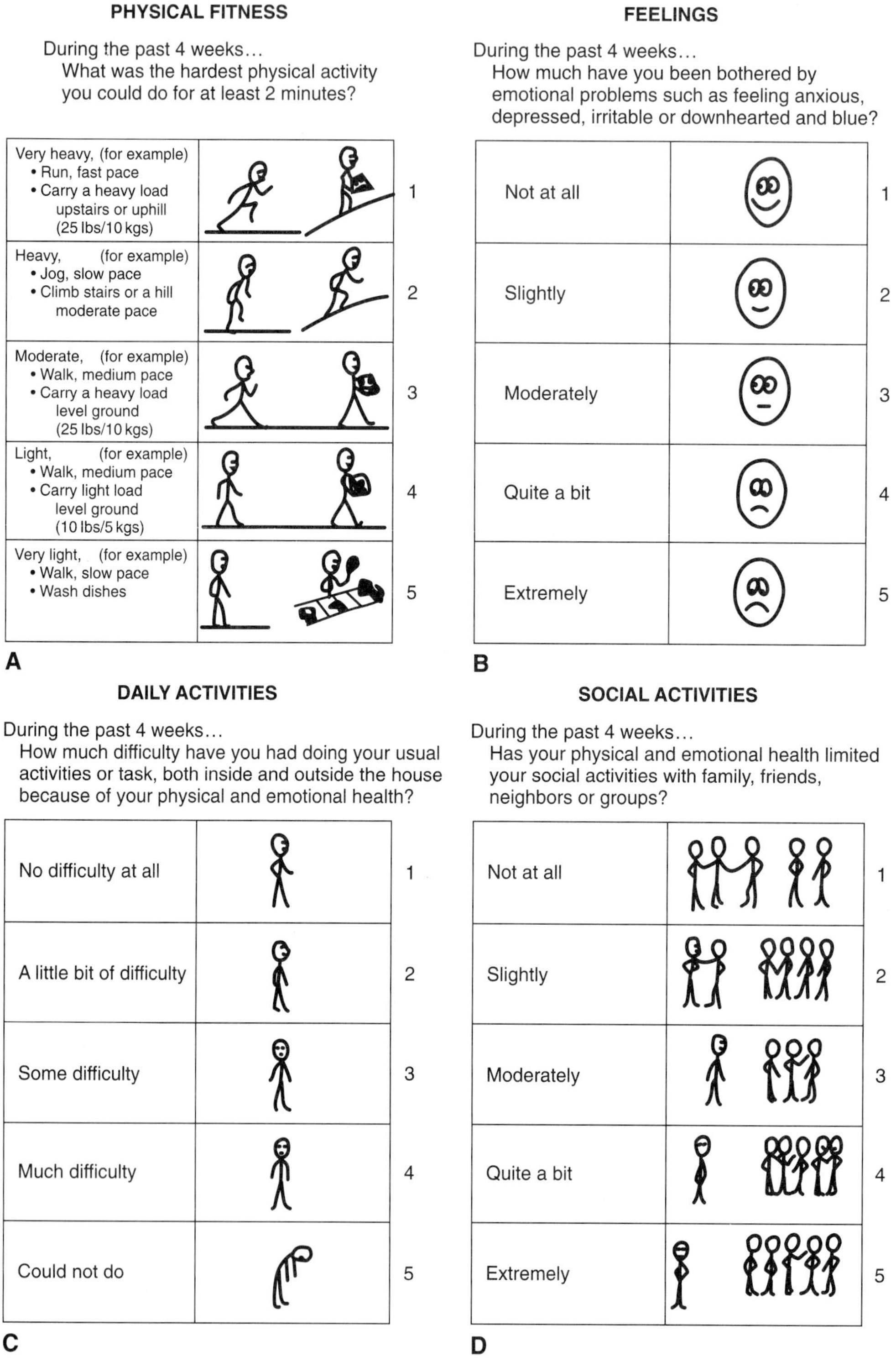

PHYSICAL FITNESS

During the past 4 weeks…
What was the hardest physical activity
you could do for at least 2 minutes?

Very heavy, (for example)
• Run, fast pace
• Carry a heavy load
  upstairs or uphill
  (25 lbs/10 kgs)
		1

Heavy, (for example) • Jog, slow pace • Climb stairs or a hill moderate pace		2

Moderate, (for example)
• Walk, medium pace
• Carry a heavy load
  level ground
  (25 lbs/10 kgs)
		3

Light, (for example)
• Walk, medium pace
• Carry light load
  level ground
  (10 lbs/5 kgs)
		4

Very light, (for example) • Walk, slow pace • Wash dishes		5

A

FEELINGS

During the past 4 weeks…
How much have you been bothered by
emotional problems such as feeling anxious,
depressed, irritable or downhearted and blue?

Not at all		1
Slightly		2
Moderately		3
Quite a bit		4
Extremely		5

B

DAILY ACTIVITIES

During the past 4 weeks…
How much difficulty have you had doing your usual
activities or task, both inside and outside the house
because of your physical and emotional health?

No difficulty at all		1
A little bit of difficulty		2
Some difficulty		3
Much difficulty		4
Could not do		5

C

SOCIAL ACTIVITIES

During the past 4 weeks…
Has your physical and emotional health limited
your social activities with family, friends,
neighbors or groups?

Not at all		1
Slightly		2
Moderately		3
Quite a bit		4
Extremely		5

D

Fig. 10-1 Dartmouth COOP chart system. (Copyright © 1995, Trustees of Dartmouth College/COOP Project.)

CHANGE IN HEALTH

How would you rate your overall health now compared to 4 weeks ago?

Much better	⬆⬆ ➕➕	1
A little better	⬆ ➕	2
About the same	⬅➡ ═	3
A little worse	⬇ ➖	4
Much worse	⬇⬇ ➖➖	5

E

OVERALL HEALTH

During the past 4 weeks…
How would you rate your health in general?

Excellent		1
Very good		2
Good		3
Fair		4
Poor		5

F

SOCIAL SUPPORT

During the past 4 weeks…
Was someone available to help you if you needed and wanted help? For example if you
- felt very nervous, lonely or blue
- got sick and had to stay in bed
- needed someone to talk to
- needed help with daily chores
- needed help just taking care of yourself

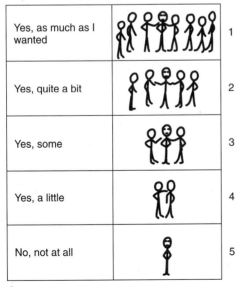

Yes, as much as I wanted		1
Yes, quite a bit		2
Yes, some		3
Yes, a little		4
No, not at all		5

G

QUALITY OF LIFE

How have things been going for you during the past 4 weeks?

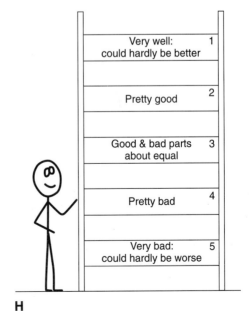

Very well: could hardly be better	1
Pretty good	2
Good & bad parts about equal	3
Pretty bad	4
Very bad: could hardly be worse	5

H

Fig. 10-1, cont'd.

enzyme (ACE) inhibitors did little to improve their quality of life even though life was prolonged with the use of these drugs (Jenkinson et al., 1997).

DIAGNOSTIC STUDIES FOR CHF

According to the practice guideline on evaluation and management of heart failure written by the American College of Cardiology (ACC)/AHA Task Force on Practice Guidelines (1995), the following diagnostic studies are indicated:

1. Complete blood count and urinalysis
2. Determination of serum electrolyte, blood urea nitrogen, creatinine, glucose, phosphorus, magnesium, calcium, and albumin levels
3. Chest radiograph and ECG
4. Thyroid studies (especially in those patients with atrial fibrillation and unexplained heart failure)
5. Transthoracic two-dimensional Doppler echocardiography
6. Noninvasive stress testing (in patients with previous history of MI)
7. Cardiac catheterization in patients with angina or large areas of ischemic myocardium

DISEASE MANAGEMENT IN CHF

The aim of therapy for the older adult with heart failure is symptom management and, when possible, improvement of cardiac output. Symptom management is imperative in order to improve quality of life. Nurses are vital to the education and ongoing assessment of general measures that will improve symptoms for these patients.

General counseling and education of the elder in strategies that will limit the progression of the disease requires an interdisciplinary approach. Important areas to address are listed in Box 10-3. Nurses, dietitians, social workers, pastoral care workers, physical therapists, occupational therapists, case managers, pharmacists, and physicians must take part in a coordinated team approach in counseling and educating patients with end-stage heart disease, and the plan should be maintained across all settings. For the older adult, aggressive use of nonpharmacologic measures is vital, because drug therapy can often cause unpleasant side effects. Recommended general treatment measures are outlined in Box 10-4.

Pharmacologic Approach

Before discussing the evidence-based pharmacologic treatment of CHF, it is important to review how cardiovascular drugs can be altered pharma-

---

Box 10-3 Patient Education for Managing Congestive Heart Failure

- Explanation of heart failure and its symptoms
- Symptoms of worsening failure
- Self-monitoring activities
- Explanation of the prescribed treatment plan
- Identification of risk factors with goals that are achievable (especially in the elder client)
- Value of support groups
- Importance of vaccinations
- Advance directives
- Dietary recommendations (individualized) and medication review

---

Box 10-4 General Treatment Measures for Congestive Heart Failure

- Decreasing more or new cardiac injury by reducing risk factors
- Advising patient to limit alcohol use to 2 glasses/day
- Maintaining fluid balance by restricting patient's salt intake (2 g/day)
- Helping patient to improve physical conditioning
- Avoiding use of calcium channel blockers (except amlodipine) and nonsteroidal antiinflammatory drugs
- Carefully managing comorbid conditions
- Educating patient regarding self-care
- Advising patient to receive influenza vaccination every fall
- Advising patient to receive pneumococcal immunizations after diagnosis and revaccination every 5 years
- Ensuring that care of patients with heart failure is across settings and by interdisciplinary team

Data from Makalinao, J. (2000). Chronic heart failure: examining consensus recommendations for patients' management. *Geriatrics, 55,* 53-58.

EVIDENCE-BASED PRACTICE

Reference: A specialist-nurse intervention reduced readmissions in patients hospitalized with chronic heart failure. (2002). *ACP Journal Club,* 136(3), 87. Research Problem: Can a specialist-nurse intervention reduce mortality and morbidity in patients hospitalized with chronic heart failure?

Design: Randomized (allocation concealed), blinded (outcome assessors) controlled trial with follow-up at 1 year.

Sample and Setting: 165 patients (mean age 75 years, 58% men) who were admitted on an emergency basis at a teaching hospital in Glasgow, Scotland, with heart failure caused by left ventricular systolic dysfunction. Exclusion criteria were inability to comply with the intervention, acute myocardial infarction, comorbidity likely to lead to death or readmission in the near future, planned discharge to long-term residential care, or residence outside of the hospital catchment area. Follow-up at 1 year was 95%.

Methods: Eighty-four patients were allocated to usual care plus a specialist-nurse intervention, which consisted of planned home visits of decreasing frequency supplemented by telephone contact as needed. The aim was to educate patients about heart failure and its treatment, optimize treatment, monitor electrolyte levels, teach self-monitoring and management, encourage treatment adherence, liaise with other health care providers, and provide psychological support. Nurses were given training and followed written protocols on the use of specific

drugs. Patients were given a pocket-sized booklet that included information about heart failure and its treatment; contact information for nurses; a list of their drugs, weight, and blood test results; and details of planned visits. Eighty-one patients were allocated to usual care and managed by the admitting physician and subsequently the general practitioner. They did not see the specialist nurses after discharge.

Results: The primary outcome was combined death or readmission for heart failure (emergency or elective). Secondary outcomes included combined death or readmission for any reason, death, readmission for worsening chronic heart failure, and readmission for any reason. At 1 year, fewer patients in the specialist-nurse group than in the usual-care group had the combined outcome of death or readmission for heart failure, and fewer were readmitted for worsening chronic heart failure. The groups did not differ on combined death or readmission for any reason (62% vs. 75%, $p=0.075$), death (30% vs. 31%, $p=0.81$), or readmission for any reason (56% vs. 60%, $p=0.27$).

Implications for Nursing Practice: Planned home visits and telephone contact by specialist nurses should be considered to reduce mortality rates and readmission to the hospital for patients with chronic heart failure.

Conclusion: A specialist-nurse intervention reduced readmissions for heart failure in patients admitted to the hospital with chronic heart failure.

codynamically in the elder patient. There can be many adverse reactions to cardiovascular medications when used in the older adult population. Physiologically, changes in the metabolism and excretion of drugs occur with age. It is well known that, with age, there is a decrease in glomerular filtration and tubular secretion (Nolan & Marcus, 2000). Cardiac medications that are dependent upon the kidney for excretion should be titrated appropriately; digoxin and ACE inhibitors are drugs in this category. The hepatic metabolism of drugs also decreases

with age. The commonly used medications for relief of symptoms in CHF can therefore have a delayed and variable absorption in the elder patient. Careful dosing and titration of these drugs on an individual basis is imperative. The recommendations in Box 10-5 should be considered when prescribing cardiac medications for older adults.

Guidelines for treatment of CHF are available from several sources. The Agency for Health Care Policy and Research published heart failure care guidelines in 1994, and the ACC/AHA

Box 10-5 Prescribing Cardiac Medications for Older Adults

1. Always begin with the smallest effective dose; titrate up in small increments, keeping in mind the patient's comorbid conditions that could influence the pharmacokinetics of the drug(s).
2. As dose adjustment is made, clinical evaluation should occur.
3. Review each medication the patient is currently taking, even over-the-counter medications and herbal remedies, and be aware of contraindications or adjustments needed.
4. Avoid empirical treatment of symptoms. Have a diagnosis before initiating drug therapy.
5. Keep it simple! Adherence decreases as the number of medications and frequency of dosing increases.
6. Make sure that the patient can read the labels; if not, a family member or home care nurse should set up a weekly pill dispenser.
7. Patient education is key. Make sure that each patient understands the adverse reactions to watch for and knows when to call for assistance.

Task Force also published guidelines in 1995. The *American Journal of Cardiology* ("Consensus Recommendations," 1999) published guidelines for the management of heart failure taking into account recent advances in pharmacologic management. Finally, the Heart Failure Society of America (HFSA) published guidelines that are addressed in the following sections as they relate to the elder patient with chronic heart failure ("HFSA Guidelines," 1999).

Agents approved by the HFSA for the management of heart failure include diuretics, ACE inhibitors, aldosterone antagonists, beta-adrenergic receptor blockers (in selected cases), and inotropes (medications that increase contractility of the heart). The recommendations below address primarily the treatment of chronic left ventricular systolic dysfunction, which accounts for the majority of heart disease in the older adult population. These recommendations do not apply to patients with aortic stenosis because a decrease in afterload and diuresis pre-

cipitate heart failure in these patients. In those patients with aortic stenosis, valvular surgery is the only option when heart failure is diagnosed.

Diuretics

Loop diuretics are the preferred class of drugs for use with older adult patients. These are recommended because they are efficacious in sodium and water excretion even when renal function is compromised. Loop diuretics provide immediate relief of symptoms associated with fluid overload, but should not be used as the only pharmacologic agent because they lose effect over an extended period. Diuretics used on a chronic basis can increase renin, which magnifies the activation of the renin–angiotensin system, and therefore should be combined with ACE inhibitors (Goldstein, 2001). Common loop diuretics used in CHF are furosemide (Lasix), torsemide (Demodex), and bumetanide (Bumex). Because loop diuretics cause loss of essential electrolytes (resulting in hypokalemia, hypomagnesemia, hyponatremia, glucose intolerance, and hyperlipidemia), careful ongoing assessment of the elder patient is recommended.

Determination of the proper initial dose and readjustment of doses require ongoing evaluation of symptoms, especially in the older adult population. As heart failure increases, the absorption of loop diuretics in the gastrointestinal tract decreases, and increased dosage may be necessary (Goldstein, 2001). In end-stage disease, the addition of metolazone (Zaroxolyn) may be necessary, especially in patients with renal insufficiency (Arling, 1997). According to Aronow (1996), hydrochlorothiazide (a thiazide diuretic) is recommended for mild CHF, but with caution, because the thiazide diuretics can cause hyperkalemia when combined with ACE inhibitors.

ACE Inhibitors

ACE inhibitors have been studied extensively over the last 10 years in many large trials (Table 10-2). ACE inhibitors were introduced initially as treatment for hypertension. It was believed that, because these agents dilate the peripheral blood vessels by inhibiting the renin–angiotensin system, there might be an indication for use in CHF. Extensive studies found that not only did these agents decrease afterload and preload as expected, but also, more importantly, they had

Table 10-2 **Trials of ACE Inhibitors**

Trial	Inclusion Criteria	Therapy	Results
SOLVD*	EF≤35%	Enalapril vs. placebo	16% reduction in mortality
CONSENSUS[†]	NYHA IV	Enalapril vs. placebo	40% reduction in mortality at 6 mo, 31% reduction at 1 yr
SAVE[‡]	NYHA I-II, EF≤35%	Captopril vs. placebo	20% reduction in mortality
AIRE[§]	EF≤40%	Ramipril vs. placebo	27% reduction in all-cause mortality
ELITE[k]	Age>65, CHF	Losartan vs. captopril	Losartan well tolerated, 46% reduction in mortality in 15 mo
RESOLVD[¶]	NYHA II-IV, EF≤40%	Candesartan+enalapril vs. enalapril alone	EF increased, prevention of LV remodeling with cardesartan+enalapril
V-HeFT-II**	NYHA II-III	Hydralazine/isosorbide vs. enalapril	28% reduction in mortality with enalapril vs. hydralazine/isosorbide

CHF, congestive heart failure; EF, ejection fraction; LV, left ventricular; New York Heart Association.

*Data from The SOLVD investigators: Effect of enalapril on survival in patients with reduced left ventricular ejection fraction and congestive heart failure. (1991). *New England Journal of Medicine, 325,* 293-302.

[†]Data from Effects: Results of the of enalapril on mortality in severe congestive heart failure. Results of the Cooperative North Scandinavian Enalapril Survival Study (CONSENSUS). The CONSENSUS Trial Study Group. (1987). *New England Journal of Medicine, 316,* 1429-1435.

[‡]Data from St. John Sutton, M., Pfeffer, M. A., Moye, L., Plappert, T., Rouleau, J. L., Lamas, G., et al. (1997). Cardiovascular death and left ventricular remodeling two years after myocardial infarction: baseline predictors and impact of long-term use of captopril. Information from the Survival and Ventricular Enlargement (SAVE) trial. *Circulation, 96,* 3294-3299.

[§]Data from Effect of ramipril on mortality and morbidity of survivors of acute myocardial infarction with clinical evidence of heart failure. The Acute Infarction Ramipril Efficacy (AIRE) Study Investigators. (1993). *Lancet, 342,* 821-827.

[k]Data from Pitt, B., Segal, R., Martinez, F. A., Meurers, G., Cowley, A. J., Thomas, I., et al. (1997). The ELITE study investigators. Randomised trial of losartan versus captopril in patients over 65 with heart failure (Evaluation of Losartan in the Elderly Study, ELITE). *Lancet, 349,* 747-752.

[¶]Data from McKelvie, R., S., Yusuf, S., Pericak, D., Avezum, A., Burns, R. J., Probstfield, J., et al. (1999). Comparison of candesartan, enalapril, and their combination in congestive heart failure: Randomized Evaluation of Strategies for Left Ventricular Dysfunction (RESOLVD) pilot study. The RESOLVD Pilot Investigators. *Circulation, 100,* 1056-1064.

**Data from Cohn, J. N., Johnson, G., Ziesche, S., Cobb, F., Francis, G., Tristani, F., et al. (1951). A comparison of enalapril with hydralazine-isosorbide dinitrate in the treatment of chronic congestive heart failure. *New England Journal of Medicine, 325,* 303-310.

a significant effect on ventricular remodeling. Through the mechanisms of decreasing aldosterone secretion and response of the sympathetic nervous system, symptoms dramatically improved almost immediately. There continues to be concern regarding hypotension and the use of ACE inhibitors, especially in elders, and further large-scale studies should be done with patients over age 65. Enalapril, one of the earliest ACE inhibitors studied, has been to shown benefit elder patients (Arling, 1997). Gillespie, Darbar, Struthers, and McMurdo (1998) believe that

ACE inhibitors would be better tolerated if patients were hydrated and electrolytes were within normal limits. ACE inhibitors should not be used in patients with a history of angioedema or anuria with prior ACE inhibitor use. Also, cautious use of ACE inhibitors is warranted in those patients with high serum creatinine levels (>3 mg/dL), bilateral renal stenosis, high serum potassium levels (>5.5 mmol/L), and low systolic blood pressure (Makalinao, 2000). Many patients complain of an irritating dry cough, a common side effect caused by the ability of ACE inhibitors to increase bradykinin release, and this can be a major reason for treatment failure.

Studies since 1997 have examined agents that block angiotensin by a different mechanism than that of ACE inhibitors, such as angiotensin II receptor blockers (ARBs). These agents block angiotensin II and aldosterone at the receptor level. Hemodynamic effects are the same as those of the ACE inhibitors as far as reducing preload and afterload and increasing cardiac output, but these agents do not increase bradykinin levels, thus diminishing the side effect of cough (Gillespie et al., 1998). The first of these agents, losartan, was found to be well tolerated by elder patients.

Early data from clinical trials in progress have demonstrated that use of ACE inhibitors and ARBs can improve survival of CHF patients. They have also brought symptomatic relief and functional improvement. According to Goldstein (2001), ACE inhibitors have also decreased the recurrence of CHF in patients who were asymptomatic. Current practice guidelines from the HFSA (1999) recommend either an ACE inhibitor or an ARB as standard therapy in both symptomatic and nonsymptomatic patients with an LVEF less than 40%. Table 10-3 details the recommended initial and target doses for ACE inhibitors and ARB agents.

Pharmacologic recommendations and practice guidelines for ACE inhibitors are as follows ("HFSA Guidelines," 1999):

1. In the absence of contraindications, all patients with or without symptomatic heart failure should be considered for treatment with an ACE inhibitor.
2. ACE inhibitors rather than ARBs continue to be agents of choice.

Table 10-3 Pharmacologic Agents Used In Heart Failure

Classification/Agent	Recommended Starting Dose*	Target Doses[†]
LOOP DIURETICS		
Furosemide (Lasix)	20-40 mg/day	Titrated until u/o increases
Bumetanide (Bumex)	0.5-2 mg/day	
Metolazone (Zaroxolyn)	5-20 mg/day	
ACE INHIBITORS		
Captopril (Capoten)	6.25 mg tid	150 mg tid
Enalapril (Vasotec)	2.5 mg bid	20-40 mg bid
Ramipril (Altace)	2.5 mg bid	5 mg bid
Lisinopril (Zestril)	2.5 mg/day	20-40 mg/day
ANGIOTENSIN RECEPTOR BLOCKERS		
Losartan (Cozaar)	25 mg/day	50 mg/day
Valsartan (Diovan)	80 mg/day	80-320 mg/day
Candesartan (Atacand)	4 mg/day	4-32 mg/day
Irbesartan (Avapro)	75 mg/day	150-300 mg/day
BETA-ADRENERGIC BLOCKERS		
Carvedilol (Coreg)	3.125 mg bid	25-50 mg/day
Metoprolol (Lopressor)	12.5 mg/day (XL)	200 mg/day
Bisoprolol (Zebeta)	12.5 mg bid	150 mg/day
	1.25 mg/day	10 mg/day

*Data from *PDR Electronic Library* (Version 5.20a). (2001). Montvale, NJ: Medical Economics Company.
[†]Data from Lonn, E. (2000). Drug treatment in heart failure. *British Medical Journal, 320*, 1188-1192.

3. If intolerance to ACE inhibitors develops, agents to be considered are either ARBs or hydralazine and isosorbide dinitrate.

Aldosterone Antagonists

Spironolactone, an aldosterone antagonist, has been found helpful at low doses (12.5 to 25 mg/day) in patients with NYHA class IV disease or severe heart failure. The aldosterone antagonists block aldosterone, which causes diureses, resulting in decreased preload. Patients on aldosterone antagonists should have normal serum potassium levels (<5.0 mEq/L) and adequate renal function (creatinine <2.5 mg/dL) ("HFSA Guidelines," 1999). It is also important that serum potassium levels be monitored at regular intervals.

Beta-Adrenergic Blocking Agents

Use of beta-blockers in patients with chronic heart failure has been studied in 20 clinical trials with over 10,000 patients. These trials have shown that use of these agents reduces the risk of sudden death by 40% to 50%, decreases the need for hospital admission, and improves overall functional capacity (Lonn, 2000). The beneficial effects of beta-blockers in heart failure are related to the blocking of adrenergic stimulation of the heart, specifically that of norepinephrine, which in CHF is related to increased mortality (Goldstein, 2001). Beta-blockade has a negative inotropic effect, and was for many years contraindicated in heart failure patients. In clinical trials, however, it was shown that this decrease in cardiac output was transient, and that, in fact, beta-blockade was shown to increase LVEF. This benefit was found in patients who were experiencing therapeutic responses to diuretics and ACE inhibitors.

Patients with NYHA class II through IV disease were studied in multiple trials; one trial was able to show a decrease in mortality of 35% (MERIT-HF Study Group, 1999). The studies looking at beta-blockers in heart failure examined three agents; carvedilol, bisoprolol, and metoprolol (continuous and extended release formulations). The first Cardiac Insufficiency Bisoprolol Study (CIBIS I) trial found that there was a 34% reduction in hospital admission rates for patients who were on bisoprolol, and many showed improvements in overall quality of life

(CIBIS Investigators and Committees, 1994). In the second trial, CIBIS II, there was a 34% reduction in mortality and a 20% reduction in hospital admissions in patients with NYHA class III and IV disease treated with bisoprolol (CIBIS Investigators and Committees, 1999). In the Metoprolol CR/XL Randomized Intervention Trial in Congestive Heart Failure (MERIT-HF), it was found that metoprolol not only had a vasodilatory effect (as a result of its alpha-adrenergic properties), but also had antioxidant effects (MERIT-HF Study Group, 1999).

Beta-blockers are contraindicated in patients with bronchospastic disease, advanced heart block, or symptomatic bradycardia, and should be used with caution in those with low systolic blood pressure. Beta-blockers should generally be added once diuretics and ACE inhibitors have been optimized and clinical stability is obtained.

Pharmacologic recommendations and practice guidelines for beta-blockers are as follows ("HFSA Guidelines," 1999):
1. Beta-blocker therapy should be routinely administered to clinically stable patients with a LVEF less than 40% and those with mild to moderate heart failure (NYHA classes II and III) who are on standard therapy (ACE inhibitors, diuretics, and digoxin).
2. Beta-blocker therapy should be considered for patients who have a LVEF less than 40% and are asymptomatic (NYHA class I) and on standard therapy (ACE inhibitors).
3. Clinical stability on standard therapy should be achieved before beta-blockers are started.
4. Beta-blockers should be initiated at low doses and titrated slowly (every 2 weeks), with clinical reevaluation at each point of titration.
5. Beta-blockers are indicated in high-risk patients after an acute MI.

Digitalis

Digitalis glycosides (positive inotropic agents) have been a part of the medical regimen for patients in heart failure for over 200 years. These agents are indicated for use in patients with symptomatic heart failure in combination with ACE inhibitors and diuretic therapy. In a study on the effects of digoxin ("The Digitalis Investigation Group," 1997), patients with mild to moderate heart failure on digoxin experienced a decrease in the progression of heart failure

EVIDENCE-BASED PRACTICE

Reference: Treating isolated systolic hypertension prevented major cardiovascular events across strata of risk in older patients. (2002). *ACP Journal Club,* *137*(1), 4.

Research Problem: In older patients with isolated systolic hypertension (ISH), is blood pressure (BP)–lowering treatment more effective than placebo for preventing major cardiovascular disease (CVD) events in those at high risk than in those at low risk?

Design: Randomized (allocation concealed), blinded (outcome assessors), placebo-controlled trial with 4.5-year follow-up (subgroup analysis of the Systolic Hypertension in the Elderly Program [SHEP] trial).

Sample and Setting: 4736 community-dwelling patients who were 60 years of age or older and had ISH (systolic BP 160 to 219 mm Hg and diastolic BP <90 mm Hg assessed and averaged over two visits), no atrial fibrillation, and no history of myocardial infarction (MI) or stroke in the past 6 months. Patients taking antihypertensive medications were eligible if their BPs met the entry criteria for ISH after medication withdrawal. Also, 4189 patients (88%) (64% age≥70 years, 58% women) who did not report previous CVD or stroke at baseline and who had complete CVD risk factor data were included in the analysis reported here. The study was conducted at five clinical centers in the United States.

Methods: Patients were allocated to treatment (n= 2365) or placebo (n=2371). ISH treatment was a stepped-care approach: step 1 consisted of chlorthalidone, 12.5 mg/day, and step 2 consisted of addition of atenolol, 25 mg/day, or reserpine, 0.05 mg/day, if atenolol was not tolerated. Treatment in both groups was increased by doubling the dosage or adding a second-step drug until the BP goal (systolic BP decreased to <160 mm Hg or by ≥20 mm Hg) was reached, side effects precluded an additional step up, or the highest step was reached.

Results: The study outcome was first-occurring major CVD event (stroke, MI, or congestive heart failure). (Analysis was by intention to treat.) Patients were stratified by sex-specific quartiles of global cardiovascular risk scores. The rate for any major CVD event across strata of risk was lower in the treatment group than in the placebo group ($p < 0.001$). The beneficial trend for treatment across strata was also seen ($p < 0.001$) when MI, stroke, and heart failure were analyzed separately.

Implications for Nursing Practice: BP lowering therapies should be considered for older patients with isolated systolic hypertension and at high risk for cardiovascular events (stroke, MI, CHF) to lower such risk.

Conclusion: In older patients with isolated systolic hypertension, BP-lowering treatment prevented major cardiovascular events across strata of risk.

and had decreased hospital admissions (28%), but had no overall decrease in mortality. Digoxin is indicated in patients with heart failure and those with atrial fibrillation with uncontrolled ventricular response.

Pharmacologic recommendations and practice guidelines for digoxin are as follows ("HFSA Guidelines," 1999):

1. Digoxin should be considered for patients who have symptoms of heart failure (NYHA classes II through IV), while receiving standard therapy.

2. In the majority of patients, the dosage of digoxin should be 0.125 to 0.25 mg/day.

Anticoagulation in Heart Failure

Atrial fibrillation complicating heart failure contributes to an increased incidence of stroke, and the appropriateness of anticoagulation therapy for these patients is well established. Routine use of anticoagulation in heart failure patients without atrial fibrillation has not been confirmed by randomized controlled trials. Secondary analysis of the Study of Left

Ventricular Dysfunction (SOLVD) ("The SOLVD Investigators," 1992) supported the use of warfarin (Coumadin) in these patients. It was found that those who received warfarin had a 25% risk reduction in all-cause mortality.

Medications to Avoid Prescribing for Elder Patients with Heart Failure

As outlined above, there are well-established guidelines related to therapeutic agents in CHF; however, certain classes of pharmacologic agents should be avoided. According to the latest practice guidelines (Zoler, 2000):

- Antiarrhythmics (other than beta-blockers) are not recommended to suppress asymptomatic ventricular arrhythmia or ectopy.
- Most calcium channel blockers should not be used in patients with systolic dysfunction.
- Nonsteroidal anti-inflammatory drugs should be avoided (because of the sodium and water retention resulting from prostaglandin inhibition).

Electrical Therapy

Because the pharmacologic agents have fallen short in improvement of quality of life and prognosis, especially in those patients with chronic ventricular dysfunction, recent consideration has been given to interventional therapies in heart failure. These therapies include biventricular pacing and implantable cardioverter–defibrillators (ICDs).

Biventricular Pacing

Since the early 1990s, numerous approaches have been implemented to improve left ventricular function in patients with CHF by means of cardiac pacing. In the last 2 years, the most promising of these approaches has been biventricular pacing, or ventricular resynchronization therapy.

Normally, electrical impulses arise in the sinoatrial node of the heart, travel down through the atrioventricular node to the bundle of His, and then through the left and the right bundle branches to the Purkinje fibers, where simultaneous depolarization of the right atrium and the ventricles occurs. This coordinated conduction enables stroke volume to be maximized. If one or more of these conduction pathways (left bundle or right bundle) is damaged or blocked, the

impulse will reach one ventricle before the other, causing an asynchrony of the ventricular contraction known as intraventricular conduction defect (IVCD). This can be seen in the QRS complex (measurement of time for ventricular depolarization) of the ECG, which becomes prolonged (>120 msec). IVCD has been found in 30% to 50% of patients with CHF (Naccarelli, 2001). These conduction delays cause inefficient ventricular contraction, with segments of the ventricle contracting at different times. Short diastole occurs with overlapping of systole and diastole and decrease in cardiac output (Bald, 2000). If the patient already has a failing left ventricle, ICVD with decrease in cardiac output leads to further dysfunction and increased symptoms.

The biventricular pacemaker looks like other pacemakers, but it has three leads instead of two. Electrical leads are threaded into both the left and right ventricles and the right atrium. This device provides electrical stimulation that is programmed precisely to synchronize and coordinate the right and left ventricular contractions (Barold, 2000).

Early evidence in the use of biventricular pacing with CHF patients came from small observational studies (Dresing & Natale, 2001). Larger clinical trials (VIGOR-CHF, MIRACLE, and PATH-CHF) have been done in the last 2 years on the efficacy of this treatment. Most patients in these trials had NYHA class II through IV disease and prolonged QRS duration (>150 msec) and were on optimum medical therapy (Naccarelli, 2001). Primary end points for these trials were 6-minute walk tests, quality of life, and O_2 consumption at peak exercise (Dresing & Natale, 2001). Consistently it was found that there was an almost immediate increase in cardiac output, a positive effect on left ventricular remodeling, and an improvement of diastolic function.

Combination ICDs and Ventricular Resynchronization Therapy

Sudden death occurs in 30% to 59% of patients in NYHA class IV (Daubert et al., 2000). Because of these alarming statistics, the role of combined ICD and ventricular resynchronization devices in chronic heart failure patients has been investigated. ICD implantation is a life-saving option for the patient who is at risk for sudden cardiac death as a result of lethal ventricular arrhythmia. The combined use of ICDs and biventricular pacemakers has been investigated in the VENTAK CHF, Insync ICD, and COM-PANION trials (Dresing & Natale, 2001). The difference in the inclusion criteria for these patients as compared with those in the biventricular pacemaker studies was that the subjects in these trials also had an indication for ICD implantation (ventricular tachycardia) (Dresing & Natale, 2001). Preliminary reports of the results of these studies have indicated an improvement of symptoms, increased quality of life, and decreased incidence of sudden death. The efficacy of combined biventricular pacing and ICDs in patients with CHF and IVCDs in the general CHF population has yet to be determined; the Food and Drug Administration is currently reviewing these data (Naccarelli, 2001).

Complementary Therapies

People are becoming increasingly interested in holistic modalities for the prevention and treatment of disease. Natural treatments—use of vitamins, herbs, antioxidants, and other nontraditional therapies—are used by many patients to complement or even replace drugs and other interventions. Adjunctive healing modalities can be a benefit to traditional medicine, and specific homeopathic remedies have shown some efficacy for the elder patient with CHF.

Antioxidants

Oxygen-derived free radicals, the by-products of oxygen metabolism, have been found to cause damage to cells and are considered to be among the causes of many chronic diseases, including CHF (Weglicki, Kramer, & Mak, 1999). Antioxidants have been shown to inhibit atherogenesis and thrombosis in the coronary arteries by interfering with the oxidation of low-density lipoproteins, which prevents the formation of foam cells, a major cause of atherosclerosis (Anderson & Kessenich, 2001). Antioxidants are found naturally in a wide variety of foods and plants, including many fruits and vegetables, and they are available as nutritional supplements (vitamin C, vitamin E, and beta-carotene). The foods that contain the greatest amounts of

antioxidants are carrots, tomatoes, yams, leafy greens, blueberries, garlic, and green tea. Tribble (1999) reviewed the evidence regarding the use of antioxidants for the Nutrition Committee of the AHA and found that most of the studies have been observational and the evidence thus far is insufficient to recommend antioxidants in coronary heart disease.

Vitamin E, along with vitamin C and selenium, have been found to promote cardiovascular health. In animal models, oxidant injury to cardiac membranes, which in part leads to the pathologic changes that occur in cardiomyopathy, was decreased by these compounds (Weglicki et al., 1999). It was also found (Weglicki et al., 1999) that magnesium deficiency produced a proinflammatory condition resulting in overproduction of free radicals that caused cardiovascular cell injury. The U.S. Department of Agriculture recommended dose for vitamin E is 30 to 400 IU/day; however, the Cambridge Heart Antioxidant Study showed that doses of 400 to 800 IU/day were more effective (Tribble, 1999).

Ubiquinone (coenzyme-Q10), a fat-soluble vitamin-like compound, is an endogenous antioxidant that protects against free radical damage in the mitochondria (Skidmore-Roth, 2001). Ubiquinone is a nutrient needed for cells to produce energy. A small study by Hofman-Bang, Rehnquist, Swedberg, Wiklund, and Astrom (1995) found that ubiquinone reduced hospitalizations and serious complications in patients with heart failure. It is indicated for use in ischemic heart disease, angina, hypertension, and CHF. The recommended dose is 300 mg/day, and the drug should be avoided in patients taking beta-blockers or cholesterol-lowering preparations.

Hawthorn, an herb, has been indicated for use in heart failure patients. According to Starbuck (1999), hawthorn is rich in flavonoids, which have been shown to benefit patients with heart disease. Patients who have taken this herb as a treatment noted improvement in exercise tolerance, shortness of breath, ankle edema, nighttime urination, and mental well-being. The dose is 100 to 250 mg/day. Side effects may include hypotension, and hawthorn should not be used with antihypertensives or cardiac glycosides because it may increase the effects of each (Skidmore-Roth, 2001).

Other Complementary Therapies

Other complementary therapies for CHF may include slow breathing exercises, meditation, prayer, biofeedback, and yoga. Slow breathing, according to Bernardi et al. (2002), improves oxygen saturation and exercise tolerance in heart failure patients by increasing the arterial barore-flex sensitivity.

Stress reduction techniques also have shown promise in the prevention and treatment of coronary artery disease. Transcendental meditation is associated with decreased hypertension and atherosclerosis (King, Carr, & D'Cruz, 2002).

Spirituality influences the manner in which a patient adjusts to a chronic illness. Patients with end-stage heart disease often reflect on their past and attempt to nurture hopes for the future. Westlake and Dracup (2001) looked at how spirituality affected patient adjustment in end-stage heart failure. Eighty-seven patients were interviewed using a semistructured questionnaire, and a three-step process was identified in which they adjusted to or came to terms with their illness. The three steps were development of regret regarding past behaviors and lifestyles, the search for meaning within the present experience of heart failure, and the search for hope and optimism.

PALLIATIVE CARE FOR PATIENTS WITH END-STAGE HEART DISEASE

The end of life for elder patients with heart disease does not have to be one that is breathless, painful, frightening, and isolated. Palliative care is finally coming into practice when patients are at this point in their life. Oncology medicine paved the way, and there is much that can be learned from its history of caring for advanced cancer patients. It was unheard of, only a decade ago, to apply palliative care principles to cardiac patients. Patients' only option was to come into a critical care unit, be intubated, and die in the hands of strangers. Older adult patients with heart disease rarely had a voice as to how their death would occur, who would be a part of it, and in what environment they would spend their last days. Now, these patients can expect more health care practitioners whose goals are to improve the quality of life until its end. The holistic care provided by nurses is exactly what makes the "last" days as important as the "birth" days.

Comfort care, or palliative care, is directed toward providing quality of life and quality of dying. The Ethics Committee of the American Geriatrics Society (AGS) ("The Care of Dying Patients," 1995) identified 10 domains in which one can measure quality of life (Box 10-6). Assessment of these 10 domains can be applied to all patients, including those with end-stage heart disease. According to the AGS, most people who are in this end stage of life desire to be treated respectfully, in comfort, and among their loved ones. To achieve a level of comfort, symptom management continues to be key, along with consistent support. The preferences of the individual at death should be respected, which can be a quandary for health care providers, especially if the chosen path is different from what the health care provider believes is best. Our duty as health care providers is to assure the patient and family that appropriate steps will be taken in fulfilling the treatment options the patient and family have chosen. The goal of providing this care is to bring about as good a death as possible.

As with all patients in this stage of life, ongoing communication is the key in achieving the goal of dying well. Communication skills needed for the discussions necessary in this phase of life are often lacking in the education of health care providers. After all, we spent hours learning the curative model of care, and dying and death was not part of that construct. In fact, to many

---

Box 10-6 Domains to Measure Quality of Life

1. Physical and emotional symptoms
2. Support of function and autonomy
3. Advance care planning
4. Aggressiveness of care near death
5. Patient and family satisfaction
6. Global quality of life
7. Family burden
8. Survival time
9. Provider continuity and skill
10. Bereavement

From The care of dying patients: A position statement from the American Geriatrics Society. AGS Ethics Committee. (1995). *Journal of the American Geriatrics Society, 43*, 577-578.

health care professionals, patient death is viewed as a failure. Sharing of bad news and discussion of advance directives, living wills, and care options for the end of life are rarely approached, and often left to discuss when it is too late.

In a qualitative study done in Britain by Rogers (2000), it was found that patients with chronic heart failure were given little information about not only the disease process, but also the likely prognosis. Depression was prominent, and was partly attributed to the fact that there was a lack of open communication between the patient and the physician. Rogers also found that patients wanted to ask questions about their illnesses but felt reluctant to do so. Patients believed that their doctors were averse to discussing dying and death, whereas, overall, patients would welcome frank discussions about their prognosis.

Programs that enhance end-of-life communication between health care providers and their patients are needed (Heffner, 2000). In a study of 415 patients in cardiac rehabilitation programs, Heffner (2000) found that patients want more end-of-life information and wanted physicians to initiate the discussion in the office setting. Ninety percent of the patients in this study did not believe that physicians understood their end-of-life wishes.

When patients want and need to discuss wishes for this stage of their lives, they often depend on their health care provider to initiate the conversation. Explanation of the normal process of dying and goals of palliative care are important because many patients have never directly experienced a death, and the process that occurs in dying. These discussions need to happen before the patient becomes too ill to participate, because they affect not only his or her own life, but also the lives of his or her loved ones.

According to the AGS position statement ("The Care of Dying Patients," 1995), optimal care requires an interdisciplinary approach so that the needs of both the patient and family can be met. The ACC/AHA Task Force (1995) also recommended that multidisciplinary disease management programs be developed for patients at risk for hospital admission or clinical deterioration. This care should be provided in the patient's home if that is where the patient wishes

to die. The ACC/AHA Task Force (1995) also published practice guidelines for the care of patients with end-stage heart failure:

1. Ongoing patient and family education regarding prognosis for function and survival
2. Patient and family education about options for formulating and implementing advance directives
3. Continuity of medical care between inpatient and outpatient settings
4. Components of hospice care that are appropriate in the relief of suffering

When heart failure becomes intolerable, resuscitation may no longer be desired. If management at home with hospice care is desired, the symptoms of breathlessness will require potent opioids and anxiolytics (ACC/AHA Task Force, 1995), as well as the use of complementary therapies.

Older adult patients dying from heart disease are usually taking the maximum doses of diuretics and ACE inhibitors, yet may still have episodes of pulmonary edema and breathlessness. It is believed that, when heart failure progresses to this stage, the absorption of the medications that previously controlled the symptoms decreases, requiring increased doses (Taylor, 2001). In order to provide comfort to the elder patient, doses of up to 600 mg of furosemide may be required and combinations of diuretics may be necessary in order to control fluid overload. Morphine is also indicated at doses that provide rest and comfort and relieve suffering in the elder patient with CHF by decreasing preload and relieving pain. Because of the vasodilator effects of these drugs, there is less venous return, which decreases further overload in the heart. There is no ceiling dose for opioids, so the appropriate dose is whatever is needed to relieve pain and dyspnea for patients with CHF.

When dying from heart failure, the patient's cardiac output eventually decreases to a point where he or she has multiple organ dysfunction with involvement of the liver, kidneys, and lungs. Secondary to biventricular failure, the right-sided failure causes liver engorgement, which leads to not only nausea and vomiting, but also ascites and the inability to eat. Pulmonary edema from left ventricular failure causes respiratory acidosis, which cannot be compensated by the kidneys because renal failure and azotemia also occur. As azotemia increases, metabolic acidosis develops and the patient dies from both respiratory and metabolic acidosis.

Case Study Conclusion

Mrs. C. wanted to talk about her future, and this is the time to explore this topic with her. If treatment options have not already been outlined, it would be important to do so at this point. In talking with her about the management of her symptoms, it is important to explain what she can expect with each choice.

There are some additional adjustments to therapy that may help in relieving Mrs. C.'s symptoms. Maximizing her diuretics (dosing in the morning so she can sleep at night) would help to relieve her dyspnea. Her ACE inhibitor should be slowly titrated up to a dose that is more beneficial. Home oxygen therapy would also help, even when oxygen saturation levels are within normal range. General measures that could help alleviate some of her breathlessness should be reviewed, and referrals to home care regarding nutrition and physical therapy can be arranged. Advance directives and living wills should be explained and forms made available for her to complete if she so desires. When her condition becomes such that she needs intravenous medication, Mrs. C. needs to know what that therapy involves, and how hospice or home care can help. Goals need to be outlined so she can be reassured that a peaceful death is achievable.

After all the above options are examined with both Mrs. C. and her family, her wish to "give up" should be explored. Antidepressants may be helpful at this point, and, if acceptable to her, a selective serotonin reuptake inhibitor (SSRI) may be an important part of the plan. SSRIs are well tolerated by older adults. A list of support groups for those in heart failure may be helpful, and she may want to see a psychologist or a social worker; referrals should be made.

Mrs. C. can be reassured that she does not have to be readmitted to the hospital. Explain to her that it is always an option, and that she can change her mind on this, or any other choice, at any time.

The plan that Mrs. C. has decided upon should be detailed in her chart. All colleagues in the practice should be aware of the plan so that continuity of care can be maintained. Most practices have a problem list in the front of each patient's chart that is continually updated, and her plan needs to be outlined there where it is always accessible. Above all, Mrs. C. must be empowered to make the decisions that feel right for her at this time in her life, and her decision respected. She must know that she can depend on the health care team . . . and that her quality of life, in death, matters.

CONCLUSION

As one can see, there are many new pharmacological agents and interventional devices that have become the mainstay in the treatment of heart failure. Symptom relief can be achieved for a time, but despite these advances our clients will eventually die of this disease. The option of when to stop treatment and what is needed to proceed with a "good death" is an individual and family decision. Our goal as nurses should be to facilitate the process, not interfere with its eventuality.

RESOURCES
- American Heart Association (*www.americanheart.org*): very helpful in assessing data regarding statistics, patient information, and risk factor identification; publications/brochures for patient education
- National Guideline Clearinghouse (*www.guideline.gov*): searchable database of latest evidenced-based guidelines on the care of patients with heart disease
- National Heart, Lung and Blood Institute (*nhlbi.nih.gov*): health information on cardiac risk factors with guidelines for management
- Framingham Heart Study (*framingham.com/heart*): score sheet for estimating risk of development of heart disease; good patient educational materials
- Center to Advance Palliative Care (*www.capcmssm.org*): publications, resources, conferences on palliative care
- Geriatric Medicine, Community Internal Medicine Division, Department of Internal Medicine, Mayo Clinic (*www.mayo.edu/geriatrics-rst/Card_ToC.html*): "Topics in Geriatrics: Cardiovascular Disease in the Elderly" web page, helpful for patient and provider information on geriatrics

REFERENCES

Agency for Health Care Policy and Research. (1994). *Heart failure evaluation and care of patients with left ventricular systolic dysfunction.* Rockville, MD: Author.

American College of Cardiology/American Heart Association Task Force on Practice Guidelines, Committee on Evaluation and Management of Heart Failure. (1995). Guidelines for the evaluation of heart failure. *Circulation, 92,* 2764-2784.

American Heart Association. (2002). *Heart and stroke statistical update.* Dallas: Author.

Anderson, J., & Kessenich, C. (2001). Cardiovascular disease and micronutrients therapies. *Topics in Advanced Practice Nursing Journal 1*(2). Retrieved from www.medscape.com/viewarticle/408410

Arling, M. (1997). Management of heart failure in nursing facility residents according to AAMDA guidelines. *Nursing Home Medicine, 5,* 374.

Aronow, W. S. (1996). Therapy of congestive heart failure in older patients. *Nursing Home Medicine, 4,* 61-67.

Bald, S. (2000). Promising new therapy for congestive heart failure. *Chest, 118,* 1819-1821.

Barefoot, J., Helms, M., & Mark, D. (1996). Depression and long-term mortality risk in patients with coronary artery disease. *American Journal of Cardiology, 78,* 613-617.

Barold, S. (2000). Biventricular cardiac pacing: Promising new therapy for congestive heart failure. *Chest, 118,* 1819-1821.

Bernardi, L., Porta, C., Scpicuzza, L., Bellwon, J., Giammario, S., Frey, A., et al. (2002). Slow breathing increases arterial baro-reflex sensitivity in patients with chronic heart failure. *Circulation, 105,* 143-145.

The care of dying patients: A position statement from the American Geriatrics Society. AGS Ethics Committee. (1995). *Journal of the American Geriatrics Society, 43,* 577-578.

CIBIS Investigators and Committees. (1994). A randomized trial of beta-blockade in heart failure: The Cardiac Insufficiency Bisoprolol Study (CIBIS). *Circulation, 90,* 1765-1773.

CIBIS Investigators and Committees. (1999). The Cardiac Insufficiency Bisoprolol Study II (CIBIS II): A randomized trial. *Lancet, 353,* 9-13.

Consensus recommendations for the management of chronic heart failure. On behalf of the membership of the Advisory Council to Improve Outcomes Nationwide in Heart Failure. (1999). *American Journal of Cardiology, 83*(2a), 1A-38A.

Criteria Committee of the New York Heart Association. (1964). *Diseases of the heart and blood vessels: Nomenclature and criteria for diagnosis* (6th ed.). New York Heart Association.

Daubert, J., Leclercq, C., Alonso, C., Walker, S., & Cazeau, S. (2000). Long-term experience with biventricular pacing in refractory heart failure. In I. E. Ovsyshcher (Ed.), *Cardiac arrhythmia and device therapy: Results and perspectives for the new century.* Armonk, NY: Futura.

The Digitalis Investigation Group: The effect of digoxin on mortality and morbidity in patients with heart failure. (1997). *New England Journal of Medicine, 336,* 525-533.

Dresing, T. J., & Natale, A. (2001). Congestive heart failure treatment: The pacing approach. *Heart Failure Reviews, 6,* 15-25.

Ducas, J., Madger, S., & McGregor, M. (1983). Validity of hepatojugular reflux as a clinical test for congestive heart failure. *American Journal of Cardiology, 52,* 1200-1303.

Ferketich, A. K., Schwartzbaum, J. A., Frid, D. J., & Moeschberger, M. L. (2000). Depression as an antecedent to heart disease among women and men in the NHANES I study. *Archives of Internal Medicine, 160,* 1261-1268.

Frasure-Smith, N., Lesperance, F., & Talajic, M. (1995). Depression and 18-month prognosis after myocardial infarction. *Circulation, 91,* 999-1005.

Gillespie, N. D., Darbar, D., Struthers, A. D., & McMurdo, M. E. (1998). Heart failure: A diagnostic and therapeutic dilemma in elderly patients. *Age and Ageing, 27,* 539-543.

Goldstein, S. (2001). Heart failure therapy at the turn of the century. *Heart Failure Review, 6,* 7-14.

Heart Failure Society of America (HFSA) practice guidelines: HFSA guidelines for management of patients with heart failure caused by left ventricular systolic dysfunction—pharmacological approaches. (1999). *Journal of Cardiac Failure, 5,* 357-382.

Heffner, J. E. (2000). End-of-life care preferences of patients enrolled in cardiovascular rehabilitation programs. *Chest, 117,* 1474-1481.

Ho, K. K. L., Pinsky, J. L., Kannel, W. B., & Levy, D. (1993). The epidemiology of heart failure: The Framingham Study. *Journal of the American College of Cardiology, 22,* 6a-13a.

Hofman-Bang, C., Rehnquist, N., Swedberg, K., Wiklund, I., & Astrom, H. (1995). Coenzyme Q 10 as an adjunctive in the treatment of chronic congestive heart failure. The Q 10 Study Group. *Journal of Cardiac Failure, 1,* 101-107.

Hudak, C., Gallo, B., & Morton, P. (1998). *Critical care nursing* (7th ed.). Philadelphia: Lippincott.

Jaarsveld, C., Sanderman, R., Miedema, I., Ranchor, A., & Kempen, G. (2001). Changes in health-related quality of life in older patients with acute myocardial infarction or congestive heart failure: A prospective study. *Journal of the American Geriatrics Society, 49,* 1052-1058.

Jenkinson, C., Jenkinson, D., Shepperd, S., Layte, R., & Petersen, S. (1997). Evaluation of treatment for congestive heart failure in patients aged 60 and older using generic measures of health status (SF-36 and COOP charts). *Age and Ageing, 26,* 7-13.

Jonas, B. S., Franks, P., & Ingram, D. D. (1997). Are symptoms of anxiety and depression risk factors for hypertension? Longitudinal evidence from the National Health and

Nutrition Examination Survey I Epidemiological Follow-up Study. *Archives of Family Medicine, 6,* 43-49.

Kannel, W. (2000). Incidence and epidemiology of heart failure. *Heart Failure Reviews, 5,* 167-173.

King, M. S., Carr, T., & D'Cruz, C. (2002). Transcendental meditation, hypertension and heart disease. *Australian Family Physician, 31,* 164-168.

Kubzansky, L., & Ichiro, K. (2000). Going to the heart of the matter: Do negative emotions cause coronary heart disease? *Journal of Psychosomatic Research, 48,* 323-337.

Lamb, D. R. (1984). *Physiology of exercise: Responses and adaptations.* New York: Macmillan.

Laurent-Bopp, D. (2000). Heart failure. In S. L. Woods, E. S. Froelicher, & S. Motzer (Eds.), *Cardiac nursing* (pp. 560-570). Philadelphia: Lippincott Williams & Wilkins.

Lonn, E. (2000). Drug treatment in heart failure. *British Medical Journal, 320,* 1188-1192.

Makalinao, J. (2000). Chronic heart failure: Examining consensus recommendations for patients' management. *Geriatrics, 55,* 53-58.

Mann, D. L. (2001). The role of inflammatory mediators in the failing heart. *Heart Failure Review, 6,* 385-388.

MERIT-HF Study Group. (1999). The effect of Metoprolol CR/XL in chronic heart failure: Metoprolol CR/XL Randomized Intervention Trial in Congestive Heart Failure (MERIT-HF). *Lancet, 353,* 2001-2007.

Micheals, A., & Frances, C. (2001). *Saint Frances guide to cardiology.* Philadelphia: Lippincott Williams & Wilkins.

Naccarelli, G. V. (2001, March 20). *Biventricular pacing in congestive heart failure: A post-ACC meeting perspective.* Presented at the 50th Annual Scientific Session of the American College of Cardiology, Orlando, FL.

National Center for Health Statistics. (2000). *National nursing home survey, 1997.* Hyattsville, MD: Author.

National Heart, Lung and Blood Institute. (1996). *Data fact sheet: Congestive heart failure in the United States: A new epidemic.* Bethesda, MD: Author.

Neither prevention nor cure: Managed care for women with chronic conditions. (1999). Supplement from *Jacobs Institute of Women's Health, 9*(2), 68s-78s.

Nelson, E. C., Wasson, J. H., Johnson, D., & Hays, R. (1996). Dartmouth COOP functional health assessment charts: Brief measures for clinical practice. In B. Spilker (Ed.), *Quality of life and pharmacoeconomics in clinical trials* (pp. 3331-3338). Philadelphia: Lippincott–Raven.

Nolan, P., & Marcus, F. (2000). Cardiovascular drug use in the elderly. *American Journal of Geriatric Cardiology, 9,* 127-129.

O'Mahoney, P.G. (1998). Is the SF-36 suitable for assessing health status of older stroke patients? (form used for self-reporting on health status in the United Kingdom). *Age and Ageing, 27,* 19-22.

Rogers, A. E. (2000). Knowledge and communication difficulties for patients with chronic heart failure: Qualitative study. *British Medical Journal, 321,* 605-607.

Rossen, E. K., & Buschmann, M. T. (1995). Mental illness late in life: The neurobiology of depression. *Archives of Psychiatric Nursing, 9,* 130-136.

Shamsham, F. (2000). Essentials of the diagnosis of heart failure. *American Family Physician, 61,* 1319-1328.

Skidmore-Roth, L. (2001). *Handbook of herbs & natural supplements.* St. Louis: Mosby.

Starbuck, J. (1999). *Better Nutrition, 61*(7), 52.

The SOLVD Investigators: Effects of enalapril on mortality and the development of heart failure in asymptomatic patients with reduced left ventricular ejection fraction. (1992). *New England Journal of Medicine, 327,* 575-576.

Taylor, G. (2001). *Primary care management of heart failure.* St. Louis: Mosby.

Tribble, D. L. (1999). Antioxidant consumption and risk of coronary heart disease: Emphasis on vitamin C, vitamin E, and beta-carotene. A statement for healthcare professionals from the American Heart Association. *Circulation, 99,* 591-595.

Ware, J. E., & Sherbourne, C. D. (1992). The MOS 36-Item Short-Form health survey (SF-36): I: Conceptual framework and item selection. *Medical Care, 30,* 473-483.

Weglicki, Kramer, & Mak (1999). The role of antioxidant drugs in oxidative injury of cardiovascular tissue. *Heart Failure Reviews, 4,* 183-192.

Westlake, C., & Dracup, K. (2001). Role of spirituality in adjustment of patients with advanced heart failure. *Progress in Cardiovascular Nursing, 16,* 119-125.

Woods, S., Froelicher, E. S., & Motzer, S. (2000). *Cardiac nursing* (4th ed.). Philadelphia: Lippincott Williams & Wilkins.

Zoler, M. (2000, April 15). New drug recommended for heart failure. *Family Practice News,* 1-2.

11 CANCER

Amy E. Guthrie and Polly Mazanec

Case Study

Mr. B., 81, presented with a persistent cough and 1 week of hemoptysis. His past medical/surgical history included a 20-year history of hypertension, coronary artery disease (two coronary artery bypass surgeries and carotid stenosis treated with left carotid endarterectomy), type 2 diabetes mellitus for 3 years, osteoarthritis of the knees, and degenerative disk disease of the spine. His social history is significant for smoking three packs per day for 35 years until the age of 50. He worked as a store manager for 45 years, retiring 15 years ago. He lives with his wife of 55 years and has 4 grown children and 10 grandchildren, all living within the community. Mr. B. has been active in his retirement, volunteering weekly at his church, playing bridge and golf, and vacationing to Florida each winter.

Physical exam revealed a slightly overweight elder male in no acute distress. Mr. B.'s vital signs were as follows: blood pressure 140/82 mm Hg; pulse 82 beats/min, regular rate and rhythm; respirations 16 breaths/min; and afebrile. Lung sounds were diminished on the right upper lobe, with dullness to percussion and positive egophony; the left lung was clear to auscultation. Cardiovascular examination revealed a positive S_4 and no S_3 heart sound, no edema, pulses of 2+ throughout, and no bruits. Abdominal examination was unremarkable. Musculoskeletal examination revealed full range of motion and upper and lower extremity strength of 5+. On his neurologic examination, Mr. B. was grossly intact, alert, and oriented, with a Mini-Mental State Examination score of 29/30. His current medications are isosorbide, enalapril (Vasotec), diltiazem (Cardizem), clopidogrel (Plavix), metformin (Glucophage), glyburide, aspirin, and over-the-counter (OTC) acetaminophen for osteoarthritis. Chest radiography and computed tomography revealed a right hilar mass, highly suspicious for lung cancer.

A definitive diagnosis by bronchoscopy revealed non–small cell lung cancer, a squamous cell carcinoma, with no evidence of distant metastasis. The presence of positive hilar lymph nodes suggests that the cancer is stage IIA.

Questions that the nurse should consider are

What lung cancer treatment options does Mr. B., an elder male with multiple comorbid illnesses, have?

What pain and symptom management issues may arise in the course of his disease trajectory?

What support is needed to help Mr. B. and his family/caregivers cope with his diagnosis, treatment, and disease progression?

What model of end-of-life care would best support Mr. B.'s physical, psychological, social, and spiritual needs throughout the disease trajectory?

INTRODUCTION

The incidence of cancer increases with age so that preventive oncology becomes more imperative for those 65 years of age and older. In addition, aggressive curative treatments, with new drugs to treat toxicities, will become increasingly available for the population ages 75 to 85 years (Bailes, 1997). It is essential to provide quality cancer care for the older population throughout the entire disease trajectory.

INCIDENCE AND PREVALENCE OF CANCER

Approximately 77% of all cancers are diagnosed at the age of 55 or older. By the end of the year

2002, approximately 1,284,900 newly diagnosed invasive cancer cases will be identified. Cancer is second to heart disease as a leading cause of death in the United States in both men and women. It is the leading cause of death in men and women ages 60 to 80 and the second leading cause of death in those ages 80 and older (American Cancer Society [ACS], 2002). Approximately 555,500 Americans are expected to die of cancer in the year 2002, averaging more than 1500 deaths each day. The greatest impact of cancer is seen in the older adult population because 60% of new cancer incidences and 69% of all cancer deaths occur in individuals 65 years and older (Repetto & Comandini, 2000). Cancers of the lung and bronchus, breast, colon and rectum, and prostate are the most common malignancies affecting older adults (Fig. 11-1).

The relationship between increasing age and the development of cancer is attributed to cancer growth characteristics and the biophysical environment. First, cancer cells take time to proliferate; this growth may not be apparent until the later stages of life. Second, a changing physical environment contributes to the programmed death of healthy cells and the propagation of cancer cells (Balducci & Extermann, 1998). As a result, elders are at increased risk for cancer.

Even though age is a well-known risk factor for cancer, age alone is an imperfect indicator of outcomes. Functional ability is the most significant factor in treatment options and disease prognosis of the older adult (Weissman, 2000). Prognostication is impacted not only by functional capability, but also by type, severity, and

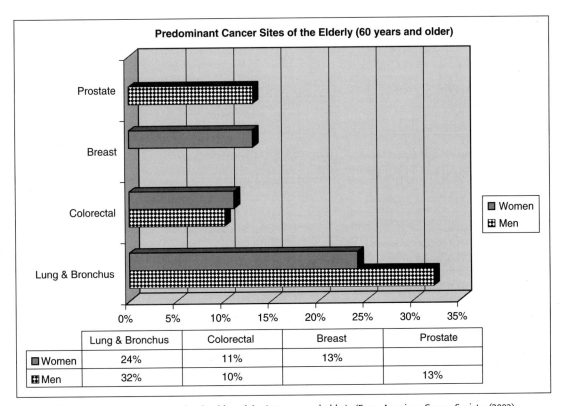

Fig. 11-1 Predominant cancer sites in older adults (60 years and older). (From American Cancer Society. (2002). *Cancer facts and figures 2002.* Atlanta: Author.)

number of coexisting illnesses (Lazarro & Comandini, 2000). The elder's functional status and cognitive ability to withstand the disease and the treatment need to be considered regardless of whether the goal is curative or palliative (Carbone, 2000).

COMORBIDITY

Critical assessment of the older adult is important when determining life expectancy, treatment tolerance, and palliation. Physical reserve, psychosocial support, economic support, and comorbidity impact treatment outcomes (Repetto & Comandini, 2000). The Karnofsky Performance Scale (KPS) is the most widely used assessment tool in the field of oncology (Repetto, Comandini, & Mammoliti, 2001). The KPS (Table 11-1) evaluates physical function, and draws a close parallel with mortality (Repetto et al., 2001).

Geriatric terminology categorizes elders as "young-old" (70 to 74 years), "old-old" (75 to 84 years), and "oldest old" (85 years and older). These age-related categorizations should be considered when developing a treatment plan because aging involves a progression of organ systems decline, coexisting physical conditions, cognitive impairment, social isolation, functional dependence, and economic limitations (Balducci & Extermann, 1999). Natural changes associated with age often lead to a greater susceptibility to chronic and acute disease, yet a comprehensive evaluation of the older adult's day-to-day mental and physical functional status, social supports, and personal resolve give a more accurate definition of age in relation to physical capabilities, cognitive status, and treatment tolerance.

Another commonly used geriatric classification of the older adult is the "frail elder." This term is used when the older adult lacks physical functional tolerance in response not only to minimal stress, but also to aggressive treatment (Balducci & Extermann, 1999). In addition, the term is associated with the presence of more than one geriatric syndrome, a limited life expectancy (not much beyond 2 years), and the inability to maintain homeostasis in nonstressed conditions; also, there is greater risk of developing treatment-

Table 11-1 Karnofsky Performance Scale

Definition	Rating	Criteria
Able to carry on normal activity and to work; no special care needed	100%	Normal; no complaints; no evidence of disease
	90%	Able to carry on normal activity; minor signs or symptoms of disease
	80%	Normal activity with effort; some signs or symptoms of disease
Unable to work; able to live at home and care for most personal needs; varying amount of assistance	70%	Cares for self; unable to carry on normal activity or to do active work
	60%	Requires occasional assistance, but is able to care for most of personal needs
	50%	Requires considerable assistance and frequent medical care
Unable to care for self; requires equivalent of institutional or hospital care; disease may be progressing rapidly	40%	Disabled; requires special care and assistance
	30%	Severely disabled; hospital admission is indicated although death is not imminent
	20%	Very sick; hospital admission necessary; active supportive treatment necessary
	10%	Moribund; fatal processes progressing rapidly
	0%	Dead

From McDonald, N. (1993). Principles governing the use of cancer chemotherapy in palliative medicine. In D. Doyle, G. Hanks, & N. MacDonald (Eds.), *Oxford textbook of palliative medicine* (p. 109). Oxford: Oxford University Press.

related toxicities with the loss of functional independence (Repetto & Comandini, 2000).

Geriatric syndromes should be included in a comprehensive assessment in order to determine accurately the elder's stage of life and functional capabilities. Geriatric syndromes that have been defined and used in treatment planning within the last 10 years include dementia, depression, abuse/neglect, incontinence, osteoporosis, failure to thrive, and risk for falls (Balducci & Extermann, 1999). Activities of daily living (ADLs) and instrumental activities of daily living (IADLs) are useful tools for assessing functional ability (Box 11-1). Limited independence in ADLs and IADLs closely parallels limited life expectancy. In addition, limited independence in IADLs correlates with treatment intolerance (Balducci & Monfardini, 1999). Comorbidity is predominantly a normal process of age, and is known to complicate cancer diagnosis, prognosis, and treatment (Lazzaro & Comandini, 2000). Comorbidity is associated with decreased survival rates, and merits attention during a comprehensive assessment.

LUNG CANCER

Lung cancer is the most significant cause of cancer mortality in men and women in the United States, and the leading cause of cancer death in people 60 years of age and older (ACS, 2002; Lutz et al., 2001). In 1999, cancers of the lung comprised 36% of cancer deaths in persons ages 60 to 79 and 23% of deaths in those over the age of 80 (ACS, 2002). The estimated number of new cases of lung cancer in 2002 was 169,400, with an estimated death rate of 154,900, reflecting the poor prognosis associated with this disease (ACS, 2002). The average annual incidence and mortality rates between 1992 and 1998 were highest among African Americans (ACS, 2002). The number of older people who will develop lung cancer is expected to rise in the coming years, as smoking exposure effects become more evident, and as the U.S. population continues to age (Yancik & Reis, 1994).

Pathogenesis

Lung cancer is divided into two main groups, non–small cell lung cancer (NSCLC) and small cell lung cancer (SCLC). NSCLC comprises 75% to 80% of all lung cancers and includes squamous cell carcinoma, large cell carcinoma, and adenocarcinoma (Blackwell & Crawford, 1997). The incidence of squamous cell cancer increases with age, especially in older males. Squamous cell cancer may be detected at an earlier stage than other NSCLCs; however, it has a 5-year survival rate of only 25% (Blackwell & Crawford, 1997; Nally, 1996). SCLC has a very aggressive clinical course and poorer prognosis. It is usually detected at a more advanced stage, growing rapidly and metastasizing early in the course.

Signs, Symptoms, and Staging

More than 95% of patients with lung cancer are symptomatic at the time of diagnosis (Blackwell & Crawford, 1997; Kraut & Wozniak, 2000). Common symptoms such as cough, dyspnea, dysphagia, hoarseness, fatigue, and weight loss are frequently attributed to comorbid illnesses. The elder may dismiss these symptoms as part of aging, or as the effects of other comorbid diseases. For example, cough may be attributed to chronic bronchitis in elder smokers; dyspnea or chest pain may be linked to a history of heart disease. This assumption may result in a delay in cancer diagnosis, consequently affecting treatment options and outcomes. Unfortunately, with lung cancer, these common symptoms usually are the result of locally advanced or metastatic disease.

Tissue diagnosis is usually made by bronchoscopy. Once the lung cancer diagnosis has been confirmed, staging is essential to determine the extent of disease. In NSCLC staging, the

---

Box 11-1 ADLs and IADLs	
ACTIVITIES OF DAILY LIVING (ADL)	**INSTRUMENTAL ACTIVITIES OF DAILY LIVING**
Bathing	Telephone use
Dressing	Housekeeping
Toileting	Meal preparation
Eating	Shopping
Continence	Managing money
Able to get in and out of bed	Taking prescribed medications

From Fratinino, L., Serraino, D., & Zagonel, V. (1998). The impact of cancer on the physical function of the elderly and their utilization of health care. *Cancer, 83,* 589-592.

TNM classification groups patients according to size and extent of the tumor (T), lymph node involvement (N), and the presence or absence of metastatic disease (M) (Blackwell & Crawford, 1997). Surgical staging with mediastinoscopy is essential in the older adult to determine the nodal status of the patient before recommending surgical options (Blackwell & Crawford, 2000). Seventy percent of patients with NSCLC have locally advanced or unresectable stage IV disease at the time of diagnosis (Lutz et al., 2001).

SCLC is considered a systemic disease at diagnosis and therefore has its own staging system. Sixty percent to 70% of SCLC patients have metastatic disease at diagnosis (Lutz et al.,

2001). More than 90% of patients have stage III or IV disease (Feld, Sagman, & LeBlanc, 2000). Limited-stage disease in patients with SCLC has a median survival of 12 to 16 months; extensive disease has a median survival of 7 to 11 months.

Once staging is completed, the treatment plan is based on staging classification, the patient's ability to tolerate treatment, and the patient's performance status. Performance status is a critical factor in determining treatment options. Patients who are symptomatic but have a KPS status of 80% to 90% tolerate treatment better, and live longer, than those with a poor performance status (Blackwell & Crawford, 1997).

EVIDENCE-BASED PRACTICE

Reference: Kurtz, M., Kurtz, J. C., Stommel, M., Given, C., & Given, B. (2000). Symptomatology and loss of physical functioning among geriatric patients with lung cancer. *Journal of Pain and Symptom Management, 19*(4), 249-256.

Research Problem: The researchers examined how symptom severity in geriatric patients with lung cancer varied according to the type of treatment received. The staging of the disease and gender; the relationship of change in physical functioning to symptomatology, prior physical functioning, comorbidity, and age; and the differences according to treatment, staging, and gender were also of interest.

Design: Descriptive cohort study.

Sample and setting: 133 lung cancer patients, ages 65 and older, recruited from a larger multicenter longitudinal cancer study in southern Michigan.

Methods: Data were collected through patient interviews and chart audits and analyzed using analysis of variance and analysis of covariance. Interviews were conducted posttherapy. Patients were asked to complete a physical functioning status assessment retrospectively relative to their status 3 months prior to their diagnosis. Physical functioning was measured using a subscale of the Short Form 36. Symptom

severity was measured using the Symptom Experience Scale.

Results: The most common symptoms identified were fatigue, dyspnea, pain, night urination, weakness, and cough. Symptoms were more frequent in patients with aggressive treatment and late-stage disease. Loss of physical functioning was found to be positively correlated with prior physical functioning and negatively correlated with age. There were no significant differences in loss of physical functioning or symptom severity according to treatment, staging, or gender.

Implications for Nursing Practice: Patients' prediagnosis physical functioning is an important factor when considering risk for suffering loss of function. The impact of the disease and treatment is likely to be more severe for patients with higher levels of functioning and lower age prediagnosis. Nurses need to provide support to help patients deal with decreased physical functioning.

Conclusion: The researchers described a profile for elder patients with lung cancer who are at high risk for suffering significant losses in physical functioning early in their treatment. Identifying those at risk and instituting support may improve quality of life.

Disease Management

Surgery

It is inappropriate to assume that all elders prefer "quality of life" to "quantity of life" when making treatment decisions. All options should be presented to patients who want choice in treatment (Blackwell & Crawford, 2000). Surgical resection remains the only potential curative treatment for patients with NSCLC presenting with surgically resectable disease. Despite this knowledge, older adults often are not treated as aggressively as younger patients (Brown, Eraut, Trask, & Davison, 1996; Lima, Herndon, Kosty, Clamon, & Green, 2002). Younger patients, even those with more extensive disease, are more likely to be offered surgical resection than older patients. In the past, age greater than 70 was considered a risk factor for thoracotomy. However, operative mortality and postoperative complication rates decreased in the 1990s, and newer minimally invasive surgical techniques have improved surgical outcomes (Blackwell & Crawford, 1997).

Radiation Therapy

Radiation therapy is an important treatment modality in inoperable regional NSCLC. It is also used as an alternative for older patients who are not considered surgical candidates because of comorbid disease states, or for those who decline surgery. The median survival for patients undergoing radiation therapy is less than 1 year. Combined-modality treatment with radiation therapy and chemotherapy in patients with non-resectable stage III NSCLC and limited-stage SCLC is the standard of care for physiologically fit elders (Blackwell & Crawford, 2000).

Chemotherapy

Chemotherapeutic options are often limited in elders as a result of unwarranted fears that they cannot tolerate treatment. In fact, studies done over the past 15 years have demonstrated that older adults cope as well as, and sometimes better than, younger patients, often experiencing lower levels of emotional distress and life disruption (Blackwell & Crawford, 2000; Walsh, Begg, & Carbone, 1989). A prospective, randomized, multicenter trial found a statistically significant 7-week improvement in survival in elder patients receiving chemotherapy as compared to best supportive care. The chemotherapy group had fewer disease-related symptoms but more treatment toxicity than the supportive care group. Current studies targeting chemotherapeutic toxicities in older adults have suggested that monotherapy with agents that have a favorable side effect profile (e.g., vinorelbine, gemcitabine) is tolerated well (Brown et al., 1996; "Effects of Vinorelbine," 1999; Shepard et al., 1997; Veronesi, Crivellari, & Magri, 1996).

The role of chemotherapy and the treatment of advanced NSCLC is controversial. Conversely, recent studies have suggested that adjuvant chemotherapy in advanced NSCLC does not improve survival (Carney, 2002). Combination chemotherapy and radiation therapy in the greater-than-70 age group with locally advanced NSCLC showed no benefit in median survival when compared with radiation therapy alone (Langer et al., 2000). It is difficult to fully evaluate treatment options for elders because this age group continues to be largely underrepresented in clinical studies and study results remain controversial (Lima et al., 2002).

SCLC is widely metastatic; therefore, treatment options are usually limited to chemotherapy and/or radiation therapy. With combination chemotherapy, patients who have limited-stage SCLC have a median survival of about 15 months, and those with extensive disease about 9 months. The debate continues as to whether highly toxic combination chemotherapy is appropriate for elders. Studies of elder patients to date suggest that they can derive benefit from treatment for SCLC; however, the limited data available support the need to include this age group in large clinical trials.

Palliative Care for Lung Cancer

Palliative care is best initiated for elder patients with cancer at the time of diagnosis. Palliative care can help the patient and family with complex decision making during the staging process. Supportive care can be provided throughout diagnosis, staging, and treatment, as well as at the time of disease progression and in the dying process. About one third of surgically resected NSCLCs follow the same pattern of recurrence: metastasis to the brain, followed by bone, ipsilateral and contralateral lung, liver, and adrenal gland. More than 80% of recurrences occur within 2 years and are complicated by distressing symptoms.

Palliative care can provide symptom management throughout the disease trajectory. Pain, dyspnea, fatigue, weight loss, and cough are commonly associated with lung cancer. Pain may occur as a result of tumor infiltrating the brachial plexus, bone metastasis, or brain metastasis, producing headache (Hoskin & Makin, 1998). Dyspnea occurs in as many as 40% of patients, and in 70% of patients in the last 6 weeks of life (Abrahm, 1998). Interventions to alleviate fatigue and other physical symptoms are important for improving quality of life regardless of the life expectancy.

COLORECTAL CANCER

The estimated number of new cases of colorectal cancer in the United States for the year 2002 was 152,200, with an estimated death rate of 57,100 (ACS, 2002). Colorectal cancer ranks as the third leading cause of cancer death overall and in those over the age of 80. It is the second leading cause of cancer death in persons ages 60 to 79 (ACS, 2002). As with lung cancer, the average annual incidence and mortality rates between 1992 and 1998 were highest among African Americans (ACS, 2002). Colorectal cancer is a disease associated with aging, with the exception of those cases resulting from inflammatory bowel disease or inherited polyposis syndromes (Forman, 1997). Ninety percent of all cases of colorectal cancer occur in people ages 50 and older (Kennedy-Malone, Fletcher, & Plank, 2000). In the elder population, the risk for developing colorectal cancer is increased in the presence of a previous history of colorectal, breast, ovarian, and/or endometrial cancer.

Pathogenesis

Colon cancer includes more than half of all cancers of the large bowel, with 70% of cancers occurring on the right side. Rectal and anal cancers, seen more frequently in men, comprise the remaining large bowel cancers (Saddler & Ellis, 1999). Most cancers of the bowel are moderately or well-differentiated adenocarcinomas. These cancers usually develop as a result of progressive colonic polyp mutations (Ahlgren, 1999; Saddler & Ellis, 1999). Screening for and

removal of potentially malignant polyps can prevent development of metastatic disease.

Signs, Symptoms, and Staging

Colorectal cancer is difficult to diagnose at an early stage because patients are usually asymptomatic early in the disease process (Saddler & Ellis, 1999). Diagnosis of colorectal cancer in the older adult is especially challenging because many of the common changes of aging in the gastrointestinal tract can prevent early detection. For example, constipation, common in elders, is associated with cancer of the descending and sigmoid colon (Forman, 1997). Changes in bowel patterns, generalized weakness, and fatigue may be inaccurately attributed to the aging process. Patients often present with bowel obstruction as the disease progresses (Forman, 1997). Diagnostic work-up includes physical exam, ultrasound, colonoscopy, chest radiography, computed tomography of the abdomen and pelvis, magnetic resonance imaging, and computed tomography portography to identify small focal hepatic metastases (Saddler & Ellis, 1999).

The Dukes classification system for TNM staging has been modified to correspond with the Astler-Coller classification system. This staging process evaluates the depth of bowel wall penetration by the tumor, lymph node involvement, and metastasis. Obstruction is associated with a poor prognosis and increased perioperative mortality in elders (Forman, 1997). The pathologic stage is the major prognostic finding for survival, with stages III and IV associated with poorer prognoses (Baker, 2001). Spread to the liver occurs in about 50% of patients, and spread to the lung in about 10% (Baker, 2001).

In conducting the best preoperative evaluation of the elder person with suspected colorectal cancer, consideration of comorbid conditions is essential. Postoperative sepsis and other complications have been associated with the presence of comorbid disease rather than chronologic age (Ahlgren, 1999).

Disease Management
Surgery

Disease-specific survival is equivalent in elders and younger patients. In fact, age greater than 65 has been associated with prolonged time to tumor progression and increased survival (Douillard et al., 2000; Mulay, 2001). In older adult patients with probable colorectal cancer, surgery remains the standard treatment. Tumor location, blood supply, and lymph node patterns in the area of the cancer determine the extent of the resection. Laparoscopic advances have allowed the use of minimally invasive surgical procedures to resect colon cancers. Early mobility, return of pulmonary function, and decreased ileus and adhesion formation have made this procedure desirable for many patients, especially those with advancing age and comorbid illnesses (Baker, 2001). A conclusion regarding the efficacy of laparoscopic technology awaits the outcome of several large prospective, randomized trials (Blumberg & Ramanathan, 2002).

Surgical management of rectal cancer involves resection with preservation of anorectal sphincter function, and sexual and urinary function whenever possible (Saddler & Ellis, 1999). Patients with rectal cancer who develop local recurrence are rarely helped by additional surgery. At this point in the disease trajectory, palliative management of bone and nerve pain, hemorrhage, pelvic sepsis, and bowel and urinary obstruction is the cornerstone of care (Saddler & Ellis, 1999).

Radiation Therapy

Radiation therapy is not a primary treatment modality for colorectal cancer (Forman, 1997). Debate over the value of pre- or postsurgical radiation therapy continues. Although preoperative radiation therapy has been shown to reduce local recurrence, a higher postoperative mortality was noted in those over the age of 75 receiving preoperative therapy ("Preoperative Short-Term Radiation," 1990; Saddler & Ellis, 1999).

Chemotherapy

Patients with advanced colorectal cancer may benefit from chemotherapy. The goal of chemotherapy in metastatic colorectal cancer is quality of life and palliation of symptoms (Ahlgren, 1999; Baker, 2001). Modest prolongation of survival may be seen with newer chemotherapeutic regimens and agents. Symptomatic relief occurs in about 30% of patients, with a mean duration of response of 6 to 12 months (Ahlgren, 1999). The cornerstone of colorectal cancer chemotherapy has been 5-fluorouracil (5-FU); however, studies have demonstrated superior response and survival rates with a combination 5-FU/leukovorin/irinotecan (5FU/LV) regimen. Lower doses of 5FU/LV can minimize toxicity in older adults (Ahlgren, 1999). Newer chemotherapeutic agents such as oral fluoropyrimidine (a 5-FU prodrug), oxaliplatin, and specific thymidylate synthase inhibitors are currently in clinical trials (Blumberg & Ramanathan, 2002).

Palliative Care for Colorectal Cancer

Over half of all colorectal cancers are diagnosed in the advanced stages; most recurrences develop within 3 years (Hoskin & Makin, 1998). Because the portal vein drains the blood supply from the colon, the liver is the most common site of metastasis in advanced disease. The lungs are usually the first site of metastasis for rectal cancer (Earle & Stern, 2001). Comfort measures to manage metastatic disease and bowel obstruction are essential for quality of life.

BREAST CANCER

Breast cancer is the most frequently occurring female malignancy in the United States. More than 50% of all new cases occur in women 65 years and older. The frequency of breast cancer is 300 in 100,000 in women over the age of 70, and 430 in 100,000 in women over 80 years of age (Mackay, 2000). Breast cancer is directly related to age in 75% of cases. At the age of 50, the risk of developing breast cancer is 1 in 50, with the risk increasing to 1 in 8 at 80+ years (Robinson & Huether, 1998b). Probable factors increasing the risk of breast cancer are classified as reproductive, hormonal, environmental, obesity, and familial. Physiologic factors favorable to breast cancer growth in the elder can be attributed to postmenopause fat tissue replacing glandular breast tissue (Van Dijck, Broeders, & Verbeek, 1997).

Pathogenesis

Ductal carcinoma in situ (DCIS) is the most frequently occurring (70%) breast cancer in older adults (Mackay, 2000). Although DCIS is not known for large tumor size, it is likely to metastasize at an early stage. Pathogenesis involves DNA mutation by genetic alterations or environmental agents, probably occurring early in life. Growth factors then increase the growth rate of those mutated cells, and, finally, progressive alteration of specific oncogenes, or the loss of suppressor genes, leads to advanced metastatic disease (Robinson & Huether, 1998b). The environment for breast cancer growth in elder women is not as favorable as that in younger women because of the decrease of stimulating growth factor specifically for breast cancer and diminishing mononuclear cell reactions. Breast cancer in older women tends to be more differentiated and rich in hormone receptors than that in young women. This renders nonmetastatic tumors more receptive to treatment. Thus, rather than treating the cancer based on the patient's age, it is essential to treat each tumor individually, addressing the characteristics of the tumor and the desires of the patient (Balducci & Extermann, 2001).

Signs, Symptoms, and Staging

Most generally, breast cancer presents as a painless lump; other signs include palpable axillary nodes, dimpling, or bone pain resulting from metastasis. Breast cancer is evaluated with mammography, percutaneous needle aspiration, biopsy, and hormone receptor assays. Treatment, like that for many other cancers, is geared toward the stage of the tumor. Staging uses the primary tumor size (TX to T4), regional lymph nodes (NX to N3), and distant metastasis (MX to M1) system. Stage grouping from 0 to IV is used in addition to the TNM status. Staging levels increase with tumor size and node involvement; stage IV is the only stage that represents metastasis (Robinson & Huether, 1998b).

Disease Management

Treatment is based on the individual's physical condition, the stage of the disease, hormonal responsiveness to therapy, and personal preferences. The number of coexisting conditions strongly correlates with decreased survival rates. Cardiovascular disease, dementia, delirium, stroke, failure to thrive, and lack of social and financial supports are common in the 70-year-old and older age group (Mackay, 2000).

Surgery

Surgical procedures for breast cancer include lumpectomy, quadrant excision, partial mastec-

tomy, total or simple mastectomy, modified radical mastectomy, and radical mastectomy (Robinson & Huether, 1998b). Options available for the surgical management of stage I or II breast cancer are lumpectomy with removal of axillary lymph nodes, mastectomy with the removal of the axillary lymph nodes, radiation therapy, chemotherapy, and hormone therapy. The treatment is typically multimodal.

Axillary node involvement is the most important prognostic indicator for the breast cancer patient. Historically, many medical authorities have suggested testing at least four nodes at the time of surgery; however, others recommended testing only the sentinel node to accurately indicate lymph node involvement. Adequate nodal removal is not commonly offered to elders, which may lead to inadequate adjuvant therapy (Mackay, 2000). Treatment for DCIS includes excision of the tumor, radiation, and/or tamoxifen. High-dose chemotherapy has been shown to increase survival rates up to 6 months; however, it is not considered a curative treatment option at this time for the elder with multiple comorbidities (Coyne, Lyckholm, & Smith, 2001). Treatment for stage III (locally advanced) tumors does not usually involve curative surgery because of the poor prognosis associated with this stage. Conversely, a combination of surgery, chemotherapy, and radiation would be an option for local control of the tumor, because many locally advanced tumors carry the likelihood of metastasis (Hunter-Dorcas, 1991).

Radiation Therapy

In older women, local recurrence after partial mastectomy is reduced with or without irradiation, yet the occurrence of nonvisceral metastases is greater. Older women assessed to have adequate functional reserves tolerated radiation as well as their younger counterparts (Balducci & Extermann, 2001). Radiation therapy can be problematic for the elder patient with cognitive impairment. The procedure requires immobilization, which could concern the patient to the point of anxiety.

Hormonal Therapy

The addition of tamoxifen, a nonsteroidal antiestrogen, to the breast cancer treatment regimen provides positive results with regard to longevity, and therefore is considered first-line treatment for the elder, regardless of nodal involvement (Mackay, 2000). When tamoxifen was used in postmenopausal women for 2 years or longer, the recurrence rate dropped 25% and the mortality rated dropped 16%. There is no evidence to date that shows any advantages to extending the therapy to 5 years or longer (Balducci & Extermann, 2001). Systemic adjuvant hormonal treatment of breast cancer is most useful for women with a life expectancy of 2 or more years. Because tamoxifen therapy extends over a 2-year period, it is not considered an option for the frail elder (Balducci & Extermann, 2001).

Chemotherapy

Factors to be evaluated when considering chemotherapy for breast cancer include physical well-being, staging, tumor type, comorbidity, patient preference, and drug efficacy in the older adult. Guidelines (Box 11-2) provide criteria that are useful when evaluating an elder patient for chemotherapy (Balducci & Extermann, 2001). Tumors rich in hormone receptors are less sensitive to chemotherapy than tumors poor in

hormone receptors. The International Breast Cancer Study Group concluded that overall survival benefits from chemotherapy decreased as age increased, and were nonexistent in women over 65 years of age (Balducci & Extermann, 2001). However, Carbone (2000) reported that chemotherapy increased survival rates of elders significantly when compared to those who were not treated, as long as frequent dose adjustments were made for toxicity. Low-dose taxines, capecitabine, vinorelbine (Navelbine), and gemcitabine have low toxicity indices when dosed appropriately (Balducci & Extermann, 2001). The controversy over chemotoxicity in elders is a result of the heterogeneous population and the underrepresentation of older adults in clinical trials.

Palliative Care for Breast Cancer

The 5-year survival rate for localized breast cancer is currently 96%, a 24% increase since 1940. If the tumor has not metastasized, comorbidity is most generally the cause of death in the elder woman with breast cancer (Gajdos, Tartter, Bleiweiss, Lopchinsky, & Bernstein, 2001). Metastatic breast cancer is incurable, with a life expectancy, most generally, of 18 to 24 months. The treatment goal for metastatic breast cancer is to maintain quality of life through symptom management and lengthening survival (Mackay, 2000). Many frail elders have advanced breast cancer, and they present with symptoms requiring aggressive palliation. Bisphosphonates are effective for bone metastases, and new antitumor agents such as capecitabine, low doses of taxines, liposome-encapsulated doxorubicin, vinorelbine, and gemcitabine may be beneficial for palliation of symptoms while producing minimal toxicity (Carbone, 2000).

Regional and distant metastases reduce survival rates to 78% and 21%, respectively. However, these numbers do not take into account the effect of comorbid conditions and patient choice of treatment (ACS, 2002). Prognostic accuracy is limited for all cancers because of the impact of physical, functional, cognitive, and emotional conditions within the elder population. Clinical trials are needed to study the outcomes of treatment options in terms of quality of life and survival in the older adult population (Mackay, 2000).

Box 11-2 NCCN Summarized Guidelines for the Management of Chemotherapy for Breast Cancer in Older Adults

- Patients 70 years and older should undergo a geriatric assessment.
- Drugs whose metabolites are excreted by the kidneys should have dose adjustment according to the GFR.
- Hemopoietic growth factors used as a prophylactic measure for patients 70 years and older who are receiving dose intensity chemotherapy equal to cyclophosphamide, doxorubicin, vincristine, and prednisone (CHOP).
- Maintain hemoglobin levels >12 g/dl.

From Balducci, L., & Extermann, M. (2001). Management of breast cancer in the older woman. *Cancer Control, 8,* 431-441.

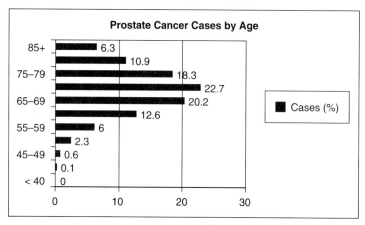

Fig. 11-2 Prostate cancer cases by age. Data from San Jose-Monterey and Los Angeles for 1988 through 1995. (From The National Cancer Institute Seer Reports, 1988-1995.)

PROSTATE CANCER

Prostate cancer is the second leading cause of cancer death in men. The ACS (2002) estimated 189,000 newly diagnosed men with prostate cancer and 30,200 deaths for the year 2002. Over 70% of all prostate cancer cases are diagnosed in men ages 65 years or older (Fig. 11-2) (Stanford et al., 1999). Prostate cancer is common in North America and northwestern Europe; conversely, it is rare in Asian, African, and South American populations. Incidence rates remain highest in African American men. Risk factors for prostate cancer include age, race, family history, and dietary factors (ACS, 2002; National Cancer Institute [NCI], 2002).

Pathogenesis

Over 95% of prostate malignancies are adenocarcinomas, primarily occurring in the periphery of the prostate. Grading systems use the glandular pattern, the degree of differentiation, or a combination of the two (Robinson & Huether, 1998a). The cancer cells metastasize via posterior local extension, the lymphatic system, and blood vessels to distant lymph nodes, bone, liver, lungs, and adrenal glands. The most common sites of bone infiltration are the pelvis, lumbar and thoracic spine, femur, and ribs. The 5-year survival rate for localized prostate cancer is 98%, and that for all prostate cancers is 78%. These figures do not take into account coexisting conditions that may affect prognosis (Robinson & Huether, 1998a).

Signs, Symptoms, and Staging

Elders with early and localized stages of prostate cancer generally do not present with symptoms. Hallmark symptoms that occur more frequently in advanced-stage cancer are usually associated with urinary outlet obstruction: frequent urination, urinary hesitancy or inability to urinate, nocturia, and dysuria. Impotence, painful ejaculation, bloody urine or semen, frequent pain, and stiffness in the lower back, hips, or upper thighs are additional symptoms signifying malignancy. Because many of these symptoms can be caused by other factors, it is common for men to postpone medical consultation. Symptoms of malignant prostate disease usually do not subside, which distinguishes prostate cancer from benign disease. In advanced disease, upper urinary tract (ureter) and rectal obstructions are possible. If rectal obstruction occurs, bowel obstruction or difficult defecation will follow (NCI, 2002).

Digital rectal exams and prostate-specific antigen blood tests are the two most effective screening procedures. Diagnosis of prostate cancer is by transrectal ultrasonography, intravenous pyelogram, and possibly cystoscopy. When cancer is suspected, biopsy is completed after the tumor has been visualized.

Box 11-3 Prostate Cancer Staging

- **Stage A or I (very early)**—confined to prostate gland, impalpable, visualization only possible through a microscope. Treatment includes local excision and regular follow up.
- **Stage B or II (localized)**—cancer is palpable and is limited to the prostate gland; asymptomatic; PSA levels are elevated.
- **Stage C or III (regionalized)**—spread is evident to surrounding tissues. Symptoms are present. Palpation and visualization is most definite.
- **Stage D or IV (advanced)**—reoccurrence of cancer to prostate and other parts of the body.

From American Cancer Society (1995). In *Cancer response system document #10028*. New York, The Society: Cancer Net: Prostate cancer, National Cancer Institute, 1998. Available at www.cancernet.nci.nih.gov/wyntle_pubs/ prostate.

Box 11-4 Treatment Options for Prostate Cancer

- No treatment—*careful observation as symptoms present*
- Prostactomy—*total or partial excision of tumor, radical perineal prostatectomy, or transurethral resection of the prostate (TURP)*
- Hormonal therapy—*otherwise known as systemic therapy*
- Radiation therapy—*otherwise known as local therapy*
- Chemotherapy
- Cryosurgery
- Combination

From Robinson, K. M., & Huether, S. (1998). Structure and function of the reproductive systems. In K. L. McCance & S. L. Huether (Eds.), *Pathophysiology: The biologic basis for disease in adults and children* (3rd ed., pp. 788-790). St. Louis: Mosby.

Disease Management

Treatment depends on age, health status, and the life expectancy of the individual. If factors appear favorable, the stage (Box 11-3) of the neoplasm determines the treatment (Box 11-4). Stage I and II treatments have increased curative rates in many men with early and localized tumors, whereas Stage III and IV treatments are more beneficial to shrink tumors larger in size, palliate symptoms, and possibly prolong life (Robinson & Heuther, 1998a).

Observation alone, known as "watchful waiting" or "deferred treatment," is also an option. At the onset of symptoms, hormonal treatment is initiated. Deferring treatment postpones the undesirable side effects of hormonal therapy, but is only beneficial for Stage I and II cancers. In order to lengthen survival rates, hormonal treatment following a radical prostatectomy should be done immediately (Pignon et al., 1997).

Surgery

Surgical options include total or partial excision (prostatectomy) of the tumor, radical perineal prostatectomy, or transurethral resection of the prostate. Surgery for prostate cancer could result in loss of urinary control, which rebounds anywhere from weeks to months after treatment is complete. Urethral scarring, associated with surgery, interferes with patency. This results in urinary stream changes, incomplete bladder emptying, and incontinence; permanent incontinence occurs in less than 3% to 5% of all men after surgery (Robinson & Heuther, 1998a).

Another adverse effect of surgical treatment is that of sexual dysfunction. It is a common societal belief in America that elders are no longer sexually active (Robinson & Heuther, 1998a). An assessment of the older adult's sexual activity is important when developing a treatment plan, especially if preexisting conditions are absent. Treatment planning should involve the spouse or significant other in order to enhance emotional coping and physical healing (Willert & Semans, 2000).

Radiation Therapy

Radiation therapy is considered the treatment of choice for Stage I and II prostate cancers. Huguenin, Bitterli, Lutolf, Bernhard, and Glanzmann (1999) suggested that healthy elder men with localized prostate cancer should be offered radiation therapy. This study also agrees with current data from the literature that treatment should be urgently implemented. Hormonal treatment can be offered instead of radiation therapy in the same immediate fashion. Disparity in outcomes at the 5- and 7-year marks was attributed to coexisting disease or tumor-associated complications (Huguenin et al., 1999).

It is important to note that the effects of radiation therapy to the pelvis can be severe and unyielding. During pelvic irradiation, diarrhea is expected and nausea and vomiting are common. These manifestations can alter the older recipient's ability and desire to maintain proper dietary intake; however, symptom management with antiemetics, antispasmodics, or anticholinergic drugs can enable a physiologically healthy older adult to tolerate this treatment. Patients with hypertension, diabetes mellitus, and pelvic inflammatory disease are not considered candidates for radiation therapy (Pignon et al., 1997). Radiation therapy may also cause fatigue, skin irritation, localized hair loss, and temporary incontinence (NCI, 2002). Nonetheless, treatment options, including information concerning controversies of treatment, should be shared with the older adult so that informed decisions can be made.

Chemotherapy

Combination therapy with cytotoxic agents has been beneficial in improving survival for men with relapsed prostate cancer. Recommended cytotoxic drugs are mitoxantrone, paclitaxel, estramustine, and vinblastine; cytotoxic therapy can also be used for symptom management. Mitoxantrone reduces bone pain in nearly 30% of elders with metastatic prostate cancer (Balducci & Extermann, 1999). Triptorelin (Trelstar) is a luteinizing hormone–releasing hormone (LHRH) agonist that is recommended by the Food and Drug Administration for palliation of symptoms in advanced cancer. Side effects are similar to those of other hormone agonist agents (Finkelstien, 2000). Hormonal therapy, such as an LHRH agonist, may produce impotence, hot flushes, and lack of libido as a result of the inhibition of testosterone production. These side effects are temporary and are referred to as "flares" (NCI, 2002). Palliative chemotherapy with mitoxantrone and prednisone has been proven to improve quality of life, but did not increase survival rates (Coyne et al., 2001).

The aim in management of prostate cancer in the older adult is diagnosis, effective treatment, and quality of life, balanced with length of life, and thorough palliation of symptoms. Aggressive screening and detection of early-phase confined disease is not considered for the frail elder with a life expectancy of less than 10 years because of the latency of most prostate tumors (Kirk, 1998).

CANCER TREATMENT OPTIONS IN OLDER ADULTS

Treatment decisions should be determined based on shared decision making among the elder patient, his or her family, and the multidisciplinary team. Informed choice is essential for quality cancer care. When the treatment options are presented, patients need to be informed of the benefits and risks. In addition, elder patients should be afforded the opportunity to participate in clinical trials if they so choose.

Surgical options for older adults are based on evidence that the number of comorbid conditions, rather than chronologic age, has the greatest impact on outcome (Berger & Rosalyn, 1997). Postoperative management should focus on pain management, wound care, fluid and electrolyte balance, bowel and bladder function, and preventing cardiac and pulmonary complications (Berger & Rosalyn, 1997).

Radiation therapy for elders is effective for both curative and palliative care, with limited systemic toxicity (Olmi, Cerafo, Balzi, Becciolini, & Geinitz, 1997). Radiation therapy for cancer of the breast, head and neck, and prostate is generally well tolerated; however, radiation therapy for cancer of the bladder and rectum may cause toxicity in older patients. Radiation therapy is especially valuable in the palliative care management of pain, bleeding, bone metastases, and obstruction.

Although it is thought that elder patients are more susceptible to the toxicities of chemotherapy, studies are conflicting (Baker & Grouchow, 1997). It is recognized that elder patients with cancer have diminished hematopoietic reserve, which may make them more susceptible to chemotherapy-induced myelosuppression. It has been shown that bleomycin induces pulmonary toxicity, and doxorubicin induces cardiotoxicity, in this population. Symptomatically, mucositis appears to be more severe in the older adult.

Avoiding severely toxic agents or decreasing the dose may minimize toxicity in the elder (Baker & Grouchow, 1997).

DYING TRAJECTORY

The main causes of death in cancer patients are infection (sepsis and pneumonia), thromboembolism, cachexia, hemorrhage, and multisystem organ failure (Hoskin & Makin, 1998). Only about 50% of deaths are due to disease progression. Treatment-related complications may occur in the first year and include postoperative mortality, chemotherapy-related side effects such as cardiotoxicity, and radiation-induced damage.

The most common cause of death is infection. Pneumonia may result from weakness and wasting of respiratory muscles, dysphagia, or ineffective cough. Organ failure is the second most common cause of death. This may be due to infiltration by the tumor. Cancers of the ovary and extrahepatic biliary duct and stomach cancers are associated with an increased risk of thromboembolism. Extreme cachexia is responsible for about 20% of deaths. Clotting abnormalities occur in about 50% of patients with advanced cancer and can result in disseminated intravascular coagulation or a massive bleed (6%). Sudden death may occur from obstruction by tumor, metabolic crisis, or increased intracranial pressure (Hoskin & Makin, 1998).

Regardless of age, disease progression resulting from metastases is regarded as the cause of death in lung, colorectal, urinary bladder, pancreas, stomach, and kidney cancers. Physical function and coexisting disease have very little effect on mortality rates in these cancer types. In more indolent cancers, such as metastatic breast and prostate cancers, comorbidity and functional ability tend to have a more prominent role in the death of the elder (Repetto et al., 2001).

ONCOLOGIC EMERGENCIES
Malignant Bowel Obstruction

Malignant bowel obstruction occurs in 3% of all terminally ill cancer patients, with the greatest incidence occurring in ovarian malignancies and colorectal cancers (Rousseau, 1995). Obstruction is the presenting symptom in up to 40% of patients with colorectal cancer and ovarian cancer (Fainsinger, Spachynski, Hanson, &

Bruera, 1994). Obstruction occurs when normal passage of stool is blocked by partial or complete obstruction by tumor or loss of normal bowel propulsion (Murphy-Ende, 2001). Elder patients with cancer who are at risk for developing malignant bowel obstruction are those with tumor progression, radiation to the abdomen or abdominal surgery, immobility, or decreased oral intake or who are taking medications that cause severe constipation.

Signs and symptoms are dependent on the level of occlusion. Abdominal pain is usually continuous and colicky, intensifying with perforation or strangulation. In large bowel obstruction, nausea occurs after the pain starts and the emesis is foul and fecal. In gastric outlet or small intestinal obstruction, vomiting develops early after the onset of pain, and the emesis is biliary and odorless.

Physical exam findings vary depending on the acuity of obstruction. Distention, absent or hyperactive high-pitched bowel sounds, and peritoneal signs, including rebound tenderness and rigidity, are often present.

Management of malignant bowel obstruction is determined by the goals of patient care and the patient's expected life span. Surgical intervention is appropriate for patients with early disease and an anticipated life expectancy of 2 months or more (Rousseau, 1998). The mortality is 12% to 40%, and complications of infection, dehiscence, and fistula formation are high (Rousseau, 1995). In patients with advanced disease, the benefits versus risks need to be discussed with the patient and family (Murphy-Ende, 2001). Surgical risks include advanced age, comorbid disease, poor nutritional status, previous obstruction/surgeries, and previous radiation therapy (Rousseau, 1995).

For the frail elder, medical management may be the best option. Comfort care is aimed at decreasing abdominal pain and managing nausea and vomiting. Decompression of the bowel with percutaneous endoscopic gastrostomy provides comfort to patients whose symptoms have responded to nasogastric decompression. This procedure has few complications, prevents the discomfort of a nasogastric tube, and allows patients to eat and drink as they wish. Parenteral nutrition is of limited benefit (Rousseau, 1998).

Somatostatin analogues, such as octreotide, may decrease gastrointestinal secretions.

Corticosteroids, such as dexamethasone, may reduce inflammation, thereby improving comfort. There are no controlled trials evaluating efficacy, but clinical benefits have been described (Rousseau, 1998). Pharmacologic interventions for nausea and vomiting, intestinal colic, and pain need to be administered via the transdermal, rectal, sublingual, or parenteral route (Murphy-Ende, 2001). Frequent mouth care is imperative. Nonpharmacologic interventions such as distraction and guided imagery may also be helpful in managing symptoms.

Hypercalcemia

Hypercalcemia, or serum calcium levels greater than 12 mg/dL (Huether, 1998), is the most commonly occurring metabolic complication of cancer. It occurs in about 10% of all cancer patients, with a 16% to 35% incidence in advanced NSCLC and a 30% to 40% incidence in breast cancer. It is also highly prevalent in prostate cancer and multiple myeloma (Hoskin & Makin, 1998). Early symptoms include excessive thirst, polyuria, anorexia, abdominal cramping, nausea and vomiting, and constipation. As dehydration progresses, confusion, orthostatic hypotension, and loss of deep tendon reflexes occur. Patients may be asymptomatic if the calcium levels are gradually increasing; however, if the rise is rapid, death from coma, renal failure, or cardiac arrest may occur (Morton & Ritch, 2002).

Treatment of hypercalcemia is aimed at fluid and electrolyte balance. Increased fluid intake, often in the form of intravenous fluids at a rate of 2 to 3 L/day, is the mainstay of acute treatment (Bower, Brazil, & Coombes, 1998). However, fluid replacement to correct dehydration and promote calcium excretion should be done with caution in the older adult. Bisphosphonates, such as pamidronate, can be used to restore calcium homeostasis within a few days, decrease bone pain related to metastatic disease, and prevent the recurrence of hypercalcemia (Hoskin & Makin, 1998). Encouraging mobility (which decreases serum calcium level), managing bone pain from metastases, and preventing falls (which could result in fracture) are important nursing considerations for improving quality of life for elders with advancing disease.

CARDINAL SYMPTOMS AT THE END OF LIFE

At the end of life, elder patients with advanced cancer have a median number of 11 symptoms, with a range of 1 to 27 (Donnelly & Walsh, 1995). More than 90% of patients with advanced cancer who are near death have more than three distressing symptoms (Donnelly & Walsh, 1995). Symptoms may be attributed to disease progression, treatment, debilitation, poor nutritional status, or comorbid disease (Sheehan & Forman, 1997).

Pain, dyspnea, and confusion are common in the last week of life (Fainsinger, Miller, Bruera, Hanson, & Maceachern, 1991). Studies continue to indicate that pain is prevalent and often undertreated despite current research-based guidelines for pain management. Bereaved family members reported that greater than 40% of those who died of colon or lung cancer had severe pain in the last 3 days of life (SUPPORT Principal Investigators, 1995).

As cancer progresses, metastatic disease can compromise quality of life in elder patients. Bone, liver, pleural, and brain metastases can cause distressing symptoms that affect the patient and the family. Bone metastases may develop in any bone in the skeleton, but most commonly are found in the vertebrae, pelvis, ribs, and long bones (Hoskin & Makin, 1998). Bone metastases are often seen in cancers of the breast, prostate, and lung. Bone pain and neuropathic pain associated with bone metastases can affect mobility and comfort; aggressive pain management is essential. Palliative radiation therapy, chemotherapy, or hormonal manipulation may be of help with some tumor types. The goal is comfort and prevention of pathologic fractures.

Liver metastasis is present in up to 50% of patients dying with cancer (Hoskin & Makin, 1998). Tumors that typically metastasize to the liver are those of the colon, lung, and breast. The development of symptomatic liver metastases is a poor prognostic sign, usually associated with steady physical decline and increasing cachexia. Death typically occurs within weeks or months (Hoskin & Makin, 1998). Symptomatic management will improve quality of life but not survival. Enlargement of the liver often causes nausea, dull aching pain, and shortness of breath.

The presence of pulmonary metastases is indicative of incurable disease and reduced life expectancy (Hoskin & Makin, 1998). They are commonly associated with breast, colorectal, and lung cancer. The development of a malignant pleural effusion suggests a median survival of 2 to 3 months for all cancers (Hoskin & Makin, 1998). Large effusions cause significant shortness of breath, which may be temporarily relieved with drainage of fluid. Sclerosing agents may be used to prevent reaccumulation in 70% to 80% of cases (Hoskin & Makin, 1998).

Brain metastases develop in over 25% of lung cancer patients and nearly 25% of breast cancer patients (Hoskin & Makin, 1998). Brain metas-tases may cause focal neurologic changes, mood and cognitive functional changes, and seizure activity. Persistent headache is present in 50% of patients. Treatment is aimed at reducing cerebral edema, decreasing pain and symptoms, and maintaining or improving neurologic functioning (Hoskin & Makin, 1998). High-dose steroids will alleviate symptoms. A short course of radiation therapy improves neurologic symptoms and functioning in over 70% of patients.

IMPROVING PALLIATIVE CARE FOR THE OLDER ADULT WITH CANCER

The case study at the beginning of this chapter is fairly typical of an elder patient confronted with

---

EVIDENCE-BASED PRACTICE

Reference: Kiely, M. T., & Alison, D. L. (2000). Palliative care activity in a medical oncology unit: The implications for oncology training. *Clinical Oncology, 12,* 179-181.

Research Problem: This study examined the implications of a previous report recommending the integration of specialized palliative care medicine within all areas of cancer care provision.

Design: A prospective survey.

Sample and Setting: A convenience sample of 111 patients admitted to the Medical Oncology Unit of St. James's University Hospital within a 4-week period.

Methods: Observation with category system upon admission and continuous daily clinical activity assessment. Analyzed with frequency distribution to evaluate frequency of events. Because of a paucity of evidence to support the benefits of the inclusion of palliative specialists in cancer treatment, this study compared the activity in a medical oncology unit with recent recommendations for cancer care provision.

Results: Reasons for admission to the oncology unit included chemotherapy alone, chemotherapy with another aspect of care (without palliative care), palliative care alone, palliative care with another aspect of care, chemotherapy and palliative care, toxicity, and other reasons. Subjects were not placed in more than one category. Administration of chemotherapy alone or with other treatments was the most common reason for admission (42%). Palliative care admissions alone or combined with other treatment modalities accounted for 23% of admissions into the unit. However, palliative care bed-day usage (34%) on the unit was greater than that for either chemotherapy or toxicity, at 32% and 14%, respectively.

Implications for Nursing Practice: As palliative care plays a more vital role in the treatment of cancer, it is imperative for nurses to be familiar with the precepts of palliative care and treatments. Nurses play an important part within the palliative care interdisciplinary team in order to provide "seamless care" for patients with cancer.

Conclusion: Collaboration between palliative care specialists and medical and clinical oncologists is essential for the provision of expert clinical care. The revision of medical training to incorporate a palliative care rotation is indicated by the need to provide optimal symptom control as well as psychosocial and spiritual support in the care of cancer patients.

a new diagnosis of cancer. Conflicting medical opinions, based on age rather than functional status, confuse patients and families during the decision-making process. Health care professionals assume that quality of life rather than quantity of life is most important to the elder facing a life-threatening disease.

It is vital to determine the goals of care of the patient and family; shared decision making is critical to quality care. Patients and families need time and support from the interdisciplinary team to make the best decision. Clinical trials should be offered as a treatment option. Advancing age is not a reason to assume that a patient does not want to pursue curative treatment.

Most importantly, throughout the disease trajectory, the elder patient with cancer and the family need a supportive interdisciplinary team with palliative care expertise to help manage symptoms and to help in establishing individual goals of care. Having this expertise available will help the older adult with cancer navigate the complex health care system, and find support for his or her choices in the plan of care.

Family Considerations

In addition to the physical care of the elder with advanced cancer, comprehensive care requires family support. Palliative care includes physical, emotional, and spiritual comfort of the patient and family. Spouses, adult children, extended relatives, and neighbors account for the 7 million Americans who consider themselves caregivers. Approximately 15% of those 7 million Americans care for elders with serious illness and disability. Spouses represent roughly 62% of these caregivers, with women comprising 72% of this number (Derby & O'Mahony, 2001). Often, primary caregivers are spouses with their own health care needs that many make them susceptible to depression, fatigue, and frequent acute illnesses. Other caregiving relationships involve adult children as dual-role caregivers to parents and their own children, or the staff at the elder's nursing facility or assisted living environment. Researching the use of home medical/social services by elders in the last 6 months of life, Kobayashi (2000) found that the focus of care needed by the patient and family is that of medical and psychosocial treatment. Symptom management is more intense and requires regular

evaluation. A large part of the advanced stage of illness may require more physical symptom monitoring; however, the psychosocial needs of the patient and family are just as important. Utilization of the palliative care team is vital at the end of life (Kobayashi, 2000).

End-of-life decisions place additional burdens on the family and the elder patient with cancer. Those decisions include where the final days will be spent, what impact there will be on loved ones, and whether the family can afford the care involved. The preference of most elders is to die in the comfort of their home. Family members often take a leave of absence from their jobs to care for a dying loved one; those that do not have that option may experience feelings of remorse for taking a more peripheral role in the care of the older adult (Meiner, 1999).

When the terminal phase of cancer is reached, conflict may occur among the elder patient, his or her family members, and health care workers. Conflict at the end of life transpires because of the disparity between patient/family expectations and the patient's functional and symptom status. As the disease progresses, symptoms and physical function are in flux. Family members attempt to adjust to the changes; however, in advanced cancer, the changes can occur quickly, which provokes conflict (Neuenschwander, Bruera, & Cavalli, 1991).

Family concerns throughout the course of advanced illness are directed toward the physical comfort of the patient, the emotional impact on the family, and the desire for accurate information. Vachon, Kristjanson, and Higginson (1995) reported that most families feel that information concerning their loved ones' illness is difficult to obtain, and that support is inadequate. It is commonly perceived by family members that, once the terminal prognosis is discussed, health care professionals do not feel the need to provide additional information. Because of the rapid change in physical and cognitive status, however, information updates are just as significant as before. Of 22 terminally ill patients interviewed, Kutner, Steiner, Corbett, Jahnigen, and Barton (1999) found that 98.2% requested information concerning changes in their disease status. It is interesting to note that, even though most patients and families request the truth, they still want health care providers to be optimistic and maintain a sense of hope (Kutner et al., 1999).

Initially, the family's focus of hope is often on cure. It is also the hope and goal of the family to provide comfort and support to their loved one as death becomes imminent. The palliative care team assists caregivers to develop the physical, emotional, and mental reserves that are required to maintain hope (Borneman, Stahl, Ferrell, & Smith, 2002). As the family's focus of hope changes with the changing status of the patient's physical condition, family members may strengthen the connection with their faith system, as well as their relationship to the patient and others. The connection made prior to the death of the loved one is integral in the grieving process (Brant, 1998).

Case Study Conclusion

Even though Mr. B. is physically active, and has a geographically close support system, he has multiple concurrent illnesses. Normally, a physically active, mentally intact, 81-year-old man with a localized NSCLC tumor staged at IIA would be a candidate for surgical resection. However, it is important to remember that his comorbid illnesses of hypertension and coronary artery disease and history of cardiac surgeries put him in a high-risk category for surgery. Knowing this, it is important to offer all options available, with adequate information regarding the risks involved. Allowing Mr. B. and his family to make treatment decisions is an important palliative care measure. That having been said, palliative care treatment should begin at the time of diagnosis. Mr. B. and his family benefited from the palliative care interdisciplinary team expertise and support, and symptom management began before symptoms presented.

Symptom management for Mr. B. consisted of management of pain resulting from tumor growth and excessive coughing caused by chronic bronchitis. Combined radiation and chemotherapy is the standard treatment for nonresectable NSCLC. This treatment modality has the potential to hamper tumor growth, which, as a result, will diminish pain. Symptom management intensifies as the treatment progresses and the disease advances.

Education and follow-up was offered to Mr. B.'s wife. Mr. B. and his family directed the course of treatment and follow-up care with the assistance of the palliative care team. The entire team assisted Mr. B. and his family in making informed decisions on treatment choices, as well as providing psychosocial and spiritual support necessary to find meaning and direction in a time of uncertainty.

CONCLUSION

Older patients with cancer may experience multiple symptoms throughout their disease trajectory. These symptoms increase in frequency and severity in the advanced stages of cancer (Foley & Gelband, 2001). Clinical practice guidelines for improving symptom management in end-of-life care are needed and are in the developmental stage.

In addition to suffering with physical symptoms, older patients with cancer may experience psychosocial and/or spiritual distress. Distress is defined as

an unpleasant experience of an emotional, psychological, social, or spiritual nature that interferes with the ability to cope with cancer treatment. It extends along a continuum, from common normal feelings of vulnerability, sadness, and fear, to problems that are disabling, such as true depression, anxiety, panic, and feeling isolated or in a spiritual crisis. (Holland & Chertkov, 2001, p. 207)

Measurement of distress and implementation of interventions to alleviate it are essential to quality cancer care.

In an effort to improve all dimensions of care for patients with cancer, and to promote quality of life, the National Cancer Policy Board has recommended that palliative care begin at the time of cancer diagnosis and increase in amount and intensity throughout the course of a patient's illness, until death (Foley & Gelband, 2001). Teno's (2001) model of patient-focused, family-centered medical care identifies quality end-of-life care focused on physical comfort, emotional support, and shared decision making. Emphasis on the patient, the needs of the caregivers before and after death, coordination and continuity of care, and education are hallmarks of this model, which is useful in the care of the older adult and his or her family. Measurement of quality of life and quality care at the end of life with the "Toolkit of Instruments to Measure End-of-Life Care" (Teno, 1999) will provide much-needed data for supporting elder patients and their caregivers throughout the disease trajectory.

RESOURCES
National Cancer Institute Websites
- Surveillance, Epidemiology, and End Results (*seer.cancer.gov*): general information on cancer incidence and survival in the United States
- Cancer Mortality Maps and Graphs (*www3.cancer.gov/atlasplus*): maps, graphs, text, tables, and figures of geographic patterns and time trends of cancer death rates for more than 40 types of cancer
- "Prostate Cancer Home Page" (*www.nci.nih.gov/cancer_information/cancer_type/prostate*): information on all aspects of prostate cancer for patients and professionals

Centers for Disease Control and Prevention Websites
- National Center for Chronic Disease Prevention and Health Promotion, Cancer Prevention and Control, National Cancer Data (*www.cdc.gov/cancer/natlcancerdata.htm*): provides links to various cancer data resources on the World Wide Web
- National Center for Chronic Disease Prevention and Health Promotion, Cancer Prevention and Control, State/Territory Cancer Data (*www.cdc.gov/cancer/dbdata.htm*): state cancer burden fact sheets and National Program of Cancer Registries state/territory profiles for lung, colorectal, breast, and prostate cancer
- National Center for Health Statistics (*www.cdc.gov/nchs*): searchable database of government statistics

Other Websites
- National PACE Association (*www.NPAonline.org*): information on health care services for elders provided through Programs of All-inclusive Care for the Elderly (PACE)
- Nursing, Midwifery and the Allied Health Professions, University of Sheffield, UK (*nmap.ac.uk*): offers a free tutorial on use of the Internet for nurses, midwives, and other health professionals

Nursing Links and Listserves
Note to readers: E-mail message information provided below uses quotation marks to designate the content of the message and angle brackets (⟨ and ⟩) to indicate that the information noted within is to be added by the reader. Neither the quotation marks nor the angle brackets should be typed into the message.
- NP Info discussion group (electronic mailing lists for nurse practitioners on the NP Central website: *www.npcentral.net/lists.shtml*).
- FLORENCE. To subscribe, send an e-mail to *majordomo@ualberta.ca*. In the message section, type "Subscribe florence."
- NURSENET. To subscribe, send an e-mail to *Listserv@listserv.utoronto.ca*. In the message section, type "sub nursenet ⟨your first name⟩ ⟨your last name⟩."
- The NURHIS-L Listserv (an international forum for the discussion of nursing history). To subscribe, send an e-mail to *LISTSERV@UCONNVM.UCONN.EDU*. Leave the subject line BLANK. In the message section, type "SUB NURHIS-L ⟨your name⟩."
- CAPHIS (Consumer and Patient Health Information Section, Medical Library Association). To subscribe, send an e-mail to *LISTSERV@SHRSYS.HSLC.ORG*. Leave the subject line BLANK. In the message section, type "Subscribe CAPHIS ⟨your first name⟩ ⟨your last name⟩."
- Web Nursing List (a discussion list for nurses using the Internet and World Wide Web as a means of communication). To subscribe, send an e-mail to *LISTSERV@ITSSRV1.UCSF.EDU*. Leave the subject line BLANK. In the message section, type "subscribe Web-Nsg-L ⟨your name⟩.".
- Selected Nursing Links (provided by the Virtual Nursing College of Langara College, Vancouver, British Columbia, Canada): *www.langara.bc.ca/vnc/links.htm*

REFERENCES
Abrahm, J. (1998). Promoting symptom control in palliative care. *Seminars in Oncology Nursing, 14*(2), 95-109.

Ahlgren, J. (1999). Gastrointestinal cancer in the elderly. *Clinics in Geriatric Medicine, 15*(6), 627-635.

American Cancer Society. (2002). *Cancer facts and figures 2002.* Atlanta: Author.

Bailes, J. S. (1997). Health care economics of cancer in the elderly. *Cancer, 80,* 1348-1350.

Baker, D. (2001). Current surgical management of colorectal cancer. *Nursing Clinics of North America, 36,* 579-591.

Baker, S., & Grouchow, L. (1997). Pharmacology of cancer chemotherapy in the older person. *Clinics in Geriatric Medicine, 13,* 169-185.

Balducci, L., & Extermann, M. (1998). Cancer in the elderly. *Clinical Geriatrics, 6*(3), 51-60.

Balducci, L., & Extermann, M. (1999). Management of cancer in the elderly. Home Health Care Consultant Oncology. *Clinical Geriatrics, 6*(3), 2-3, 7-10.

Balducci, L., & Extermann, M. (2001). Management of breast cancer in the older woman. *Cancer Control, 8*(5), 431-441.

Balducci, L., & Monfardini, S. (1999). A comprehensive geriatric assessment (CGA) is necessary for the study and management of cancer in the elderly. *European Journal of Cancer, 53,* 1771-1772.

Berger, D., & Roslyn, J. (1997). Cancer surgery in the elderly. *Clinics in Geriatric Medicine, 13,* 119-141.

Blackwell, S., & Crawford, J. (1997). Lung cancer. In C. Cassel, H. Cohen, E. Larson, D. Meier, N. Resnick, L. Rubenstein, et al. (Eds.), *Geriatric medicine* (3rd ed., pp. 73-80). New York: Springer.

Blackwell, S., & Crawford, J. (2000). Treatment of non-small cell lung cancer in the elderly patient. In H. Pass, J. Mitchell, D. Johnson, A. Turrisi, & J. Minna (Eds.), *Lung cancer: Principles and practice* (2nd ed., pp. 1071-1080). Philadelphia: Lippincott Williams & Wilkins.

Blumberg, D., & Ramanathan, R. (2002). Treatment of colon and rectal cancer. *Journal of Clinical Gastroenterology, 34,* 15-26.

Borneman, T., Stahl, C., Ferrell, B., & Smith, D. (2002). The concept of hope in family caregivers of cancer patients at home. *Journal of Hospice and Palliative Nursing, 4*(1), 21-33.

Bower, M., Brazil, L., & Coombes, R. C. (1998). Endocrine and metabolic complications of advanced cancer. In D. Doyle, G. Hanks, & N. MacDonald (Eds.), *Oxford textbook of palliative medicine* (2nd ed., pp. 709-725). New York: Oxford University Press.

Brant, J. M. (1998). The art of palliative care: Living with hope, dying with dignity. *Journal of Hospice & Palliative Care Nursing, 25,* 995-1003.

Brown, J. S., Eraut, D., Trask, C., & Davison, A. G. (1996). Age and treatment of lung cancer. *Thorax, 51,* 564-568.

Carbone, P. P. (2000). Advances in the systemic treatment of cancers in the elderly. *Critical Reviews in Oncology/Hematology, 35,* 201-218.

Carney, D. (2002). Lung cancer: time to move on from chemotherapy. *New England Journal of Medicine, 346,* 126-128.

Coyne, P., Lyckholm, L., & Smith, T. J. (2001). Clinical interventions, economic outcomes, and palliative care. In B. Ferrell & N. Coyle (Eds.) *Textbook of palliative nursing* (pp 73-80). New York: Oxford University Press.

Derby, S., & O'Mahony, S. (2001). Elderly patients. In B. Ferrell & N. Coyle (Eds.), *Textbook of palliative nursing* (p. 437). New York: Oxford University Press.

Douillard, J. Y., Cunningham, D., Roth, A. D., Navarro, M., James, R. D., Karasek, P., et al. (2000). Irinotecan combined with fluorouracil compared with fluorouracil alone as first-line treatment for metastatic colorectal cancer: A multicentre randomised trial. *The Lancet, 355,* 1041-1047.

Donnelly, S., & Walsh, D. (1995). The symptoms of advanced cancer. *Seminars in Oncology, 22*(Suppl. 3), 67-72.

Earle, C., & Stern, H. (2001). Colorectal cancer therapy. In E. J. Irvine & R. Hunt (Eds.), *Evidence-Based Gastroenterology* (pp. 280-306). London: BC Decker.

Effects of Vinorelbine on quality of life and survival of elderly patients with advanced non-small-cell lung cancer. The Elderly Lung Cancer Vinorelbine Italian Study Group. (1999). *Journal of the National Cancer Institute, 91,* 66-72.

Fainsinger, R., Miller, M. J., Bruera, E., Hanson, J., & Maceachern, T. (1991). Symptom control during the last week of life on a palliative care unit. *Journal of Palliative Care, 7*(1), 5-11.

Fainsinger, R., Spachynski, K., Hanson, J., & Bruera, E. (1994). Symptom control in terminally ill patients with malignant bowel obstruction. *Journal of Pain and Symptom Management, 9,* 12-18.

Feld, R., Sagman, U., & LeBlanc, M. (2000). Staging and prognostic factors in small cell lung cancer. In H. Pass, J. Mitchell, D. Johnson, A. Turrisi, & J. Minna (Eds.), *Lung cancer: Principles and practice* (2nd ed., pp. 612-627). Philadelphia: Lippincott Williams & Wilkins.

Finkelstien, J. B. (2000). *Prostate cancer drug approved to ease symptoms of advanced disease.* Retrieved February 23, 2002, from http://www.oncology.com/v2_MainFrame

Foley, K., & Gelband, H. (2001). Background and recommendations. In K. Foley & H. Gelband (Eds.), *Improving palliative care for cancer* (pp. 9-61). Washington, DC: National Academy Press.

Forman, W. (1997). Colon cancer and other gastrointestinal malignancies. In C. Cassel, H. Cohen, E. Larson, D. Meier, N. Resnick, L. Rubenstein, et al. (Eds.), *Geriatric medicine* (3rd ed., pp. 281-291). New York: Springer.

Gajdos, C., Tartter, P. I., Bleiweiss, I. J., Lopchinsky, R. A., & Bernstein, J. L. (2001). Breast cancer in the elderly. *Journal of the American College of Surgeons, 192,* 698-707.

Holland, J., & Chertkov, L. (2001). Clinical practice guidelines for the management of psychosocial and physical symptoms of cancer. In K. Foley & H. Gelband (Eds.), *Improving palliative care for cancer* (pp. 199-232). Washington, DC: National Academy Press.

Hoskin, P., & Makin, W. (1998). *Oncology for palliative medicine.* New York: Oxford University Press.

Huether, S. (1998). The cellular environment: Fluids and electrolytes, acids and bases. In K. L. McCance & S. L. Huether (Eds.), *Pathophysiology: The biologic basis for disease in adults and children* (3rd ed., p. 99). St. Louis: Mosby.

Huguenin, P. U., Bitterli, M., Lutolf, U. M., Bernhard, J., & Glanzmann, C. (1999). Localized prostate cancer in elderly patients: Outcome after radiation therapy compared to matched younger patients. *Strahlentherapie und Onkologie, 175,* 554-558.

Hunter-Dorcas, R. (1991). Cancer and sexuality. In S. Baird, M. Donehower, V. Lindquist-Stalsbroten, & T. Ades (Eds.), *A cancer source book for nurses* (6th ed., pp. 220-227). Atlanta: American Cancer Society.

Kennedy-Malone, L., Fletcher, K., & Plank, L. (2000). *Management guidelines for gerontological nurse practitioners.* Philadelphia: F.A. Davis.

Kirk, D. (1998). Prostate cancer in the elderly. *European Journal of Surgical Oncology, 24,* 379-383.

Kobayashi, N. (2000). Formal service utilization by the frail elderly at home during the last 6 months of life. *Nursing and Health Sciences, 2*(4), 201.

Kraut, M., & Wozniak, A. (2000). Clinical presentation. In H. Pass, J. Mitchell, D. Johnson, A. Turrisi, & J. Minna (Eds.), *Lung cancer: Principles and practice* (2nd ed., pp. 521-534). Philadelphia: Lippincott Williams & Wilkins.

Kutner, J. S., Steiner, J. F., Corbett, K. K., Jahnigen, D. W., & Barton, P. L. (1999). Information needs in terminal illness. *Social Science & Medicine, 48,* 1341-1352.

Langer, C., Scott, C., Buhart, R., Movasa, B., Sause, W., & Komaki, R. (2000). Effect of advanced age on outcome in radiation therapy oncology group studies of locally advanced NSCLC. *Lung Cancer, 29,* 104.

Lazzaro, R., & Comandini, D. (2000). Cancer in the elderly: Assessing patients for fitness. *Critical Reviews in Oncology/Hematology, 35,* 155-160.

Lima, C., Herndon, J., Kosty, M., Clamon, G., & Green, M. (2002). Therapy choices among older patients with lung carcinoma: An evaluation of two trials of the Cancer and Leukemia Group B. *Cancer, 94,* 181-187.

Lutz, S., Norrell, R., Bertucio, C., Kachnic, L., Johnson, C., Arthur, D., et al. (2001). Symptom frequency and severity in patients with metastatic or locally recurrent lung cancer: A prospective study using the Lung Cancer Symptom Scale in a community hospital. *Journal of Palliative Medicine, 4,* 157-164.

Mackay, H. J. (2000). Metastatic and advanced breast cancer in the elderly. *Clinical Geriatrics.* Retrieved on April 10, 2002, from http://www.mmhc.com/engine.pl?station=mmhc&template=cgfull.html&id=1179

McDonald, N. (1993). Principles governing the use of cancer chemotherapy in palliative medicine. In D. Doyle, G. Hanks, & N. MacDonald (Eds.), *Oxford textbook of palliative medicine* (p. 109). Oxford, UK: Oxford University Press.

Meiner, S. E. (1999). Essentials of home-based cancer care of the elderly. *Geriatric Nursing, 20*(5), 275-277.

Morton, A. R., & Ritch, P. S. (2002). Hypercalcemia. In A. Berger, R. Portenoy, & D. Weissman (Eds.), *Principles in practice of palliative care & supportive oncology* (2nd ed., pp. 497-498). Philadelphia: Lippincott Williams & Wilkins.

Mulay, M. (2001). Treatment decision-making. In D. Berg (Ed.), *Contemporary issues in colorectal cancer: A nursing perspective* (pp. 81-104). Boston: Jones & Bartlett.

Murphy-Ende, K. (2001). Palliation of gastrointestinal obstructive disorders. *Nursing Clinics of North America, 36,* 761-778.

Nally, A. (1996). Critical care of the patient with lung cancer. *AACN Clinical Issues, 7*(1), 79-94.

National Cancer Institute. (2002). *What you need to know about prostate cancer: Information about detection, symptoms, diagnosis, and treatment of prostate cancer* (NIH Publication No. 00-1576; Posted: 12/05/00, Updated 1/22/02). Retrieved from http://www.cancer.gov/cancer_information/wyntk/prostate

Neuenschwander, H., Bruera, E., & Cavalli, F. (1991). Matching the clinical function and symptom status with the expectations of patients with advanced cancer, their families, and health care workers. *Supportive Cancer Care, 4,* 252-256.

Olmi, P., Cerafo, G., Balzi, M., Becciolini, A., & Geinitz, H. (1997). Radiotherapy in the aged. *Clinics in Geriatric Medicine, 13,* 143-159.

Pignon, T., Horiot, J., Michel, B., van Poppel, H., Barelink, H., Roelofson, F., et al. (1997). Age is not a limiting factor for radical radiotherapy in pelvic malignancies. *Radiotherapy and Oncology, 42,* 107-120.

Preoperative short-term radiation in operable rectal carcinoma: A prospective randomized trial. Stockholm Rectal Cancer Study Group. (1990). *Cancer, 66,* 49-55.

Repetto, L., & Comandini, D. (2000). Cancer in the elderly: Assessing patients for fitness. *Critical Reviews in Oncology/Hematology, 35,* 155-160.

Repetto, L., Comandini, D., & Mammoliti, S. (2001). Life expectancy, co-morbidity, and quality of life: The treatment equation in the older cancer patient. *Critical Reviews in Oncology/Hematology, 37,* 147-152.

Robinson, K. M., & Huether, S. (1998a). Structure and function of the reproductive systems. In K. L. McCance & S. L. Huether (Eds.), *Pathophysiology: The biologic basis for disease in adults and children* (3rd ed., pp. 788-790). St. Louis: Mosby.

Robinson, K. M., & Huether, S. (1998b). Structure and function of the reproductive systems. In K. L. McCance & S. L. Huether (Eds.), *Pathophysiology: The biologic basis for disease in adults and children* (3rd ed., pp. 796-805). St. Louis: Mosby.

Rousseau, P. (1995). Non pain symptom management in terminal care. *Clinics in Geriatric Medicine, 12,* 313-327.

Rousseau, P. (1998). Management of malignant bowel obstruction in advanced cancer: A brief review. *Journal of Palliative Medicine, 1,* 65-72.

Saddler, D., & Ellis, C. (1999). Colorectal cancer. *Seminars in Oncology Nursing, 15*(1), 58-69.

Sheehan, D., & Forman, W. (1997). Symptomatic management of the older person with cancer. *Clinics in Geriatric Medicine, 13,* 203-217.

Shepard, F., Abratt, A., Anderson, H., Gatzemeier, U., Anglin, G., & Iglesias J. (1997). Gemcitabine in the treatment of elderly patients with advanced non-small cell lung cancer. *Seminars in Oncology, 24,* 50-55.

Stanford, J. L., Stephenson, R. A., Coyle, L. M., Cerhan, J., Correa, R., Eley, J. W., et al. (1999). *Prostate Cancer Trends 1973-1995.* SEER Program, National Cancer Institute. (NIH Pub. No. 99-4543). Bethesda, MD: National Cancer Institute.

SUPPORT Principal Investigators. (1995). A controlled trial to improve care for seriously ill hospitalized patients: The Study to Understand Prognoses and Preferences for Outcomes and Risks of Treatments (SUPPORT). *Journal of the American Medical Association, 274,* 1591-1598.

Teno, J. (2001). Quality of care and quality indicators for end-of-life cancer care: Hope for the best, yet prepare for the worst. In K. Foley & H. Gelband (Eds.), *Improving palliative care for cancer* (pp. 96-131). Washington, DC: National Academy Press.

Teno, J. (1999). *TIME: Toolkit of Instruments to Measure End of Life Care.* Retrieved on March 6, 2002, from http://www.chcr.brown.edu/pcoc/Choosing.htm

Vachon, M. L., Kristjanson, L., & Higginson, I. (1995). Psychosocial issues in palliative care: The patient, the family, and the process and outcome of care. *Journal of Pain and Symptom Management, 10,* 142-150.

Van Dijck, J. A., Broeders, M. J., & Verbeek, A. (1997). Mammographic screening in older women: Is it worthwhile? *Drugs and Aging, 10*(2), 69-79.

Veronesi, A., Crivellari, D., & Magri, M. (1996). Vinorelbine treatment of advanced non-small-cell lung cancer with special emphasis on elderly patients. *European Journal of Cancer, 32,* 1809-1815.

Walsh, A., Begg, C., & Carbone, P. (1989). Cancer chemotherapy in the elderly. *Seminars in Oncology, 16,* 66-69.

Weissman, D. (2000). *Fast Fact and Concepts #13: Determining prognosis in advanced cancer.* Retrieved April 12, 2002, from the End-of-Life/Palliative Education Resource Center Web site: www.eperc.mcw.edu

Willert, A., & Semans, M. (2000). Knowledge and attitudes about later life sexuality: What clinicians need to know about helping the elderly. *Contemporary Family Therapy, 22*(4), 415-435.

Yancik, R., & Reis, L. A. (1994). Cancer in older persons—magnitude of the problem. How do we apply what we know? *Cancer, 74*(Suppl. 7), 1995-2003.

STROKE, COMA, AND BRAIN DEATH

Barbara Evans

Mrs. C., an 86-year-old artist, mother, and pet lover, was admitted to the nursing home for rehabilitation following an ischemic stroke 10 days ago. Her poststroke deficits include left-sided weakness (upper extremity more than lower), neglect, mild cognitive impairment (short-term memory and impulsivity), and urinary incontinence. Her hospital admission was extended for treatment of atrial fibrillation and a urinary tract infection, and regulation of her diabetes. Prior to admission, Mrs. C. lived with her cat in an assisted living facility and required assistance with her medications. She ambulated around her apartment, but required a wheelchair for distances because of lower extremity weakness, arthritic pain in her knees, and a history of falls.

Mrs. C. often spent her mornings painting. Her family consists of a daughter and two grandsons who live out of state, but are with the patient upon admission. During the initial assessment, Mrs. C. is assessed to be at a high risk for falls based on her history of falls, hemiparesis with neglect of the affected limb, mild cognitive impairment with impulsivity, knee pain, and poor endurance. Her daughter adds that her mother rarely complained of pain, but took acetaminophen for her arthritis. Mrs. C. is tearful in response to several questions during the interview, and her daughter is concerned that she is not eating and resistant to getting out of bed. She has no previous psychiatric history, but two close friends recently died. In the past, she relied on family and her faith for support. At times of stress, she often lost herself in her art.

Mrs. C. states that she hopes to regain continence and return to her apartment and cat. Her daughter has a copy of Mrs. C.'s living will, which outlines her previous wishes not to be resuscitated or intubated or to have her life prolonged by artificial nutrition. Plans are to continue to pay the rent on her apartment, but her daughter is aware that Mrs. C. may require long-term placement at the nursing home. The cat will go to her daughter's home, but can come in with the daughter when she visits.

Physical therapy also evaluates Mrs. C. and notes that her potential for stroke recovery could be impacted by her advanced age, poor endurance prior to stroke, and cognitive impairment. Her left heel has a small intact blister, and her coccyx is reddened and needs nursing intervention with pressure-relieving techniques. The patient's left upper extremity is partially flexed, with increased tone and reduced range of motion. There is some mild left footdrop developing; however, Mrs. C. is able to transfer and walk short distances with a walker and assistance. She complains of increased knee pain and fatigue after physical therapy.

STROKE

The term *stroke* refers to the sudden onset of a focal or global neurologic deficit that lasts longer than 24 hours and is caused by disrupted cerebral vascular circulation. Signs of impairment may be perceptual, motor, cognitive, or speech related. Risk factors include hypertension, hyperlipidemia, cardiac disease, diabetes, family history, and tobacco and alcohol abuse (Aminoff, 2001). Strokes have been classified into two categories based on the underlying pathologic process. Ischemic or nonhemorrhagic strokes are the most common, comprising approximately 80% (Weisberg, 1996), and can be the result of a buildup of plaque (thrombus) or a clot (embolus). Hemorrhagic strokes, caused by bleeding into the brain, comprise the remaining 20%. Key to initiating any treatment is establishing the underlying cause.

Incidence and Prevalence

Strokes are currently the third leading cause of death in the United States, with over 600,000 people experiencing a stroke each year (American Heart Association [AHA], 2001). After age 55, the incidence more than doubles each decade. Over the past two decades, the number of patients surviving their strokes has increased; currently, there are an estimated 4.6 million stroke survivors in the United States (AHA, 2001). This is partially attributed to improved management of acute stroke, as well as better identification and treatment of risk factors, particularly hypertension (Wolf, Cobb, & D'Agostino, 1992). Mortality rates are highest during the first 30 days and increase with advancing age. In general, patients are more likely to survive an ischemic stroke than a hemorrhagic stroke. Approximately 30% to 40% of patients surviving ischemic strokes will have severe disabilities (Adams & Biller, 1996). This represents a significant challenge to the provision of continuous and coordinated health care to stroke patients. Knowing when and how to incorporate palliative care interventions from the acute care setting through rehabilitation to long-term care or home requires a knowledge of common stroke-related symptoms and expected outcomes.

Disease Trajectory and Prognosis

It is important to have an understanding of the general time frame for poststroke recovery. This can facilitate more appropriate, stepwise care planning and provide a method by which to evaluate treatment interventions. It can also assist patients and families in setting realistic goals and expectations during the months of recovery. As they assess the benefit versus the burden of various treatment options, guidance needs to be based on clinical information that is intertwined with the values of the patient and his or her family. The following are general guidelines in terms of recovery from stroke.

Up to 20% of patients with acute stroke do not survive the first week (Volpe, 2001). The major-

ity of these deaths are attributed to the direct effect of the stroke damage, specifically herniation or brainstem injury (Longstreth et al., 2001). Advanced age is a predictor of decreased ability to survive a stroke. In addition, African Americans are more likely to die from a stroke (AHA, 2001). After the initial few days to weeks, complications from immobility, such as infection and blood clots, also impact mortality rates.

Given the multiple variables of age, type of stroke, and comorbidities, there is variation in the literature regarding recovery time frames for survivors. Within hours to days of stroke onset, muscle tone can begin to return to paralyzed extremities. Overall, there is agreement that the majority of recovery occurs within the first 2 to 3 months, with less functional gain after 4 to 6 months and minimal gains beyond 6 months (Kwakkel, Wagenaar, Kollen, & Lankhorst, 1996). Research has focused on identifying variables that best predict prognosis and outcomes in stroke patients, as well as which patients are most likely to benefit from the acute rehabilitation setting. A review of the literature by Kwakkel et al. (1996) found that age, previous stroke, disability on admission, urinary incontinence, degree of paralysis, level of consciousness within the first 48 hours, orientation to time and place, sitting balance, and level of social support were all valid prognostic indicators for stroke recovery.

In order to guide clinicians as they assess stroke patients for hospice eligibility, the National Hospice Organization (1996) developed criteria for determining prognosis in stroke and coma patients (Box 12-1). In the acute poststroke phase, they have listed coma beyond 3 days associated with age over 70 years, renal impairment, and absent verbal and withdrawal responses as some of the predictors of poor prognosis and early mortality. For chronic-phase patients, age over 70 years, poor functional status (Karnofsky Performance Status scale score <50%), poststroke dementia, poor nutritional status, and medical complications (e.g., infection, pressure ulcers) are potential correlates of poor survival rates. (See Table 11-1 for the Karnofsky Performance Status scale.)

For those elders who do survive their stroke, several factors influence the recovery of lost function and the extent of their disabilities. The size

---

Box 12-1 Medical Guidelines for Determining Prognosis: Stroke and Coma

After stroke, patients who do not die during the acute hospitalization tend to stabilize with supportive care only. Continuous decline in clinical or functional status over time means that the patient's prognosis is poor.

Conversely, steady improvement in the patient's functional or physiologic status may indicate that the patient is not terminally ill. Care should be taken to distinguish true recovery of performance and physiologic function from the improvement in symptoms and subjective well-being that can accompany hospice intervention.

I. *During the acute phase immediately following a hemorrhagic or ischemic stroke*, any of the following are strong predictors of early mortality:
   A. Coma or persistent vegetative state secondary to stroke, beyond three days' duration.
   B. In post-anoxic stroke, coma or severe obtundation, accompanied by severe myoclonus, persisting beyond three days past the anoxic event.
   C. Comatose patients with any 4 of the following on day 3 of coma had 97% mortality by two months:

     1. Abnormal brain stem response
     2. Absent verbal response
     3. Absent withdrawal response to pain
     4. Serum creatinine >1.5 mg/dl
     5. Age >70
   D. Dysphagia severe enough to prevent the patient from receiving food and fluids necessary to sustain life, in a patient who declines, or is not a candidate for, artificial nutrition and hydration.

II. *Once the patient has entered the chronic phase*, the following clinical factors may correlate with poor survival in the setting of severe stroke, and should be documented.
   A. Age greater than 70.
   B. Poor functional status, as evidenced by Karnofsky score of <50%.*
   C. Post-stroke dementia, as evidenced by a FAST score of greater than 7.
   D. Poor nutritional status, whether on artificial nutrition or not:
     1. Unintentional progressive weight loss of greater than 10% over past six months.
     2. Serum albumin less than 2.5 gm/dl may be a helpful prognostic indicator, but should not be used by itself.

*See Table 11-1.
From National Hospice Organization. (1996). *Medical guidelines for determining prognosis in selected non-cancer diseases* (2nd ed.). Arlington, VA: National Hospice Organization.

---

and location of the stroke and the associated neurologic deficits are directly related to the potential for recovery, as well as to the length of time to maximum recovery. Each stroke patient is unique in presentation relative to the extent and combination of any motor, sensory, cognitive, perceptual, and speech deficits. The greater the initial damage, the longer and more difficult the recovery. Prestroke factors must also be considered; these refer to the age and overall health status of patients prior to their stroke. Studies have found that increased age is associated with poorer outcomes poststroke (Ween, Alexander, D'Esposito, & Roberts, 1996). Brandstater (1998) cautioned that this may be due to the effect of

comorbidities that increase with age, particularly heart disease and diabetes, rather than to age alone. There is some speculation that older adults may not receive rehabilitation that is as intensive as that provided to younger stroke patients, and that this may also contribute to poorer outcomes. It makes sense that those patients who are less functional prestroke will have more difficulty regaining function poststroke.

A study by Longstreth et al. (2001) looked at predictors of stroke death and after controlling for age and type of stroke; the strongest predictor of death after stroke was poor performance on a timed walking exercise measured prior to the stroke. This may imply that slow walking reflects prestroke frailty and less reserve for recovery. Similarly, in a study by Sharma, Fletcher, and Vassallo (1999), younger stroke patients (<75 years old) were compared with older stroke patients (>75 years old), and higher mortality rates were found for those over age 75 during the acute poststroke phase and up to 3 months after their stroke. The findings from this study indicate that older stroke patients are unique from their younger cohorts, as is their disease trajectory. In addition, educational level, financial assets, and premorbid personality can also impact stroke recovery (Gresham, 1992). Preexisting cognitive impairments further compromise a patient's ability to participate in his or her rehabilitation.

A number of poststroke factors also affect the recovery process. How soon patients seek treatment, the incidence of medical complications, the availability and quality of services, the amount of family/community support, and the level of motivation can all influence eventual outcomes. Depression, for example, has been shown to develop in at least 30% of stroke patients (Gustafson, Nilsson, Mattsson, Astrom, & Bucht, 1995). Untreated depression can delay and reduce functional recovery; Kauhanen et al. (1999) reported depression in 50% of patients 3 months poststroke.

Acute Stroke

The first 30 days following an acute stroke are associated with the highest mortality rates as a result of the direct effects of the stroke and/or resulting complications. Patients who present with a change in level of consciousness or coma are at highest risk because of potential respiratory and circulatory compromise and require immediate medical management. Early recognition of symptoms and timely diagnostic evaluations are key. For example, thrombolytic therapy to reverse the obstruction from thrombus or embolism in an ischemic stroke should be initiated within the first 3 hours. This demonstrates the importance of seeking rapid evaluation and treatment and why the term *brain attack* has been used to promote this concept. In addition, monitoring for signs and symptoms of deteriorating neurologic status, stabilizing vital signs, and managing other medical complications are priorities. Efforts to protect the patient's airway, provide fluids and nutrition, and maintain bowel and bladder

function are critical. During the acute phase, infection (especially pneumonia), pulmonary embolism (PE), and deep vein thrombosis (DVT) can all contribute to morbidity and mortality. Anticoagulation therapy (with ischemic strokes only), support stockings, and intermittent pneumatic calf compression have all been used to reduce the likelihood of both DVT and PE. Aspiration resulting from an impaired swallow reflex or decreased level of consciousness is a common finding, and patients should have their swallow evaluated by a speech therapist when this is suspected.

Multiple comorbidities place elders at a higher risk for complications, and medical management can be complex. During these first few days, if the elder patient continues to decline medically rather than stabilize or improve, his or her likelihood of surviving is diminished. Mental status changes can pose additional problems for the patient's safety and ability to communicate and cooperate with treatment. Attributing these changes solely to the stroke could overlook additional contributing factors. The patient may be delirious from medications, hypoxemia, infection, metabolic abnormalities, or other potentially reversible causes (see Chapter 18 for information on evaluating delirium). Maintaining a safe environment for the patient is vital during any episodes of acute confusion.

Comorbidities

Care of the older adult who has had a stroke requires a systematic review of the medical/surgical history and a complete physical and psychosocial assessment. Sources for information should include the elder, the family, and available records to ensure the most accurate medical profile. As previously stated, the risk of stroke increases with age, and the older patient is also more likely to have coexisting chronic illnesses. A survey of community-dwelling people over 65 years of age indicated that arthritis, hypertension, hearing impairments, and heart disease were the most common chronic disabilities (U.S. Bureau of the Census, 1993). In addition, the most common comorbidities found in stroke survivors in the Framingham study (Gresham et al., 1979) were hypertension, coronary heart disease, obesity, diabetes, arthritis, congestive heart failure, and chronic lung disease.

EVIDENCE-BASED PRACTICE

Reference: Barba, R., Morin, M., Cemillan, C., Delgado, C., Domingo, J., & Del Ser, T. (2002). Previous and incident dementia as risk factors for mortality in stroke patients. *Stroke, 33,* 1993-1998.

Research Problem: Do patients who have dementia prior to their stroke or develop it within 3 months after their stroke have a higher risk of mortality than stroke patients without dementia?

Design: A prospective study of patients admitted to an acute care hospital with stroke, who underwent clinical, functional, and cognitive assessments at admission and at 3, 6, 12, and 24 months.

Sample and Setting: 324 patients, diagnosed with ischemic or hemorrhagic stroke, were enrolled upon admission to a large urban hospital and then followed at a neurology clinic.

Methods: Patients admitted with acute stroke underwent a medical history, and clinical interviews were done with proxy relatives per protocol to assess cognition during the 5 years before their stroke. The presence or absence of dementia was determined based on criteria in the *Diagnostic and Statistical Manual of Mental Disorders (Third Edition–Revised)*. At 3 months poststroke, 251 survivors continued in the study and underwent neuropsychological testing,

with the diagnosis of poststroke dementia being made using the criteria in the *Diagnostic and Statistical Manual of Mental Disorders, Fourth Edition*. Follow-up visits were then scheduled at 6, 12, and 24 months.

Results: Forty-nine of 324 patients (15.1%) were found to have dementia up to 5 years prior to their stroke. At 3 months, 75 of 251 survivors were diagnosed with dementia, including 25 patients with "prestroke" dementia and 50 patients who developed dementia following or "incident to" their stroke. Thirty-two percent of the sample ($n = 105$) died. The proportion of survivors was 20.4% in patients with prestroke dementia versus 72.6% in those without prestroke dementia. Similarly, the proportion of survivors was 58.3% in patients who developed dementia following their stroke versus 95.4% in those who did not.

Implications for Nursing Practice: Understanding the relative risks and challenges that cognitive impairment adds to the stroke patient's potential for recovery is important to establishing goals of care.

Conclusion: Dementia that is either present prestroke or appears within 3 months following a stroke is a significant prognostic factor and increases the risk for mortality.

Many of the predisposing factors for stroke overlap with those for cardiovascular disease, and up to 75% of stroke patients have been shown to have concomitant heart disease (Brandstater, 1998). This can lead to complications with unstable blood pressure, angina, congestive heart failure, myocardial infarction, and arrhythmias. Any functional limitations associated with these comorbidities can impede stroke rehabilitation. For example, admission criteria to an acute inpatient rehabilitation unit include the ability to participate in 3 hours of therapy per day. Patients with significant heart or lung disease may not have that level of endurance. Underlying demen-

tia may make it difficult for patients to participate in or cooperate with their treatment modalities. Patients may also be resistive to therapy if they have been inadequately treated for pain from osteoarthritis, osteoporosis, or other musculoskeletal disorders. Addressing the stroke-related deficits while managing concurrent comorbidities will help to maximize each patient's ability to survive and to recover lost function.

Stroke Deficits and Related Complications

After reviewing the literature, Dombovy (1991) found that, within the first week after a stroke,

73% to 88% of patients have some hemiparesis, 23% to 33% have some language impairment, 67% to 84% have visual-perceptual disturbances, 13% to 32% have dysphagia, and 29% are incontinent. Three months poststroke, 35% to 60% continue to have impaired memory and cognition. There is much heterogeneity in the presentation and combination of these stroke-related deficits.

The risk of complications varies; in a study by Langhorne et al. (2000), the majority occurred within the first 6 weeks. Up to 85% of hospitalized stroke patients, with an average age of 76 years, developed at least one complication. The most prevalent complications were confusion (36%), pain (34%), falls (25%), urinary tract infection (24%), and chest infection (22%). On a long-term basis, coping with residual deficits appeared to present additional challenges. These same patients were followed for up to 30 months, at which time the most common complications were depressive symptoms (54%), anxiety symptoms (49%), falls (45%), and pain (37%). This particular study included symptomatic complications and revealed that over half of the poststroke patients were expressing self-reported symptoms of depression and anxiety. The impact of these symptoms on function and quality of life can be significant and is discussed later in this chapter.

Immobility increases the risk of pneumonia, skin breakdown, clotting disorders, contractures, and falls. Stroke patients have shown a higher rate of falls, as evidenced by up to a fourfold increased risk of hip fracture (Ramnemark, Nilsson, Borssen, & Gustafson, 2000). This risk is associated with hospital admission (Langhorne et al., 2000) and continues for noninstitutionalized stroke patients. Jorgensen, Engstad, and Jacobsen (2002) found that stroke patients in the community were twice as likely to fall at least once when compared to controls. Interestingly, depressive symptoms were related to this increased risk of falling. Stroke is clearly a risk factor for falls, and an increased awareness should lead to more preventive strategies.

Following a stroke, some patients develop neglect or a loss of awareness of their affected limbs. This is associated with right hemispheric strokes and, in the extreme, can result in patients being completely unaware of the left side of their body or of stimuli coming from the left side of their environment. Patient safety is compromised because neglect can increase the risk of injury and falls. Therapy focuses on techniques to compensate, for example, by adapting the environment to promote use of the neglected side and teaching the patient to visually scan from side to side.

Strokes occurring in the left hemisphere, in particular, can impair the ability to communicate. Those elders with expressive aphasia may comprehend spoken language, but are unable to express themselves verbally to varying degrees. Receptive aphasia is the result of deficits in receiving the message/auditory perception or retaining it. It is important to differentiate true aphasia from other possible disorders such as delirium or dementia that may also affect cognition and language. Treatment needs to be individualized to utilize whatever communication abilities remain. As a result of difficulty expressing their needs or interpreting what is going on around them, aphasic patients may become noncompliant, angry, fearful, or withdrawn.

Patients with swallowing disorders are at risk for aspiration pneumonia. Simple bedside testing can be done by a speech therapist when this is suspected, and more formal testing (modified barium swallow) done as indicated. Whether or not to insert a feeding tube to maintain nutrition may need to be addressed early on when the dysphagia is severe. A review of the literature by Finucane, Christmas, and Travis (1999), although focused on end-stage dementia patients, indicates that tube feeding does not prevent aspiration pneumonia because patients can still aspirate their oral secretions or gastric reflux. Therefore, the decision regarding the use of feeding tubes is not a simple one and should be guided by appropriate clinical input regarding potential for stroke recovery as well as patient and family preferences. (See Chapter 23 for a discussion regarding hydration and nutrition.)

Seizures occurring within the first 24 hours are not associated with higher mortality (Yatsu, DeGraba, & Hanson, 1992). They have been found in approximately 8% of stroke patients (Dombovy, 1991) and may require anticonvulsant therapy. A neurologist should periodically review long-term use of anticonvulsant medications.

Urinary incontinence and retention are additional complications poststroke and can be related to immobility, the location of the lesion, and other contributing factors. Therefore, efforts to prevent skin breakdown and promote bladder emptying through medication, intermittent catheterization (preferred to indwelling catheters in rehabilitative settings), or prompted toileting are possible interventions. Monitoring for signs and symptoms of urinary tract infection is important given the above risk factors.

Mental status changes can be evidenced by reduced level of consciousness, attention deficits, problems with memory and cognition, and changes in affect and behavior. Cognitive impairment can negatively impact the elder's ability to participate in rehabilitative programs and his or her final outcome. It is imperative to rule out additional factors that may be contributing to changes in mental status.

In conclusion, elders who have had a stroke remain at high risk for recurrent stroke for the rest of their lives. Reducing risk factors by controlling blood pressure, hyperlipidemia, weight, and concomitant diabetes and treating cardiac arrhythmias (particularly atrial fibrillation) continues to be important, based on the goals of care.

Common Symptoms Associated with Stroke

Fatigue

Fatigue, depression, and specific pain syndromes are symptoms that have been found to occur commonly in stroke patients. Fatigue is a subjective feeling of early exhaustion that impacts an individual's ability to interact mentally or physically with his or her environment. It is a commonly reported symptom poststroke, and yet few studies have looked at the frequency of poststroke fatigue and its impact on function (Staub & Bogousslavsky, 2001). In addition, research is only beginning to investigate a possible correlation between fatigue and location of stroke damage, such as brainstem and thalamic regions that impact the reticular activating system. An understanding of the relationship between fatigue and depression, sleep disturbances, and specific stroke deficits is needed in order to better recognize and treat fatigue.

Poststroke fatigue may be underreported and undertreated if it is attributed to depression and not evaluated independently.

One survey matching stroke survivors and an elder control group, both living in the community, found that 68% of the stroke group, compared to 35% of the control group, listed fatigue as a symptom (Ingles, Eskes, & Phillips, 1999). Up to 13 months after their stroke, these elders continued to describe fatigue as contributing to their functional limitations. In a pilot study by Staub, Annoni, and Bogousslavsky (2000), 42 stroke patients were evaluated between 3 months and 3 years after their stroke. Thirteen (31%) of the subjects reported disabling fatigue that did not appear to correlate with depression, age, gender, or time interval poststroke. These studies support the high incidence of complaints of fatigue poststroke.

Patients should be carefully evaluated for factors that could be contributing to their fatigue, such as anemia, pain, occult infections, hypothyroidism, medications, malnutrition, and sleep apnea. (Refer to Chapter 20 for further discussion of fatigue.) Adapting the environment to promote sleep, pacing activities, treating pain, and eliminating or reducing any offending medications should all be considered as possible interventions. Relaxation techniques such as breathing exercises, massage, imagery, or music also may promote sleep and reduce fatigue.

Depression

In contrast to fatigue, there are more published studies regarding poststroke depression. The development of depression associated with stroke is often multidimensional. Lesion location (i.e., frontal lobe) and disturbed neurotransmitter metabolism from the stroke damage can increase a patient's susceptibility to depression. Also, adapting to the loss of physical or cognitive abilities can be overwhelming, and the individual's premorbid personality, coping skills, and resources are all factors in making this adaptation. Medications can contribute to depressive symptoms as well.

There is concern that depression is underdiagnosed in stroke patients because of communication and cognitive impairments, as well as assumptions that it is a normal reaction to a serious, life-changing event (Gustafson et al.,

1995). The prevalence of poststroke depression varies in the literature depending upon methodologic procedures, diagnostic criteria, and timing of the evaluation. Overall, it is estimated that at least 30% of patients experience depression during the acute or chronic phase of their stroke (Gustafson et al., 1995). The scope of the problem may not be fully appreciated because of cases that go unrecognized or unreported. Kauhanen et al. (1999) evaluated 106 stroke patients at 3 and 12 months poststroke. Neurologic and psychological testing revealed that 53% of the patients at 3 months and 42% of the patients at 12 months were diagnosed with depression using the criteria in the *Diagnostic and Statistical Manual of Mental Disorders (Third Edition–Revised)* (American Psychiatric Association, 1987). Their study also revealed that cognitive impairment and dependency in activities of daily living (ADLs) were associated with higher rates of depression.

From another perspective, Ramasubbu, Robinson, Flint, Kosier, and Price (1998) looked at the impact of depression on function in acute poststroke patients with a mean age of 63 years. Their findings documented greater functional impairments in self-reported depressed stroke patients than in nondepressed stroke patients. The relationship between depression and functional impairment poststroke is not yet understood. To what extent is depression a response to stroke-related deficits? In turn, to what extent does depression cause further functional impairment as a result of related fatigue or lack of motivation?

These studies emphasize the importance of assessing all stroke patients for depression throughout the course of their disease. It is important to understand that the risk extends well beyond the acute poststroke period and increases with the severity of any cognitive and functional deficits. For severely aphasic or cognitively impaired patients who are exhibiting physiologic symptoms consistent with depression (sleep disturbances, appetite changes, and low energy), it may be appropriate to offer an empirical trial of an antidepressant and monitor response. Choosing the most appropriate antidepressant may require the input of a specialist in geriatric psychology, and ongoing supportive counseling may be beneficial as well. (Refer to Chapter 18 for further information on the treatment of depressed older adults.)

Stroke-Related Pain Syndromes and Treatments

The consequences of untreated pain are far reaching, and assessing for pain and treating it early will help to improve psychosocial and functional outcomes. Spasticity resulting from increased muscle tone presents as resistance to passive range of motion. Brain lesions poststroke can interfere with the descending central nervous system pathways that regulate muscle tone. The flexor muscle groups of the upper extremities and the extensor muscle groups of the lower extremities are most likely to be involved. The arms flex and pronate and the legs extend and adduct. When the spasticity is severe enough to interfere with the ability to perform ADLs, or if secondary complications such as pressure ulcers, contractures, or pain develop, then treatment should be considered (Gelber, 2002).

Early and continued range-of-motion exercises done at least twice daily to the affected areas and individualized splinting may reduce the risk of contractures. Given the risk of sedation and mental status changes, particularly in the older adult, the decision to treat pain pharmacologically must be weighed carefully. Drugs such as baclofen, tizanidine, benzodiazepines, and dantrolene each work slightly differently, but all patients using them must be closely monitored for side effects. Baclofen can also be administered intrathecally for spasticity. Nerve blocks with phenol or botulinum toxin to focal areas of spasticity can be effective for a number of weeks to months, but need to be repeated for sustained symptom relief. In order to restore a functional position or facilitate hygiene, surgical tendon release or lengthening can also be an option in extremities with no voluntary movement. Nondrug treatments that may be helpful include the application of heat or cold to areas of spasticity, but not if there is reduced sensation, given the risk of injury. Gentle massage and relaxation techniques such as imagery or music may also promote comfort.

Shoulder pain after stroke is common, affecting from 16% to 72% of patients (Walsh, 2001). Both flaccidity and spasticity in the paretic arm can cause subluxation (partial separation), instability of the shoulder joint, pain, and increased risk of subacromial bursitis. Eventually, if preventive techniques such as external support for the affected limb when seated, proper positioning when in bed, and passive and active range-of-motion exercises are not instituted, contractures occur. Establishing the underlying cause of the shoulder pain is necessary to choosing the appropriate intervention. Reinforcing to staff, patients, and families that long-term compliance with these interventions will help to prevent or reduce shoulder deformities, pain, and contractures is important. The concerns regarding medications to treat spasticity have already been mentioned. To date the effect of electrical stimulation on shoulder pain is inconclusive (Price & Pandyan, 2001), but it may offer relief for some patients. Intra-articular steroid injections can be helpful, especially with bursitis. Shoulder pain resulting from spasticity has also responded to intramuscular botulinum toxin injections.

Shoulder-hand syndrome, or reflex sympathetic dystrophy, is due to autonomic dysfunction in the affected upper extremity. Paresis in the shoulder and arm can lead to joint instability and trauma that may trigger overstimulation of the sympathetic nervous system. It develops in stages, and, typically, there is vasoconstriction in the affected arm with complaints of burning pain. If it progresses beyond 3 months, the limb may develop trophic changes with decreased hair, thin shiny skin, increased or decreased sweating, edema, and bone demineralization. Movement and touch usually cause pain, and patients tend to guard the limb, leading to further dysfunction. After 9 months, atrophy and contractures may also occur. Diagnosis is supported by a triple-phase bone scan revealing osteopenia or osteoporosis. Treatment options available include a short course of rapidly tapered oral steroids, oral analgesics, tricyclic antidepressants, and gabapentin (Neurontin) (DuPen & McCaffery, 1999). A stellate ganglion block at C6 may also be effective in relieving symptoms (Walsh, Dumitru, Schoenfeld, & Ramamurthy, 1998). Nonpharmacologic treatments such as ice, heat, transcutaneous electrical nerve stimulation, and ultrasound may also relieve pain in some patients. Range-of-motion exercises, proper positioning, and techniques to manage edema should be initiated immediately poststroke in the affected limb.

Central poststroke pain (CPSP) is described as a neuropathic pain in all or the part of the body affected by the stroke that may develop immediately or up to 2 years after the initial stroke (Bowsher, 1999). It is associated with sensory deficits and tactile allodynia (pain elicited by a normally nonpainful stimulus). This often prompts patients to lie perfectly still in order to avoid discomfort. One survey of 80-year-old stroke survivors revealed 11% with symptoms related to CPSP (Bowsher, 1999). Treatment options used for neuropathic pain can include anticonvulsants (e.g., gabapentin) and tricyclic antidepressants (e.g., amitriptyline and nortriptyline). The risk versus the benefit of a trial of a tricyclic antidepressant in an older adult must be carefully considered given the anticholinergic side effect profile.

Opiates play a relatively small role in the management of neuropathic pain. Vestergaard, Anderson, Gottrup, Kristensen, and Jensen (2002) tested the anticonvulsant lamotrigine on patients with CPSP (median age 59 years). Pain scores were reduced by 30%, and, at 200 mg/day, the drug was well tolerated. Further study with older age groups and different doses may prove lamotrigine to be a promising new treatment alternative. Adapting relaxation techniques to assist patients in coping with this pain syndrome can be helpful as well.

Palliative Care Nursing for Stroke Patients

In order to improve both immediate and sustained quality of life of elders who have had a stroke, a holistic and interdisciplinary response is important throughout the disease process. Opening the lines of communication with the patient and family is critical to establishing trust, relaying clinical information, and promoting shared decision making. Active listening to older adults and their families promotes the opportunity to understand what brings meaning and quality to the life of each patient. This will help to set appropriate and mutual treatment goals throughout the acute and rehabilitative phases and at the end of life.

The initial assessment of the elder's clinical condition and prognostic indicators may indicate a high risk of morbidity and mortality. When the prognosis is poor—for example, as a result of a massive stroke from which the patient is not likely to recover—decisions need to be made regarding treatment goals. The patient's quality of life prior to the stroke and any advance directives should be considered during these discussions. Immediate issues could include whether or not to intubate the elder if he or she develops respiratory failure or to initiate or continue resuscitation efforts in those patients profoundly compromised by the stroke. These are very common issues in palliative care and require staff comfortable in discussing them and knowledgeable about the potential risks and benefits. Reassuring family members that palliative care measures are in place throughout the acute phase of the stroke, no matter the outcome, may offer comfort.

Families should understand that the risk of mortality remains relatively high for up to 30 days poststroke. Once the patient is stabilized, interventions to maximize function, reduce complications, and prevent disability become priorities. Dysphagia increases the risk of aspiration pneumonia, and virtually all stroke patients should be evaluated by a speech therapist to determine if feeding by mouth is safe, and if aspiration pre-

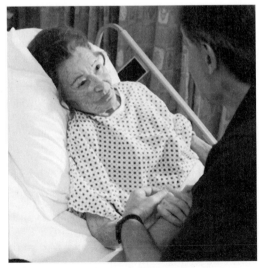

Addressing the needs of older patients through the illness trajectory. (Courtesy Mathy Mezey.)

cautions are needed. Patients with dysphagia should be reevaluated periodically to see if their swallow improves and whether or not inserting a percutaneous endoscopic gastrostomy tube to maintain nutrition will need to be addressed. (Issues regarding enteral nutrition are reviewed in Chapter 23.) Based on the patient's prognosis and potential for recovery, enteral feedings may be seen as a temporary intervention to allow time to assess outcomes or as a permanent intervention to prolong life.

For the elder who has had a stroke, the recovery period can be prolonged, with continued functional gains up to 6 months or longer. Elders who have had a stroke may live for years with their deficits; however, stroke rehabilitation tends to focus on the immediate poststroke period. This has particular relevance to the philosophy of palliative care and its focus on quality of life for patients living with chronic, incurable illnesses. Stroke recovery may continue for months at home, virtually outside of the health care system. Coping with stroke-related deficits over the long term requires active efforts by patients and caregivers to maintain function and adapt to perceived losses.

Stroke-related pain syndromes and depression are two symptoms that may not be exhibited for months to years poststroke. Without medical management that is continuous and comprehensive and incorporates palliative care measures, untreated symptoms may lead to a spiral of decline. As time passes, and if functional recovery diminishes, accepting the reality of stroke deficits may be difficult, especially if expectations were unrealistic or never addressed. At any point during the recovery process, acknowledging and reinforcing the continued strengths and talents of each stroke patient can help maintain and validate his or her sense of self. Allowing elders who were at least 6 months poststroke to "tell their story" was described as a positive experience in a study by Secrest and Thomas (1999). To bear witness to any such story should be seen as a privilege, an opportunity to understand this individual better, and the chance to show respect for his or her humanity.

Being aware of common symptoms and complications associated with a stroke, nurses are more prepared to recognize, intervene, and com-

EVIDENCE-BASED PRACTICE

Reference: Secrest, J., & Thomas, S. (1999). Continuity and discontinuity: The quality of life following stroke. *Rehabilitation Nursing, 24*(6), 240-246.

Research Problem: How do stroke survivors describe their quality of life following rehabilitation?

Design: A phenomenological study to analyze the transcripts of interviews with stroke patients, during which they are asked about their daily experiences postrehabilitation.

Sample and Setting: 14 participants (7 men and 7 women), with a median age of 67, were recruited from three inpatient rehabilitation units. All were living at home and were at least 6 months poststroke. Interviews occurred in their homes or at the researchers' offices.

Methods: Interviews lasting $1\frac{1}{2}$ to 2 hours were transcribed verbatim and analyzed by a research group from the disciplines of nursing, psychology, philosophy, and education to recognize and describe patterns, themes, and interrelationships among these experiences.

Results: The quality of life of stroke survivors was found to be grounded in the experiences of loss and the effort needed to participate in everyday life. Within this structure, three more themes emerged: independence-ability/dependence-disability, being in control/out of control, and connection/disconnection with others. The opportunity to tell their stories was described positively by the participants.

Implications for Nursing Practice: Nursing assessments that include the opportunity for patients to share the meaning of their stroke experience and the impact it has had on their quality of life should help to establish individualized treatment goals and interventions that reflect the values of each patient. The act of empathic listening to the ongoing experiences of stroke survivors may be an important part of their rehabilitation process.

Conclusion: Offering stroke patients the chance to "tell their story" may reveal not only what we want to know, but what they may need to tell us. The issues of loss and effort impact the poststroke experience.

municate them to the appropriate disciplines. Early identification of dysphagia, depression, and pain syndromes can improve functional outcomes and limit complications. Patients who are receiving rehabilitative services, but are unable to tolerate them because of depression, fatigue, or pain, may have them discontinued prematurely. Nursing input regarding patient comfort levels, mood, and behavior early in the disease process will help to maximize each patient's potential for recovery.

Nursing interventions to reduce the risks of immobility may be ongoing for some patients, and much creativity and interdisciplinary effort may be required to maintain function and prevent further disability. With or without ongoing rehabilitative services, nurses should monitor the plan of care for adequacy in promoting and maintaining the highest level of independence. Dependency in ADLs may require patient education and support in using adaptive equipment and adjusting to losses in autonomy. Incontinence, dysphagia, aphasia, cognitive impairment, and hemiplegia are consequences requiring lifelong changes and can result in institutional placement, financial burdens, and family stresses.

The disease trajectory and cause of death are quite variable among stroke survivors and vary over time for each individual survivor. The most common cause of death within the first week following a stroke is from the direct insult to the brain. These elders tend to present with a deteriorating level of consciousness and die in the acute care setting. During the following weeks to months, it is the secondary complications such as blood clots and infection that contribute to poststroke mortality rates; this reinforces the importance of preventive nursing interventions. Some patients may appear to be improving after their stroke and then suddenly die from complications. Long-term stroke survivors may die from recurrent stroke, complications of immobility, their comorbidities, or other acute conditions.

Family/Caregiver Issues

The extent of family support clearly impacts the ability of elders to return to and remain in the community after their strokes. In a study by Ween et al. (1996), patients' discharge to home was also strongly affected by their age. The rate of return home after a stroke was 77% for patients ages 55 to 75, 68% for those ages 75 to 85, and 57% for those over age 85. The absence of a committed caregiver decreased the likelihood of discharge to home; the oldest stroke patients are more likely to be widowed or have spouses too frail to be active caregivers, or their children may themselves be of advanced age. Families of patients who are admitted to a nursing home may have issues related to loss, guilt, and finances. There may be continued uncertainty as to how well the elder is going to tolerate the rehabilitative process. If he or she improves enough to return to the community, what future role will the family have? The nursing assessment of the strengths and weaknesses of the patient-family unit can facilitate timely and appropriate referrals for medical and community resources.

For stroke patients living in the community, their level of dependency may or may not require a caregiver. The care of stroke patients with moderate to severe disabilities may entail physical exertion and 24-hour responsibility. Long-term caregiving may cause physical, emotional, spiritual, and financial strain; this is particularly true for the older adult caregiver. The caregiver may neglect his or her own personal needs and become isolated as a result of his or her overwhelming responsibilities. Nurses are likely to be the primary source of elder and caregiver education on providing personal care, symptom monitoring, and medication management. Monitoring the health and well-being of the caregivers should be incorporated into the plan of care for stroke patients in the acute care setting, the community, and long-term care facilities. Referral to support groups, educational seminars, or Internet resources may help stroke survivors and their caregivers to learn new coping strategies and to feel less isolated.

Research Implications Related to Stroke

More clinical research is needed that studies the oldest stroke patients and how they differ from younger stroke patients. Asplund, Carlberg, and Sundstrom (1992) compared patients over 85 years of age with patients younger than 85 years poststroke and found differences in risk factor profiles, severity of neurologic deficits on admission, and fatality rates during the first month. They concluded that decision making can be more complicated for very old stroke patients and that a better understanding is needed regarding their unique clinical characteristics and prognostic indicators. These should help guide clinicians, elders, and families as they determine goals of treatment and the appropriate role of palliative care measures. More studies exploring the impact that specific comorbidities have on stroke recovery could lead to novel interventions and improved outcomes. Fatigue and depression are both common symptoms in the poststroke patient, but more data are needed on their relationship to stroke location, specific stroke deficits, and factors associated with onset. Identifying those patients who are most susceptible and intervening earlier could help to prevent or reduce the severity of these symptoms and their negative impact on function.

COMA AND BRAIN DEATH
Coma

Another neurologic condition that may occur in the older adult is coma. Comatose patients exhibit a sleeplike state from which they cannot be aroused. Those in the deepest coma are not conscious of self or their environment; they show no sleep-wake cycles or auditory or visual responses and have reflex and postural responses only to external stimuli (Giacino et al., 2002). To date, valid estimates of the incidence and prevalence of severe disorders of consciousness are not available (Giacino et al., 2002). The differential diagnosis for coma includes a structural lesion (stroke, head trauma, or tumor), meningeal irritation (infection or bleeding), metabolic encephalopathy (organ failure or drugs), and seizure (Simon, 2000). Getting a history from witnesses or significant others is helpful in making a differential diagnosis. If the coma was preceded by a period of confusion or delirium, this is more consistent with infectious or metabolic etiologies, whereas sudden loss of consciousness suggests an intracranial bleed or infarct.

The initial priority in the emergency management of comatose patients is to evaluate and maintain respiratory and circulatory function and then to establish the underlying disease process. Timely diagnosis will improve the likelihood of reversing the coma, when this is possible, and reducing mortality. The Glasgow Coma Scale (Box 12-2) is often used to assess and score the level of consciousness. Eye opening, verbal response, and motor response to stimuli are evaluated. The scores range from 3 to 15, and patients with scores between 3 and 8 are said to be in a coma.

Determining prognosis is dependent upon the underlying cause of the coma. Poor prognostic signs are when the coma follows cardiac arrest or if the patient has not regained pupillary function or purposeful movement after 72 hours. Coma resulting from traumatic head injury has a worse prognosis in older patients, with patients over 60 years old being three times more likely to die than patients less than 60 years old (Simon, 2000). Most comatose stroke patients do not survive. Medical comorbidities, advanced age, and complications all negatively affect survival. Box 12-1 presents the National Hospice Organization's criteria for determining prognosis in coma patients.

Overall, metabolic causes of coma imply a more favorable outcome (Strub, 1996). The length of time that an individual remains in a comatose state also reflects the severity of the brain injury. The majority of coma patients will die in the acute care setting, except for those whose coma is persistent; they are transferred to a long-term care facility for supportive nursing care. As with stroke, they may die from the initial damage to the brain that precipitated the coma or from subsequent complications or comorbidities.

Brain Death

Improved medical technology capable of sustaining life and current organ transplantation protocols have created circumstances in which the older adult may have cardiopulmonary functions but is brain dead. In response to the need to define and determine brain death, the President's Commission (1981) developed the Uniform Determination of Death Act, which allowed brain death to be a legal definition of death. Declaring a person dead requires that either his or her heart function has ceased or his or her

---

Box 12-2 Glasgow Coma Scale*

EYE OPENING (E)	BEST MOTOR RESPONSE (M)	BEST VERBAL RESPONSE (V)
Spontaneous: 4	To verbal command: obeys: 6	Oriented and converses: 5
To speech: 3	To painful stimulus: localizes pain: 5	Disoriented and converses: 4
To pain: 2	flexion—withdrawal: 4	Inappropriate words: 3
No response: 1	flexion—abnormal: 3	Incomprehensible sounds: 2
	extension: 2	No response: 1
	no response: 1	

*Coma is defined as (1) not opening eyes, (2) not obeying commands, and (3) not uttering understandable words. The Glasgow Coma Scale score is the sum of the best scores (E+M+V), ranging from 3 (no response) to 15 (normal response). Implications of specific scores are as follows: ≤8: 90% are in coma; ≥9: not in coma; 8: severe injury; ≤8 at 6 hours: 50% die; 9-11: moderate severity of injury; ≥12: minor injury.
Adapted from Teasdale, G., & Jennet, B. (1974). Assessment of coma and impaired consciousness: a practical scale. *Lancet, 2,* 81-84.

brain no longer functions because of irreversible damage. There is continued controversy and ongoing research to improve accuracy in determining irreversible brain death, and a variety of confirming tests have been suggested. These include electroencephalography, cerebral angiography, magnetic resonance imaging, and testing of cerebrospinal fluid. Clinical findings, however, continue to be the gold standard for the diagnosis of brain death. Brain dead patients exhibit the following findings on physical examination (Wijdicks, 1995):

1. Unresponsive coma with no response to noxious stimuli (pressure to supraorbital ridge or nail beds)
2. Absence of brainstem reflexes (e.g., pupillary, oculocephalic, vestibulo-ocular, corneal, and pharyngeal)
3. Apnea, for which there are specific testing guidelines

Direct damage to the brainstem (from head trauma, intracranial hemorrhage, infarcts, or mass lesions) or diffuse damage to neuronal metabolism (from drugs, renal failure, or hypoglycemia) are the mechanisms by which irreversible brain death may occur. Clinical diagnosis of brain death in a comatose patient should proceed in the following stepwise manner (Wijdicks, 2001):

1. Exclude possible confounding factors (hypothermia, drugs, and metabolic disturbances)
2. Establish a cause (usually a computed tomography scan or lumbar puncture will provide this information)
3. Ascertain that the condition is irreversible
4. Accurately test brainstem reflexes at all levels

There should be an interval of at least 6 hours of observation with repeat testing before diagnosing brain death, although no definitive time frame is documented in the literature (Sullivan, Seem, & Chabalewski, 1999). When an elder is determined to be brain dead, it is futile to continue life-sustaining medical treatment. Asystole from systemic injury usually occurs within 4 days even with continued life support (Wijdicks, 2002).

More than likely, this scenario will unfold in the intensive care unit or emergency room. Families will need significant education and support throughout the diagnostic evaluation and the process of treatment withdrawal. If brain death has occurred as the result of a long illness with multiple organ failure, as opposed to a sudden unpredictable trauma, they may have had time to absorb information and develop realistic expectations about their loved one's survival. It is important to have staff available who are comfortable discussing the implications of brain death, the need for withdrawal of treatment, and how to incorporate any previous wishes of the patient and requests by the family.

Truog et al. (2001) recommended that families be given a very straightforward but compassionate explanation that the patient died when his or her brain died, and that treatment is being withdrawn from someone who is already dead. This may relieve feelings of guilt that withdrawal of treatment contributed to the patient's death. Because of the extent of the brainstem injury, brain dead patients do not feel pain. Reassurance that they are not suffering and that measures to ensure patient dignity are in place is important, as is incorporating any cultural or spiritual rituals. Nurses can help to establish an environment in which the family feels supported and valued.

Before withdrawing life support, families should be offered adequate time to process and cope with the information they have been given and to spend time with the patient if requested. Discussion of any possible organ donation should be separate from the notification of brain death. The United Network for Organ Sharing requires that, in cases of potential organ donation, all patients determined to be brain dead be referred to the local organ procurement organization (OPO) before pronouncement to determine suitability for donation (McCoy & Argue, 1999). Nurses in the critical care or palliative care setting must work collaboratively with the OPO and the medical team to support families as they make these difficult decisions.

Palliative Care Nursing for Comatose and Brain Dead Patients

Assessing for signs and symptoms of discomfort in patients who are in a coma is difficult because of the lack of response to stimuli. Depending upon the depth of the coma, it is possible that some comatose patients may feel painful stimulation but be unable to respond in any meaningful way.

Physiologic responses such as changes in blood pressure, heart rate or respiratory rate and rhythm, diaphoresis, and decreased oxygen saturation levels may be possible cues of pain sensation. Monitoring of facial electromyography and electroencephalographic tracings have both been used, but they remain unvalidated measures. Bispectral analysis using encephalographic signals to assess level of consciousness and comfort during withdrawal of life support has been attempted (Truog et al., 2001). This technology may assess level of arousal, but is not able to quantify pain. The use of opiates to relieve potential pain in unresponsive patients with diagnoses consistent with pain or undergoing painful procedures should be initiated.

Although brain dead patients, by definition, do not feel pain, they should be treated with the intent to maximize their physical integrity and minimize discomfort. Families may be comforted by touching and speaking to them and should be offered privacy to do so. Attention should be focused on the physical and emotional needs of the family members throughout these events.

Withdrawal of Life Support

By the time it is determined that any meaningful recovery is unlikely, health care providers may have had the opportunity to process the implications. Families, however, may require additional time and counseling to reconcile with the poor prognosis and the option of treatment withdrawal. It is always a difficult and emotionally charged issue to begin discussing the withdrawal of life support from a patient. Having consistent staff members communicating with families and providing ongoing opportunities to discuss diagnosis, prognosis, and quality-of-life issues should help to prepare them for potential outcomes.

Information regarding the actual process for withdrawal of treatment can be reviewed to the extent that the family requests, and input from all appropriate disciplines should be encouraged. The actual process of withdrawal needs to incorporate any preferences for timing, those who will be present, and religious and cultural rituals. This promotes the family's ability to infuse personal meaning into the experience. Ideally, this should occur in a calm environment with respect for privacy.

Protocols vary between institutions, and more evidence-based data are needed to determine the optimum management of patients during the withdrawal of life support. Prior to discontinuing mechanical ventilation, all other treatments that do not contribute to the patient's level of comfort and all unnecessary electronic monitoring should be discontinued. An intravenous line should be maintained in order to administer medications. Rubenfeld and Crawford (2001) recommended that, given the uncertainty regarding the potential for pain and suffering in comatose patients, clinicians administer an appropriate level of sedation. However, because of the extent of their neurologic injuries, sedation is not required in brain dead patients. Opioids and benzodiazepines are the primary drugs used for sedation and analgesia in comatose patients before and during the withdrawal of life support (von Gunten & Weissman, 2001), and these should be titrated up to effect or comfort.

After removing all other life support equipment, ventilator withdrawal in comatose or brain dead patients can be done by simply removing the endotracheal tube (extubation), or by gradually reducing the ventilator settings (terminal weaning). Terminal weaning may take several minutes or longer depending on the pace of the process that causes hypoxia and hypercarbia. For unconscious patients unlikely to experience discomfort, Truog et al. (2001) suggested rapidly withdrawing ventilator support by removing the artificial airway or disconnecting the ventilator rather than using the process of terminal weaning. For any distress during or after extubation, Pendergast (2002) recommended midazolam (2 to 5 mg intravenously [IV] every 7 to 10 minutes) or diazepam (5 to 10 mg IV every 3 to 5 minutes) and/or morphine (5 to 10 mg IV every 10 minutes) or fentanyl (100 to 250 µg IV every 3 to 5 minutes).

Following the withdrawal of supportive measures, the family may need time to share their feelings and have their decisions reaffirmed. Information on grief counseling should be offered to all who were involved in the elder's care. Staff members should also have opportunities to debrief after withdrawing a patient from life support. Discussing reactions with co-workers can be therapeutic and lead to quality improvement initiatives.

Research Implications Regarding Care of Comatose and Brain Dead Elders

Future research is needed to develop technology that could better assess pain perception in unconscious patients. This same technology might be applied to patients with impairments in cognition or communication as well. Currently, protocols for withdrawal of life support vary within and among institutions. Analysis of staff competencies, perceived patient comfort, and family acceptance of different protocols would support evidence-based clinical guidelines for the care of comatose and brain dead patients. Putting the available resources of the health care system to the most appropriate use takes on added meaning with patients who require advanced technology for life support.

Case Study Conclusion

Following Mrs. C.'s stroke, the interdisciplinary team had many issues to address. Because of her left-sided neglect, her room was changed to encourage people to approach her from the left and increase her awareness of the left side of her environment. Despite frequent reminders with signs, verbal reinforcement, and alarms, Mrs. C. tended to get up unassisted and experienced several falls. A fall mat was also placed next to her bed. Given her issues related to grieving, her mood, and her reduced appetite, a psychiatrist was consulted and an antidepressant was started. Arrangements were made for her local chaplain to visit for spiritual support. Occupational therapy and activities staff obtained appropriate art supplies, and her daughter hung her favorite painting on the wall across from her bed.

Mrs. C.'s left shoulder developed increased tone and the potential for contractures. Pillows were positioned for support in the bed, and her wheelchair was fitted with an adaptive arm trough. Range-of-motion exercises by physical therapy and nursing staff continued twice daily. So far, Mrs. C. has not developed any left shoulder pain, but her condition is an ongoing concern requiring vigilance to protect and support the left upper extremity. An EZ boot was used on her left leg to relieve pressure on the heel, and the blister resolved without complication. For the arthritic pain in her knees, she did not experience relief from acetaminophen (Tylenol) four times a day,

but reported improvement on a cyclooxygenase-2 inhibitor. Hydrocodone (Vicodin), 2 tablets every 6 hours, as needed, relieved the moderate pain she experienced with therapy and at the end of the day. For the first few weeks she was encouraged to premedicate prior to therapy sessions. An aggressive bladder training program was initiated. The nutritionist worked on food preferences and supplements to reverse some earlier weight loss.

After 8 weeks at the nursing home, and 10 weeks following her stroke, Mrs. C. was discharged from rehabilitative services because her functional gains had reached a plateau. At this point, she transferred independently but required assistance and a rolling walker with left arm support for ambulation. She had been fitted for an ankle-foot orthosis and wore a soft splint on her left arm at night to reduce contractures. Mrs. C. continued on a prompted toileting schedule, which maintained her continence. Her weight stabilized and she was beginning to paint.

Mrs. C.'s frequent falls resulted in the assisted living facility determining that Mrs. C. was not safe to return to her apartment. Her goal of urinary continence was achieved; however, the loss of her apartment, cat, and supportive neighbors was devastating. She was beginning to consider moving to a nursing home closer to her family because she knew it was hard for them to visit and that she could visit her cat at her daughter's home. The social worker was helping her to investigate appropriate facilities. Mrs. C. did request a final visit to her apartment and to participate in any decisions regarding her belongings.

CONCLUSION

Older adult patients and their families who are dealing with the consequences of stroke, coma, or a diagnosis of brain death face enormous challenges. These challenges may occur over a period of hours in the acute care setting, with immediate decisions to be made regarding prognosis and life support, or they may be experienced for years following a stroke and require lifelong coping strategies. The need for palliative care is evident throughout the health care continuum, beginning in the emergency room and following elders to their homes, the long-term care facility, or a hospice unit. From a palliative care perspective, nurses in all these settings need to combine knowledge of the disease, its trajectory, and related symptoms with appreciation of the values and goals of the elder patient and his or her family. Understanding the potential complications and symptoms following a stroke can lead to better preventive care, a reduction in post-stroke disabilities, and improved quality of life in the acute rehabilitation setting and beyond. For the older adult, it is particularly important to factor in the impact that comorbidities and cognitive/functional status can have on post-stroke survival and recovery and mobilize the appropriate resources and expertise of the palliative care interdisciplinary team. For families whose loved one is in a coma or determined to be brain dead, palliative care nursing can provide information and support along the illness trajectory and into the bereavement period. Such support is central in assisting families to cope effectively with illness and to find strength in facing their loss.

RESOURCES
Stroke

- National Stroke Association (*www.stroke.org*): National Stroke Association website: Resource center for patients and health care professionals on stroke prevention, treatment, and recovery.
- American Stroke Association (*www.strokeassociation.org*): American Stroke Association website: A division of the American Heart Association offering information on research, education, fundraising, and advocacy for consumers and health care providers.
- Internet Stroke Center (*www.strokecenter.org*): educational resources provided by the Stroke Center at Washington University School of Medicine, St. Louis
- The Stroke Information Directory (*www.stroke-info.com*): website maintained by family members of stroke survivors to provide consumers, clinicians, and researchers with a source for online stroke resources
- National Institute of Neurological Disorders and Stroke (*www.ninds.nih.gov/health_and_medical/disorders/stroke.htm*): NINDS Stroke Information page

- StrokeHelp.com (*www.strokehelp.com*): rehabilitation information for clinicians, families, and stroke survivors
- "Depression and Stroke" (*www.nimh.nih.gov/publicat/stroke.cfm*): National Institute of Mental Health fact sheet on poststroke depression
- "Stroke and Cerebrovascular Diseases: A Guide for Patients and their Families" (*www.stanford.edu/group/neurology/stroke/strokeinfo.html*): Stanford Stroke Center's guide for stroke patients and families

Brain Death and Coma
- International Network for the Definition of Death (*www.changesurfer.com/BD/Brain.html#1*): brain injury and brain death resources listing
- University of Buffalo Center for Clinical Ethics and Humanities in Health Care (*www.buffalo.edu/faculty/research/bioethics/man-bdg.html*): Determination of Death Consensus Conference: Voluntary consensus guidelines for determination of death. (Ethics Committee Core Curriculum document)
- Harley, D. H., & Pallis, C. (1999). *ABC of brain stem death*. London: BMJ Books.
- Wijdicks, E. (Ed.). (2001). *Brain death*. Philadelphia: Lippincott Williams & Wilkins.

Organ Transplantation
- United Network for Organ Sharing (UNOS) (*www.unos.org*): United Network for Organ Sharing website: Provides access to data and resources on organ transplantation to recipients, donor families, and health care professionals.

REFERENCES

Adams, H., & Biller, J. (1996). Ischemic cerebrovascular disease. In W. Bradley, R. Daroff, G. Fenichel, & C. Marsden (Eds.), *Neurology in clinical practice: The neurological disorders* (pp. 993-1031). Boston: Butterworth-Heinemann.

American Heart Association. (2002). *Heart and stroke statistical update*. Dallas, TX: Author.

Aminoff, M. (2001). Nervous system. In L. Tierney, S. McPhee, & M. Papadakis (Eds.), *Current medical diagnosis and treatment* (40th ed., pp. 983-990). New York: Lange Medical Books/McGraw-Hill.

American Psychiatric Association. (1987). *Diagnostic and statistical manual of mental disorders* (*third edition–revised*). Washington, DC: Author.

Asplund, K., Carlberg, B., & Sundstrom, G. (1992). Stroke in the elderly: Observations in a population-based sample of hospitalized patients. *Cerebrovascular Disease, 2,* 152-157.

Bowsher, D. (1999). Central post-stroke ('thalamic syndrome') and other central pains. *American Journal of Hospice and Palliative Care, 16,* 593-597.

Brandstater, M. (1998). Stroke rehabilitation. In J. DeLisa & B. Gans (Eds.), *Rehabilitation medicine principles and practice* (pp. 1165-1189). Philadelphia: Lippincott–Raven.

Dombovy, M. (1991). Stroke: Clinical course and neurophysiologic mechanisms of recovery. *Physical and Rehabilitation Medicine, 2,* 171-188.

DuPen, A., & McCaffery, M. (1999). Reflex sympathetic dystrophy/causalgia: In M. McCaffery & C. Pasero (Eds.), *Pain clinical manual* (2nd ed., pp. 581-584). St. Louis: Mosby.

Finucane, T., Christmas, C., & Travis, K. (1999). Tube feeding in patients with advanced dementia: A review of the literature. *Journal of the American Medical Association, 282,* 1365-1370.

Gelber, D. (2002). Management of stroke-related spasticity in the long-term care setting. *CNS/LTC, 1*(1), 33-37.

Giacino, J. T., Ashwal, S., Childs, N., Cranford, R., Jennett, B., Katz, D. I., et al. (2002). The minimally conscious state: Definition and diagnostic criteria. *Neurology, 58,* 349-353.

Gresham, G. (1992). Rehabilitation of the stroke survivor. In H. Barnett, J. Mohr, B. Stein, & F. Yatsu (Eds.), *Stroke: Pathophysiology, diagnosis, and management* (pp. 1189-1201). New York: Churchill Livingstone.

Gresham, G., Phillips, T., Wolf, P., McNamara, P., Kannel, W., & Dawber, T. (1979). Epidemiological profile of long-term stroke disability: The Framingham study. *Archives of Physical Medicine and Rehabilitation, 60,* 487-491.

Gustafson, Y., Nilsson, I., Mattsson, M., Astrom, M., & Bucht, G. (1995). Epidemiology and treatment of post-stroke depression. *Drugs & Aging, 7,* 298-309.

Ingles, J., Eskes, G., & Phillips, S. (1999). Fatigue after stroke. *Archives of Physical Medicine and Rehabilitation, 80,* 173-178.

Jorgensen, L., Engstad, T., & Jacobsen, B. (2002). Higher incidence of falls in long-term stroke survivors than in population controls: Depressive symptoms predict falls after stroke. *Stroke, 33,* 542-547.

Kauhanen, M., Korpelainen, J., Hiltunen, P., Brusin, E., Mononen, H., Maatta, R., et al. (1999). Post-stroke depression correlates with cognitive impairment and neurological deficits. *Stroke, 30,* 1875-1880.

Kwakkel, G., Wagenaar, R., Kollen, B., & Lankhorst, G. (1996). Predicting disability in stroke—a critical review of the literature. *Age and Ageing, 25,* 479-489.

Langhorne, P., Stott, D., Robertson, L., MacDonald, J., Jones, L., McAlpine, C., et al. (2000). Medical complications after stroke. *Stroke, 31,* 1223-1229.

Longstreth, W., Bernick, C., Fitzpatrick, A., Cushman, M., Knepper, L., Lima, J., et al. (2001). Frequency and predictors of stroke death in 5,888 participants in the Cardiovascular Health Study. *Neurology, 56,* 368-375.

McCoy, J., & Argue, P. (1999). The role of critical care nurses in organ donation: A case study. *Critical Care Nurse, 19*(2), 48-52.

National Hospice Organization. (1996). *Medical guidelines for determining prognosis in selected non-cancer diseases* (2nd ed.). Arlington, VA: Author.

Pendergast, T. (2002). Palliative care in the intensive care unit setting. In A. Berger, R. Portenoy, & D. Weissman, (Eds.), *Principles and practice of palliative care and supportive oncology* (2nd ed., pp. 1086-1104). Philadelphia: Lippincott Williams & Wilkins.

President's Commission for the Study of Ethical Problems in Medicine and Biomedical and Behavioral Research. (1981). *Defining death: A report on the medical, legal, and ethical issues in the determination of death.* Washington, DC: Author.

Price, C., & Pandyan, A. (2001). Electrical stimulation for preventing and treating post-stroke shoulder pain: A systematic Cochrane review. *Clinical Rehabilitation, 15,* 5-19.

Ramasubbu, R., Robinson, R., Flint, A., Kosier, T., & Price, T. (1998). Functional impairment associated with acute poststroke depression: The Stroke Data Bank Study. *Journal of Neuropsychiatry and Clinical Neurosciences, 10,* 26-33.

Ramnemark, A., Nilsson, M., Borssen, B., & Gustafson, Y. (2000). Stroke, a major and increasing risk factor for femoral neck fracture. *Stoke, 31,* 1572-1577.

Rubenfeld, G., & Crawford, S. (2001). Principles and practices of withdrawing life-sustaining treatment in the ICU. In J. Curtis & G. Rubenfeld (Eds.), *Managing death in the intensive care unit* (pp. 127-147). New York: Oxford University Press.

Secrest, J., & Thomas, S.(1999). Continuity and discontinuity: The quality of life following stroke. *Rehabilitation Nursing, 24*(6), 240-246.

Sharma, J., Fletcher, S., & Vassallo, M. (1999). Strokes in the elderly—higher acute and 3-month mortality—an explanation. *Cerebrovascular Diseases, 9,* 2-9.

Simon, R. (2000). Coma and disorders of arousal. In L. Goldman (Ed.), *Cecil textbook of medicine* (21st ed., pp. 2023-2026). Philadelphia: Saunders.

Staub, F., Annoni, J., & Bogousslavsky, J. (2000). Fatigue after stroke: A pilot study. *Cerebrovascular Diseases, 10*(Suppl. 2), 62.

Staub, F., & Bogousslavsky, J. (2001). Fatigue after stroke: A major but neglected issue. *Cerebrovascular Diseases, 12,* 75-81.

Strub, R. (1996). Stupor and coma. In L. Weisberg, C. Garcia, & R. Strub (Eds.), *Essentials of clinical neurology* (3rd ed., pp. 226-247). St. Louis: Mosby.

Sullivan, J., Seem, D., & Chabalewski, F. (1999). Determining brain death. *Critical Care Nurse, 19*(2), 37-46.

Truog, R., Cist, A., Brackett, S., Burns, J., Curley, M., Danis, M., et al (2001). Recommendations for end-of-life care in the intensive care unit: The Ethics Committee of the Society of Critical Care Medicine. *Critical Care Medicine, 29,* 2332-2348.

U.S. Bureau of the Census. (1993). *Statistical abstract of the United States.* Washington, DC: Author.

Vestergaard, K., Andersen, G., Gottrup, H., Kristensen, B., & Jensen, T. (2002). Lamotrigine for central poststroke pain. *Neurology, 56,* 184-190.

Volpe, B. T. (2001). Palliative treatment for stroke. *Neurologic Clinics, 19,* 903-920.

von Gunten, C., & Weissman, D. (2001). *Fast Facts and Concepts #34: Symptom control for ventilator withdrawal in the dying patient.* Retrieved from the End-of-Life/Palliative Education Resource Center Web site: *www.eperc.mcw.edu*

Walsh, K. (2001). Management of shoulder pain in patients with stroke. *Postgraduate Medical Journal, 77,* 645-649.

Walsh, N., Dumitru, D., Schoenfeld, L., & Ramamurthy, S. (1998). Treatment of the patient with chronic pain. In J. DeLisa & B. Gans (Eds.), *Rehabilitation medicine principles and practice* (pp. 1385-1421). Philadelphia: Lippincott-Raven.

Ween, J., Alexander, M., D'Esposito, M., & Roberts, M. (1996). Factors predictive of stroke outcome in a rehabilitation setting. *Neurology, 47,* 388-392.

Weisberg, L. (1996). Cerebrovascular disease. In L. Weisberg, C. Garcia, & R. Strub (Eds.), *Essentials of clinical neurology* (3rd ed., pp. 251-305). St. Louis: Mosby.

Wijdicks, E. (1995). Determining brain death in adults. *Neurology, 45,* 1003-1011.

Wijdicks, E. (2001). Clinical diagnosis and confirmatory testing of brain death in adults. In E. Wijdicks (Ed.), *Brain death* (pp. 61-90). Philadelphia: Lippincott Williams & Wilkins.

Wijdicks, E. (2002). Brain death worldwide: Accepted fact but no global consensus in diagnostic criteria. *Neurology, 58,* 20-25.

Wolf, P., Cobb, J., & D'Agostino, R. (1992). Epidemiology of stroke. In H. Barnett, J. Mohr, B. Stein, & F. Yatsu (Eds.), *Stroke: Pathophysiology, diagnosis and management* (pp. 3-27). New York: Churchill Livingstone.

Yatsu, F., DeGraba, T., & Hanson, S. (1992). Therapy of secondary medical complications of strokes. In H. Barnett, J. Mohr, B. Stein, & F. Yatsu (Eds.), *Stroke: Pathophysiology, diagnosis and management* (pp. 995-1004). New York: Churchill Livingstone.

13

DEMENTIA AND NEURODEGENERATIVE ILLNESSES

Christine R. Kovach

Case Study

Mrs. C., 84, is in the late stages of Alzheimer's disease. Her dementia has severely impaired her short- and long-term memory as well as her functional ability. She lives in a nursing home and spends most of her day in her bed repetitively grunting and tapping the side of the bed rails. She verbalizes few intelligible words, continually picks at her clothes, grimaces, and rocks her body. When approached, she yells out fearfully; when bathed, she screams and exhibits aggressive behavior. Attempts to bring her to the dining room or to therapeutic activities are met with resistance and screaming. Staff have responded by leaving her alone in the room, providing stimulation by keeping the television on in her room and hanging a mobile of flowers in her line of vision.

INTRODUCTION

The chronic neurologic disorders (CNDs), although unique and individualized in many respects, share a cluster of common symptoms and treatment needs. People with CNDs often exhibit unresponsiveness or only slight responsiveness to curative treatments. Symptoms associated with CNDs are amenable to palliative treatment, and a growing body of evidence supports the belief that quality of life is increased for patients with CNDs from an array of palliative care interventions.

This chapter presents a description of common symptoms experienced during the final stages of Alzheimer's disease (AD) and related disorders, Parkinson's disease (PD), multiple sclerosis (MS), and amyotrophic lateral sclerosis (ALS). Comorbid conditions that frequently accompany the latter stages of these illnesses are described along with interventions aimed to provide symptom management.

INCIDENCE AND PREVALENCE

The prevalence of dementia in people over age 85 is 23%, with an increase to 58% in those over the age of 95. It is estimated that dementia of the Alzheimer's type affects 3% to 5% of adults over age 65, and that the number of people with the disease doubles every 5 years beyond age 65 (National Institute on Aging, 2000). The prevalence of PD is approximately 1.5 per 1000 people (Snow, 1997). The peak of incidence of PD is between the ages of 60 and 69 years (Brummel-Smith, 1997). The incidence of ALS is 1 to 2 per 100,000, with more men affected and the peak age of incidence in the sixth or seventh decade (Krieger & Eisen, 1999). Onset of MS occurs at younger years than the other CNDs discussed in this chapter, commonly between the ages of 20 and 40 years. The prevalence of MS in the northern United States and Canada is approximately 1 per 1000, with women more commonly affected (Richert, 1999; Ebly, 1994).

DYING TRAJECTORY

Chronic neurologic illnesses often have a less predictable course than other chronic progressive illnesses. Patients with CNDs generally have a decreased life expectancy, but mortality tabulations are unreliable estimates because the death of people with CNDs is often attributed to coexisting medical conditions. Palliative treatment of these conditions has been associated in some instances with significantly increasing length of life (Borasio, 2001; Miller, 2001). PD and AD progress slowly, but, in the late stages, people are severely disabled by these illnesses. ALS is a relatively rare but rapidly fatal illness. Indicators of poor prognosis in ALS include older age at time of onset, early pulmonary dysfunction, and predominance of lower motor neuron disease at diagnosis (Cartner, Bednar-Butler, Abresch, & Ugalde, 1999).

There are several typical patterns to the progression of MS. A rare acute form of the illness results in rapid progression of the illness over a period of months, resulting in death from severe brain cell dysfunction. The chronic relapsing form of the illness is most common (40%). There is a pattern of exacerbations and remissions, but each exacerbation becomes more severe, with more debilitating symptoms presenting and remaining. The chronic progressive form of MS occurs in approximately 15% of cases and is not associated with remissions (Lublin & Reingold, 1996).

While the course of CNDs is less predictable than that of many other illnesses that lead to death in the older adult population, common causes of death are acute or chronic hypoventilation and pneumonia and other severe infections, including aspiration pneumonia. In the

acute form of hypoventilation, weakness of the respiratory muscles causes rapid reduction in vital capacity and symptoms of respiratory failure. In the chronic form, impairment of the respiratory muscles decreases the ability to clear secretions and may eventually affect the respiratory centers in the brain (Sivak, Shefner, & Sexton, 1999). The earliest symptoms of alveolar hypoventilation may be disturbances in sleep. If people with ALS are not ventilated, they will commonly die in their sleep as a result of the insurgence of hypercapnic coma.

The use of palliative care interventions that provide improved comfort while also lengthening the late stage of the illness trajectory has posed new ethical and economic challenges for patients, caregivers, and the health care system. The long trajectory of illness and cognitive and communication deficits associated with many CNDs suggests the need for appropriate timing for decision making, which may change with disease progression.

LATE-STAGE NEURODEGENERATIVE DISEASES
AD and Related Disorders

Neuropathologists often classify neurodegenerative illnesses by three predominant dementing processes: AD, vascular dementias, and dementias associated with Lewy body disease. The hallmarks of AD are neurofibrillary tangles and neuritic plaques. These are often seen early in the illness in the hippocampus, an area that controls short-term memory. As the tangles and plaque accumulation become evident throughout more areas of the cerebral cortex, more severe cognitive deficits, as well as severe sensory and motor symptoms, are manifested. Vascular dementia involves multiple small areas of vascular insufficiency or infarct. There is often a sudden onset of deficits, more variability in deficits than in AD, and a stepwise progression of deterioration in cognition, sensation, and function. Lewy bodies are described as pathologic intracellular material that, when present in the brain, has been associated with dementia. Lewy bodies may be found in only specific areas of the brain or may be diffuse. PD is one illness associated with Lewy bodies. Much of the research on late stages of

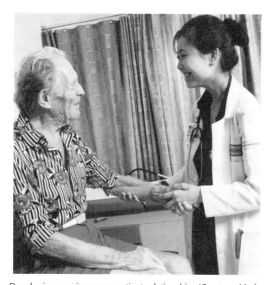

Developing a caring nurse-patient relationship. (Courtesy Mathy Mezey.)

dementia involves people with AD or a mix of AD and vascular dementia.

During late-stage dementia, the person has severe impairment of all cognitive functions. He or she may no longer recognize family members. Attention, orientation, and short- and long-term memory are impaired; both receptive and expressive aphasia is present. The number of words in the person's vocabulary is usually limited to 20 or fewer. Muscles become rigid, movement is slowed, and gait disturbances progress so that the person becomes more chair-bound or bed-bound (Kurlan, Richard, Papka, & Marshall, 2000). Resting tremor is rarely present (Wilson et al., 2000).

Primitive reflexes such as hand grasping, sucking reflexes, and paratonia may be present (Mayeux & Schofeld, 1994). Paratonia is the involuntary resistance of an arm or leg to movement of the limb by another person. This may be misinterpreted by a caregiver as aggressive behavior but is actually a reflexive process. Appetite decreases, and impairments in swallowing can lead to aspiration. Bowel and bladder incontinence is present, and caregivers need to complete most or all activities of daily living for the person. Immune system function is impaired, and infections are the most frequent cause of death for patients in the terminal stage of dementia (Kukull et al., 1994).

Various manifestations of changes in circadian rhythm are present. The sleep-wake cycle is greatly altered, and the person may spend increasing periods of time dozing, socially withdrawn, and less aware of the surrounding environment or activities (Pollack & Stokes, 1997). Sundown syndrome, an increase in agitation in the late afternoon or evening, is often present (Volicer, Harper, Manning, Goldstein, & Satlin, 2001).

People with dementia are very sensitive to and reactive to stressful stimuli in the environment, though this behavioral response is somewhat less evident in later stages. Behaviors associated with dementia should be considered signs of unmet need. The need may be physical, such as pain or feeling hungry, or may be psychosocial, such as feeling fearful, alone, or disturbed by confusing events or visual hallucinations. The elder may have active hands and may exhibit repetitive movements or vocalizations (i.e., perseverance). Delusions and hallucinations may be present, and the person may display agitation, aggressive outbursts, and spontaneous screaming.

Pain experienced by elders with AD and related disorders may arise from the medical conditions commonly prevalent in the older age group, or as a result of comorbid conditions such as pressure ulcers, constipation, and contractures. The most common reported causes of pain in nursing home residents with cognitive impairment are arthritis (70%), old fractures (13%), neuropathies (10%), and malignancies (4%) (Ferrell, Ferrell, & Rivera, 1995).

Parkinson's Disease

PD involves degeneration of cells in the basal ganglia, the primary structure in the brain that is involved is the substantia nigra. This structure makes and stores the neurotransmitter dopamine, so the degenerative process results in depletion of dopamine. The loss of dopamine alters the balanced functioning of neurotransmitters in the basal ganglia and creates the classic triad of motor symptoms: bradykinesia (i.e., slow movement), rigidity, and tremor. Other areas of the brain and extrapyramidal system can be involved, and diffuse degeneration of neurons occurs in severe stages of the illness. The cause of PD is usually not known, although some environmental trigger may be involved.

A person with late-stage PD experiences severe functional impairment as a result of the disease process and as an adverse effect of antiparkinsonian drugs. Motor problems late in the illness that result from drug therapy include dyskinesias (involuntary movements), shorter duration of benefit or lack of benefit from medication, and end-of-dose deterioration of effect. Severe muscle rigidity and bradykinesia contribute to the person becoming more bed-bound or chair-bound. When movement does occur, the person often needs physical help initiating the movement. Akinesia, or freezing of movement, becomes debilitating. Involuntary movements during the night can greatly impair sleep.

Muscle rigidity moves from the cogwheel to the pipelike variety. Cogwheel rigidity is a "ratchety" catch of the limb when moved and is a manifestation of both rigidity and tremor. In severe

PD, the resistance to passive movement of the limb is constant whether the limb is moved slowly or quickly (i.e., like trying to bend a lead pipe) (Kurlan et al., 2000). Painful muscle spasms are common, particularly in the feet and legs. Dysphagia and aspiration are both problematic late in the illness. Drooling and an inability to control oral secretions are troublesome to the older adult.

Autonomic nervous system symptoms occur with degeneration of cells in the basal ganglia and depletion of the neurotransmitter dopamine, as well as from the drug therapy. Postural hypotension and constipation may be severe; bowel dysfunction may result from both a delay in colon transit time and impaired muscle coor-dination in the anorectal area (Pfeiffer, 2000). Delayed gastric emptying is caused by reduced parasympathetic activity and can affect timing of drug response. Heartburn, nausea, early satiety, and epigastric pressure may be felt (Jost, 1997). Urine retention, urgency, and incontinence are common.

A frequently cited statistic is that 30% of people with PD also have dementia, but reports have ranged from 8% to 93% (Bine, Frank, & McDade, 1995). Depression is common and is associated with impaired serotonin and norepi-nephrine levels. Drug-induced confusion and psy-chosis are major problems in trying to manage severe cases. A variety of sleep difficulties are reported.

EVIDENCE-BASED PRACTICE

Reference: Bailey, B., Aranda, S., Quinn, K., & Kean, H. (2000). Creutzfeldt-Jakob disease: extend-ing palliative care nursing knowledge. *International Journal of Palliative Nursing, 6*(3), 131-139.

Research Problem: Creutzfeldt-Jakob disease (CJD) is a rare neurodegenerative disease associated with severe cognitive deterioration and with a rapid course, usually resulting in death within a few months of onset. Nursing care needs of people with this illness are poorly understood.

Design: Exploratory descriptive design.

Sample and Setting: There were three samples: (1) six cases in one hospice; (2) respondents to an invi-tation to participate that was posted on an Internet site for people with experiences with CJD; and (3) nursing staff.

Methods: The study included a retrospective chart review, Internet chat group, and focus group of nursing staff with experience caring for the six cases in the hospice.

Results: The mean age of the six cases was 61 years and the average duration of illness was 5.5 months.

The subjects had moved through an average of four care settings before being admitted to the hospice. Fever was a common symptom, with wide fluctua-tions in temperature occurring even in the absence of a diagnosed infection. All subjects experienced dysphagia, myoclonic jerking, incontinence, consti-pation, and heightened sensitivity to touch and noise. Assessment of pain and psychosocial needs was impeded by impaired communication and cognition. Shortness of breath was common and was exacer-bated by muscle spasms in the neck and face. Family distress was high in all cases.

Implications for Nursing Practice: Minimizing touching, turning, and movement is suggested as an intervention to decrease myoclonic jerking and heightened sensation. In addition, environments should be calm, and muscle relaxants may be admin-istered. Opioids were used effectively for control of pain, anxiety, and dyspnea.

Conclusion: Providing palliative nursing care to people with CJD is complex and requires continuity of care. Families require intense support.

Multiple Sclerosis

Inflammation, demyelination, and scarring (gliosis) of nerves results in the chronic neurologic disorder known as MS. This scar tissue forms hard sclerotic plaques in multiple regions of the central nervous system. The pathology is believed to involve an immune-mediated inflammatory process that may be triggered by a virus in genetically susceptible individuals. Early in the illness the myelin sheath is affected, but the nerve fiber is not affected and nerve impulses are still transmitted. As the damage to nerves progresses, nerve axons become destroyed and nerve impulses are totally blocked, resulting in permanent loss of function (Ozuna, 2000). The symptoms of MS depend on the area of the nervous system involved. Motor, sensory, emotional, cognitive, and autonomic nervous system symptoms are common.

Fatigue may be severe in the late stage of the illness. Loss of mobility may result from weakness, spasticity, and defective muscle coordination. Spasticity may be severely disabling, can be accompanied by painful spasms, and is associated with the development of muscle contractures. Upper limb function is also impaired as a result of spasticity, weakness, and lack of ability to coordinate muscle movements. Impairments in muscle function also cause dysarthria, making verbal communication increasingly difficult. Dysphagia becomes a problem as the illness progresses.

Damage to the sensory system causes or contributes to a variety of problems. Visual dysfunction is common, including diplopia, vision loss, and nystagmus. A variety of changes in bladder function can occur, and the severity of bladder symptoms is associated with the severity of other neurologic symptoms. People with severe MS commonly have incontinence and/or urine retention. Bowel dysfunction occurs in over 50% of patients (Hindis, Eidelman, & Wald, 1990). Symptoms may include constipation, urgency, and fecal incontinence. Loss of sensation leads to sexual dysfunction, and women may also experience a loss of vaginal lubrication (Thompson, 1996).

Cognitive dysfunction is also estimated to occur in 40% to 60% of cases, but deficits primarily impact short-term memory, attention, and speed of processing. Mood and anxiety disorders are common. The extent to which these symptoms are a consequence of the disease process as opposed to the individual's emotional reaction to the illness is unclear (Minden, 2000). Frontal lobe symptoms of euphoria and pathologic laughing and weeping may result from demyelination (Minden, 2000). Psychosis is uncommon (Feinstein, du Boulay, & Ron, 1992).

People with MS may experience the acute onset of paroxysmal symptoms that last 2 minutes or less. These symptoms can include seizures, dysarthria, speech disturbance, sensory disturbance, or uncoordinated movement. Occasionally a person will have many of these episodes of paroxysmal symptoms in a day (Thompson, 1996).

Approximately half of the patients who have MS will die of complications of MS, with pneumonia being the most common cause (Midgard, Riise, Kvale, & Nyland, 1996; Sadovnik, Eisen, Ebers, & Paty, 1991). Weakness of the respiratory muscles produces a restrictive ventilatory defect with resulting atelectasis and a feeling of dyspnea or increased work of breathing. Expiratory weakness is more prominent than inspiratory and may contribute to impaired coughing, aspiration, and the development of pneumonia (Gosselink, Kovacs, & Decramer, 1999). Acute respiratory failure can also occur in MS secondary to demyelinating lesions of the cervical spinal cord or the respiratory centers of the medulla (Carter & Noseworthy, 1994).

Pain in MS occurs as a consequence of both the disease process and the resulting disability. Acute pain in MS may originate from trigeminal neuralgia, headache, facial pain, tonic seizures, and limb pain. The pain may indicate an underlying inflammatory process or a demyelinating lesion affecting a pain pathway (D'Aleo et al., 1999). Subacute pain in MS has been defined as pain that occurs because of worsening symptoms or as a result of treatments (Moulin, Foley, & Ebers, 1988). Causes of subacute pain include optic neuritis, infection, urinary retention, urinary incontinence, and decubitus ulcer. Pain associated with optic neuritis is caused by traction on the meninges surrounding the swollen optic nerve (Maloni, 2000).

Of the people with MS who experience pain, 70% have chronic pain (Indaco, Iachetta, Nappi, Socci, & Carrieri, 1994). Sources of chronic pain in MS include muscle spasms, dysesthetic extremity pain, and musculoskeletal pain (Maloni, 2000). Muscle spasms of the legs are common, particular when hypertonicity of muscles is pronounced. Spasm results from the reaction of the spinal cord to an irritated neural site. Sources of irritation include a distended bladder, decubitus ulcer, or tactile sensation (Clanet & Azais-Vuillemin, 1997). Dysesthetic extremity pain is a result of demyelinating lesions and is described as persistent and burning. The legs and feet are most commonly affected, but the upper extremities and trunk can also be affected. Pain is often worse at night and after exercise, and may be precipitated by changes in temperature, particularly the use of warm water. Joint pain and back pain are common, resulting from the disease process, steroid-induced osteoporosis, postural changes, immobility, and weakness with improper use of compensatory muscles (Maloni, 2000).

Amyotrophic Lateral Sclerosis

ALS, although relatively rare, is a fatal and rapidly progressive motor neuron disease; death usually occurs within 2 to 6 years after diagnosis (Ozuna, 2000). People with ALS have a degeneration of motor neurons in the brain and spinal cord, while remaining cognitively intact. The main symptoms are weakness (particularly of upper limbs), muscle wasting, dysarthria, and dysphagia. The person loses muscle strength, muscle mass, and mobility, finally becoming completely dependent. Approximately 50% of patients in the late stage of the illness report pain as a result of immobility, ligament laxity, spasticity, fasciculations and muscle cramps, and associated problems (Miller, 2001). Hypoventilation and dyspnea are major problems and sources of discomfort in the late stages. Aspiration is also prevalent, thick respiratory secretions are difficult to manage, and uncomfortable, excessive drooling is common.

MANAGEMENT OF COMMON NEEDS AND COMORBID CONDITIONS IN ELDERS WITH CNDS

Specific chapters in this book that cover management of symptoms such as dyspnea, pain, immobility, and gastrointestinal symptoms should be consulted for an overview of treatment options. This section focuses on some of the palliative care issues and their management for elders with CNDs, such as cognition and communication, affect and behavior, pain, eating and swallowing, dyspnea and air hunger, sleep, and infection.

Cognition and Communication

Difficulty communicating severely reduces quality of life for elders with CNDs. The nurse should develop a plan for providing meaningful communication and socialization that considers the wishes of the elder and the accommodations needed because of dysarthria, aphasia, or cognitive impairment.

People with dysarthria use a wide variety of augmentative communication devices. However, as the elder's condition deteriorates, there may be less ability to use the device. A consistent caregiver or family member is often able to understand speech that others consider unintelligible. Supporting the remaining demonstrations of attempts to communicate enables the patient to feel connected and accepted; he or she may begin using many more nonverbal cues to communicate needs. The older adult also may use the behaviors listed in Box 13-1 to communicate to the caregiver that there is an unmet need such as pain or hunger, or the need to eliminate or change positions.

Anticipating physical needs decreases frustration for the elder who is unable to clearly or consistently verbalize needs. Nonverbal communication through touch, massage, and eye contact should be used. Gestures are a three-dimensional language of communication; waving hello, pointing, beckoning with outstretched hands, and hugging, used judiciously by the caregiver, may be effective communication tools. Presence of a family member or caregiver conveys to the elder that he or she is not alone and that he or she is respected.

When cognitive impairment is present, the strategies outlined in Box 13-2 may be useful to facilitate communication. A calm, gentle voice communicates safety and security. Listening to the person, even if the message is unclear, communicates respect. Compared to those with mild cognitive impairment, the elder who is severely impaired may require more focused stimulation to elicit a response. Making a compassionate and

---

Box 13-1 Behavioral Symptoms of Unmet Needs in People with Impaired Communication and/or Cognition

- Any change in behavior
- Restless movement
- Moaning
- Tense muscles
- Facial grimace
- Agitation
- Combative/angry
- Pulling away
- Changes in mobility
- Rubbing/holding/bracing of a body part
- Crying/tears in eyes
- Change in sleep
- Increased confusion
- Change in appetite
- Verbal perseveration
- Withdraw/quiet
- Increased pulse, respiration

Box 13-2 Communication Strategies with the Cognitively Impaired

- Make sure the person knows you are present before communicating to avoid startling or frightening the person.
- Touching the person gently may be used to begin the communication. A conventional handshake may be well tolerated. Assess the person's reaction and gradually increase the use of appropriate touch, if tolerated.
- Keep voice, facial expression, and body movements calm, slow, clear and positive.
- Use short, simple, adult sentences.
- Use the name of the person that is most familiar to him or her. Avoid the use of pronouns.
- Use visual cues to augment verbal message.
- Limit choices to two options to avoid overwhelming the person's cognitive ability.
- Avoid "why" questions, which may be perceived as threatening.
- Avoid negative feedback statements such as "don't. . . ."
- Avoid working to teach or orient the person. Because short-term memory is severely impaired, this is ineffective.
- Listen to the person's verbal message attentively and allow enough time for the person to communicate with you.
- Validate the feelings behind the words: for example, "I hear that you are upset and I am here to help," or "I'm glad you're okay."
- Tapes of family members may be used to provide simulated presence therapy.
- End all interactions with positive feedback such as "I appreciate this time with you," or "It was nice to visit with you today."

---

meaningful connection with a person who has severe dementia will often soothe a troubled, anxious state.

Affect and Behavior

Elders with CNDs may also experience mood disorders, depression, and anxiety, which impact their quality of life. When cognitive impairment is present, the older adult may become increasingly frightened by a world that seems more and more unfamiliar. The literature suggests that people with CNDs are both underdiagnosed and inadequately treated for mood and anxiety disorders (Minden, 2000). People with neuromuscular problems may appear less animated at baseline, so flat affect and decreased involvement in activity are not useful cues for depression or mood disorders. Geropsychiatry consultations are often needed to competently assess and treat elders with more complicated symptomatology. There are few systematic studies of psychotherapy and pharmacotherapy in elders with CNDs. Evidence supports that newer selective serotonin reuptake inhibitors are the drugs of choice for depressive disorders, and anxiety disorders may be treated effectively with combined drug and nonpharmacologic therapy.

The person who has decreased competence, particularly cognitive competence, is more affected by stressors from the environment and has a decreased threshold for such stressors (Kovach, 2000). Consideration of this environmental vulnerability creates the need for two foundational interventions:

- Providing a positive environment with few environmental stressors
- Balancing sensory-stimulating and sensory-calming activity throughout the day

Health professionals should conduct a noise assessment by listening at various times of the day for sources of noxious or extraneous noise. Helpful changes include eliminating echo, background conversations, and television used for background sound. The elder may enjoy brief periods of music listening with selections that are pleasing to him or her. The visually accessible environment may be quite circumscribed, so it is important that it be pleasant and as stress-free as possible. Fluorescent lighting often creates a glare and should be avoided. Some items that are familiar to the elder should be kept in the immediate area; for example, pictures, afghans, and pillows may convey home and familiarity. Spaces that are too big or too small and cluttered areas should be avoided. One or two plants or flower arrangements are preferred to an overwhelming clutter of flora. Keeping the room temperature comfortable removes a possible tactile stressor. Itchy skin can be prevented by keeping the skin well lubricated and treating with medicated emollients; flannel sheets and silk pillowcases also may provide some comfort.

In addition to decreasing environmental stress, there is a need to balance sensory-stimulating and sensory-calming activity. As the illness progresses, there may be a need for more sensory calming time; the elder will probably tolerate less than 1 hour of activity before needing a decrease in environmental stimulation. Often only brief visits of 10 minutes or less will be tolerated. The person may need to engage in frequent inner retreat by withdrawing from others. This need should be explained to family, so they do not feel shunned; if the elder shuns socialization, allow him or her some solitary time and approach again later.

There is also a need for focused, therapeutic stimulation. Stimulation of multiple senses enhances engagement in the activity (Kovach & Magliocco, 1998). Friendly visiting, hand massage, music listening, and pet therapy are just a few examples of therapeutic activities. Multiple activity therapy books provide suggestions for therapeutic activities that accommodate any

level of cognitive or functional deficit and enhance quality of life (Bowlby, 1993).

Perseverant behavior, defined as repetitive movement or verbalization, may also occur in elder patients with CNDs. Perseverance may indicate boredom, discomfort, or an unmet need, or it may be a simple tension reduction mechanism. Calm repetitive movements or verbalizations may be a coping mechanism and do not require treatment. It is important to determine if environmental stress needs to be decreased or, alternatively, if stimulating activity should be provided. Health professionals should assess for basic comfort needs: offer a drink, be certain elimination needs have been met, provide a warm blanket or sweater, and check for pressure points and good positioning. If pain is suspected, an analgesic should be administered.

Aggression and resisting care may also be present. Resisting care may indicate that pain control is inadequate. This behavior is often temporary, so the caregiver should repeat the attempt to provide care following a short break. Paratonia, a primitive reflex that may be present, is involuntary resistance of an extremity in response to sudden passive movement. A caregiver who moves a patient's arm or leg may evoke this response, which appears to be resistance to care. Slow and gentle touch decreases the likelihood of inducing paratonia.

Delusions and hallucinations, when present, are a real part of the person's mental life and can be very discomforting. These alterations in perception often respond well to psychotropic drugs. Caregivers should not agree or disagree with the false perception, but there is a need to provide comforting intervention. For example, saying, "I hear that you are afraid and I will keep you safe," validates feelings and provides reassurance. Distraction or provision of a comforting intervention such as friendly visiting will often soothe the person's troubled state. Also, the caregiver should check to be sure the person's glasses and hearing aid are in place and functioning properly. Many suspected delusions in older adults are actually mixed messages resulting from impaired hearing.

Recognizing and Treating Pain

It may be difficult to recognize pain in the elder who has dementia and/or communication impairment. The elder's response to pain medication may be used as a part of assessment; if the older adult appears agitated or has a change in behavior that is not ameliorated by usual interventions, a trial of analgesics can be administered, and the response monitored. For people with dementia, the Assessment of Discomfort in Dementia (ADD) Protocol has been developed to provide a systematic process for assessing and treating both physical pain and affective discomfort in people who can no longer clearly or consistently communicate their needs (Kovach, Noonan, Griffie, Muchka, & Weismann, 2002).

In one study of 104 people with end-stage dementia, use of the ADD Protocol was associated with a significant decrease in discomfort ($t=6.56$, $p=0.000$) and a significant increase in the use of pharmacologic ($t=2.56$, $p=0.012$) and nonpharmacologic ($t=3.37$, $p=0.001$) comfort interventions (Kovach, Weismann, Griffie, Matson, & Muchka, 1999). In another study conducted in long-term care, for 84% of the 161 ADD Protocols initiated, behavioral symptoms improved following use of the protocol, and 83.5% of the 91 subjects who received analgesics as a part of the protocol experienced improved symptoms (Kovach et al., 2001). Findings from these studies suggest that increased analgesic use for people with late-stage dementia may be warranted.

Use of the ADD Protocol is triggered by behavioral or verbal symptoms that have not been ameliorated by basic interventions, such as changing an incontinence product or providing fluids. The five steps of the ADD Protocol are briefly described below and outlined in Figure 13-1.

Step 1: A physical assessment should be conducted to look for physical causes of discomfort—infection, inflammation, respiratory congestion, pressure points, spasticity, body misalignment, and the like.

Step 2: The person's history should be reviewed for potentially painful conditions. Does the person have an old fracture site that could be causing pain, or a history of arthritis or other relevant pain symptoms? If the source of discomfort is identified from the physical assessment or history (i.e., Steps 1 or 2), interventions or consultation with the appropriate health care provider should be instituted accordingly.

Step 3: If the history and physical assessment are negative, Step 3 involves conducting an affective assessment and implementing nonpharmacologic comfort interventions. For people with dementia, at least three fundamental areas are assessed: environmental stressors, pacing of activity so that there is a balance between sensory-stimulating and sensory-calming activity, and quantity and quality of meaningful human interaction (Kovach, Noonan, Griffie, Muchka, & Weismann, 2002). Based on the results of the affective assessment, nonpharmacologic comfort interventions are implemented. Common nonpharmacologic interventions used are therapeutic communication, providing more or less stimulation, exercise, repositioning, massage, and distraction techniques such as music listening.

Step 4: If nonpharmacologic comfort interventions are ineffective, an analgesic (e.g., acetaminophen) that is prescribed to be given as needed (prn) is administered. It is at this point that, in the past, nurses have often administered a psychotropic drug. In the ADD Protocol, a prn analgesic is given *as a part of the assessment process.* Nurses have not commonly given analgesics for the purpose of assessment and will need instruction and support in utilizing this step. The choice of analgesic is dependent on what analgesics the person is currently receiving. For example, if the person were taking no analgesics, a common order would be acetaminophen, 500 mg twice a day. If the person were already taking acetaminophen with codeine, the analgesic chosen for the assessment during Step 4 would need to be either a stronger analgesic or stronger dosage than the current prescription. The nurse should observe for a positive response to a trial of prn analgesics. If the response is positive, the nurse should determine if an order for a scheduled analgesic is needed. If there is not a positive response, the nurse should either go to Step 5 of the Protocol, or consider seeking orders to escalate either the dose or the category of analgesic administered.

Step 5: If a trial of analgesics is not effective in relieving the behavioral symptoms, the nurse should consult with the physician or other

> **Complete for: a) observed behavioral changes; _OR_ b) if behavior/pain symptoms are coded on the MDS (Sections E4A or J2a). Report appropriate sections to the prescriber.**

Resident's Name: _____ Date: _____

Behavioral Symptoms: Circle all that apply

Facial Expression   Grimacing, frowning, blinking, tightly closed or widely open eyes, frightened, weepy, worried, sad

Mood   Irritability, confusion, withdrawal, agitation, aggressiveness

Body Language   Tense, wringing hands, clenched fists, restless, rubbing/holding body part, hyperactive or hypoactive, guarding body part, noisy breathing

Voice   Moaning, mumbling, chanting, grunting, whining, calling out, screaming, crying, verbally aggressive

Behavior   Change in appetite, sleep, mobility, gait, function, participation, exiting, wandering, elopement, physically aggressive, socially inappropriate or disruptive, resists cares

Other

_____

☐ When **all basic needs met** (toileting, thirst, hunger, glasses & hearing aids in place)

Steps of the ADD Protocol

Notes: Assess, RX, and Response

STEP 1: Assessment	*+	*−	N/A	
↑ BP, P, sweating				
↑ T				
Eyes, Nose, Mouth				
Skin				
Heart/Lungs				
Abdomen				
BM/Rectal Check				
Extremities				
Multistix Urine				
Other S&S				

* A + indicates a positive assessment finding or change from baseline. A − indicates no change in assessment from baseline.

Fig. 13-1 Assessment for Discomfort in Dementia (ADD): Long-Term Care Protocol. (Copyright Christine R. Kovach, 1997.)

Notes: Assess, Rx, and Response

STEP 2: ✔'d if behaviors possibly R/T current or past history of pain	✔ if done	
STEP 3: If Steps 1 and 2 are negative, ASSESS • environmental press (i.e., stress) • pacing of activity/stimulation • meaningful human interaction and **INTERVENE** • nonpharmacologic treatments		
STEP 4: If unsuccessful, medicate with analgesic per written order	✔ if done	
STEP 5: If symptoms persist, consult with physician/other health professional or medicate with prn psychotropic per written order		

Nurse's Signature: _____ Date: _____

*If new nursing/medical interventions initiated, complete below:

Evaluate effectiveness of new nursing and/or medical intervention on behavioral symptoms. (Be Specific)

_____

_____

_____

Plan of Care Updated (if appropriate)

Nurse's Signature: _____ **Date:** _____

Fig. 13-1, cont'd.

health care professional, or give an ordered prn psychotropic drug.

The ADD Protocol is based on the assumption that behaviors associated with dementia are often symptoms of unmet needs that may originate from physiologic and/or nonphysiologic sources. The Protocol is unique in using prn analgesics as a part of a systematic assessment process. The dualistic perspective, in which physical and affective needs are considered in tandem, is an essential and innovative feature.

People with MS, as described earlier in this chapter, can have multiple sources of pain, may experience episodic or continuous pain, and need treatment for several different types of pain. Muscle spasticity may be quite painful in MS and PD. Incorrect body alignment and noxious stimuli such as infections, hot water, or uncomfortable orthotics can increase spasticity (Thompson, 1996).

Pharmacologic agents used to treat pain include oral, intramuscular, and intrathecal agents and nerve blocks. Muscle relaxants are commonly administered, including intrathecal baclofen, which allows the administration of lower dosages and thus has fewer side effects (Azouvi, Mane, & Thiebaut, 1996; Teddy, 1995). Botulinum toxin injections have also been used to produce a temporary block of nerve conduction (Snow, Tsui, & Bhatt, 1990). A variety of surgical procedures are available if baclofen is ineffective and the pain cannot be controlled (Smyth & Peacock, 2000). Gabapentin, lamotrigine, capsaicin, tricyclic antidepressants, counterstimulating elastic stockings, and cold compresses are used to treat dysesthetic extremity pain (Maloni, 2000). Pain may also occur from altered muscle tone around joints or may be skin pressure pain from inactivity (Oliver, 1993). Nonopioid and opioid analgesics may be used. Opioids may be particularly effective in decreasing feelings of anxiety, dyspnea, and pain.

Eating and Swallowing

The swallowing mechanism is quite complex, involving 26 sets of muscles and six nerves, and is dependent on critical timing of several phases and highly coordinated movement (Kulpa & DePaul, 1997). Older adults in the late stages of neurodegenerative diseases will have dysphagia

and be at risk for aspiration and malnutrition. Techniques commonly used to assist elders with dysphagia to swallow safely are reviewed here. Other options for managing eating problems also are discussed, including tube feeding, use of a sucking apparatus, and the use of neuroleptics to improve appetite.

Prior to the meal, several interventions may be helpful. For example, oral hygiene is important in maintaining a normal viscosity to the saliva. If the person is taking medications that dry the mouth, artificial saliva products should be used. For the person with dementia, providing some cueing that mealtime is coming is helpful. For example, on units for elders with late-stage CNDs in a long-term care setting, a tablecloth and vase of flowers can be placed on each table in the late afternoon to signal that it is the start of evening mealtime. The residents and staff can enjoy a glass of nonalcoholic wine together while listening to relaxing music. It is important to reduce distractions during mealtime, so that the focus is on eating and swallowing. If the person is in a long-term care facility, the dining room should optimally seat 16 or fewer residents. The person must be made comfortable, and the environment should be comfortable and free from odors. The administration of neuroleptics that increase serotonergic function may improve food intake (Rohrbaugh & Siegal, 1989).

Caregivers should provide verbal cueing to assist the person to eat by saying, for example, "the food is coming," and "swallow now." The person must not be rushed to eat and swallow too quickly, but caregivers should be aware that excessive time spent at the task may lead to fatigue and decrease eating. Positive encouragement should be provided during the meal.

Plastic utensils should not be used because a biting reflex may occur, especially if the gums or teeth are touched with the utensil. Applying gentle pressure on the jaw and cheek muscles may break the biting reflex (Kulpa & DePaul, 1997). Van Ort and Phillips (1992) found that the following behaviors by persons assisting with feeding sustained eating by people with dementia: talking and reorienting the person to the meal, offering drinks between bites, holding the spoon ready for a bite, and warmly touching the resident. Behaviors that extinguished eating were failing to respond to cues and interrupting or aborting feeding attempts.

The person with dysphagia will require alterations in diet. Calorie-dense pureed diets and thickened liquids may be used. Smaller, more frequent meals may be needed, and the person will often take in more food at meals eaten earlier in the day. For some people, the stimulation of a soft bolus of food, such as mashed potatoes, may provide more stimuli for swallowing than liquids. Asplund, Norberg, and Adolfsson (1991) presented cases of people with late-stage dementia who could no longer eat food, but successfully used a sucking apparatus to take in fluid. Although many people with late-stage dementia retain the sucking reflex, if the swallowing response is impaired, aspiration of fluid may occur.

Oral feeding may eventually become impossible, and a person should never be force fed. The decision to tube feed is complex and controversial, and the courts have recognized tube feeding as a medical treatment that can be refused. Prior decision making by the patient relative to the desire to initiate assisted feeding is helpful.

There are no randomized clinical trials examining the outcomes of tube feeding. In the case of ALS, percutaneous endoscopic gastrostomy tube placement is common, and evidence suggests that survival is prolonged as a result (Mazzini et al., 1995). However, studies involving people with dementia have actually found an increase in aspiration pneumonia in tube-fed patients (Peck, Cohen, & Mulvihill, 1990) and little or no increase in length of life (Finucane, Christmas, & Travis, 1999; Volicer et al., 1989). Other possible problems associated with tube feeding include diarrhea, surgery risks and burdens of hospitalization associated with tube placement, the need for physical restraints if tubes are pulled, wound infection, and skin breakdown.

Dyspnea/Air Hunger

In people with CNDs involving motor systems, respiratory insufficiency may cause chronic nocturnal hypoventilation and sleeplessness. (This is not a usual problem for elders with AD.) Patients and families need to be given information regarding the mechanism of terminal hypercapnic coma

and the resulting peaceful death, so that fear is decreased. Medications discussed in Chapter 17 need to be administered skillfully to successfully prevent the feeling of "choking to death." The reader should consult Chapter 17 for further information on dyspnea.

Noninvasive intermittent ventilation (NIV) is an option chosen by some patients, particularly those with ALS, to decrease feelings of dyspnea. NIV delivers air through a mouthpiece instead of a tracheostomy; this mouthpiece or "sip" intermittent positive-pressure ventilation system is attached to the standard ventilatory tubing and machinery and positioned close to the elder's face by a bracket on the wheelchair or bed frame. The elder turns toward the mouthpiece and grabs it with the lips, which triggers the ventilator to send the breath (Northwest Regional Spinal Cord Injury System, 1998). NIV is recommended as an effective initial therapy to improve quality of life (Miller, 2001). If the person does not want NIV to prolong his or her life, it can be stopped at any time (Borasio & Voltz, 1997). Mechanical ventilation is another option, but may lead to prolonged life and decreased quality of life.

Sleep/Activity

A variety of pathophysiologic mechanisms are involved in the sleep disorders of elders living with CNDs. Light and fragmented sleep does impair quality of life. Nocturnal hypoventilation is discussed above under "Dyspnea/Air Hunger." For people with PD who have nocturnal akinesia, a slow-release formulation of levodopa/carbidopa (Sinemet CR) may be helpful (Stocchi, Barbato, Nordera, Berardelli, & Ruggieri, 1998). It is important to keep a consistent schedule so that the diurnal rhythm is encouraged. Most people will need an afternoon nap, but keeping the person engaged in some activities during the daytime might help to improve nighttime sleep.

An increase in agitated behavior in the late afternoon or early evening, called sundown syndrome, occurs in some people with dementia. This often indicates a need to improve the balance between sensory-stimulating and sensory-calming activity earlier in the day. Specifically, there may be a need for more physical activity early in the day, followed by an afternoon nap. Then, during the usual sundowning period, the person can be engaged in a quiet one-on-one activity. Also, because of the severe sleep variations experienced by people with CNDs, caregivers should try to keep diurnal rhythms intact by keeping lighting low during the night and up during the day. This may require increasing use of artificial light beginning in the late afternoon.

Infection

Severe infection, commonly pneumonia and septicemia arising from the urinary tract, may be the cause of death in elders with CNDs. Delayed diagnosis of infection because of both altered clinical presentations and the patient's inability to clearly report symptoms may contribute to the severity of infection. Nurses should work to prevent infection through common practices such as good handwashing, skin care, and adequate hydration. As the illness progresses, the question of how vigorously to treat infection or if one should treat infection at all is commonly raised. One study found similar levels of comfort and survival when patients with late-stage dementia were treated with antibiotics or with comfort measures only (Hurley, Volicer, Mahoney, & Volicer, 1993).

PALLIATIVE CARE ISSUES

Unlike cancer, the illness trajectory for elder patients with CNDs is often longer and more

---

EVIDENCE-BASED PRACTICE

Reference: Travis, S. S., Bernard, M., Dixon, S., McAuley, W. J., Loving, G., & McClanahan, L. (2002). Obstacles to palliation and end-of-life care in a long-term care facility. *The Gerontologist, 42,* 342-349.

Research Problem: To examine end-of-life experiences in long-term care, focusing on obstacles to palliative and end-of-life care.

Design: Exploratory design with quantitative and qualitative methodologies.

Sample and Setting: 41 nursing home residents, 61% with dementia, with a mean age of 87.

Methods: Retrospective chart reviews were done using four obstacle constructs derived from the literature and earlier work of the researchers. Obstacles to palliation and end-of-life care begin with a lack of recognition of the futility of restorative, rehabilitative, or curative treatment for the person. Three additional obstacles follow sequentially: lack of communication among decision makers, no agreement on a course of care, and failure to implement a timely plan of care.

Results: In this sample, 46% of subjects had no obstacles to their palliative and end-of-life care. Failure to recognize treatment futility occurred in 17% of cases, lack of communication among decision makers occurred in 22%, no agreement on a course of care in 35%, and failure to implement a timely plan of care in 54% of the cases. Residents who had been hospitalized in the previous year were significantly more likely to have one or more obstacles identified in their end-of-life care.

Implications for Nursing Practice: Findings from this study suggest that agreeing on and implementing a course of end-of-life care is a major difficulty. The authors suggested that a scheduled team meetings should regularly consider explicit palliative care discussions with key decision makers.

Conclusion: Aggressive palliative care needs to become a standard for end-of-life care for residents in long-term care. Understanding the obstacles to providing end-of-life care in these settings may help to bring about needed changes.

Box 13-3 **Medical Guidelines for Determining Prognosis: Dementia**

The term *dementia* refers here to chronic, primary and progressive cognitive impairment of either the Alzheimer or multi-infarct type. Although most research on prognosis in dementia is done with Alzheimer's patients, the vascular (multi-infarct) dementias appear to progress to death more quickly. These guidelines do *not* refer to acute, potentially reversible or secondary dementias, i.e., those due to drug intoxication, cancer, AIDS, major stroke, or heart, renal or liver failure.

I.   Functional Assessment Staging
    A.   Even severely demented patients may have a prognosis of up to two years. Survival time depends on variables such as the incidence of co-morbidities and the comprehensiveness of care.
    B.   The patient should be at or beyond stage 7 of the Functional Assessment Staging Scale. The factors listed below should be understood explicitly, since many patients do not progress in an orderly fashion through the substages of stage 7.
    C.   The patient should show *all* of the following characteristics:
        1.   Unable to ambulate without assistance.
             This is a critical factor. Recent data indicate that patients who retain the ability to ambulate independently do not tend to die within six months, even if all other criteria for advanced dementia are present.
        2.   Unable to dress without assistance.
        3.   Unable to bathe properly.
        4.   Urinary and fecal incontinence.
            a.   Occasionally or more frequently, over the past weeks.
            b.   Reported by knowledgeable informant or caregiver.
        5.   Unable to speak or communicate meaningfully.
            a.   Ability to speak is limited to approximately a *half dozen or fewer intelligible and different words*, in the course of an average day or in the course of an intensive interview.

II. Presence of Medical Complications
    A.   The presence of medical co-morbid conditions of sufficient severity to warrant medical treatment, documented within the past year, *whether or not the decision was made to treat the condition*, decreases survival in advanced dementia.
    B.   Co-morbid conditions associated with dementia:
        1.   Aspiration pneumonia.
        2.   Pyelonephritis or other upper urinary tract infection.
        3.   Septicemia.
        4.   Pressure ulcers, multiple, stage 3-4.
        5.   Fever recurrent after antibiotics.
    C.   Difficulty swallowing food or refusal to eat, sufficiently severe that patient cannot maintain sufficient fluid and calorie intake to sustain life, with patient or surrogate refusing tube feedings or parenteral nutrition.
        1.   Patients who are receiving tube feedings must have documented impaired nutritional status as indicated by:
            a.   Unintentional, progressive weight loss of greater than 10% over the prior six months.
            b.   Serum albumin less than 2.5 gm/dl may be a helpful prognostic indicator, but should not be used by itself.

From Reisberg, B. (1988). Functional Assessment Staging (FAST). *Pschopharmacalogy Bulletin, 24*, 653-659; National Hospice Organization. (1996). *Medical guidelines for determining prognosis in selected non-cancer diseases* (2nd ed.). Arlington, VA: National Hospice Organization.

unpredictable. This prognostic uncertainty is associated with a host of patient, family, caregiving, and reimbursement challenges. Patients with CNDs have heavy physical and emotional care needs. Care in a hospice or long-term care facility may reduce the caregiving required of the family, but may lead to feelings of loss of control as well as feelings of isolation. Deciding on the preferred setting for end-of-life care is complex, with many factors to consider; family members may disagree with each other or with the elder. The nurse can serve as a nonjudgmental listener, help to explore options, and facilitate working through the process of decision making with family members.

Regardless of the setting of care, people with CNDs do not receive enough palliative or hospice care. In one study of 98 people with advanced ALS living at home, only 16 received hospice home care, 24 received nonhospice home care, and the remaining 58 received no in-home care services (Krivickas, Shockley, & Mitsumoto, 1997). Underutilization of home care and hospice services is a common finding in people with CNDs.

Physicians and other health care providers often do not understand that hospice services are extremely helpful to those with noncancer diseases, nor do they understand the criteria or mechanisms for establishing hospice services in their agencies or in patients' homes. The National Hospice Organization (1996) has established guidelines for determining prognosis in selected noncancer diseases, including dementia (see Box 13-3) and ALS. These guidelines are designed to predict 6-month mortality so that the person can be entered into Medicare/Medicaid-reimbursed hospice services. The accuracy of these guidelines at predicting mortality is debated.

Some long-term care facilities are opening special care units specifically for the elder person with late-stage dementia. The focus of these units is on comfort, quality of life, and human dignity. Therapeutic activities are brief, often one-on-one, and involve more use of simple sensory stimulation and human connection through touch. In one experimental study in long-term care, there was a statistically significant difference in discomfort between the people with end-stage dementia receiving hospice-oriented care and those receiving standard long-term care (Kovach, Wilson, & Noonan, 1996).

Family members should optimally be a part of a continued process of decision making throughout the illness trajectory. In the case of illnesses that are associated with dementia, early discussions and assignment of trusted family members to decision-making roles when capacity is compromised are essential. A lot of anticipatory grieving occurs with these illnesses, and family members need to be supported in accepting their feelings. Acknowledging conflicting feelings, particularly both the dread of the family member's death and the desire for the death to occur, as common and natural can be helpful. Early discussions about the typical course of the illness that are honest but sensitive are needed.

Coping with the late stages of chronic neurodegenerative illness is both physically and emotionally demanding. The patient's stress should not be amplified by an awareness of the burden on family or professional caregivers. Discussions about the burdens or problems of caregiving should be held away from the patient. The person should feel cared for and safe.

Case Study Conclusion

Mrs. C.'s case is unfortunately not atypical for elders with late-stage AD. The physical assessment of Mrs. C. was unremarkable, except for stiff inflexible muscles, arthritic changes, and the start of some contractures. Her history revealed arthritis of the hands and knees, though she currently was not taking any pain medication. Acetaminophen, 500 mg, was started on a twice-a-day schedule. The effect was a decrease in screaming and agitated behaviors, but she still was resistant and agitated by physical contact. The television was turned off and the mobile was removed to decrease extraneous and potentially confusing environmental stimulation. Mrs. C. had a new activity plan that included two 10-minute sessions of friendly visiting, soft massage and gentle range-of-motion exercises, music therapy for 15 minutes, and pet therapy twice each week. She was also given a small silk pillow that she enjoyed feeling on her skin. Flannel sheets were placed on her bed to keep her joints warm.

Eventually, since the fearful behaviors persisted, Mrs. C. was started on a psychotropic drug because of the awareness that paranoid delusions are common during the late stages of dementia. Mrs. C. was also transferred to a comfortable chair each day and ate at least one meal a day in the dining room. Though she did not participate, she watched the sing-a-long after lunch each day. Following these interventions, her appetite improved, her verbalization was more coherent, her gaze often tracked events in the room, and she would smile in response to activities such as pet therapy and massage. Her agitated behavior and repetitive vocalizations significantly decreased.

Mrs. C. had pain, delusions, social isolation, and boredom, and was receiving environmental stimulation that exceeded her stress threshold. All of these factors were compromising the quality of her life. Even though Mrs. C. was at the end of her life and would die soon, she could still engage in a variety of positive activities and stay socially connected. Although Mrs. C. did not have complex comorbid physical conditions, she clearly needed comprehensive nursing interventions to improve her comfort and quality of life.

CONCLUSION

Older adults with dementia and other CNDs are ideal candidates for palliative care. Comfort and quality-of-life interventions have been found to greatly assist people with CNDs to cope with an array of debilitating symptoms. Although nursing spends a good deal of time focused on pain management and symptom control, nurses are also responsible for addressing the quality-of-life needs of older adults who are at the end of their lives. Elders with CNDs can still experience pleasure and feelings of being socially connected. Warm conversation, music and pet therapy, massage, and activities designed to share beauty in the world and to maintain social connections should be a part of everyday life. Family members may need help learning how to avoid just sitting at the bedside in a "death watch" and instead share meaningful moments with their loved one.

Because elders with significant CNDs are often not able to advocate for themselves, it is the nurses' responsibility to continue to work to improve the care delivered to this population who are nearing the end of their lives. There is a need for the profession of nursing to develop a host of evidence-based interventions to meet the palliative care needs of older adults with CNDs.

RESOURCES
Grief and Loss
- ThirdAge.com (*www.thirdage.com/family/ caregiving/bibliography/grief.html*): caregiving bibliography on grief and loss
- Journey of Hearts (*www.journeyofhearts.org/ jofh/about/kirstimd/resa-d.htm*): extensive list of links for loss and coping resources involving numerous diseases and conditions

Alzheimer's Disease
- Alzheimer's Disease Education & Referral Center, National Institute on Aging (*www. alzheimers.org/pubs/adfact.html*): Alzheimer's Disease Fact Sheet. Information, education, and resources.
- Alzheimer's Association (*www.alz.org*): information and services for patients, caregivers, friends, and family; phone: 1-800-272-3900
- HealingWell.com (*www.healingwell.com/ alzheimers*): Alzheimer's Disease Resource Center

Amyotrophic Lateral Sclerosis (Lou Gehrig's Disease)
- ALS Association (*www.alsa.org*): up-to-date educational information for professionals, patients, and family
- "ALS Information" (*www.avalon.net/ ~kboyken/als.html*): facts and information on care, organizations, research for a treatment, death and dying
- "Reflections on Living with ALS for 11 Years" (*www.rideforlife.com/MT/archives.cover_ story/000547.html#547*): a personal narrative by Ed White detailing life with ALS
- "ALS Resources" (*www.etriloquist.com/ alslinks.html*): communication aids, assistive software and hardware, and links to other resources on ALS

Multiple Sclerosis

- Multiple Sclerosis Association of America (*www.msaa.com*): phone: 1-800-532-7667. A comprehensive overview of the programs and services of the Multiple Sclerosis Association of America. Education and referral.
- HealingWell.com (*www.healingwell.com/ms*): Multiple Sclerosis Resource Center. Information, education, and resources.
- International Multiple Sclerosis Support Foundation (*www.msnews.org*): Information, education, and resources.

Parkinson's Disease

- Parkinson's Disease Foundation, Inc. (*www.pdf.org/index.cfm*): phone: 1-212-923-4700 or 1-800-457-6676; e-mail: *info@pdf.org* Get answers to your pressing questions from Parkinson's Disease Foundation physicians and scientists.
- Somerset Pharmaceuticals Inc. (*www.parkinsonsinfo.com*): general information on PD, including drug therapy
- Adrienne Coles Memorial Trust (*james.parkinsons.org.uk/parkinsons.htm*): lots of links to specific PD websites
- Healing Well.com (*www.healingwell.com/parkinsons*): Parkinson's Disease Resource Center. Education, information, chat room, and resources.

REFERENCES

Asplund, K., Norberg, A., & Adolfsson, R. (1991). The sucking behavior of two patients in the final stage of dementia of the Alzheimer type. *Scandinavian Journal of Caring Science, 5*(3), 141-147.

Azouvi, P., Mane, M., & Thiebaut, J. B. (1996). Intrathecal baclofen administration for control of severe spinal spasticity: Functional improvement and long-term follow-up. *Archives of Physical Medicine and Rehabilitation, 77*, 35-39.

Bine, J. E., Frank, E. M., & McDade, H. L. (1995). Dysphagia and dementia in subjects with Parkinson's disease. *Dysphagia, 10*, 160-164.

Borasio, G. D. (2001). Palliative care in ALS: Searching for the evidence base. *ALS and Other Motor Neuron Disorders, 2*(Suppl. 1), S31–S35.

Borasio, G. D., & Voltz, R. (1997). Palliative care in amyotrophic lateral sclerosis. *Journal of Neurology, 244*(Suppl. 4), S11–S17.

Bowlby, C. (1993). *Therapeutic activities with persons disabled by Alzheimer's disease and related disorders.* Gaithersburg, MD: Aspen.

Brummel-Smith, K. (1997). Rehabilitation. In C. K. Cassel et al. (Eds.), *Geriatric medicine* (3rd ed., pp. 211-226). New York: Springer.

Carter, G. T., Bednar-Butler, L. M., Abresch, R. T., & Ugalde, V. O. (1999). Expanding the role of hospice care in amyotrophic lateral sclerosis. *American Journal of Hospice & Palliative Care, 16*, 707-710.

Carter, J. L., & Noseworthy, J. H. (1994). Ventilatory dysfunction in multiple sclerosis. *Clinics in Chest Medicine, 15*, 693-703.

Clanet, G. M., & Azais-Vuillemin, C. (1997). What is new in the symptomatic management of multiple sclerosis. In A. J. Thompson, C. Polman, & H. Reinhard (Eds.), *Multiple sclerosis: Clinical challenges and controversies* (pp. 235-241). London: Martin Dunitz.

D'Aleo, G., Sessa, E., D'Aleo, P., Rifici, C., DiBella, P., Petix, M., et al. (1999). Nociceptive R3 reflex in relapsing-remitting multiple sclerosis. *Functional Neurology, 14*, 43-47.

Ebly, E. M., Parhad, I. M., Hogan, D. B., & Fung, T. S. (1994). Prevalence and types of dementia in the very old: Results from the Canadian Study of Health and Aging. *Neurology, 44*, 1593-1560.

Feinstein, A., du Boulay, G., & Ron, M. (1992). Psychotic illness in multiple sclerosis: A clinical and MRI study. *British Journal of Psychiatry, 161*, 680-685.

Ferrell, B. A., Ferrell, B. R., & Rivera, L. M. (1995). Pain in cognitively impaired nursing home patients. *Journal of Pain & Symptom Management, 10*, 591-598.

Finuncane, T. E., Christmas, C., & Travis, K. (1999). Tube feeding in patients with advanced dementia. *JAMA, 282*, 1365-1370.

Gosselink, R., Kovacs, L., & Decramer, M. (1999). Respiratory muscle involvement in multiple sclerosis. *European Respiratory Journal, 13*, 449-454.

Hall, G. R., & Buckwalter, K. C. (1987). Progressively lowered stress threshold: A conceptual model for care of adults with Alzheimer's disease. *Archives of Psychiatric Nursing, 1*, 399-406.

Hindis, J. P., Eidelman, B. H., & Wald, A. (1990). Prevalence of bowel dysfunction in multiple sclerosis: A population survey. *Gastroenterology, 98*, 1538-1542.

Hurley, A. C., Volicer, B., Mahoney, M. A., & Volicer, L. (1993). Palliative fever management in Alzheimer's patients: Quality plus fiscal responsibility. *Advances in Nursing Science, 16*, 21-32.

Indaco, A., Iachetta, C., Nappi, C., Socci, L., & Carrieri, P. B. (1994). Chronic and acute pain syndromes in patients with multiple sclerosis. *Acta Neurologica, 16*, 97-102.

Jost, W. H. (1997). Gastrointestinal motility problems in patients with Parkinson's disease. *Drugs & Aging, 10*, 249-258.

Kovach, C. R. (2000). Sensoristasis and imbalance in persons with dementia. *Journal of Nursing Scholarship, 32*, 379-384.

Kovach, C. R., & Magliocco, J. (1998). Late-stage dementia and participation in therapeutic activities. *Applied Nursing Research, 11*(4), 167-173.

Kovach, C. R., Noonan, P. E., Griffie, J., Muchka, S., & Weismann, D. E. (2001). Use of the Assessment of Discomfort in Dementia Protocol (ADD). *Applied Nursing Research, 14*(4), 193-200.

Kovach, C. R., Noonan, P. E., Griffie, J., Muchka, S., & Weismann, D. E. (2002). The Assessment of Discomfort in Dementia (ADD) Protocol. *Pain Management Nursing, 3*(1), 16-27.

Kovach, C. R., Weismann, D., Griffie, J., Matson, S., & Muchka, S. (1999). Assessment and treatment of discomfort for people with late-stage dementia. *Journal of Pain & Symptom Management, 18*, 412-419.

Kovach, C. R., Wilson, S. A., & Noonan, P. E. (1996). The effects of hospice interventions on behaviors, discomfort, and physical complications of end-stage dementia in nursing home residents. *American Journal of Alzheimer's Disease, 11*(4), 7-10, 12-15.

Krieger, C., & Eisen, A. A. (1999). Amyotrophic lateral sclerosis. In W. N. Kelly (Ed.), *Textbook of internal medicine* (pp. 2394-2396). Philadelphia: Lippincott.

Krivickas, L. S., Shockley, L., & Mitsumoto, H. (1997). Homecare of patients with amyotrophic lateral sclerosis. *Journal of Neuroscience, 152*(Suppl. 1), S82–S89.

Kukull, W. A., Brenner, D. E., Speck, C. E., Nochlin, D., Bowen, J., McCormick, W., et al. (1994). Causes of death associated with Alzheimer's disease: Variations by level of cognitive impairment before death. *Journal of the American Geriatrics Society, 4*, 723-726.

Kulpa, J., & DePaul, R. (1997). Strategies for eating, swallowing, and dysphagia. In C. Kovach (Ed.), *Late-stage dementia care: A basic guide* (pp. 85-100). Washington, DC: Taylor & Francis.

Kurlan, R., Richard, I. H., Papka, M., & Marshall, F. (2000). Movement disorders in Alzheimer's disease: more rigidity of definition is needed. *Movement Disorders, 15*, 24-29.

Lawton, M. P. (1986). *Environment and aging.* Albany, NY: Center for the Study of Aging.

Lublin, F. D., & Reingold, S. C. (1996). Defining the clinical course of multiple sclerosis. *Neurology, 46*, 907-915.

Maloni, H. W. (2000). Pain in multiple sclerosis: An overview of its nature and management. *Journal of Neuroscience Nursing, 32*, 139-144.

Mayeux, R., & Schofeld, P. W. (1994). Alzheimer's disease. In W. R. Hazzard, E. L. Bierman, J. P. Blass, W. H. Ettinger, & J. B. Halter (Eds.), *Principles of geriatric medicine and gerontology* (pp. 1035-1050). New York: McGraw-Hill.

Mazzini, L., Corra, T., Zaccala, M., Mora, G., DelPiana, M., & Galante, M. (1995). Percutaneous endoscopic gastrostomy and enteral nutrition in amyotrophic lateral sclerosis. *Journal of Neurology, 242*, 695-698.

Midgard, R., Riise, T., Kvale, G., & Nyland, H. (1996) Disability and mortality in MS in western Norway. *Acta Neurologica Scandinavica, 93*, 307-314.

Miller, R. G. (2001). Examining the evidence about treatment in ALS/MND. *ALS and Other Motor Neuron Disorders, 2*, 3-7.

Minden, S. L. (2000). Mood disorders in multiple sclerosis: diagnosis and treatment. *Journal of Neurology, 6*(Suppl. 2), S160–S167.

Moulin, D., Foley, K., & Ebers, G. (1988). Pain syndromes in multiple sclerosis. *Neurology, 38*, 1830-1834.

National Hospice Organization. (1996). *Medical guidelines for determining prognosis in selected non-cancer diseases* (2nd ed.). Arlington, VA: Author.

National Institute on Aging. (2000). *Progress report on Alzheimer's disease: Taking the next steps* (NIH Publ. No. 00-4859). Rockville, MD: Author.

Northwest Regional Spinal Cord Injury System. (1998, Spring). Non-invasive ventilator. *Spinal Cord Injury Update, 7*(1). *Retrieved from http://depts.washington.edu/rehab/sci/updates/98sp_noninvasivehtml*

Oliver, D. (1993). Ethical issues in palliative care—an overview. *Palliative Medicine, 7*(Suppl. 2), 15-20.

Ozuna, J. M. (2000). Chronic neurological problems. In S. M. Lewis, M. M. Heitkemper, & S. R. Dirksen (Eds.) *Medical-surgical nursing: Assessment and management of clinical problems* (pp. 1672-1712). St. Louis: Mosby.

Peck, A., Cohen, C. E., & Mulvihill, M. N. (1990). Long-term enteral feeding of aged demented nursing home residents. *Journal of the American Geriatrics Society, 38*, 1195-1198.

Pfeiffer, R. F. (2000) Gastrointestinal dysfunction in Parkinson's disease. *Clinical Neuroscience, 5*, 136-146.

Pollak, C. P., & Stokes, P. E. (1997) Circadian rest-activity rhythms in demented and non-demented community residents and their caregivers. *Journal of the American Geriatrics Society, 45*, 446-452.

Richert, J. R. (1999). Demyelinating illness. In W. N. Kelly (Ed.), *Textbook of internal medicine* (pp. 2385-2388). Philadelphia: Lippincott.

Rohrbaugh, R. M., & Siegal, A. P. (1989). Reversible anorexia and rapid weight loss associated with neuroleptic administration in Alzheimer's disease. *Journal of Geriatric Psychology and Neurology, 2*, 45-47.

Sadovnik, A. D., Eisen, K., Ebers, G. C., & Paty, D. W. (1991). Cause of death in patients attending multiple sclerosis clinics. *Neurology, 41*, 1193-1196.

Sivak, E. D., Shefner, J. M., & Sexton, J. (1999). Neuromuscular disease and hypoventilation. *Current Opinion in Pulmonary Medicine, 5*, 355-362.

Smyth, M. D., & Peacock, W. J. (2000). The surgical treatment of spasticity. *Muscle & Nerve, 23*, 153-163.

Snow, B. J. (1997). Extrapyramidal disorders. In W. N. Kelly (Ed.), *Textbook of internal medicine* (pp. 2388-2390). Philadelphia: Lippincott.

Snow, B. J., Tsui, J. R. C., & Bhatt, M. H. (1990). Treatment of spasticity with botulinum toxin: A double blind study. *Annals of Neurology, 28*, 512-515.

Stocchi, F., Barbato, L., Nordera, G., Berardelli, A., & Ruggieri, S. (1998). Sleep disorders in Parkinson's disease. *Journal of Neurology, 245*(Suppl. 1), S15–S18.

Teddy, P. J. (1995). Implants for spasticity. *Bailliere's Clinical Neurology, 4*, 95-114.

Thompson, A. J. (1996). Multiple sclerosis: Symptomatic treatment. *Journal of Neurology, 243*, 559-565.

Van Ort, S., & Phillips, L. (1992). Feeding nursing home residents with Alzheimer's disease. *Geriatric Nursing, 13*, 249-253.

Volicer, L., Harper, D. G., Manning, B. C., Goldstein, R., & Satlin, A. (2001). Sundowning and circadian rhythms in Alzheimer's disease. *American Journal of Psychiatry, 158*, 704-711.

Volicer, L., Seltzer, B., Rheume, Y., Karner, J., Glennon, M., Riley, M. E., et al. (1989). Eating difficulties in patients with probable dementia of the Alzheimer type. *Journal of Geriatric Psychiatry and Neurology, 2*, 188-195.

Wilson, R. S., Bennett, D. A., Gilley, D. W., Beckett, L. A., Schneider, J. A. & Evans, D. A. (2000). Progression of Parkinsonian signs in Alzheimer's disease. *Neurology, 54*, 1284-1289.

14

END-STAGE RENAL DISEASE AND DISCONTINUATION OF DIALYSIS

Lynn H. Simpkins and Lynn R. Noland

Case Study

Mr. G. lost his renal function from hypertensive nephrosclerosis. Years of poor blood pressure control caused irreversible scarring of the kidneys and finally end-stage renal disease (ESRD). He initially declined dialysis because he simply could not see how, at age 62, he could tolerate being tied to any sort of technological life support, but later agreed to a trial. He would ultimately spend 10 years on dialysis.

He and his family adjusted to the 4-hour treatments three times a week. His wife became an expert in managing the various aspects of therapy required to compensate for loss of renal function. Both were kind and supportive to the other patients undergoing dialysis at the same time. They were deeply religious people who brought a sense of grace and peace to the dialysis setting.

Last August, when Mr. G. told his family and the staff that he could no longer tolerate dialysis, it was understandable but emotionally difficult. Because of progressive severe peripheral vascular disease, he was in constant pain. The cause of the increasingly intense pain seemed to have been related to a revision of his hemodialysis graft, which necessitated stopping the warfarin (Coumadin) that he took to treat chronic deep venous thrombosis. As his prothrombin time drifted into a nontherapeutic range (as measured by the international normalized ratio), he began having problems with thrombosis and leg pain that did not resolve even after the Coumadin was resumed. Soon he was no longer able to participate in church and family events, and this made his quality of life unacceptable to him. Each time he had to come in for dialysis, he experienced more pain than was tolerable, and he was now wheelchair-bound with leg and foot ulcerations from ischemia. It became clear from his lab values that he was not eating adequately (albumin, 3.1 g/dL; blood urea nitrogen, 30 mg/dL; potassium, 3.0 mg/dL—these values should be higher in dialysis patients).

The dialysis care team arranged for him to be seen by the palliative care team. Mr. G., his wife, and the dialysis nurse went to the appointment. The doctor skillfully questioned him about what he found intolerable. He determined that Mr. G. was not amenable to amputation and that his pain and subsequent inactivity were the reasons for his desire to withdraw support. He was offered a trial of several different types of pain-control medications, including oxycodone and fentanyl lozenges for breakthrough pain. Mr. G. agreed to try these therapies for 1 month. If there was no relief at the end of that period, he wanted to withdraw from treatment. He also said that he only wanted to dialyze twice weekly. All understood and sadly agreed.

Miraculously, by the end of the month, the pain had lessened greatly with the help of the powerful analgesics. Circulation to his legs also improved sufficiently for the ulcers to begin to heal. Mr. G. was able to resume some of his church and family activities. He even decided to dialyze three times weekly. A good prognostic indicator was that his appetite and his lab values improved.

Questions that the nurse should consider are

What is the incidence and prevalence of ESRD, as well as access and barriers to care, in the over-60 age group?

What are the manifestations of ESRD in the older adult and the associated etiology?

What are the treatment options for ESRD in older adults?

What are common indicators of prognosis and quality of life for patients with ESRD?

What can patients and families expect when dialysis is withdrawn?

What comfort measures did Gene's family and health care team implement to make his death more tolerable?

What else can be done to make patients comfortable in the home or the hospital at the end of life?

How could a supportive home environment have been simulated if Gene had not had such a capable family?

INTRODUCTION

A diagnosis of ESRD is an ominous sign that a patient has severe end-organ kidney damage and failure. With ESRD, pathology is so extensive that the normally resilient kidneys finally reach a point where they no longer function well enough to remove fluid, balance electrolytes, stimulate red blood cell production, or accomplish a myriad of physical and chemical processes necessary to sustain life. ESRD requires dialysis therapy or death will occur within a relatively short time, usually 7 to 10 days.

Care of older adults with ESRD is exceedingly complex. Patients with ESRD typically have at least two disabling comorbidities that result in frequent, often serious complications. On average, however, the older patient with ESRD has four significant comorbidities or complications that could result in death, but often not before a spiral of worsening symptoms and chronic overall decline.

When faced with the medical complexity of ESRD patients, the temptation for the health care professional is to focus primarily on correcting laboratory values or dwelling on the numerous physical manifestations of ESRD. This approach is too simplistic, resulting in a less than satisfactory experience for patient and provider. The goal for elders with ESRD cannot be simply to preserve life, but must include preservation of quality of life—two goals that are often in conflict, which adds to the complexity of care. The broader goal that incorporates quality of life

necessitates a holistic team-oriented approach, the importance of which is discussed later in the chapter.

Although the lifespan of an individual with ESRD cannot be reliably known, data are available for the group as a whole. Five-year survival rates for the ESRD dialysis population are 31% (U.S. Renal Data System [USRDS], 2001), which are worse than those for many cancer diagnoses, including breast (73%), colon (53%), and leukemia (38%). The death rate among ESRD patients is lower only than that in patients with the deadliest cancers (lung, liver, and pancreas) (United States Cancer Statistics Working Group, 2002). After 30 years of caring for ESRD patients treated with renal replacement therapy, we know that the disease trajectory involves brief stable periods followed by intervals of steady decline, and finally death. Realistically, death is seen as a frequent and expected occurrence when caring for patients with ESRD. Cognizance of these less than optimistic statistics can guide the health care team to make more appropriate therapy decisions.

The grim prognostic picture associated with ESRD justifies a conservative treatment approach. Excluding those patients who have the option of a living kidney donation, the most realistic way for clinicians to think about ESRD is as a terminal disease for which palliative care is often the most effective form of therapy. Quality end-of-life care is an important goal for those who care for elders with ESRD—a goal consistent with a palliative care approach.

The care of patients with ESRD can be thought of as care of two main groups: (1) the chronically ill and (2) the older adult. ESRD is increasingly becoming a disease of older adults, with 65 years being the average age at the initiation of dialysis. Kidney failure is often caused by and then added to the common health problems that older people tend to have, such as diabetes and hypertension. These other baseline disorders do not resolve when renal replacement therapy is provided. They continue their course and synergistically add complexity to the treatment. To confound ESRD care further, the general aspects of interventions associated with geriatric care of the older adult add additional challenges for providers. Vulnerability, frailty, disability, chronic pain, chronic anemia, bone disease, malnutrition, and other issues all enter into the complex algorithm of care for the older patient with ESRD.

The older demographic profile of ESRD is the result of a combination of factors such as improved nutrition and public health practices as well as improved treatment outcomes for some of the diseases prevalent in older people. The cornerstone of the American health care system is treatment of disease rather than prevention, so as people live longer, they are also living sicker. The result is that end-stage diseases of all types now have a higher incidence and prevalence, especially in older age groups. ESRD is no exception. Aggressive cardiovascular risk factor and blood glucose management may simply delay ESRD changes long enough for these patients to live into their 60s, 70s, and beyond, thus adding the element of increased age to the multitude of variables that have to be considered when providing care for patients on dialysis.

This chapter emphasizes the unique qualities and needs of elders with ESRD and their families at the end of life and the most current clinical thinking regarding their care.

FUNCTION OF THE KIDNEYS

The main functions of the kidneys are (Schena, 2001)

1. Maintenance of body composition. The kidneys regulate the volume of fluid in the body and its osmolarity, electrolyte content, concentration, and acidity by varying urine excretion of ions and water. Electrolytes that are excreted by the kidneys include sodium, potassium, chloride, calcium, magnesium, and phosphate. Numerous functions in the body are dependent upon maintenance of optimal body fluid composition and volume, such as
   a. Cardiac output
   b. Blood pressure
   c. Enzymes (most function best within a narrow range of pH)
   d. Cell membrane potentials (directly affected by potassium concentration)
   e. Membrane excitability (depends on calcium concentration in the body fluid)

2. Excretion of metabolic end products and foreign substances. The kidneys excrete metabolic end products such as urea as well as many drugs and toxins.
3. Production and secretion of enzymes and hormones:
   a. Renin is a catalyst in the formation of angiotensin and is a potent vasoconstrictor that is involved in sodium balance and blood pressure regulation.
   b. Erythropoietin stimulates the maturation of erythrocytes in the bone marrow and, when absent, causes anemia of chronic renal disease.
   c. 1,25-Dihydroxyvitamin D_3 is a steroid that is integral in regulating calcium and phosphorus in the body.

COMMON SYMPTOMS OF RENAL DISEASE (Box 14-1)

Early in the disease course, there may be few or no symptoms of renal failure. Patients have time to adjust to their renal failure because it is a chronic process, and often do not realize how badly they have been feeling until they have been on dialysis for several weeks. The symptoms increase in severity as renal function decreases. Different patients develop symptoms at varying glomerular filtration rates (GFRs). Many older renal patients do not develop symptoms of chronic renal disease until their GFR is below 10 mL/min.

INCIDENCE AND PREVALENCE

The word "epidemic" is increasingly used to describe the current incidence and prevalence of renal disease. The greatest rate of change is in the 65 and over age group. As expected, ESRD rates are increasing proportionate to the overall rate of increase in kidney disease. From 1986 to 1996, the incidence (new cases) reported per year of ESRD increased from 600 million to 1200 million in the 65- to 74-year-old age group (USRDS, 2001). This has been compared statistically to the almost flat rate of change in incidence of ESRD for the 20- to 64-year-old age group.

The increase in ESRD is not simply a U.S. health problem. For example, in Sweden, the number of those 65 years or older diagnosed with ESRD increased from 45% of the total number of

---

Box 14-1 Symptoms of Chronic Renal Disease

Early Symptoms
- Anemia
- Hypertension
- Leg cramps, joint pain, gout, arthritis, muscular pains, muscle weakness
- Edema
- Gains in weight with fluid retention
- Weakness and fatigue

Late Symptoms
- Dry, scaly skin and pruritus
- Frequent headaches
- Heat or cold intolerance
- Ammonia or urine smell to breath
- Metallic taste in mouth
- Poor healing of cuts, abrasions
- Chest pain or palpitations
- Dyspnea, orthopnea, paroxysmal nocturnal dyspnea
- Easy bruising, purpura, bleeding
- Losses in weight if anorexic or having problems with nausea and vomiting
- Fainting, seizures, peripheral neuropathy, decreased concentration and memory, mood swings and depression
- Grayish-bronze color with underlying pallor, uremic frost
- Coma, death

From Henrich, W. L. (1999). *Principles and practice of dialysis* (2nd ed.). Philadelphia: Lippincott Williams & Wilkins.

---

cases of ESRD in 1991 to 60% in 1997 (Hagren, Pettersen, Severinsson, Lutzen, & Clyne, 2001). This is consistent with the overall increase in the number of persons worldwide living longer (to 65 years and older). As noted previously, with increasing age comes increased susceptibility to all forms of illness, including ESRD.

Even though ESRD is becoming an international health problem, dialysis is predominantly a phenomenon of highly industrialized societies, with the United States, Great Britain, and Japan accounting for almost 80% of all dialysis treatments worldwide. Developing nations cannot begin to afford the price tag attached to providing renal replacement therapy when even access to basic food and shelter is a daily challenge (Iglehart, 1993).

Access and Barriers to Care

In the United States, older adults have not been excluded from access to the benefits (and burdens) of technologic innovation. Once the decision was made by the U.S. Congress and signed into law in 1972 by President Nixon to provide public funding for dialysis through the Medicare system, all patients with kidney failure who needed renal replacement therapy were considered eligible regardless of age, making it the most expensive medical entitlement in U.S. history (Iglehart, 1993).

The reason for this landmark public policy decision is complex. Medicare financing was made available as a result of public anxiety and pressure that arose when it became clear that dialysis was allocated by committees deciding who should live (by being provided dialysis) and who would die (by withholding dialysis). These committees often took social criteria into consideration, such as marital status, occupation, and dependents. Unable to tolerate rationing based on these types of subjective parameters, legislators sought a funding solution based on medical need alone. The sponsor of the amendment, Senator Vance Harks, justified funding by asking his colleagues at a hearing how society would explain that the difference between life and death was a matter of dollars (Iglehart, 1993).

This equanimity of access was not universal. In Great Britain, age was initially used as a criterion for the initiation of dialysis. Those over age 50 were not eligible for publicly funded dialysis or transplantation. The age criterion was eliminated in the 1970s as the costs associated with dialysis decreased and public pressure to change the rule increased. Logically, older members of British society were opposed to age-based rationing. Elders typically expected the same care that would be offered to younger patients, if medically indicated. In a British survey of 50 people age 65 years of age or older, patients were asked if they would opt for dialysis if their kidneys failed and 84% said yes. Eighty-three percent said they would want to be dialyzed even if they were severely physically limited (Cohen, McCue, Germain, & Kjellstrand, 1995).

Not only is age used as a criterion for withholding or providing dialysis, but ability to pay is also used to determine if someone is offered treatment for ESRD. Regardless of how health care access systems are designed, more financially secure citizens can avail themselves of both dialysis and transplantation, often regardless of age. In the case of transplantation, if one can afford to pay, the only limiting factors are physical health as it relates to surgical survival and willingness to donate on the part of a living matched donor. This raises ethical questions for providers who make decisions about allocation of dialysis and transplant resources. Should a scarce lifesaving resource only be offered to those who can afford to pay for it themselves, or should there be more equitable means available to provide these types of therapies?

Most providers agree that dialysis and transplantation should not be withheld solely for reasons of age or ability to pay. Their thinking is partially colored by individual experience and reinforced by research. For example, one study that compared patients age 60 years or older with younger patients undergoing renal replacement therapy indicated that psychosocial well-being reported by older patients is as good as, and in some instances better than, that of younger patients (Kutner, 1994). Consensus is that need or medical necessity should be the primary determining factor, and then secondary factors such as comorbidities, relative mortality risk, and quality of life on dialysis should be taken into consideration. Age should be a distant consideration to the degree that it affects medical outcomes. In a just society, ability to pay simply should not enter into decision making when it comes to dialysis or transplantation.

Many older patients who are suitable candidates are not referred to a nephrologist and thus are denied dialysis. Sekkarie, Cosma, and Mendelssohn (2000) conducted a prospective study of 76 primary care physicians and 22 nephrologists. The primary care physicians withheld dialysis from 22% of ESRD patients compared to 7% withheld by nephrologists. The primary care physicians did not refer these patients 25% of the time, and 60% cited age as a reason not to refer. Increasing numbers of comorbidities also decreased referrals for dialysis. Other factors noted in physician nonreferral were distance from the dialysis center, lack of transportation, and overcrowding of the nearest dialysis center. Given that these problems exist across age groups, it is perhaps illogical to withhold treatment from elders based on this general issue alone.

MANIFESTATIONS OF ESRD IN THE OLDER ADULT

Diagnosis of kidney disease in the older adult is elusive. Changes of aging occur in the kidney just as they do in all other organ systems. Structural changes include loss of renal mass, sclerosis of vessels, and reduction in the number and functional capacity of glomeruli; GFR also declines. Estimated renal function (GFR) as measured by 24-hour urine collection for creatinine clearance generally declines as well. However, it is also observed that at least one third of all older persons experience little or no decline in clearance (Oreopoulos, Hazzard, & Luke, 2000).

In spite of this fact, some providers rely heavily on one measurement, serum creatinine, which is a measurement that can often convey an inaccurate estimate of kidney function. Serum creatinine levels are linked to muscle mass, and muscle mass often declines in older adults. The lower the muscle mass, the lower the creatinine production. This gives health care providers a false impression of adequate kidney function because serum creatinine is low. As people age, creatinine production falls at nearly the same rate that renal clearance of creatinine declines (Lindeman, Tobin, & Shoch, 1985). This makes serum creatinine a particularly unreliable indicator of the degree and severity of renal disease in older adults. For example, an elder with low muscle mass and a creatinine of 2.0 mg/dL might have more advanced renal disease than another patient who has a creatinine of 4.0 mg/dL with near-normal muscle mass.

Providers expect changes to occur in structure and function of the kidneys of older patients; therefore, kidney disease may not be identified as early in the older patient as in a younger population group and may be well advanced by the time it is finally diagnosed. It is difficult to distinguish age-related changes in estimated function from those of chronic kidney disease. In fact, several recent studies suggested that there are no completely precise ways of estimating kidney function. For this reason, practice guidelines published by the National Kidney Foundation's (NKF's) Dialysis Outcomes Quality Initiative (NKF-DOQI) (NKF, 1997b) suggested further work-up and evaluation if the estimated renal clearance (creatinine clearance) is measured at less than 90 mL/min. A value of 90 mL/min may be completely normal, but, because of the confusing and conflicting clinical picture associated with the evaluation of renal function in older adults, the practice guidelines recommend erring on the side of caution and assessing older patients more thoroughly, with higher cutoff points for clearances (Oreopoulos et al., 2000).

Recently, one method of measuring renal function has seemed to be more accurate than others for the purpose of estimating an elder's renal function. This is a formula that was developed from the Modification of Diet in Renal Disease (MDRD) study, designed to evaluate the influence of dietary factors on manifestations of renal disease (Kopple et al., 2000). The MDRD formula correlated 91% of the time to within 30% of the values obtained with iothalamate measurement of GFR. Iothalamate is considered the most accurate (but expensive) way to measure kidney function. The MDRD abbreviated formula is as follows:

$$186 \times Scr^{-1.154} \times age^{-0.203} \times 0.742 \text{ (if female)}$$
$$or \times 1.210 \text{ (if African American)}$$

where Scr is the serum creatinine level. Alternatively, the calculator on the Nephron Information Center website (*nephron.com/cgi-bin/mdrd.cgi*) can be utilized.

ETIOLOGY OF ESRD IN THE OLDER ADULT

Older patients may be affected by any of the same kidney diseases as those seen in other age groups. However, there are several diseases that are more prevalent with advancing age. Glomerular diseases are the most common cause of end-stage disease in any age group. The most common glomerular disorders in older adults are membranous glomerulonephritis and glomerular sclerosis secondary to diabetes and hypertension. Incidence rates for specific kidney diseases are not thought to be completely accurate primarily

because the rates are dependent upon biopsy results. However, biopsies are only done in those patients for whom diagnosis is unclear. The result is that biopsies are rarely done if diabetes or hypertension is believed to be the etiology of kidney disease, and they are done less frequently in older patients overall. This means that there is more likelihood of diagnostic uncertainty for older adults (Oreopoulos et al., 2000).

SYMPTOMS AND TREATMENT OPTIONS

Treatment options for ESRD include peritoneal dialysis, hemodialysis, kidney transplant, and supportive care with eventual death. The overall goal of treatment for an older patient should be maintenance of health status at an optimal level of functioning. The older patient and his or her family should be informed about the advantages and disadvantages of all treatment options so they can choose the method that will maximize the patient's and family's quality of life. It is important to consider the psychosocial impact of the illness and its treatment on the daily lives of the patient and his or her family (Henrich, 1999).

Uremia may present in a different manner in older patients. There may be dementia, changes in personality, congestive heart failure, or simply a change in the patient's sense of well-being. Many of the signs and symptoms of uremia are often attributed to the aging process itself, and may be overlooked. A trial of dialysis can establish whether the symptoms are due to uremia or other disorders (Oreopoulos et al., 2000).

Indications for initiation of dialysis in the older patient are identical to those in younger patients. Uremic encephalopathy, pericarditis, gastritis, colitis, and neuropathy are indications of the need for immediate dialysis. Fatigue, lethargy, accumulation of fluid, loss of appetite, severe anemia, and hyperkalemia are some of the less acute reasons to begin dialysis in all age groups. Patients without symptoms are usually started at a GFR of 10 mL/min. Many nephrologists are more conservative with diabetics and initiate dialysis when the GFR falls to 15 mL/min (Henrich, 1999).

Indications for choosing one dialysis modality over another include lifestyle choice by the patient, physician preferences, distance to the nearest dialysis center, and concurrent illnesses. Comorbidities such as congestive heart failure or hypertension, specific contraindications to a particular dialysis modality, financial allocation of scarce resources, vascular access limitations, and age bias are also considerations. Either type of dialysis can generally be used; however, in the United States, hemodialysis is the most frequent form of renal replacement therapy for the older adult, while peritoneal dialysis is the second most common modality. In the United States, 83% percent of patients age 65 or older are treated with hemodialysis, 11% are treated with peritoneal dialysis, and only 5% have a functioning transplant. Internationally, hemodialysis and peritoneal dialysis are used in equal proportions. In the general ESRD population in Europe, 60% of the patients are on hemodialysis, 11% use peritoneal dialysis, and 25% have a functioning transplant (Henrich, 1999). Nationally only 5% of U.S. patients over age 65 are transplanted. By comparison, in Norway, 55% of patients over age 65 have transplants (Oreopoulos et al., 2000).

As noted, peritoneal dialysis is the second most common treatment modality and is actually an equally good choice, unless patients have clear contraindications. These would include dementia, inability to perform dialysis unless there is a competent partner to perform it, severe peripheral vascular disease, abdominal aortic aneurysm, active diverticular disease, blindness, physical or psychosocial inability to perform peritoneal dialysis, morbid obesity, poor skin healing, inguinal or abdominal hernias, or compromised peritoneal surface area secondary to abdominal surgery or adhesions. There are also very good reasons to use peritoneal dialysis instead of hemodialysis. It is possible that patients who do poorly on hemodialysis secondary to access problems or cardiovascular disease may improve with peritoneal dialysis.

All treatment options are replete with complications, especially for the older patient. Older patients have more complications with hemodialysis than with peritoneal dialysis. They include arrhythmias, vascular access–related infections, and gastrointestinal bleeding. Older peritoneal dialysis patients often have poor nutrition, require transfer to hemodialysis more often, and are hospitalized more frequently than younger patients. Interestingly, peritoneal dialysis access catheter infections are less frequent in elders than in the young (Oreopoulos et al., 2000).

Nontreatment Option: Withholding or Withdrawing Dialysis

A final option, and perhaps one that should be considered more seriously, is to suggest that patients may decline dialysis altogether, or that dialysis may be withdrawn after a trial if it becomes burdensome. These are valid options. Health care practitioners should be prepared to accept these decisions as long as the patient has the capacity to make a decision of this magnitude, and the decision is not the product of overwhelming clinical depression.

A "trial" of dialysis can be suggested with clear stopping points established with the patient, such as time to feel well or finish family or personal business. The patient who is not mentally competent places the provider in a more difficult situation. Finding the appropriate decision maker and involving the elder is important. Often the social worker and the ethics consult team can be helpful in wading through the legal and ethical implications of deciding for or against dialysis for patients who lack mental capacity.

The health care team should be in agreement that stopping dialysis for patients for whom it is overly burdensome and never starting dialysis are basically ethically equivalent. In fact, if there is any difference, it is that a trial of dialysis is in many ways a more compassionate and life-honoring approach. According to government data, withdrawal from dialysis is actively utilized; it is the second most common reason for death in the older dialysis population, much more common than in the younger dialysis population.

Interestingly, African American patients are 50% to 66% less likely to stop dialysis than are white patients (Oreopoulos et al., 2000). It is not known why there is such a discrepancy associated with race. The most likely patients to withdraw from dialysis are white, female nursing home residents older than 65 years of age. Furthermore, they are more likely to have chronic diseases such as dementia or malignancy. Patients who perform their own hemodialysis at home are more likely

---

EVIDENCE-BASED PRACTICE

Reference: Holley, J. L. (2002). A single center review of the death notification form: Discontinuing dialysis before death is not a surrogate for withdrawal from dialysis. *American Journal of Kidney Diseases, 40,* 525-530.

Research Problem: How do dialysis patients die? How many die because they no longer wish to be dialyzed? This should be a relatively simple question to answer. Renal replacement therapy for ESRD is 80% funded by the federal government through Medicare; therefore, a death notification form must be filled out to notify the insurer when ESRD patients die. It is logical to think that review of these forms would provide answers to questions like the one above. This is not necessarily the case.

Design: Retrospective record review.

Sample and Setting: Medicare ESRD patients who have died.

Methods: A total of 212 federal 2746 death notification forms were reviewed to determine cause of death for patients with ESRD.

Results: Few patients died because of an active decision to withdraw from dialysis, although discontinuation of dialysis was listed as the cause of death for 26%, or 56 patients. Only 8 of these 56 patients were listed as having death attributed to uremia. Most died from cancer and cardiovascular disease in hospitals, not in hospice (only two died in hospice care).

Implications for Nursing Practice: The terms *discontinuing dialysis* and *active withdrawal from dialysis by patients* do not have the same meaning, and substituting one term for the other does not allow accurate evaluation of events leading to death of dialysis patients.

Conclusion: The authors concluded that use of the 2746 form may not provide an accurate answer to the question of how dialysis patients die because there appears to be provider uncertainty about the meaning attributed to the phrase *discontinuing dialysis*. A secondary finding is the low number of ESRD patients referred for hospice care, which suggests that adequate end-of-life support may be lacking for dialysis patients.

---

to withdraw from dialysis when compared to patients who have in-center hemodialysis. Patients elect withdrawal from dialysis most commonly in their third month of treatment (Leggat, Bloembergen, Levine, Hulbert-Shearon, & Port, 1997).

Elders and Transplantation

In the early years of renal transplantation, candidates were rejected if they were over 55 years of age. Between 1988 and 1995, 27% to 34% of the recipients of cadaveric renal allografts were over 50 years of age. During the same period of time, the transplantation rate of patients over age 50 who received kidneys from living donors more than doubled from 10% to 23%. In 1997, 30% of all patients on transplant waiting lists were 50 to 64 years of age, and 7% were over age 65.

Currently, biologic age is more important than chronologic age in assessing a patient's suitability for transplant (Oreopoulos et al., 2000).

There is an initial increased mortality rate in the early post-transplant period for older patients, but the long-term mortality is lower when compared to older patients who remain on dialysis. Patients with transplants had a 5-year survival rate of 81% compared to 51% for patients remaining on dialysis. There is a lower risk of renal allograft rejection in older as compared to younger transplant patients, with the major cause of allograft loss being death resulting from cardiovascular disease or infection. Paradoxically, a senescent immune system of the older patient, in the presence of triple immunosuppressive therapy, may predispose the patient to more virulent infections, but also has the potential for decreasing the risk of graft rejection. The cytochrome P-450 microsomal enzyme system is less active in older adults, putting them at higher risk for cyclosporine toxicity, which leads to more graft failure in the first year post-transplant than do episodes of rejection (Oreopoulos et al., 2000).

Elders are transplanted infrequently; therefore, there is a lack of data available to determine prognosis. At present, they are assessed as completely as possible pretransplant for survival potential. Most centers require a cardiac catheterization, in addition to a carotid Doppler ultrasound study and echocardiogram. Peripheral Doppler studies are frequently employed as well. Colonoscopy is usually required, as is measurement of prostate-specific antigen for male candidates. Some centers require a gallbladder ultrasound to evaluate for cholelithiasis, which can be life threatening if infection occurs in the gallbladder after transplant. The geriatric transplant patient has an increased risk of cytomegalovirus infection, so pretransplant ganciclovir is recommended by many transplant centers. Rehabilitation plans for postoperative support are important in avoiding long hospitalizations after transplant (Oreopoulos et al., 2000).

Many ethical issues surround the transplantation of renal allografts in the geriatric population. There is a shortage of available kidneys for transplantation in the United States. Pundits call for justification of using kidneys from this limited pool for older patients with a shortened life expectancy. Geriatric patients with ESRD have higher rates of comorbidities and often are not medically eligible for transplant. There is a common misconception that advanced age is a barrier to transplant success. Many centers encourage older patients to find living donors. It has been suggested that a "senior citizen's pool" be developed to offer kidneys from older donors to older recipients, because the shortened long-term graft survival of these older kidneys would be a lesser issue in an older patient.

DYING TRAJECTORY
Morbidity and Mortality

As indicated previously, survival rates for ESRD are depressingly short. There is an expected 20% death rate per year, with the rate being even higher in older patients. The life expectancy of a person between the ages of 60 and 64 on dialysis is 2.7 to 3.9 years, versus 7.1 to 11.5 years for patients between the ages of 40 and 44 (USRDS, 2001). Six percent to 10% of all new ESRD patients die within the first 90 days of beginning dialysis (USRDS, 2001). ESRD patients have a mean of four comorbidities with an average of 15 hospital days per year. These data confirm what is logically expected—this is a sick population with a greatly shortened life expectancy. These are reasons enough to make quality of life a significant focal point of care.

Course and Progression of Illness

As expected, the dying trajectory for ESRD patients is characterized by symptoms of uremia, a term that literally means "urine in the blood." Toxins that the kidney normally eliminates, such as urea, excess phosphorus, potassium, acids, hormonal and protein by-products, sodium, and water, begin to accumulate. Symptoms resulting from this abnormal systemic state cause discomfort as fluid and toxins accumulate. For example, if dying ESRD patients are volume overloaded, dyspnea is almost certain. Knowing this, palliative care providers encourage fluid restriction and recommend that fluids be given only to provide comfort from thirst and dry mouth.

Uremic pruritus can become unbearable, and treatment should be used liberally (see "Pruritus" later in this chapter for specific treatment options). Anorexia, nausea, vomiting, and diarrhea are common and should be treated symptomatically as described in other chapters of this text. Hyperkalemia commonly occurs and can be the ultimate cause of death. Hyperkalemia first results in hyperreflexia and muscle fasciculation, eventually progressing to muscle weakness, paralysis, cardiotoxicity, and finally death as the cell is no longer able to sustain normal electrical activity. One rare but significant symptom that can cause extreme discomfort is hypothermia, which should be treated symptomatically (Henrich, 1999).

The final phase of the ESRD dying trajectory results from the effect of uremic toxins on the mental and behavioral state of patients. Memory deficits, including amnesia, accompanied by lethargy and drowsiness, are common early signs and symptoms. Gait disturbances, paresthesias, organic psychosis, and finally coma can be seen in the later stages of dying. Families benefit greatly by being informed of the likelihood of these symptoms prior to their occurrence (Henrich, 1999).

Quality of Life

For older patients, quality of life is an important component of care considerations. The most important information to obtain when evaluating quality of life is patient perception. Patients may be willing to accept a quality of life viewed as marginal by the health care team. As indicated previously, research indicates a surprisingly high degree of a sense of well-being in the geriatric dialysis population (Kutner, 1994). Conversely, patients may feel that their provider's view of an acceptable quality of life is intolerable. The only way to know this is to include quality of life data in routine evaluations of ESRD patients (Valderrabano Jofre, & Lopez-Gomea, 2001). Patient perception of what constitutes acceptable quality of life can be actively evaluated using one of a variety of assessment tools that measure quality of life in patients diagnosed with ESRD, such as the Kidney Disease Questionnaire (Lapaucis, Muirhead, Keown, & Wong, 1992) or the Kidney Disease Quality of Life Short Form (Hayes, Kallich, Mapes, Coons, & Carter, 1994).

PALLIATIVE CARE OF COMMON SYMPTOMS
Nausea and Vomiting

If dialysis is withdrawn (or never begun), patients eventually revert to a uremic state; uremic toxins accumulate and can cause chemically induced nausea. The mechanism of this type of nausea is stimulation of the central nervous system center referred to as the chemoreceptor trigger zone. Blocking receptors in this zone, located in the fourth ventricle of the brain, seems to be the most effective pharmacologic therapy for treatment of metabolically induced nausea and vomiting (Mannix, 1998).

Haloperidol given at 1.5 to 5 mg daily by mouth or subcutaneously is the current treatment of choice, but may cause extrapyramidal side effects such as dystonia, dyskinesia, and akathisia at higher doses. The addition of nonpharmacologic therapies, such as the relaxation techniques of guided imagery and progressive muscle relaxation, as well as concomitant use of transcutaneous electrical nerve stimulation and acupuncture, might also be of benefit (Mannix, 1998).

Pain

Pain can occur from any of several comorbidities of ESRD patients. Cancer and peripheral vascular disease are common causes of pain in this patient population and should be aggressively treated.

Respiratory Symptoms

The respiratory function of older adults is thought to be 25% of that of healthy young adults (Ahmedzai, 1998). With the addition of complicating illnesses, respiratory symptoms are not uncommon, and, as generalized systemic failure occurs at the end of life, they become more prevalent. Dyspnea, tachypnea, cough, and breathlessness may be common end-of-life symptoms experienced by elders with ESRD. These are typically the result of hypervolemia, congestive heart failure, and pleural effusion. Relief of these symptoms is crucial to providing comfort at the end of life.

One of the most potent causes of dyspnea is pleural effusion. It may be necessary to remove fluid from the chest by pleural aspiration, regardless of the phase of the dying trajectory, to relieve the feeling of air hunger and promote comfort. This procedure can effectively improve symptoms and lessen air hunger, even if death is imminent. Management of respiratory symptoms involves acknowledging one of the goals of end-of-life care, comfort through symptom management (Ahmedzai, 1998).

Pruritus

Itching from renal failure is thought to be the result of uremic toxin accumulation. The pathophysiologic mechanisms that cause the symptom are many and complex, but most typically pruritus is secondary to increased serum phosphorus. Logically, continuing to give phosphate-binding drugs such as calcium carbonate may be useful to control this uncomfortable symptom. Other interventions include a 0.5% to 2% phenol solution (Sarna) or another menthol phenol cream topically and systemic therapies such as antihistamines, thalidomide, and oral corticosteroids. It is imperative to find at least one intervention that will be effective, because pruritus is described as one of the more miserable of symptoms to endure (Oreopoulos et al., 2000).

EMERGENCY SITUATIONS
Severe Hyperkalemia

Spurious hyperkalemia should be ruled out first by consulting with the laboratory; if the specimen is noted to have hemolysis or marked thrombocytosis, the level may be inaccurate. Repeat testing should be considered in patients with risk factors for hyperkalemia. The development of severe hyperkalemia results from reduced renal excretion of potassium in combination with increased intake of potassium in the diet. Several medications also contribute to hyperkalemia; these include angiotensin-converting enzyme inhibitors, angiotensin II receptor agonists, nonsteroidal anti-inflammatory drugs, potassium-sparing diuretics, high-dose trimethoprim, and cyclosporine (Schena, 2001).

Patients may have no signs or symptoms of hyperkalemia or signs as severe as flaccid paralysis. Electrocardiogram changes parallel the degree of hyperkalemia. There can be initial tenting of the T wave, then P-wave flattening, widening of the QRS complex, and development of a deep S wave. Ventricular fibrillation is usually the cause of death when hyperkalemia is severe (Schena, 2001).

Emergency dialysis is the treatment of choice for patients who are already established on dialysis. Table 14-1 lists the choices for emergency treatment of hyperkalemia in patients who are not yet on dialysis or for dialysis patients when there will be a delay in starting dialysis (Schena, 2001).

Accelerated Hypertension

Diastolic blood pressures repeatedly above 120 mm Hg in adults may indicate accelerated hypertension. An elevated blood pressure alone without symptoms or progressive end-target organ damage rarely requires emergency treatment. Headache is common, and visual impairment with focal neurologic signs can develop. Additional signs and symptoms include generalized weakness, weight loss, and signs of heart failure (Schena, 2001).

These patients should be managed in the hospital because immediate blood pressure lowering is required to prevent or limit target-organ

Table 14-1 **Treatments for Hyperkalemia**

Triage Level Based on Clinical Status and Lab Values	Treatment	Dose	Time to Effect
Emergent	Calcium	20 ml 10% Ca gluconate IV; repeat q 15-20 min as needed	5 min
Urgent	Insulin + glucose	50 ml 50% dextrose + 5-10 U insulin, then 10% dextrose plus 20 U of regular insulin/L at 50-100 mL/h	15 min
	Bicarbonate	50-100 mEq NaHCO$_3$ IV	15 min
	Albuterol	10 mg by nebulized inhalation	15-30 min
	Hemodialysis	0 mEq/L K dialysate	30 min
Less urgent	Exchange resins	Sodium polystyrene sulfonate 30 g PO in 100 mL 20% sorbitol or 60 g rectally in 200 mL water	2 h
	Loop diuretic	Furosemide 250 mg IV	2-4 h

damage, such as hypertensive encephalopathy, intracranial hemorrhage, acute myocardial infarction, acute left ventricular failure with pulmonary edema, or dissecting aortic aneurysm. Initial drug choices include sodium nitroprusside, labetalol, or nicardipine given intravenously. The goal initially is to reduce mean arterial pressure by no more than 25% within minutes to several hours, and then toward 160/100 mm Hg within 2 to 6 hours. Rapid decreases in blood pressure can cause renal, cerebral, or coronary ischemia (Schena, 2001).

Fever
Infection of the dialysis access should always be considered in a febrile dialysis patient, and the most common cause is *Staphylococcus aureus*. Other common causes of fever must also be considered. Many dialysis patients present with chills hours before they develop a fever. Blood cultures should be obtained and evidence sought for other sources of bacterial infection. Empirical antibiotic administration should be seriously considered. Access infections, if not aggressively treated, can lead to sepsis and dialysis access failure (Henrich, 1999).

Hemorrhage
Arteriovenous fistulas or prosthetic grafts can bleed between treatments, and occasionally an aneurysm in the wall of the graft will rupture. Pressure should be exerted over the site of bleeding with enough force to stop bleeding, but not too strongly because thrombosis can result. Heavy bleeding or aneurysm rupture is a medical emergency and care should be immediately sought (Henrich, 1999).

Thrombosis
Peripheral dialysis accesses can clot for a variety of reasons. Patients are taught to check their accesses for a bruit and thrill daily and to report when these are absent or decreasing in strength. Early intervention increases the chances of saving the access. Emergency interventional radiologic or surgical therapies are the treatments of choice.

Acute Pulmonary Edema
Elders who are noncompliant with fluid restrictions or who skip dialysis sessions are most prone to develop pulmonary edema. Emergency dialysis is indicated and is often done in the inpatient setting.

Peritonitis
Patients who perform peritoneal dialysis are taught to visually inspect the fluid in each dialysate bag at exchanges for turbidity because it can be an indication of peritonitis. Other symptoms include abdominal pain, fever, and vomiting. The diagnosis is confirmed by the presence of 100 white blood cells/mm^3 of dialysate and later by peritoneal fluid cultures. Early diagnosis and treatment with antibiotics provides the best chance for cure and preserving the access. Repeated infections can cause scarring of the peritoneum that may cause failure of this dialysis method.

Leaks of Peritoneal Fluid
Peritoneal dialysis fluid can leak through many sites. Common signs are edema of the labia, scrotum, or penis, of the soft tissue planes of the catheter insertion site, or of a preexisting hernia. Hydrothorax is a rare and life-threatening complication that can occur. Peritoneal dialysis should be stopped and a work-up begun by the nephrology team. Temporary hemodialysis may

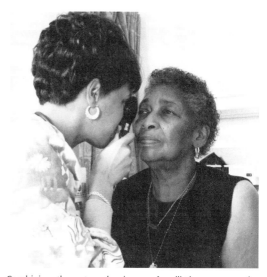

Combining the art and science of palliative care nursing. (Courtesy Mathy Mezey.)

be necessary if the work-up or treatment is prolonged.

Interdialytic Hypotension

Lower cardiac reserves and autonomic neuropathy can make ultrafiltration, or removing volume, from an older dialysis patient difficult. Rapid fluid removal from the intravascular space can exceed the plasma filling rate. In combination with a decreased ability to increase peripheral vascular resistance, abrupt hypotension can occur. Other contributors to hypotension include inadequate cardiac reserves, interdialytic hypoxemia, and medications. Postprandial hypotension is common in this population and occurs because of the patients' inability to increase cardiac output because of increased blood flow to the stomach and gut to digest food. Dialysis often interferes with mealtimes for many patients, and they must skip meals to avoid hypotension. Complications of interdialytic hypotension include seizures, cerebrovascular accidents, myocardial ischemia, aspiration pneumonia, and thrombosis of the dialysis access (Henrich, 1999).

These patients require very careful monitoring of their weight and fluid intake. Many older patients can tolerate no more than 500 to 1000 mL of volume removal per hour. Hypotensive episodes can leave the patient very weak and contribute to falls outside of the dialysis center (Henrich, 1999).

Treatment consists of immediate volume replacement, placing the patient in a recumbent position and, if necessary, using hypertonic saline. Some patients cannot take any antihypertensive medication before dialysis, even if their blood pressures are elevated, or they will have severe hypotension during treatment. Using shorter-acting antihypertensive medications in the evening prior to dialysis can help the patient arrive at treatment with a more acceptable blood pressure without the risk of hypotension during treatment (Schena, 2001).

COMORBIDITIES AND COMPLICATIONS

Many of the comorbidities and complications associated with ESRD develop because the kidneys are no longer able to fulfill their many functions. Most of the comorbidities of dialysis begin to manifest long before the kidneys fail completely, and early identification and treat-

ment of these conditions by a nephrology team can help the patient arrive at dialysis in good health. If dialysis itself is seen as a palliative treatment, then the management of these comorbidities is important to alleviate pain and suffering and also to improve quality of life. The older renal patient's care is particularly challenging because of the numerous comorbid conditions that are usually present and are superimposed upon the normal anatomic and physiologic changes that come with aging. The more comorbidities a patient has, the lower his or her survival rate. For example, diabetes mellitus effectively ages a dialysis patient by a decade (Henrich, 1999).

Renal Osteodystrophy

Aging and ESRD are characterized by low bone turnover. To complicate management, renal osteodystrophy often coexists with the osteoporosis of aging. The long-term effects of superimposing renal bone disease on senile osteoporosis are unknown because of the short survival time of this population. Thus current treatment regimens do not address the treatment of this combination. Bone disease in dialysis patients is most often related to the effects of secondary hyperparathyroidism. Hyperparathyroidism often manifests when the GFR is 50 to 70 mL/min, which is very early in the course of renal failure. The causes for an elevated parathyroid hormone (PTH) level include hypocalcemia, diminished circulating levels of vitamin D_3 (calcitriol), and phosphate retention. Calcitriol acts on cells in the parathyroid glands to reduce PTH synthesis. In uremia, the calcitriol receptors reduce in number and become less sensitive to calcitriol. Furthermore, hyperphosphatemia directly stimulates PTH secretion. Low calcium levels also stimulate the glands to produce more PTH. The glands begin to increase in size through hypertrophy and hyperplasia resulting from increased activity if medical and dietary intervention do not occur (Henrich, 1999).

There are two other forms of renal osteodystrophy, and patients may have several forms at once or move from one form to another. If PTH levels are too low, as happens in some patients, there is risk for adynamic bone disease, in which there is reduced bone activity. Aluminum-related bone disease is rare today because aluminum-based binders are less frequently used and dialysis water treatment has improved to remove aluminum almost completely from the water used in dialysis (Henrich, 1999).

Hyperparathyroid bone disease causes bone pain, joint discomfort, and pruritus. Metastatic calcification, caused by prolonged elevated levels of PTH and phosphorus, allows calcium deposits to accumulate in blood vessels, tissues, organs, and joints. In severe cases, the calcium deposits inflame the conjunctiva and also produce palpable calcium deposits under the skin. Treatment and prevention involve maintaining a good calcium and phosphorus balance in the body through diet and the use of phosphate binders. Foods high in phosphorus include dairy products, meats, legumes, nuts, whole-grain breads and cereals, and many soft drinks. PTH levels are maintained in goal ranges with the use of synthetic vitamin D_3. In severe cases in which the glands are hypertrophied from continued stimulation because serum phosphorus levels have been high for a period of time, parathyroidectomy becomes the treatment of choice. Postoperative hypocalcemia can be life-threatening and a treatment challenge for several months after surgery (Henrich, 1999).

Aluminum-related bone disease causes more severe bone pain that can be incapacitating. Fractures of the ribs and other bones occasionally occur. Anemia also worsens, and central nervous system involvement is common. Deferoxamine is used to remove aluminum from the body intravenously, and it is important to identify the dietary or drug source of aluminum and eliminate it (Henrich, 1999).

Adynamic bone disease, which can lead to osteopenia, is associated with low PTH levels and is usually asymptomatic and more common in whites than African Americans. Treatment is unclear other than preventing oversuppression of PTH levels. Adynamic bone disease is also associated with diabetes, peritoneal dialysis, age, corticosteroids, and immobilization (Henrich, 1999).

Anemia of Chronic Renal Disease

Insufficient production of erythropoietin in the kidneys is the most common cause of anemia in patients with renal disease. Without treatment, the hematocrit will often range from 18% to 24%. Before the advent of epoetin alfa, anemic dialysis patients were frequently transfused with blood products, exposing them to blood-borne diseases, transfusion reactions, viral infections, iron overload, and immune sensitization. Patients with ESRD can develop any of the other causes of anemia that are common in patients without ESRD. Treating anemia when the patient first becomes anemic is key in the prevention of left ventricular hypertrophy (LVH), which increases morbidity and mortality if present when dialysis begins. When the hemoglobin concentration drops below 10 g/dL, patients are particularly prone to develop LVH and dilated cardiomyopathy as well as congestive heart failure. Elders who are treated for anemia have an improved quality of life and overall sense of well-being. Anemia from chronic renal disease can occur a year or more before dialysis is indicated (NKF, 1997a).

Erythropoietin therapy is started in the pre-dialysis period when the creatinine clearance is below 35 mL/min and the hematocrit is between 30% and 33%. The optimal hematocrit for a dialysis patient is not known. The NKF-DOQI (NKF, 1997a) recommended a target range of 33% to 36%. Epoetin alfa can be given subcutaneously or intravenously. Side effects include worsening of hypertension, seizures, and graft clotting. Suboptimal responses to epoetin alfa are frequently due to iron deficiency secondary to rapid utilization of iron to support erythropoiesis or as the result of blood loss.

Hemodialysis patients lose blood with each dialysis treatment. Iron is replaced intravenously because oral iron is often not absorbed well from the gastric mucosa secondary to the accumulated toxins present in the systems of ESRD patients. Inflammation caused by chronic disease or infection lowers the effect of epoetin alfa and impairs release of iron from its storage sites. Hyperparathyroidism also can cause epoetin alfa resistance.

Cardiovascular Disease

Cardiac complications are the leading cause of death in the dialysis population as a whole. Older age in a dialysis patient is a risk factor for LVH, dilated cardiomyopathy, and ischemic heart disease. The prevalence of cardiovascular disease is elevated in the dialysis population because of increased risk factors for atherosclerosis. These risk factors include diabetes mellitus, hypertension, and factors associated with uremia, such as hypertriglyceridemia, hyperparathyroidism, vascular calcification, abnormal calcium and phosphorus metabolism, and elevated levels of homocysteine, urate, oxalate, and inflammatory mediators. LVH is common in the dialysis population and is a strong risk factor for cardiovascular mortality.

Cardiovascular events are the primary cause of death in the majority of dialysis patients. The morbidity of cardiovascular disease influences the quality of life for patients; thus prevention and treatment is important to maintain quality of life. Treatment includes screening for LVH and coronary artery disease (CAD), treating hyperlipidemia using goals for patients who have preexisting CAD, low-sodium and low-fat diets, fluid restrictions, maintaining a calcium/phosphorus product below 55, counseling for smoking cessation, aggressive treatment of diabetes mellitus, and measuring and treating elevations in homocysteine levels. For patients with CAD, attention to maintaining the hematocrit above 30% can help alleviate anginal symptoms. Dialysis patients also have increased risks for endocarditis, pericarditis, and arrhythmias. Sudden death risk is increased and has been linked to hyperkalemia, usually related to dietary intake (Henrich, 1999).

Vascular Access

Dialysis access procedures and complications of dialysis accesses are a major cause of morbidity, hospitalization, and cost for dialysis patients. Successful vascular access placement for dialysis can be complicated by the physiologic changes that occur with aging. Older patients frequently have peripheral vascular calcification or narrowing caused by diabetes, hyperlipidemia, high phosphorus levels, or hypertension. Placement of vascular access in calcified vessels increases the rate of ischemia and thrombosis. In many patients, more proximal and larger vessels must be used.

Complications with vascular access in the older adult are similar to those seen in younger dialysis patients. Arteriovenous fistulas are still the safest and least likely to become infected or result in arterial steal syndromes in which blood supply is decreased proximal to the access. Infection rates in patients with arteriovenous grafts are very high. These infections can be superficial or deep-seated in the graft. Infection can lead to sepsis and graft removal. Older patients who are frail with a history of long-standing atherosclerosis are more prone to steal syndromes, which can lead to amputations of fingers or hands. The "white glove syndrome" is frequently seen, in which patients wear a glove on their access hand to keep it warm. Patients with subclavian catheters or upper arm fistulas or grafts are at risk for subclavian stenosis. In patients with severe heart disease, angina and congestive heart failure can worsen during treatment with peripheral accesses, and subclavian and internal jugular sites may be the only options for dialysis access (Oreopoulos et al., 2000).

Malnutrition

Malnutrition occurs is as many as 20% of older ESRD patients. Mortality increases exponentially as the concentration of serum albumin decreases. Inadequate dialysis or incompatible dialysis membranes can be causative factors for a low albumin. There is a loss of amino acids and peptides into the dialysate at each dialysis. Acidosis and elevated PTH levels can also decrease albumin levels. These changes, combined with the changes of aging, can produce severe malnutrition. In the geriatric ESRD patient, a multidisciplinary approach utilizing home health, social work, dietary, and medical personnel provides the best chances for success. Nutritional supplementation may be necessary in many cases (Oreopoulos et al., 2000).

Nutrition is very important in maintaining the patency of dialysis accesses. Furthermore, it plays an important role in the immune system. Older patients on dialysis with high normal serum albumin levels were more than five times more likely to respond to hepatitis B vaccines than those with low-normal values of 3.01 to 3.5 g/dL (Fernandez, Betriu, Gomez, & Montooiu, 1996).

Healthy older dialysis patients with reduced serum albumin levels had an increased 3-year mortality compared to healthy older dialysis patients with high-normal albumin levels (Henrich, 1999).

Infection

Death rates from infection for older adults are double those of younger patients; septicemia is the second leading cause of death in older ESRD patients. This increased risk of infection is associated with malnutrition and the altered immune response that occurs with aging and ESRD. Sources of sepsis include pneumonia associated with aspiration, gram-positive vascular access infections, gram-negative gastrointestinal tract infections, and gram-negative genitourinary tract infections (Henrich, 1999).

Gastrointestinal Bleeding

Gastrointestinal bleeding occurs more frequently in older ESRD patients and may go undetected. Gastrointestinal bleeding should be considered when there is an unexplained drop in the hematocrit or failure of the hematocrit to respond to epoetin alfa therapy. Uremic gastritis commonly occurs in dialysis patients and is exacerbated by the use of nonsteroidal anti-inflammatory agents. Angiodysplasia, or dilation of a tubular vessel in the intestinal mucosa, can cause acute or slow bleeding. Diverticulosis with perforation associated with constipation is more common in the older patient as well. Gastrointestinal cancers

---

EVIDENCE-BASED PRACTICE

Reference: Holley, J. L., Hines, S. C., Glover, J. J., Babrow, A. S., Badzek, L. A., & Moss, A. H. (1999). Failure of advance planning to elicit patients' preferences for withdrawal from dialysis. *American Journal of Kidney Disease, 33,* 688-693.

Research Problem: Among patients with renal failure who are doing advance care planning, how many included consideration of dialysis withdrawal?

Design: Qualitative interview.

Sample and Setting: A stratified random sample of 450 adult hemodialysis patients located in two geographic areas: six dialysis units within 75 miles of Morgantown, WV, and all nine dialysis units in Rochester, NY.

Methods: Interviews were conducted by trained interviewers during a hemodialysis session with the patient and either face-to-face or by telephone with the patient's surrogate decision maker.

Results: Fifty-one percent of the patients had advanced directives. Of these, 29% had a living will and a health care proxy and 22% had a living will or

a health care proxy. Only 18% of patients had discussed stopping dialysis. This was the least often discussed intervention compared, for example, to mechanical ventilation (69%), tube feedings (55%), and cardiopulmonary resuscitation (43%). Thirty-one percent of the patients who had completed a living will and named a health care proxy had discussed withdrawal from dialysis with their surrogate decision makers, compared to 8% of the patients who had not completed an advance directive.

Implications for Nursing Practice: Patients should be made aware of their options concerning withdrawal of dialysis. Staff should help patients consider conditions under which they might want to withdraw dialysis as part of their advance care planning and help them communicate their wishes to their surrogate decision makers.

Conclusion: Withdrawal from dialysis is very common and occurs before death in at least 19% of chronic dialysis patients, but it appears that patients do not routinely discuss it with their surrogate decision makers. Furthermore, nephrologists and dialysis staff rarely discuss this issue with patients.

also cause gastrointestinal bleeding in this population (Oreopoulos et al., 2000).

Other Comorbidities

Other common comorbid conditions in the older dialysis population include diabetes, pulmonary disease, cancers, cerebrovascular disease, gastrointestinal disorders, and arthritis. The comorbid risk factors with the greatest impact on survival are hypertension, low serum albumin, and predialysis cardiac disease. Older dialysis patients spend an average of 14 to 30 days per year in the hospital compared to 11 to 12 days on average for younger patients with ESRD (Oreopoulos et al., 2000).

FAMILY CONCERNS AND CONSIDERATIONS
Caregiver Fears

ESRD and its treatment can exert a major effect on the family members of the elder patient. Family members and friends of ESRD patients may provide physical care, emotional support, companionship, transportation, housekeeping, and home management tasks. O'Brien (1980) found that the quantity of patient interactions with friends and family increased over time, but that the quality of these interactions decreased. As the patient grows older and key family members are lost, the remaining family members may not be available to help, and those who are can become easily overtaxed. It is important for nurses to identify the support systems for patients and help mobilize these resources. It is common for family members to neglect their own health when caring for the patient, and sometimes they die before the patient. The caregivers in the family need information on community resources for support and respite care.

Flaherty and O'Brien (1992) studied 50 family members of patients who were on dialysis. Five family coping styles were identified from this study: remote, enfolded, altered, distressed, and receptive. A remote family member responds as if the patient's disease has not affected him or her. Enfolded families show signs of strengthening of family bonds between family members and respond as if the disease is a family affair. The altered family shows many changes in their daily activities as a result of their family member's illness. The distressed family displays signs of grief and sorrow about the disease and the changes it has brought about in the family. The receptive family accepts the diagnosis and adjusts to it (Flaherty & O'Brien, 1992).

Many families hope that a kidney transplant will change their lives, although many express concerns about long-term immunosuppression. They also have concerns about other complications that may arise (Voepel-Lewis, Ketefian, Starr, & White, 1990). The most stressful time for families is the period of time during which the patient remains hospitalized after the transplant.

Wagner (1996) found that families identify two psychosocial needs, information and comfort, as important. They want medical staff to listen to their perspectives and want the family to be considered as the patient. Family members also indicated that they have the same needs for information, support, and comfort as the patient. Family involvement can protect the patient from increased stresses, so it is important for medical staff to address frustrations and unmet needs of family members.

Most of the research done in this area to date has been on white, middle-class families; therefore, these study results may not be generalizable to other populations. Nursing strategies may need to change with families from other cultural groups. More research is needed in this area.

Education

The best possible time for education is early in the disease course. As the disease progresses, patients undergo changes in information processing. Early education can review lifestyle choices and treatment options that patients can adopt to slow the progression of their disease. As renal failure advances, patients typically have a more depressed mentation and may require repetition of information. Renal patients often have altered perceptual states and need frequent clarification. Concentration can be decreased, and stimulation and repetition can aid the educational process.

When teaching the older patient with ESRD, there is a need to look at the patient, the environment, and the instructional design. Because of difficulties with transportation, classes are often several hours in length with large amounts of information. Written information can supplement the education, but older patients may have difficulty with vision. It is best for family members and friends to be included in the educational process so they can discuss treatment options and other choices with the patient.

DISCONTINUATION OF RENAL DIALYSIS

Candor associated with death is regrettably somewhat rare institutionally and culturally. This is partially because American patients and families have an idealized view of the capabilities of medicine. As ethicist Daniel Callahan wrote,

> We expect medicine to devise ever more ingenious ways to save our lives. That is why the NIH budget has always risen, budget crisis or not. . . . Why should anyone be astonished . . . that the other message many are trying to deliver—the need to stop treatment—has such a hard time getting through? (Callahan, 1987)

Candor regarding prognosis and life expectancy would perhaps be useful not only to patients who are considering withdrawal of dialysis, but also to those patients who would possibly opt not to begin treatment in the first place, if they knew that, for the geriatric population, overall survival is exceedingly poor.

Openness with patients and families who are considering ending dialysis is a deeply important part of the holistic care of a chronically ill older adult with ESRD. When the limits of medicine and technology are reached, patients are best served when they and all those who are significant to them work toward agreement on a plan of care. This may mean beginning the important therapy and work of care and comfort both for the dying elder and for those who remain after the patient's death. The ability to adjust thinking from preservation of life to care of the dying is crucial for the provision of full-spectrum therapy, especially when working with a highly morbid population, such as elder patients with a diagnosis of ESRD. Any lag time in this transition from thought to deed can create both psychological and physical suffering for all involved. When patients indicate a readiness to think of and speak about their death, providers must be willing to listen and discuss their issues or concerns. The proper therapy at that point is support and therapeutic presence.

Nurses can be helpful by acknowledging the devastating nature of the disease. Discussions regarding prognosis can be guided by the National Hospice Organization (1996) standards for determining prognosis for patients with renal failure (Box 14-2). It is also beneficial to present a palliative care approach to the older adult and his or her family that includes candid communication and a willingness to discuss withdrawal of therapy of all types, including dialysis, when therapy becomes more of a burden than a benefit.

In 2000, the Renal Physicians Association and the American Society of Nephrology (RPA/ASN) responded to an earlier request by the Institute of Medicine to issue guidelines for evaluating patients for whom the burdens of renal replacement therapy may substantially outweigh benefits. The report is an important document intended to provide direction to nephrologists, who, as the population ages and the incidence of ESRD increases, frequently find themselves confronting end-of-life issues (Levine, 2001). At the core of the report is the belief that initiation and withdrawal of dialysis should be a decision that the patient actively participates in (RPA/ASN, 2000). The discussion has to be broached in the context of an interactive mutual relationship between patient and provider.

Case Study Conclusion

Mr. G.'s turnaround continued for approximately 3 months, until after Christmas. He then began to experience nosebleeds from the Coumadin, deterioration in the perfusion to his legs as the Coumadin dose was reduced, and a resumption of the pain. Mr. G. told his family that he was ready to stop dialysis, because he was unwilling to tolerate the current symptoms; the pain and disability were just too great. He wanted to die at home, and his family was committed to granting this last request.

The palliative care team engaged home hospice services to provide comfort and supportive care. The dialysis team agreed to provide dialysis for fluid removal and comfort purposes on an as-needed basis. This provision proved unnecessary because Mr. G. never returned to the dialysis center. Those health care providers who had cared for him over the years stayed in touch with his wife during the 10-day process of his

Box 14-2 **Medical Guidelines for Determining Prognosis: Renal Disease**

I. Laboratory criteria for renal failure.

These values may be used to assess patients with renal failure who are not dialyzed, as well as those who survive more than a week or two after dialysis is discontinued. Patients with this degree of renal failure can be expected to die shortly without dialysis. Bearing in mind individual differences in tolerance for very elevated creatinine levels, critical renal failure is defined as:

A. Creatinine clearance of less than 10 cc/min (less than 15 cc/min for diabetics) AND

B. Serum creatinine greater than 8.0 mg/dl (greater than 6.0 mg/dl for diabetics).

Notes:

1. Creatinine clearance may be estimated by using the following formula, thus avoiding a 24-hour urine collection:

$$Ccreat = \frac{(140 - \text{age in yrs.}) \cdot (\text{body wt. in kg})}{(72) \cdot (\text{serum creat in mg/dl})};$$

multiply by 0.85 for women

2. Blood urea nitrogen (BUN) values are not used in the determination of critical renal failure, since they can be extremely elevated from prerenal azotemia due to dehydration, hypovolemia or other causes.

II. Clinical signs and syndromes associated with renal failure.

The following clinical signs are used as criteria for beginning dialysis. For patients with end-stage renal disease who are not to be dialyzed, the following may help define hospice appropriateness:

A. Uremia: clinical manifestations of renal failure.

1. Confusion, obtundation
2. Intractable nausea and vomiting
3. Generalized pruritis
4. Restlessness, "restless legs"

B. Oliguria: Urine output less than 400 cc/24 hours.

C. Intractable hyperkalemia: persistent serum potassium >7.0 not responsive to medical management.

D. Uremic pericarditis.

E. Hepatorenal syndrome.

F. Intractable fluid overload.

III. In hospitalized patients with ARF, these comorbid conditions predict early mortality:

A. Mechanical ventilation.
B. Malignancy—other organ systems.
C. Chronic lung disease.
D. Advanced cardiac disease.
E. Advanced liver disease.
F. Sepsis.
G. Immunosuppression/AIDS.
H. Albumin <3.5 gm/dl.
I. Cachexia.
J. Platelet count <25,000.
K. Age >75.
L. Disseminated intravascular coagulation.
M. Gastrointestinal bleeding.

From National Hospice Organization. (1996). *Medical guidelines for determining prognosis in selected non-cancer diseases* (2nd ed.). Arlington, VA: National Hospice Organization.

dying, and some nurses visited the home to say good-bye.

Mr. G. remained committed to not having any more invasive therapy and never wavered from this final decision. He spent his last days with his family, his friends, pastors from his church, and the health care providers who knew him best. As symptoms of uremia emerged, the hospice team treated them. His family faithfully followed directions to not overload him with fluids because this would almost certainly add to his discomfort.

In the end, Mr. G. died quietly in the night with his wife of almost 40 years at his side. He had assured her that day that he was ready to die, reliant to the last on his faith. He whispered to her that he would see her again. His loss was difficult for the family, but Mr. G.'s faith and conviction eased the pain. The dialysis staff remembered him as a quiet, respectful man with a smile that illuminated the room. His family was devoted to him, as he was to them. He was 72 when he died, and the funeral was a tribute to a life well lived. Family, friends, and health care providers all gathered in the church one last time on his behalf.

Mr. G.'s case is paradigmatically significant, not only because of what happened and how events occurred, but because of what did not happen as well. He did not die in a hospital cared for by strangers, and there were no intravenous drips, tube feedings, or futile attempts to preserve life when his body was clearly unable to sustain it. All those involved talked about, agreed on, and were sad but comfortable with the decision. Essentially, this is an example of the beneficial effect of open dialogue regarding emotionally difficult topics such as death. Desirable outcomes occur when all involved are willing to speak candidly about death with patients and their families and think about death as a part of the care continuum and not as failed therapy.

CONCLUSION

Aging is associated with an increased prevalence of diabetes and hypertension, as well as a progressive loss of renal reserve. ESRD is burgeoning in the older adult population in the United States. The economic burden threatens to overwhelm the capabilities of the nephrology community and bankrupt the Medicare resources that finance ESRD care. There are also numerous ethical dilemmas involved in the allocation of resources regarding the balance of quality and quantity of life for older adults with ESRD.

A shared decision-making model facilitates explication of patient values and preferences both for the elder patient, his or her family, and the health care team. It can also be an effective way to convey care and concern to older adults as they face one of the most difficult decisions and moments of their lives. As nurses, we are often unable to deliver patients from illness and death for very long, but we can always stand with them in their struggle, and ease their suffering with effective palliative care practices.

RESOURCES
Patient Resources

- American Association of Kidney Patients (AAKP)
  3505 Frontage Road
  Suite 315
  Tampa, FL 33607
  Phone: 1-800-749-2257
  Fax: 1-813-636-8122
  Website: *www.aakp.org*
- National Kidney Foundation, Inc.
  30 East 33rd Street
  Suite 1100
  New York, NY 10016
  Phone: 1-800-622-9010
  Fax: 212-689-9261
  Website: *www.kidney.org/patients*
- United Network for Organ Sharing (UNOS)
  P.O. Box 2484
  Richmond, VA 23218
  Phone: 1-804-782-4800
  Website: *www.unos.org*
- National Institute of Diabetes & Digestive & Kidney Diseases (*www.niddk.nih.gov/health/kidney/kidney.htm*): fact sheets, educational materials, and lists of resource organizations on kidney diseases
- DialysisFinder (*www.dialysisfinder.com*): helps locate dialysis sites near where patients live or for when they travel
- Culinary Kidney Cooks (*www.culinarykidney-cooks.com*): recipes and dialysis tips for kidney patients
- American Kidney Fund (*www.akfinc.org*): information on financial assistance programs, lifestyle ideas, and kidney disease facts; phone: 1-800-638-8299
- ikidney.com (*www.ikidney.com*): general information about kidney disease

Professional Resources

- American Kidney Fund (AKF)
  6110 Executive Boulevard
  Suite 1010
  Rockville, MD 20852
  Phone: 1-301-881-3052
  Fax: 1-301-881-0898
  Website: *www.akfinc.org*

- American Nephrology Nurses Association (ANNA)
  East Holly Avenue
  Box 56
  Pitman, NJ 08071
  Phone: 1-609-256-2320
  Fax: 1-609-589-7463
  Website: *anna.iNurse.com*
- American Society of Nephrology (ASN)
  1725 I Street NW
  Suite 510
  Washington, DC 20006
  Phone: 1-202-659-0599
  Fax: 1-202-659-0709
  Website: *www.asn-online.org*
- National Kidney Foundation (NKF)
  30 East 33rd Street
  Suite 1100
  New York, NY 10016
  Phone: 1-800-622-9010
  Fax: 1-212-689-9261
  Website: *www.kidney.org/professionals*
- RENALNET Kidney Information Clearinghouse (*www.renalnet.org*): clearinghouse for information on causes, treatment, and management of kidney disease and ESRD
- MedWeb (*www.medweb.emory.edu/MedWeb*: lists links to nephrology websites
- Nephron Information Center (*www.nephron.com*): Supports the generation and dissemination of valid information relevant to the professional kidney community and the public.
- American Society of Transplantation (*www.a-s-t.org*): Offers a forum to exchange knowledge. Scientific information and expertise in the field of transplantation.

REFERENCES

Ahmedzai, S. (1998). Palliation of respiratory symptoms. In D. Doyle, G. W. C. Hanks, & N. MacDonald (Eds.), *Oxford textbook of palliative medicine* (2nd ed., pp. 583-616). Oxford, UK: Oxford University Press.

Callahan, D. (1987). *Setting limits: Medical goals in an aging society.* New York: Simon and Schuster.

Cohen, L. M., McCue, J. D., Germain, M., & Kjellstrand, C. M. (1995). Dialysis discontinuation: A good death? *Archives of Internal Medicine, 155*, 42-47.

Fernandez, E., Betriu, M. A., Gomez, R., & Montooiu, J. (1996). Response to the hepatitis B virus vaccine in hemodialysis patients: Influence of malnutrition and its importance as a risk factor for morbidity and mortality. *Nephrology, Dialysis, Transplantation, 11*, 1159-1163.

Flaherty, M. J., & O'Brien, M. E. (1992). Family styles of coping in end stage renal disease. *ANNA Journal, 19*, 345-349, 366.

Hagren, B., Pettersen, I-M., Severinsson, E., Lutzen, K., & Clyne, N. (2001). The hemodialysis machine as a lifeline: Experiences of suffering from end stage renal disease. *Journal of Advanced Nursing, 34*, 196-202.

Hayes, R. D., Kallich, J. D., Mapes, D. L., Coons, S. J., & Carter, W. B. (1994). Development of the Kidney Disease Quality of Life (KDQOL) instrument. *Quality of Life Research, 3*, 329-338.

Henrich, W. L. (1999). *Principles and practice of dialysis* (2nd ed.). Philadelphia: Lippincott Williams & Wilkins.

Iglehart, J. K. (1993). The American health care system: The End Stage Renal Disease Program. *New England Journal of Medicine, 328*, 366-371.

Kopple, J. D., Green, T., Chumlea, W. C., Hollinger, D., Maroni, B. J., Merrill, D., et al. (2000). Relationship between nutritional status and the glomerular filtration rate: Results from the MDRD study. *Kidney International, 57*, 1688-1703.

Kutner, N. G. (1994). Psychosocial issues in ESRD: Aging. *Advances in Renal Replacement Therapy, 1*, 208-210.

Lapaucis, A., Muirhead, N., Keown, P., & Wong, C. (1992). A disease-specific questionnaire for assessing quality of life in patients on hemodialysis. *Nephrology, 60*, 302-306.

Leggat, J. E. Jr., Bloembergen, W. E., Levine, G., Hulbert-Shearon, T. E., & Port, F. K. (1997). An analysis of risk factors for withdrawal of dialysis before death. *Journal of the American Society of Nephrology, 8*, 1755-1763.

Levine, D. Z. (2001). Nephrology Ethics Forum. Shared decision making in dialysis: The new RPA/ASN guideline on the appropriate initiation and withdrawal of treatment. *American Journal of Kidney Diseases, 37*, 1081-1091.

Lindeman, R. D., Tobin, J., & Shoch, N. W. (1985). Longitudinal studies in the rate of decline in renal function with age. *Journal of the American Geriatrics Society, 33*, 278-285.

Mannix, K. A. (1998). Palliation of nausea and vomiting. In D. Doyle, G. W. C. Hanks, & N. MacDonald (Eds.), *Oxford textbook of palliative medicine* (2nd ed., pp. 489-499). Oxford, UK: Oxford University Press.

National Hospice Organization. (1996). *Medical guidelines for determining prognosis in selected non-cancer diseases* (2nd ed.). Arlington, VA: Author.

National Kidney Foundation. (1997a). *National Kidney Foundation Dialysis Outcomes Quality Initiative (DOQI): Clinical practice guidelines for the treatment of anemia of chronic renal failure.* New York: Author.

National Kidney Foundation. (1997b). *National Kidney Foundation Dialysis Outcomes Quality Initiative (DOQI): Executive summaries of the NKF-DOQI clinical practice guidelines.* New York: Author.

O'Brien, M. E. (1980). Hemodialysis regimen compliance and social environment: A panel analysis. *Nursing Research, 29,* 250-255.

Oreopoulos, D. G., Hazzard, W. R., & Luke, R. (Eds.). (2000). *Nephrology and geriatrics integrated.* Dordrecht: Kluwer.

Renal Physicians Association/American Society of Nephrology. (2000).

Schena, F. P. (2001). *Nephrology.* Milan: McGraw-Hill International.

Sekkarie, M., Cosma, M., & Mendelssohn, D. (2000). Non-referral and acceptance to dialysis by primary care physicians & nephrologists in Canada and the United States. *American Journal of Kidney Disease, 38,* 36-41.

United States Cancer Statistics Working Group. (2002). *U.S. cancer statistics, 1999.* Washington, DC: National Cancer Institute/Centers for Disease Control and Prevention.

U.S. Renal Data System. (2001). *Annual data report: Atlas of end stage renal disease in the United States.* Bethesda, MD: National Institute of Diabetes and Digestive and Kidney Diseases.

Valderrabano, F., Jofre, R., & Lopez-Gomez, J. M. (2001). Quality of life in end stage renal disease patients. *American Journal of Kidney Disease, 38,* 443-464.

Voepel-Lewis, T., Ketefian, S., St arr, A., & White, M. J. (1990). Stress, coping, and quality of life in family members of kidney transplant recipients. *ANNA Journal, 17,* 427-432.

Wagner, C. D. (1996). Family needs of chronic hemodialysis patients: A comparison of perceptions of nurses and families. *ANNA Journal, 23,* 19-26, 27-28.

15

CHRONIC LUNG DISEASE

Karen Parr-Day

Case Study

Mr. P., 80, was diagnosed 5 years ago with chronic obstructive pulmonary disease (COPD). His medical history is significant for gastroesophageal reflux disease and numerous hospitalizations for pneumonia. Mr. P.'s last hospital admission for pneumonia was complicated by respiratory failure necessitating endotracheal intubation and mechanical ventilation. This admission took place 6 months ago. His surgical history is noncontributory.

He is a 70-pack-year smoker who continues to smoke against medical advice; he denies alcohol consumption. Mr. P. is a retired accountant, married for 50 years, with three adult children. On physical exam, he is pale and cachectic, with an increased anteroposterior (AP) chest diameter. There is bilateral wheezing noted upon auscultation, and he is short of breath with any physical exertion. His wife reports that he is becoming short of breath with conversation or with eating.

Mr. P. sleeps sitting up in a chair with several pillows. He reports decreased appetite and denies a cough at this time. His heart rate is tachycardic (110 beats/min) and regular; there is no peripheral edema. His medications include oxygen at 2 L/min, theophylline (Theo-Dur), albuterol nebulizers, famotidine (Pepcid), and guaifenesin (Humibid L.A.). Mr. P. and his family are aware that his disease is at the end stage with no hope of improvement. He wishes to stay at home and his family concurs. During his last hospital admission, his eldest daughter became his durable power of attorney for health care. Included in his discharge teaching was information regarding palliative and hospice care upon returning home.

In offering quality end-of-life care to Mr. P., the nurse needs to consider the following questions and acquire the related knowledge and skills for expert nursing care:

What are the physiologic changes associated with the aging process?

What are the etiologies involved in the development of COPD?

How is COPD diagnosed and what are the current medical treatment modalities?

Are there alternative/complementary therapies that can assist the older adult with COPD?

What can nurses do to assist the older adult who is at the end stage of COPD?

INTRODUCTION

Chronic lung disease, specifically COPD, is the fourth leading cause of death (American Lung Association, 2003) and is the most common cause of death from respiratory disease in the United States (Sommers & Johnson, 2002). The diseases emphysema and chronic bronchitis are included within the diagnosis of COPD. Eighty percent to 90% of COPD cases are the result of smoking (American Lung Association, 2003). Emphysema affects males slightly more often than females (57% to 43%, respectively). Symptoms of COPD may appear as early as the third or fourth decade, but usually the severity of symptoms increases in the fifth decade and beyond (Sommers & Johnson, 2002).

FUNCTION OF THE LUNGS

The lungs expand and contract in order to allow atmospheric air to enter the body. Upon inspiration, the diaphragm contracts and the lungs are pulled downward. At the same time, the rib cage is elevated (Guyton & Hall, 1996). Upon expiration, the diaphragm relaxes and the elastic recoil of the lungs, chest wall, and abdominal structures compresses the lungs (Guyton & Hall, 1996). During the expiratory phase of ventilation, the rib cage is depressed. The lungs can be described as "floating" structures within the thoracic cavity surrounded by pleural fluid (Guyton & Hall, 1996). It is this pleural fluid that contributes to the negative pressure found within the thoracic cavity.

Pleural pressure is defined as the pressure of fluid in the narrow space between the lung pleura and the chest wall pleura (Guyton & Hall, 1996). Diffusion of gases (oxygen and carbon dioxide) takes place at the alveolar-capillary junction in the lungs. The respiratory center within the medulla sends signals to the respiratory muscles when there is an increase in carbon dioxide or hydrogen (H^+) ions, resulting in increased respiratory rate and depth. When there is a decrease in oxygen in the arterial blood, however, it is the peripheral chemoreceptors located within the carotid and aortic bodies that stimulate the respiratory center in the medulla via the nervous system (Guyton & Hall, 1996).

LUNG CHANGES ASSOCIATED WITH AGING

Changes in lung function that are associated with the aging process include decreased elastic recoil and chest wall stiffening. As a result of these changes, there is a decrease in compliance resulting in decreased lung pressures and volumes (Hall, 1998; Sheahan & Musialowski, 2001). The residual volume, or air remaining in the lungs after a maximal expiration, increases (Hall, 1998). This increase in residual volume reflects the changes in lung elasticity. Airway compression occurs earlier in the expiratory phase of ventilation, resulting in air trapping and altered gas exchange (Sheahan & Musialowski, 2001). Mucociliary clearance in both upper and lower airways may be diminished (Hall, 1998). Coupled with the earlier airway compression, the older adult is predisposed to lung infection.

The partial pressure of arterial oxygen (Pao_2) also decreases with age as a result of the premature airway closure. According to Hall (1998) and Sheahan and Musialowski (2001), exercise capacity can be diminished as a result of decreased muscle mass, decreased cardiac function, and decreased level of conditioning that

may occur in some older adults. A decrease in the function of lymphocytes and a decreased humoral response also predispose the older adult to viral and bacterial infections (Hall, 1998).

CHRONIC OBSTRUCTIVE PULMONARY DISEASE

COPD is a class of chronic lung diseases that includes emphysema and chronic bronchitis. Although bronchial asthma has some similar characteristics, it is no longer considered COPD (Weinberger, 1998). Chronic bronchitis and emphysema are distinct entities and they are common comorbid conditions. Smoking is a major precursor to the development of emphysema and chronic bronchitis; a smoking history of 20 pack-years has been associated with the development of COPD (Witta, 1997). However, only 15% of smokers go on to develop COPD (Brashers, 2002). Urban living and air pollution have also been implicated in the development and the exacerbation of COPD (Brashers, 2002). Alpha-antitrypsin is a glycoprotein that appears to protect the alveolar walls from destruction; congenital deficiency of alpha-antitrypsin has been implicated in the diagnosis of COPD in persons who are young and nonsmokers (Weinberger, 1998). In the 15% of smokers who will develop COPD, a deficiency of alpha-antitrypsin is suspected (Weinberger, 1998).

Chronic bronchitis is diagnosed by history and physical exam. The individual who reports a chronic cough for 3 months of the year for 2 consecutive years is diagnosed as having chronic bronchitis (Weinberger, 1998). There is also sputum production, periods of exacerbation caused by respiratory infections, and the presence of residual disease between exacerbations (Weinberger, 1998). Upon physical examination, wheezing and rhonchi will be auscultated. With a disease exacerbation, accessory muscle use will become visible—motion of the sternocleidomastoid and trapezius muscle groups with intercostal muscle retractions is an example (Weinberger, 1998). The lungs will appear normal upon chest radiography; however, the diaphragm will appear shortened and flattened. Pulmonary function tests (PFTs) and arterial blood gases (ABGs) will exhibit alveolar air trapping. The patient will complain of fatigue and dyspnea as well as decreased appetite.

Emphysema is also diagnosed by history and physical exam. There is destruction of the respiratory walls as a result of abnormal and permanent enlargement of the terminal airways (Sommers & Johnson, 2002). Upon physical examination, wheezing and possibly crackles will be auscultated. Because of an increased AP diameter, the heart sounds may be distant. The chest radiograph will demonstrate hyperinflation, a flat diaphragm, and increased AP diameter (Weinberger, 1998). In the later stages of the disease, a mucoid cough may occur (Sommers & Johnson, 2002). The ABGs will remain fairly normal until the later stages of the disease. PFTs, when performed, will demonstrate air trapping. The patient will complain of dyspnea upon exertion as well as at rest. A decrease in appetite, or a loss of appetite, can occur as dyspneic symptoms worsen. As a result of decreased food intake, the older adult may report weight loss. Mental status changes, caused by decreased oxygenation, may be reported by family members or significant others.

The Older Adult with COPD

The older adult has both structural and functional changes of the lungs associated with the normal aging process. The changes associated with COPD may be more discrete in presentation in the older adult. However, the health impact of the disease can be enormous (Hall, 1998). Comorbid conditions such as cardiovascular disease and arthritis can cause diagnostic confusion during the history and physical examination because of the older adult's inability to perform pulmonary function and exercise testing. This age cohort is at particular risk related to the etiologic factors of cigarette smoking and environmental pollution. The current generation of older adult began smoking prior to World War II, when there was no focus on the deleterious effects of smoking (Hall, 1998). Also, because of their age and the increasing industrialization of the United States since World War II, they have had a longer exposure to adverse environmental conditions (Hall, 1998). Evaluation of the older adult may be difficult because of his or her perception that dyspnea upon exertion is just due to "old age." Also, the older adult will decrease his or her activity in order to prevent the dyspnea from occurring. In addition, dyspnea and breathless-

Box 15-1 **Modified Borg Scale**	
0	Nothing at all
0.5	Very, very slight (just noticeable)
1	Very slight
2	Slight (light)
3	Moderate
4	Somewhat severe
5	Severe
6	
7	Very severe
8	
9	Very, very severe (almost maximal)
10	Worst imaginable

From Spector, N., & Klein, D. (2001). Chronic critically ill dyspneic patients: Mechanisms and clinical measurement. *AACN Clinical Issues: Advanced Practice in Acute and Critical Care, 12,* 220-233.

ness may not appear in some elders until late in the disease course (Hall, 1998).

Taking these issues into consideration, asking the older adult about changes in his or her daily activity level is a more valuable assessment. Diagnostic studies such as PFTs and ABGs can be performed. However, most "normal" measures in PFTs are based on younger people (Hall, 1998), and ABGs may remain normal in emphysema until later in the course of the disease. Use of the modified Borg Scale (Box 15-1) and noninvasive technology, such as pulse oximetry, may also help to quantify the changes in respiratory status of the older adult (Hall, 1998).

The decreased immunologic function associated with normal aging may blunt the febrile response. Diminished cough and sputum production are also associated with advancing age. The absence of a fever and the lack of sputum production may delay the diagnosis of a respiratory infection in the older adult.

Complications of COPD

The complications of COPD can include cardiac, pulmonary, and gastrointestinal dysfunction. Examples of such dysfunction include cor pulmonale, atrial arrhythmias, pneumothorax, recurrent respiratory infections (such as pneumonia), respiratory failure, and malnutrition. Cor

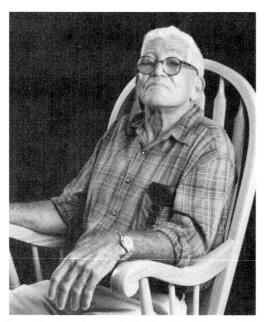

Recognizing the unique needs of older adults. (Courtesy Mathy Mezey.)

pulmonale most commonly occurs as the result of chronic bronchitis; however, it can occur as a late sign of emphysema (Marini & Wheeler, 1997). A pneumothorax can occur as a result of the rupture of bullae, which develop as the result of COPD. Recurrent respiratory infections, commonly viral in origin, can cause a transient worsening of COPD symptoms and can also decrease pulmonary function (Weinberger, 1998). Respiratory failure, a serious complication of COPD, could necessitate hospitalization, intubation, and mechanical ventilation. Malnutrition can develop as the result of decreased food intake caused by dyspnea, or the increased energy expenditure caused by the disease process (Marini & Wheeler, 1997). It may also develop as a result of the diaphragmatic changes associated with COPD. The lowering and flattening of the diaphragm can result in early satiety and gastric distention (Marini & Wheeler, 1997).

As in younger adults with COPD, complications such as cor pulmonale, respiratory failure, and malnutrition can develop in older adults. Cor pulmonale, or right-sided hypertrophy of the heart, is due to pulmonary vascular hypertension

(Sommers & Johnson, 2002). Pulmonary vascular hypertension develops as the result of hypoxia causing vasoconstriction of the pulmonary arterioles (Weinberger, 1998). The development of pulmonary hypertension can also be due to hypercarbia and polycythemia. Cor pulmonale accounts for 25% of all types of heart failure and is more common in middle-aged and older males (Sommers & Johnson, 2002). Cor pulmonale is a late sign of COPD, and there is a poor response to therapeutic interventions unless the patient is also hypoxemic (Marini & Wheeler, 1997).

The complication of respiratory failure can be due to an acute insult (such as an infection) or to a worsening of COPD (Weinberger, 1998). Hypoxemia develops and hypercarbia develops or worsens. Because of the nature of COPD, the gas exchange at the alveolar-capillary membrane is already compromised (St. John, 1998). Dyspnea is a subjective experience and may be difficult to ascertain by the presenting symptoms. In the older adult, changes in mental status, such as irritability and confusion, or a decrease in the ability to perform the activities of daily living, may signal the worsening of COPD (Hall, 1998; St. John, 1998; Weinberger, 1998).

The development of malnutrition is multifactorial in the older adult. A 20% to 50% increase in metabolic demands is associated with COPD (Witta, 1997). Changes in the diaphragm caused by COPD can contribute to anorexia. Fatigue and dyspnea can result in decreased oral intake. Depression resulting from chronic illness or changes in lifestyle and personal losses may decrease the interest in eating (Witta, 1997).

TREATMENT MODALITIES FOR COPD

Current treatment modalities for COPD include smoking cessation, prevention of infection, maximizing pulmonary function, and education (Barnes, 2001; Gaine & Terry, 1997; Witta, 1997). After the age of 65, smoking continues to be a major risk factor for death as well as a decreased quality of life (Hall, 1998). Smoking cessation in the older adult can improve quality of life, prevent the progression of COPD, and therefore reduce the development of complications resulting from COPD (Hall, 1998). The risk for the development of influenza and pneumonia decreases as the result of smoking cessation in the older adult. Therapies suggested for smoking

EVIDENCE-BASED PRACTICE

Reference: Powers, J., & Bennett, S. J. (1999). Measurement of dyspnea in patients treated with mechanical ventilation. *American Journal of Critical Care*, 8, 254-261.

Research Problem: Dyspnea is not generally measured or monitored in patients during mechanical ventilation. The evaluation of test–retest reliability of five dyspnea rating scales as well as the criterion validity of four dyspnea rating scales was the first aspect of the study. The second was the examination of the correlation between each of the five rating scales and physiologic measures of respiratory function.

Design: Experimental.

Sample and Setting: A convenience sample of 28 patients hospitalized in the intensive care units (ICUs) of a large inner-city hospital (level 1 trauma center) and treated with mechanical ventilation was used. Mean age of the patients in the sample was 48.25 years.

Methods: A visual analogue scale (VAS) was used as the standard of comparison. Dyspnea was rated twice in each patient at 30-minute intervals. Vital signs and oxygen saturation were measured within 10 minutes of administering the rating scales. Heart rate and blood pressure were recorded from the bedside cardiac monitor. Respiratory rate was measured for 1 minute. Each patient completed the VAS, the Visual

Analogue Dyspnea Scale (VADS), the modified Borg Scale, the numerical scale, and the Faces scale in random order. The patients were also asked which rating scale that they preferred. After 30 minutes, the five rating scales were then readministered.

Results: All of the rating scales had acceptable test–retest reliabilities; interclass correlation coefficients ranged from 0.81 to 0.97. Criterion validity of the four scales with Spearman rank-order correlation coefficients ranged from 0.76 to 0.96. The rating scales were not correlated with most of the physiologic variables. Also, at least half of the patients reported moderate to severe dyspnea.

Implications for Nursing Practice: Various tools are available to improve the assessment of dyspnea and the evaluation of interventions to decrease dyspnea. Also, the variety of scales enables nurses to select the rating scale appropriate to the patients being assessed. The scales are portable and can be utilized in the home with older adults who have chronic lung disease.

Conclusion: The scales demonstrated acceptable reliability and validity. Each scale can be useful in quantifying dyspnea experienced by mechanically ventilated patients. As noted, almost half of the patients reported moderate to severe dyspnea. Further work is needed in the evaluation of dyspnea in mechanically ventilated patients in order to evaluate the effectiveness of interventions.

---

cessation are nicotine replacements (gum and patches), advice from the health care provider, and community support (Barnes, 2001; Hall, 1998).

The prevention of infection is an important consideration in the older adult with COPD. Simple interventions, such as hand washing and avoidance of exposure to illness, can reduce the development of respiratory infections. Inoculation in order to prevent the development of influenza and pneumonia is also recommended to prevent disease exacerbation (Barnes, 2001).

Maximizing pulmonary function includes pharmacologic therapy, pulmonary rehabilitation, breathing retraining, and the prevention of malnutrition. Standard pharmacologic therapies include bronchodilators, steroids, and supplemental oxygen (Table 15-1). If the older adult has developed cor pulmonale or atrial arrhythmias, pharmacologic therapy is directed toward reducing the adverse cardiovascular effects that occur.

Bronchodilators may cause a reduction of dyspnea and an improvement in exercise capac-

Table 15-1 **Pharmacologic Interventions for Chronic Lung Disease**	
Medication*	Routes:
BRONCHODILATORS	
Sympathomimetics	Inhaled, oral, parenteral
Epinephrine	
Isoproterenol	
Albuterol	
Xanthines	
Theophylline	Oral
Aminophylline	Parenteral
Anticholinergics	
Ipratroprium	Inhaled
SUPPLEMENTAL O$_2$	
Nasal cannula	Compressed gas, liquid, or concentrate
STEROIDS	
Corticosteroids	
Prednisone	Oral
Methylprednisolone	Parenteral
Beclomethasone	Inhaled

*Not an inclusive list of medications.

ity. Bronchodilators can be administered via metered-dose inhalers, by nebulizer, or by oral administration. Theophylline, as an example of a bronchodilator, can be an effective therapy in the setting of COPD. Theophylline can increase the strength and effectiveness of respiratory muscles and improves blood flow to the diaphragm (Gaine & Terry, 1997). However, changes in cardiac or liver function associated with aging can decrease the clearance of theophylline (Barnes, 2001). Cigarette smoking can also negatively influence the metabolism of theophylline.

Steroids are administered by inhalation to prevent exacerbations or orally or intravenously to decrease the severity of exacerbations if they occur (Brashers, 2002). Older adults are at risk for the development of osteoporosis resulting from decreased activity and poor nutrition (Barnes, 2001). Because a potential side effect of steroid use is the development of osteoporosis, the potential benefits of therapy should be

weighed against this risk. Oxygen therapy can decrease the potentially harmful effects on the pulmonary vasculature by hypoxemia. Oxygen is utilized during acute exacerbations (Brashers, 2002), to reduce the dyspnea associated with cor pulmonale (Marini & Wheeler, 1997), and in the long-term management of COPD (Barnes, 2001). Oxygen therapy is titrated to a Pao$_2$ of 55 to 60 mm Hg in order to avoid "turning off" the hypoxic drive in patients with COPD (Weinberger, 1998).

Small breaths and a decreased respiratory rate are a COPD patient's response to exercise (Collins, Langbein, Fehr, & Maloney, 2001). As stated previously, the older adult will reduce his or her activity in order to reduce the occurrence of dyspnea. Pulmonary rehabilitation is focused on exercise and muscle reconditioning (Witta, 1997). Rehabilitation can take place in a community setting, as well as in the patient's home. By increasing physical activity, muscle atrophy may be reduced and the efficiency of oxygen uptake will be improved (Collins et al., 2001).

Breathing retraining for patients with COPD includes the techniques of pursed-lip breathing and diaphragmatic/abdominal breathing (Box 15-2). Because of the pathophysiology of COPD, air becomes trapped in the terminal airways and adequate ventilation decreases. Lung changes associated with aging can result in air trapping without the presence of COPD (Sheahan & Musialowski, 2001). Pursed-lip breathing facilitates the expulsion of air from the lungs by the patient, controlling and lengthening the expiratory phase of respiration (Collins et al., 2001; Dunn, 2001).

Diaphragmatic/abdominal breathing serves a purpose similar to that of pursed-lip breathing. The patient utilizes the diaphragmatic and abdominal muscles to control both inspiration and expiration (Dunn, 2001). Both techniques assist the patient to reduce panic and anxiety associated with dyspneic episodes (Dunn, 2001). The older adult can perform both of these exercises while seated comfortably in a chair. Utilizing a controlled-breathing technique can improve ventilation at the alveolar-capillary membrane by the reduction of air trapped at the end of expiration.

Malnutrition negatively affects the pulmonary system (Gaine & Terry, 1997; Witta, 1997) as

---

Box 15-2 **Breathing Exercises**

ABDOMINAL/DIAPHRAGMATIC
- Sit comfortably with feet on floor.
- Press one hand to abdomen, rest the other hand on chest.
- Inhale through nose slowly; use abdominal muscles.
- Hand on abdomen should rise with inspiration, drop with expiration.
- Exhale through mouth.
- Hand on chest should stay still.

PURSED-LIP
- Breathe slowly through nose.
- Hold your breath to a count of 3 seconds.
- Purse lips like you will be whistling; breathe out to a count of 3 seconds.
- By exhaling through pursed lips, air is expelled from the lungs and breathing is slowed.

From Sheahan, S. L., & Musialowski, R. (2001). Clinical implications of respiratory changes in aging. *Journal of Gerontological Nursing, 27*(5), 26-34.

---

well as the immune system (Hall, 1998; Witta, 1997) in the older adult. Because of the physiologic changes associated with aging, immunity and pulmonary function may already be compromised (Sheahan & Musialowski, 2001). If an older adult is concurrently on diuretic therapy, losses of phosphorus and potassium can contribute to further muscle weakness (Gaine & Terry, 1997). Recommendations to improve nutrition include eating smaller, more frequent meals (Sommers & Johnson, 2002; Witta, 1997); increasing protein and calories (Berry & Baum, 2001; Collins et al., 2001; Sommers & Johnson, 2002; Witta, 1997); and limiting carbohydrates to 50% of the total caloric intake (Marini & Wheeler, 1997).

Administering bronchodilators prior to meals can also facilitate intake by decreasing dyspneic episodes. Oral care prior to meals can improve the eating experience for patients who mouth-breathe or have sputum production. Improving nutritional intake can increase the lung response to hypoxemia and hypercarbia and can maintain immune function (Witta, 1997), which can be decreased as a result of the physiologic changes associated with aging as well as the pathophysiologic process of COPD.

Education is incorporated in the care of the older adult during each contact. Explanations should be given regarding smoking cessation, medication administration and potential side effects of these medications, breathing retraining and pulmonary rehabilitation, and, if necessary, home oxygen therapy. Because significant others often function as caregivers in the home, they should be included in the education sessions.

Once older adults are diagnosed with COPD, they and their significant others should be made aware of the prognosis. Death generally occurs within 5 years of diagnosis of advanced disease (Weinberger, 1998). There is no cure for COPD (Witta, 1997), only treatment of symptoms and prevention of complications and exacerbations. The end point of the disease is pulmonary hypertension and the development of cor pulmonale (Marini & Wheeler, 1997). All information regarding the diagnosis and prognosis should be delivered honestly to the elder and his or her significant others at their level of understanding (Meier, Morrison, & Ahronheim, 1998).

Once the diagnosis has been made, it is appropriate to begin discussions about advance directives. Such discussions should begin prior to the development of a life-threatening event (Meier et al., 1998). Even though predicting the exact time of death is difficult, the patient and significant others should be offered options in treatment. Information regarding palliative care can also be included in the treatment plan for patients with COPD (Meier et al., 1998).

Symptom Identification and Treatment

Dyspnea and the resultant development of anxiety are commonly associated with end-stage COPD (Meier et al., 1998). Dyspnea may also be associated with cor pulmonale, which is a late sign of COPD and a poor outcome indicator (Marini & Wheeler, 1997). However, in the older adult with COPD, dyspnea and complaints of breathlessness may be difficult to ascertain (Hall, 1998). Dyspnea is a subjective symptom of breathlessness, but the older adult may compensate for its development by decreasing his or her level of activity (Hall, 1998).

Once dyspnea has been diagnosed, the underlying cause needs to be identified. In the older adult with COPD, dyspnea can be the result of the disease process itself, the development of cor pulmonale, or a respiratory infection such as pneumonia. Nonpharmacologic interventions for symptom relief of dyspnea include repositioning the patient with his or her head up or to a position of comfort in a chair (Kazanowski, 2001; LaDuke, 2001). A cool environment can decrease the perception of dyspnea (Kazanowski, 2001; Meier et al., 1998). Balancing rest and exercise as tolerated can also assist the patient to breathe easier (Kazanowski, 2001; LaDuke, 2001). Frequent reassurance and providing a physical presence can assist in decreasing anxiety and thereby decrease dyspnea (Meier et al., 1998).

The pharmacologic interventions chosen to treat dyspnea depend upon the underlying etiology. Oxygen can be an initial adjunctive therapy for dyspnea (Kazanowski, 2001; LaDuke, 2001; Meier et al., 1998) and can be delivered via nasal cannula, face mask with cool mist, bi-level positive airway pressure (BiPAP), or mechanical ventilation. Although BiPAP is used in the acute care setting to reverse respiratory failure, it may provide some relief from dyspnea (McGowan, 1998). BiPAP may also be desirable because it may be chosen as a less invasive alternative to mechanical ventilation (McGowan, 1998).

Mechanical ventilation is an intervention that involves the creation of an artificial airway in order to deliver oxygen. In the setting of end-stage COPD, it is not an option that offers many advantages. There is an increased risk of nosocomial infection in an already compromised host, such as the older adult with COPD (Pilbeam, 1998). It is difficult to wean a patient with COPD from the ventilator because of diaphragmatic muscle weakness and, in the older adult, a decreased physiologic response to hypoxemia and hypercarbia (Phelan, Cooper, & Sangkachand, 2002). Mechanical ventilation also increases the risk of cardiac problems, aspiration, and barotrauma (Pilbeam, 1998). All oxygen delivery options should be offered to the patient and family, along with information on the risks and benefits associated with treatment. In the setting of palliative care, the least invasive and intrusive

therapies will promote comfort (Meier et al., 1998).

Opioids, such as morphine sulfate, can be administered to decrease the perception as well as the sensation of dyspnea (Kazanowski, 2001; LaDuke, 2001; Meier et al., 1998). Morphine can be administered sublingually, orally, parenterally, and via nebulizer (Box 15-3). Anxiety is also reduced because of the mood-altering effects of morphine (LaDuke, 2001; Meier et al., 1998). Somnolence is the main side effect of morphine; however, no severe respiratory compromise is noted (Kazanowski, 2001). Steroids can be administered to the patient with COPD to alleviate the inflammatory effects within the lungs (Kazanowski, 2001; LaDuke, 2001). Bronchodilators can also relieve the dyspnea associated with end-stage COPD (Kazanowski, 2001; LaDuke, 2001).

Box 15-3 Pharmacologic Interventions for Dyspnea

OPIATES
Morphine sulfate
    Nebulized (5 mg/2 mL 0.9 NS q4h)
    Parenteral (1-2 mg IV every 10-15 min; 2-5 mg
        SC initially)
    Oral or sublingual (5-10 mg, repeat 8 h prn)
    Rectal (10-20 mg q4h)

ANXIOLYTICS
Benzodiazepines
    Lorazepam (0.5 mg orally or sublingually q4h)
Phenothiazines
    Thorazine (25-100 mg PO tid or qid)

DIURETICS
Furosemide
    Administered PO, SC, IV, or IM for signs/symptoms of fluid volume excess
    20-80 mg PO (per dose)
    20-40 mg IV/IM (per dose)

From Kazanowski, M. K. (2001). Symptom management in palliative care. In M. L. Matzo & D. W. Sherman (Eds.), *Palliative care nursing: Quality care to the end of life* (pp. 327-361). New York: Springer.

EVIDENCE-BASED PRACTICE

Reference: Epstein, C. D., El-Mokadem, N., & Peerless, J. R. (2002). Weaning older patients from long-term mechanical ventilation: A pilot study. *American Journal of Critical Care, 11*, 369-377.

Research Problem: Accuracy is needed to determine the readiness for weaning from ventilatory support. A description of temporal changes in pulmonary and systemic variables in older adults was being sought. The purpose of the study was to determine whether there are differences between patients who can be weaned from long-term (3 or more days) ventilation and those who cannot be weaned.

Design: Descriptive.

Sample and Setting: A convenience sample of 10 patients admitted to the surgical intensive care unit (SICU) in a 750-bed hospital with a level 1 trauma center in Cleveland, Ohio. The study participants were 60 years of age or older; the mean age was 72.6 years.

Methods: Each patient was monitored for weaning progress. The attending physician determined weaning initiation. The study investigators defined active weaning a priori as progress in ventilatory weaning by changes in ventilator mode or decreases in rate, oxygen level, and pressure support. Patients were monitored daily until they were successfully weaned (i.e., remained extubated for 24 hours), or up to 14 days. The instrument utilized to assess readiness for weaning was the Burns Weaning Assessment

Program (BWAP), a 26-item checklist. Oxygen cost of breathing was measured by metabolic monitoring prior to and after each ventilator change. Multidimensional variables were also collected daily for each participant. Patient differences in weaning were compared by the Mann-Whitney and Wilcoxin signed rank tests.

Results: Six participants were successfully weaned. The mean age of those successfully weaned was 70 years; for those not successfully weaned, the mean age was 76 years.

Implications for Nursing Practice: Age can prolong the weaning process because of the normal physiologic changes in the pulmonary system. Older patients, because of age-related changes in physiology, may not be able to correct acid–base imbalances, metabolize sedatives and opiates, and so forth. Nurses can utilize this information to provide interventions to optimize all factors that can promote weaning from mechanical ventilation. Because chronic lung disease can prolong a patient's time being mechanically ventilated, this information can improve care for this population group.

Conclusion: Further research is needed in the older adult population. The sample size was small (10 participants), and this limits generalization to other populations. Through further studies with older adults, weaning strategies can be tailored for this population.

Dyspnea related to cor pulmonale may respond to the administration of diuretics. If the patient has tenacious secretions associated with COPD or a respiratory infection, mucolytics may be administered (Kazanowski, 2001). If a respiratory infection, such as pneumonia, has been identified as the source of dyspnea (symptoms of fever and congested cough), antibiotic therapy is appropriate (Kazanowski, 2001; LaDuke, 2001). Anxiolytics, such as benzodiazepines, barbiturates, and phenothiazines, may be prescribed

to relieve the anxiety and fear associated with the feelings of breathlessness (Kazanowski, 2001; LaDuke, 2001; Meier et al., 1998).

Complementary Therapies

Complementary therapies, when incorporated into the practice of nursing, can increase the repertoire of interventions available to older adults (Frisch, 2001). For those patients who are receiving symptom relief at the end of life, complementary therapies can positively enhance what is already being done by helping to promote rest and sleep and reduce anxiety. Such therapies enable the nurse to create care that is patient centered and holistic (Frisch, 2001). There is increasing demand by consumers to receive care that is holistic, taking into account the mind, body, and spirit (Kreitzer & Jensen, 2000). Complementary therapies are already available in the community. The use of complementary therapies can give patients and their families control over their care decisions (Kreitzer & Jensen, 2000); most can be utilized in the home. Examples of complementary therapies include guided imagery, relaxation, massage, and music therapy.

Rest is necessary in order to decrease the intensity of dyspnea, and it can also decrease the work of breathing. Promoting rest and sleep can also decrease anxiety. Assessment of the older adult's sleep habits can be a helpful starting point to the promotion of restful sleep (Tullmann & Dracup, 2000). Assisting the patient into a position of comfort can promote sleep (Tullmann & Dracup, 2000); in the case of the patient with COPD, this generally means elevation of the head of the bed, which also facilitates diaphragmatic expansion.

Guided imagery is a technique that can be utilized to promote sleep in the patient with COPD (Tusek & Cwynar, 2000). Guided imagery can also assist the patient through a stressful experience (Tusek & Cwynar, 2000). The older adult can practice guided imagery with a partner or via audiotape. Patients focus on the present, and then are taken to a safe place in their mind.

Massage can also be explored as an option for sleep promotion (Richards, Gibson, & Overton-McCoy, 2000). Prior to initiating massage, the nurse must first determine that the elder is comfortable with being touched (Richards et al., 2000). In the patient at the end stage of COPD, there are no contraindications to massage being utilized for the promotion of rest and sleep.

Music can also be added to the therapeutic plan for the promotion of rest and sleep (Chlan, 2000; Richards et al., 2000). Music therapy can be helpful in elders with COPD who tire easily; however, music should be selected to their personal preference (Chlan, 2000). Anxiety reduction can also be facilitated through the use of complementary therapies such as massage (Richards et al., 2000), guided imagery (Tusek & Cwynar, 2000), and music therapy (Chlan, 2000). Reducing anxiety can also result in the reduction of dyspnea in the patient with COPD.

Patients or their significant others may ask the nurse about the utility of natural remedies in the treatment of COPD. Several medicinal plants are used in the treatment of respiratory ailments. *Larrea tridentata* (often called "chaparral"), cinnamon, horehound (*Marrubium vulgare*), and pansy (*Viola*) have been used in the treatment of bronchitis, although *Larrea* can cause severe liver damage, and cinnamon can precipitate shortness of breath (Skidmore-Roth, 2001). Anise (*Pimpinella anisum*) and huang qi (*Astragalus membranaceus*) have been used in the treatment of COPD. For general respiratory care and cough, lobelia (*Lobelia inflata*) and wild cherry bark (*Prunus serotina*) have been used (Skidmore-Roth, 2001). Lobelia is contraindicated in a patient who has congestive heart failure or dysrhythmias, and wild cherry bark is contraindicated in a patient who has respiratory or cardiovascular depression (Skidmore-Roth, 2001). If the patient is self-medicating with ginseng (*Panax*), tachycardia and hypertension can result if he or she also ingests caffeinated beverages, such as coffee or tea (Kuhn, 2002). St. John's wort (*Hypericum perforatum*) taken in combination with theophylline can decrease the serum level of theophylline, making it less effective as a bronchodilator (Kuhn, 2002). Theophylline should not be used concurrently with the herb guarana (*Paullinia cupana*) because it also contains theophylline (Kuhn, 2002). The benefits of natural remedies should be weighed against the harmful side effects that could exacerbate COPD or the complications of cor pulmonale and respiratory failure.

More research is needed regarding the benefits of complementary therapies in the treatment plan of end-stage COPD. Palliative care of the older adult encompasses the physical, psychological, and social domains of care. In addition, spirituality plays a role in fostering a positive attitude in the patient and the maintenance of hope in family members. Complementary therapies can be incorporated with other pharmacologic and nonpharmacologic modalities in the care of the older adult with end-stage COPD.

DEATH OF THE OLDER ADULT WITH COPD

The National Hospice Organization (1996) has developed guidelines for determining prognosis in COPD (Box 15-4). The death of the elder with COPD is commonly the result of respiratory failure (Weinberger, 1998). Respiratory failure can be due to the development of either hypoxemia or hypercapnia. The older adult may initially present with dyspnea, disorientation, or confusion. Vague symptoms such as tachypnea, tachycardia, and restlessness can occur. If the respiratory failure is due to hypercapnia, the patient may become stuporous or lapse into a coma

---

Box 15-4 Medical Guidelines for Determining Prognosis: Pulmonary Disease

Determining prognosis in end-stage lung disease is extremely difficult. There is marked variability in survival. Physician estimates of prognosis vary in accuracy, even in patients who appear end-stage. Even at the time of intubation and mechanical ventilation for respiratory failure from acute exacerbation of chronic obstructive pulmonary disease (COPD), six-month survival cannot be predicted with certainty from simple data easily available to the clinician. Far less information than this is available to most hospice programs at the time of referral.

Patients who fit the following parameters can be expected to have the lowest survival rates. Although the end stages of various forms of lung disease differ in some respects, most follow a final common pathway leading to progressive hypoxemia, cor pulmonale and recurrent infections. Thus, these Guidelines refer to patients with many forms of advanced pulmonary disease. At the present time, it is uncertain what number or combination of these factors might predict six-month mortality; clinical judgment is required.

I. Severity of chronic lung disease documented by:
   A. Disabling dyspnea at rest, poorly or unresponsive to bronchodilators, resulting in decreased functional activity, e.g., bed-to-chair existence, often exacerbated by other debilitating symptoms such as fatigue and cough.
      1. Forced expiratory volume in one second (FEV1), after bronchodilator, less than 30% of predicted, is helpful supplemental objective evidence, but should not be required if not already available.
   B. Progressive pulmonary disease.
      1. Increasing visits to Emergency Department or hospitalizations for pulmonary infections and/or respiratory failure.
      2. Decrease in FEV1 on serial testing of greater than 40 ml per year is helpful supplemental objective evidence, but should not be required if not already available.

II. Presence of cor pulmonale or right heart failure (RHF).
   A. These should be due to advanced pulmonary disease, not primary or secondary to left heart disease or valvulopathy.
   B. Cor pulmonale may be documented by:
      1. Echocardiography.
      2. Electrocardiogram.
      3. Chest x-ray.
      4. Physical signs of RHF.

III. Hypoxemia at rest on supplemental oxygen.
   A. pO_2 less than or equal to 55 mm Hg on supplemental oxygen.
   B. Oxygen saturation less than or equal to 88% on supplemental oxygen.

IV. Hypercapnia.
   A. pCO_2 equal to or greater than 50 mm Hg.

V. Unintentional progressive weight loss of greater than 10% of body weight over the preceding six months.

VI. Resting tachycardia greater than 100/minute in a patient with known severe chronic obstructive pulmonary disease.

From National Hospice Organization. (1996). *Medical guidelines for determining prognosis in selected non-cancer diseases* (2nd ed.). Arlington, VA: National Hospice Organization.

(Weinberger, 1998). Cyanosis is a late sign of respiratory failure. Therapeutic interventions are based on the etiology of the respiratory failure. Supplemental oxygen may be delivered either noninvasively or via mechanical ventilation. Dyspneic symptoms are treated with opiates, bronchodilators, and anxiolytics.

In order to support the family through the death of their loved one, an honest discussion about the dying process needs to occur (Meier et al., 1998). Dyspnea is a symptom that is seen during the dying process of a patient with COPD. Family members can panic when these dyspneic episodes occur (Tarzian, 2000). Because the elder has no control over his or her breathlessness (Tarzian, 2000), including the patient's family in the management of dyspneic episodes can decrease their sense of panic and increase their sense of control.

Case Study Conclusion

Mr. P. continued to become increasingly dyspneic with minimal exertion. Morphine sulfate was added to his medication regimen to ease the dyspneic symptoms. He began to develop episodes of confusion, despite oxygen therapy. His family assisted him with activities of daily living, such as toileting and bathing. Sleep was difficult despite extra pillows, a cool room, and music prior to bedtime. Mr. P. died with his family at his bedside 4 months after entering the hospice program.

CONCLUSION

COPD is the fourth leading cause of death in the United States, and it is the leading cause of death from a respiratory cause. Development of this disease occurs as the result of cigarette smoking and exposure to environmental pollution. These factors place older patients at particular risk for developing COPD because they have been exposed to smoking and pollution for an extended period of time. In addition, the normal physiologic changes inherent in the aging process place the older adult at increased risk for the development of complications, such as cor pulmonale and pneumonia. In order to reduce the risk of developing the complications of COPD, smoking cessation is recommended to the older adult. Pharmacologic modalities focus on improving ventilation, reducing inflammation, and preventing complications. Nonpharmacologic interventions, including exercise, rest, and improved nutrition, can be valuable adjunctive therapies in the care of elder patients with COPD.

RESOURCES FOR COMPLEMENTARY THERAPIES

- Complementary and Alternative Medicine Program at Stanford (CAMPS) (*http://camps.stanford.edu/*): CAMPS is conducting scientific inquiry into the concept of successful aging, its vast array of implications for personal behavior, medical practice, and public policy, and the specific effects of selected complementary and alternative medicine therapies that could increase successful aging.
- Mind/Body Medical Institute (*www.mbmi.org*): A resource on mind/body medicine and the Mind/Body Medical Institute.
- Health World Online (*www.healthy.net/clinic/therapy/herbal/herbic*): provides extensive information on medicinal plants, including the Herbal Materia Medica and the American Herbal Pharmacopoeia.
- National Center for Complementary and Alternative Medicine (NCCAM) (*www.nccam.nih.gov*): the mission is to support rigorous research on complementary and alternative medicine (CAM), to train researchers in CAM, and to disseminate information to the public and professionals on which CAM modalities work, which do not, and why.
- American Holistic Medical Association (*www.holisticmedicine.org*): the mission of the AHMA is to support practitioners in their evolving personal and professional development as healers and to educate physicians about holistic medicine.

REFERENCES

American Lung Association. (2003). *Fact sheet: Chronic obstructive pulmonary disease (COPD)*. Retrieved from lungusa.org/diseases/copd_factsheet_html

Barnes, P. J. (2001). Modern management of COPD in the elderly. *Annals of Long-Term Care, 9*(5), 51-56.

Berry, J. K., & Baum, C. L. (2001). Malnutrition in chronic obstructive pulmonary disease: Adding insult to injury.

AACN Clinical Issues: Advanced Practice in Acute and Critical Care, 12, 210-219.

Brashers, V. L. (2002). Chronic obstructive pulmonary disease. In *Clinical applications of pathophysiology: Assessment, diagnostic reasoning and management*. St. Louis: Mosby.

Chlan, L. L. (2000). Music therapy as a nursing intervention for patients supported by mechanical ventilation. *AACN Clinical Issues: Advanced Practice in Acute and Critical Care, 11,* 128-138.

Collins, E. G., Langbein, W. E., Fehr, L., & Maloney, C. (2001). Breathing pattern retraining and exercise in persons with chronic obstructive pulmonary disease. *AACN Clinical Issues: Advanced Practice in Acute and Critical Care, 12,* 202-209.

Dunn, N. A. (2001). Keeping COPD patients out of the ED. *RN, 64*(2), 33-38.

Frisch, N. C. (2002). Nursing as a context for alternative/complementary modalities. *Online Journal of Issues in Nursing, 6*(1). Retrieve from www.nursinggworld.org/ojin/topic15/tpc15_2.htm

Gaine, S. P., & Terry, P. (1997). Treatment modalities for COPD in the institutionalized elderly. *Annals of Long-Term Care, 5*(11), 390-397.

Guyton, A. C., & Hall, J. E. (1996). *Textbook of medical physiology*. Philadelphia: Saunders.

Hall, W. J. (1998). Pulmonary disorders. In E. H. Duthrie & P. R. Katz (Eds.), *Practice of geriatrics* (pp. 494-504). Philadelphia: Saunders.

Kazanowski, M. K. (2001). Symptom management in palliative care. In M. L. Matzo & D. W. Sherman (Eds.), *Palliative care nursing: Quality care to the end of life* (pp. 327-361). New York: Springer.

Kreitzer, M. J., & Jensen, D. (2000). Healing practices: Trends, challenges, and opportunities for nurses in acute and critical care. *AACN Clinical Issues: Advanced Practice in Acute and Critical Care, 11,* 7-16.

Kuhn, M. A. (2002). Herbal remedies: Drug-herb interactions. *Critical Care Nurse, 22*(2), 22-28, 30.

LaDuke, S. (2001). Terminal dyspnea and palliative care. *American Journal of Nursing, 101*(11), 26-31.

Marini, J. J., & Wheeler, A. P. (1997). *Critical care medicine. The essentials*. Baltimore: Williams & Wilkins.

McGowan, C. M. (1998). Noninvasive ventilatory support: Use of bi-level positive airway pressure in respiratory failure. *Critical Care Nurse, 18*(6), 47-53.

Meier, D. E., Morrison, R. S., & Ahronheim, J. C. (1998). Palliative care. In E. H. Duthrie & P. R. Katz (Eds.), *Practice of geriatrics* (pp. 99-111). Philadelphia: Saunders.

National Hospice Organization. (1996). *Medical guidelines for determining prognosis in selected non-cancer diseases* (2nd ed.). Arlington, VA: Author.

Phelan, B. A., Cooper, D. A., & Sangkachand, P. (2002). Prolonged mechanical ventilation and tracheostomy in the elderly. *AACN Clinical Issues: Advanced Practice in Acute and Critical Care, 13,* 84-93.

Pilbeam, S. P. (1998). *Mechanical ventilation. Physiology and clinical applications* (3rd ed.). St. Louis: Mosby.

Richards, K. C., Gibson, R., & Overton-McCoy, A. L. (2000). Effects of massage in acute and critical care. *AACN Clinical Issues: Advanced Practice in Acute and Critical Care, 11,* 77-96.

Sheahan, S. L., & Musialowski, R. (2001). Clinical implications of respiratory system changes in aging. *Journal of Gerontological Nursing, 27*(5), 26-34.

Skidmore-Roth, L. (2001). *Handbook of herbs and natural supplements*. St. Louis: Mosby.

Sommers, M. S., & Johnson, S. A. (2002). *Diseases and disorders: A nursing therapeutics manual* (2nd ed.). Philadelphia: Davis.

St. John, R. E. (1998). The pulmonary system. In J. G. Alspach (Ed.), *Core curriculum for critical care nursing* (pp. 1-136). Philadelphia: Saunders.

Tarzian, A. J. (2000). Caring for dying patients who have air hunger. *Journal of Nursing Scholarship, 32,* 137-143.

Tullmann, D. F., & Dracup, K. (2000). Creating a healing environment for elders. *AACN Clinical Issues: Advanced Practice in Acute and Critical Care, 11,* 34-50.

Tusek, D. L., & Cwynar, R. E. (2000). Strategies for implementing a guided imagery program to enhance patient experience. *AACN Clinical Issues: Advanced Practice in Acute and Critical Care, 11,* 68-76.

Weinberger, S. E. (1998). *Principles of pulmonary medicine*. Philadelphia: Saunders.

Witta, K. M. (1997). COPD in the elderly: Controlling symptoms and improving quality of life. *Advance for Nurse Practitioners, 5*(7), 18-20, 22-23, 27, 72.

16

END-STAGE LIVER DISEASE

Robert B. Davis

Mrs. M.'s daughter, Rachel, returned home to visit her mother during the Christmas holidays. She had not seen her 70-year-old mother in several months, although they often chatted by phone. Mrs. M. had been a widow for over 10 years but insisted on living alone in her rural home.

Although Mrs. M. was normally a "tidy" person, Rachel found her mother's home in shambles. Clothing and garbage littered the kitchen and living room, where her mother had been obviously sleeping. Rachel noticed that her mother seemed confused about what day Rachel was going to visit; also, she did not seem to know when she had last eaten. In the refrigerator were several plates of partially eaten meals. Her mother's arms and legs were thin, but she had a very round belly. The backs of her hands and her neck had small open sores.

Rachel called Mrs. M.'s family doctor, only to find that he had retired and the practice had been taken over by another physician. According to the receptionist, Mrs. M. had not been seen by the new doctor and had not been to the office in the 2 years since the previous physician had retired. Faced with the options of waiting for 2 weeks for an office appointment or taking her mother to the emergency room, Rachel decided to help her mother "clean up" and fix some healthier meals and see if her confusion cleared.

Rachel helped her mother to bed and fixed her a meal. When she began cleaning, she noticed several empty vodka bottles in the trash and under the couch. Her mother and father had made "toddy time" a regular evening ritual, but Rachel had never seen her mother intoxicated. After eating, Rachel's mother came into the kitchen opened a bottle of vodka, poured a glass, and topped it off with a few ice cubes. "I don't think that is a good idea," Rachel counseled. "Helps me sleep," her mother retorted as she went off to bed.

INTRODUCTION

Each year chronic liver disease and cirrhosis kills over 25,000 people in the United States. In 1999, septicemia displaced chronic liver disease and cirrhosis as the 10th leading cause of death in the United States. Liver disease and cirrhosis, however, is the ninth leading cause of death among men and the sixth leading cause of death among Hispanics and Native Americans (Anderson, 2001). Although there is a downward trend in overall death from end-stage liver disease (ESLD) among all ethnic groups, African American men and women continue to have a higher rate of death than their white age-adjusted counterparts (Singh & Hoyert, 2000). The death rate for liver disease and cirrhosis peaks between 65 and 84 years of age, when it is responsible for approximately 32 of every 100,000 deaths in the United States (Hoyert, Arias, Smith, Murphy, & Kochanek, 2001). Deaths for those 85 and older are nearly the same as for those 55 to 64, at a rate of 24 per 100,000.

Primary cancer of the liver and bile duct accounts for 16,600 (<2%) of the new diagnoses of cancer in the United States. The annual rate of new cases in men outnumbers that in women 2:1. Each year 14,100 Americans die of primary carcinoma of the liver, with the distribution of death between men and women maintaining the 2:1 ratio. Since the mid-1970s, liver and pancreatic cancer share the dubious distinction of having the lowest survival rates of all forms of cancer, with less than 7% of these patients living beyond 5 years after diagnosis. African Americans have a slightly lower liver cancer survival rate than all other races (4% in comparison to 6%) (Jemal, Thomas, Murray, & Thun, 2002).

PHYSIOLOGY

The liver is the largest solid organ in the body and has two primary functions. First, it is an essential organ of digestion, producing chemicals that break down food; second, it is the primary organ for the recycling of red blood cells. The liver receives approximately 20% of its oxygen-rich blood flow from the hepatic artery. Critical to understanding ESLD is knowing that the remaining 80% of the flow is nutrient-rich blood from the stomach, intestines, and spleen via the portal vein (Keith, 1985).

The liver is responsible for (Ghany & Hoofnagle, 2001)

- Synthesis of most serum proteins (albumin, carrier proteins, coagulation factors, and many hormonal and growth factors)
- Production of bile and its carriers (bile acids, cholesterol, lecithin, and phospholipids)
- Regulation of nutrients (glucose, glycogen, lipids, cholesterol, and amino acids)
- Metabolism and conjugation of bilirubin and cations as well as medications, and excretion of these compounds in the bile or urine

COMORBIDITY AND COMPLICATIONS

The liver is a resilient solid organ and withstands 80% to 90% loss in function before symptoms occur (McGrew, 2001). Liver disease is usually divided into obstructive and hepatocellular types. Obstructive liver disease is most often caused by

---

EVIDENCE-BASED PRACTICE

Reference: Singh, G., & Hoyert, D. I. (2000). Social epidemiology of chronic liver disease and cirrhosis mortality in the United States, 1935-1997: Trends and differential by ethnicity, socioeconomic status, and alcohol consumption. *Human Biology, 72,* 801-820.

Research Problem: What are the extent and demographic trends in alcohol consumption and liver disease?

Design: Longitudinal.

Sample and Setting: National data on over 200,000 men and women over 25 years of age collected over a 9-year period.

Methods: The study examined data from the National Vital Statistics system and the National Longitudinal Mortality Study (NLMS).

Results: From 1973 to 1997, death from cirrhosis declined 4.5% for African American men and women, in comparison to a 2.8% decline for whites. Despite this decline, age-adjusted death rates remained 20% to 25% higher for African Americans.

Those with highest risk for death from cirrhosis were unmarried males with less than college educations who were unemployed and lived in cities. Prevalence of cirrhosis peaked between 65 and 74 years of age for men, and between 55 and 64 for women. Martial status among women was significantly associated with rates of cirrhosis, with those women who were single, divorced, or widowed having the higher rates of cirrhosis. Alcohol consumption was more likely to increase during periods of marital disruption, and to be more prevalent among women with lower income levels.

Implications for Nursing Practice: Nursing assessment should include a detailed history of alcohol consumption and patterns. Women who are in the midst of a disruption to their primary relationship are at greater risk for acquiring alcohol consumption patterns that can lead to liver disease. Older widowed women, especially those with lower incomes, are at greatest risk.

Conclusion: Socioeconomic status, gender, stress, and ethnicity are all variables for alcohol consumption and cirrhosis mortality.

stones blocking the bile duct; this is an acute problem that is corrected surgically. The causes of ESLD are hepatocellular and can be divided into (1) chemical, (2) infectious, and (3) neoplastic origins. The various forms of viral hepatitis are the primary infectious agents. Alcohol is the primary cause of cirrhosis, followed by medications such as acetaminophen and industrial chemicals such as acetone. Fatigue and pruritus are often the first sign of a failing liver's inability to process bilirubin. The excess bilirubin accumulates in the skin, first causing an itch, then later jaundice.

For these reasons, the patient with ESLD, regardless of age, may present with a number of problems that may include (Ghany & Hoofnagle, 2001)

- Malnutrition with serum albumin levels less than 3.0 g/L
- Muscle wasting with abdominal and peripheral edema
- Disseminated intravascular coagulation or extended bleeding time
- Hyperlipidemia
- Fluid, vitamin, and electrolyte imbalances
- Fatigue and mental status changes
- Chronic wounds on sun-exposed areas of the skin
- Urticaria and later, jaundice

Chemical and Alcoholic Cirrhosis

Many prescribed, herbal, and over-the-counter medications stress the aging liver. Acetaminophen, considered a benign painkiller outside the medical community, can, if used in combination with prescription drugs assimilated in the liver, be a deadly combination for the older adult.

At least 70% of adults in the United States drink alcohol to some degree, but drinking more than two drinks (22 to 30 g of alcohol) per day in women and three drinks (33 to 45 g of alcohol) in men is necessary to increase the risk for liver disease. Most patients with alcoholic cirrhosis have a much higher daily intake and have drunk excessively for 10 years or more before onset of liver disease. Clinically, issues of alcoholism are often intertwined with depression and may be described by the patient as "the blues," fatigue, social isolation, and decreased interest in social as well as physical activities.

Alcohol is the leading cause of chemical cirrhosis in the United States, and alcohol-induced cirrhosis is the primary cause of portal hypertension in the portal venous system or vena cava. This pressure increase eventually will cause an expansion of the veins surrounding the esophagus, creating hemorrhoid-like sacks (varices) that are susceptible to sudden rupture. Without intervention early in the development of esophageal varices, their eventual rupture is a life-threatening emergency. Intervention must include abstinence from alcohol and may include sclerosis of the varices.

Increased pressure in the mesenteric arms to the portal vein causes fluid to leak into the peritoneal cavity, causing ascites. Likewise, because blood is not circulated completely through the liver, toxins build up, causing encephalopathy. Ammonia is produced by the breakdown of protein either during metabolism or by bacteria in the gut. The healthy liver can break down and excrete this ammonia, but, in the late stages of liver disease, ammonia accumulates in the blood stream and leads to portal-systemic encephalopathy (PSE). Symptoms include progressive behavioral change and memory loss, and may eventually include hallucinations. Butterworth

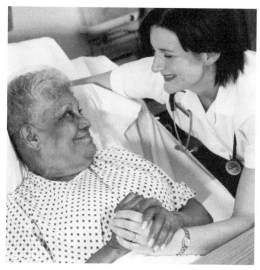

The art of palliative care nursing: a meaningful presence. (Courtesy Mathy Mezey.)

Table 16-1 **Grading of Portal-Systemic Encephalopathy (PSE) and Characteristic Signs**		
Stage of PSE	Cognitive Signs	Neuromuscular Signs
Subclinical	Abnormal psychometric test scores	None
Grade 1	Abnormal sleep patterns, shortened attention span, irritability, apathy	Tremor, incoordination
Grade 2	Personality changes, time disorientation, memory loss	Asterixis, dysarthria, abnormal muscle tone
Grade 3	Confusion, drowsiness, sleeplessness, paranoia, anger, stupor	Hyperactive reflexes, muscle rigidity
Grade 4	Coma	

From Butterworth, R. F. (1995). The role of liver disease in alcohol-induced cognitive defects. *Alcohol and Health Research World*, *19*, 122-129.

Box 16-1 **CAGE Questionniare**

- Have you ever tried to **C**ut down on your drinking?
- Have you ever been **A**nnoyed by anybody criticizing your drinking?
- Have you ever felt **G**uilty about your drinking?
- Have you ever had an "**E**ye opener" (drink) in the morning?

(1995) outlined a grading schema for PSE (Table 16-1).

Alcohol consumption patterns should be a part of the physical assessment of older adult patients. Less than 50% of primary care physicians include the diagnosis of alcohol dependence in the differential for patients who consume four or more drinks per day, and less than a third of health care professionals can effectively identify patients with substance abuse patterns (Gambert, 1997). Exacerbating the lack of consistent assessment is the reluctance of many older adults to openly discuss how much they drink. To decrease the likelihood of conflict, several questionnaires are available for patients to answer while filling out their health history. The most commonly used is the CAGE questionnaire (Box 16-1). A "yes" answer to two or more of the questions indicates alcohol dependence. The

CAGE tool may not be as valid in older adults who are retired or living alone (Fingerhood, 2000; Rigler, 2000). For example, in the case of Mrs. M., there was no one around her to "criticize" her drinking. The Alcohol Use Disorders Identification Test (AUDIT) (Box 16-2), developed by the World Health Organization, provides more detail than the CAGE questionnaire (Trotto, 2000).

Infectious Liver Disease

The primary causes of infections in the liver are an expanding cluster of viral hepatitis agents. Hepatitis is subdivided into acute and chronic disease forms. Hepatitis A is the most common acute form of hepatitis and has no chronic state. It is passed through the fecal-oral route and normally produces flulike symptoms in a non–immune-compromised population. In older adults, and immune-compromised populations, hepatitis A can be deadly because it stresses the already damaged liver.

Hepatitis B, hepatitis C, and others in this expanding list have both acute and chronic stages. The major sources of chronic hepatitis are blood, blood products, and unprotected sexual activity. A review of transfusions and other medical procedures should therefore be a part of the medical history. Hepatitis B virus infects over 1.25 million Americans and is presently the leading cause of hepatitis mortality. Infection is not restricted to the young or middle aged, and, as the overall American population ages, rates of

Box 16-2 Alcohol Use Disorders Identification Test (AUDIT)

1. How often do you have a drink containing alcohol?
   (0) Never **(1)** Monthly or less **(2)** 2-4 times a month **(3)** 2-3 times a week **(4)** 4 or more times a week
2. How many drinks do you have in a typical day when you are drinking?
   (0) 1 or 2 **(1)** 3 to 4 **(2)** 5 to 6 **(3)** 7 to 9 **(4)** 10 or more
3. How often do you have 6 or more drinks on one occasion?
   (0) Never **(1)** Less than monthly **(2)** Monthly **(3)** Weekly **(4)** Daily or almost daily
4. How often during the last year have you found that you were unable to stop drinking once you had started?
   (0) Never **(1)** Less than monthly **(2)** Monthly **(3)** Weekly **(4)** Daily or almost daily
5. How often during the last year have you failed to do what was normally expected from you because of drinking?
   (0) Never **(1)** Less than monthly **(2)** Monthly **(3)** Weekly **(4)** Daily or almost daily
6. How often within the last year have you needed a drink first thing in the morning to get yourself going after a heavy drinking session the night before?
   (0) Never **(1)** Less than monthly **(2)** Monthly **(3)** Weekly **(4)** Daily or almost daily
7. How often in the past year have you felt guilt or remorse after drinking?
   (0) Never **(1)** Less than monthly **(2)** Monthly **(3)** Weekly **(4)** Daily or almost daily
8. How often during the last year have you been unable to remember what happened the night before because you had been drinking?
   (0) Never **(1)** Less than monthly **(2)** Monthly **(3)** Weekly **(4)** Daily or almost daily
9. Have you, or has someone else, been injured as a result of your drinking?
   (0) No **(1)** Yes, but not within the last year **(2)** Yes, during the last year
10. Has a relative, friend, doctor, or other healthcare worker been concerned about your drinking or suggested that you cut down?
   (0) No **(1)** Yes, but not within the last year **(2)** Yes, during the last year

A score of 8 or more indicates alcohol dependence. High scores on the first three items and lower scores on items 4 through 10 suggests hazardous alcohol use. Higher scores on questions 4, 5, and 6 point to the presence or emergence of alcohol dependence. High scores on 7 through 10 suggest harmful alcohol use.

From World Health Organization. (1992). *AUDIT: The Alcohol Use Disorders Identification Test: Guidelines for use in primary health care*. Geneva: WHO.

all hepatitis infections among older adults will likely increase.

The nurse should never assume that an older patient is not sexually active. Although the number of sexual partners and frequency of coitus may decrease with age, being older does not mean being abstinent. Older women are at greater risk of sexually acquired hepatitis, human immunodeficiency virus, and other sexually transmitted diseases because they may not see themselves as vulnerable because of their age and in comparison to younger women (Davis, Turner, & Young, 2000). Up until the mid-1980s, condoms were primarily used as a birth control device. Therefore, the postmenopausal woman may not view condoms as an integral part of the sex act. In addition, the aging tissue of the genitalia is more susceptible to microscopic tears during coitus.

Screening for the increasing variety of hepatitis viruses will be a challenge for medical and laboratory science. As of the writing of this chapter, the alphabet of hepatitis viruses had reached "G." Because of lack of long-term experience, the natural disease history of hepatitis viruses C and beyond is unknown, but they appear deadly and increasingly widespread. Interferon alfa-2b and lamivudine (Epivir) are the treatments recommended for hepatitis B at the present time (Malik & Lee, 2000).

Liver Cancer

Primary liver cancer is significantly lower in the United State than in foreign countries, especially those in Africa and Asia; in these regions, the primary cause of liver cancer is chronic viral hepatitis infections. However, the rate of liver cancer is declining in developing countries and increasing in developed nations. This trend is due to a increase in hepatitis C infection in developed countries and an increasing use of hepatitis B vaccines in underdeveloped areas. As the incidence of viral hepatitis increases in the United States, it is also likely that liver cancer with this etiology will increase. For now, as with so many other diseases of the liver, risk of hepatic carcinoma in America increases proportionally with alcohol consumption (El-Serag, 2001; McGlynn, Tsao, Hsing, Devesa, & Fraumeni, 2001).

Primary cancer of the liver is often in an advanced stage before symptoms appear. Box 16-3 presents medical guidelines from the National Hospice Organization (1996) for determining the prognosis of advanced liver disease. The first symptom is usually liver pain. The abdomen is usually tender over the liver and a mass may be palpable; a friction rub or bruit may be heard when the abdomen is auscultated. Alkaline phosphatase and alpha-fetoprotein (AFP) may be elevated; however, AFP is not elevated in 20% to 30% of liver cancers. The average survival for all ages with primary liver cancer is 10 months (Stuart, Anand, & Jenkins, 1996). The most likely long-term survivor of primary hepatic carcinoma is someone whose cancer is detected early enough for definitive treatment by surgical resection. If the older adult patient presents symptomatically, the prognosis is poor, with an average survival between 3 and 6 months. Because it is a solid organ rich in blood, the liver's structure and function make it unsuitable for radiation therapy. Currently, surgical debulking of the tumor and chemotherapy are palliative interventions (Lau, 2000).

The liver filters blood; therefore, many of the cancers that affect the liver have their origin somewhere else in the body. The liver is second only to lymph nodes as the most common site of metastasis. Metastatic cancer in the liver is over 20 times more prevalent than primary liver carcinoma.

Other Causes of Liver Disease

Hepatic steatosis and nonalcoholic fatty liver disease (NAFL), or nonalcoholic steatohepatitis, are the outcomes of the gradual metamorphosis of liver cells from a normal structure to one of fatty tissue. Hepatic steatosis secondary to alcohol use is the primary cause of fatty liver disease. NAFL is more common in older, obese diabetic patients with hyperlipidemia or patients on long-term parenteral nutrition. Patients with fatty liver disease may show few signs of disease other than mild to moderate tenderness over the upper right abdominal quadrant. Without control of their diabetes and lipids as well as alcohol abstinence, these patients may progress to acute liver failure (Marchesini et al., 2001).

DYING TRAJECTORY

The life expectancy of a person with ESLD is difficult to predict. Fox et al. (1999) followed over 2600 patients who had been diagnosed with advanced stages of either chronic obstructive pulmonary disease, congestive heart failure, or ESLD. In this study, ESLD was defined as a diagnosis of cirrhosis and at least two of the following:

- A serum albumin of 30 g/L or less
- Cachexia
- A serum bilirubin level of 51 μmol/L (30 mg/dL) or more
- Uncontrolled ascites
- Hepatic encephalopathy
- Massive gastrointestinal bleed requiring 2 or more units of blood transfused within a 24-hour period
- Hematemesis or gross blood on endoscopic exam or nasogastric tube aspiration

Of those patients meeting these criteria and predicted to die within 6 months by their physician, over 50% were still alive 6 months later. Roth, Lynn, Zhong, Borum, and Dawson (2000) likewise found the 6-month projection of death in liver failure to be tenuous, but very predictable in the last 2 weeks, when symptoms such as significant jaundice developed.

Esophageal varices increase in size by 4% to 10% each year the alcoholic continues to drink. If varices hemorrhage, 20% to 30% of these patients die. If untreated, 70% of patients with varices will die within a year (Hegab & Luketic,

Box 16-3 Medical Guidelines for Determining Prognosis: Liver Disease

Prognosis in advanced liver disease has been widely studied to assess readiness for liver transplantation. Some of these variables, with the addition of other clinical syndromes associated with mortality, are shown below.

The following factors have been shown to correlate with poor short-term survival in advanced cirrhosis of the liver due to alcoholism, hepatitis, or uncertain causes (cryptogenic). Their effects are additive; i.e., prognosis worsens with the addition of each one. Clinical judgment is vital. The following factors should be followed and reviewed over time. Patients should have end-stage cirrhosis; those who are newly decompensated, i.e., in their first hospitalization, may improve dramatically with treatment compared to those who are in the terminal phase of a chronic process.

The patient should not be a candidate for liver transplantation.

I. Laboratory indicators of severely impaired liver function:
    Patients with this degree of impairment have a poor prognosis. The patient should show *both* of the following:
    A. Prothrombin time prolonged more than 5 sec. over control.
    B. Serum albumin <2.5 gm/dl.

II. Clinical indicators of end-stage liver disease: The patient should show *at least* one of the following:
    A. Ascites, refractory to sodium restriction and diuretics, or patient non-compliant.
        1. Maximal diuretics generally used: Spironolactone 75–150 mg/day plus furosemide ≥40 mg/day.
    B. Spontaneous bacterial peritonitis.
        1. Median survival 30% at one year; high mortality even when infection cured initially if liver disease is severe or accompanied by renal disease.
    C. Hepatorenal syndrome.
        1. In patient with cirrhosis and ascites, elevated creatinine and BUN with oliguria (400 ml/da) and urine sodium concentration <10 mEq/l.
        2. Usually occurs during hospitalization; survival generally days to weeks.
    D. Hepatic encephalopathy, refractory to protein restriction and lactulose or neomycin, or patient non-compliant.
        1. Manifested by: decreased awareness of environment, sleep disturbance, depression, emotional lability, somnolence, slurred speech, obtundation.
        2. Physical exam may show flapping tremor of asterixis, although this finding may be absent in later stages.
        3. Stupor and coma are extremely late-stage findings.
    E. Recurrent variceal bleeding.
        1. Following initial variceal hemorrhage, one third died in hospital, one third re-bled within six weeks; two thirds survived less than 12 months.
        2. Patient should have re-bled *despite therapy*, or refused further therapy, which currently includes:
            a. Injection sclerotherapy or band ligation, if available.
            b. Oral beta blockers.
            c. Transjugular intrahepatic portosystemic shunt (TIPS).

III. The following factors have been shown to worsen prognosis and should be documented if present:
    A. Progressive malnutrition
    B. Muscle wasting with reduced strength and endurance.
    C. Continued active alcoholism, i.e., >80 g ethanol per day
    D. Hepatocellular carcinoma
    E. HBsAg positivity

BUN, blood urea nitrogen; *HBsAg*, hepatitis B surface antigen.
From National Hospice Organization. (1996). *Medical guidelines for determining prognosis in selected non-cancer diseases* (2nd ed.). Arlington, VA: National Hospice Organization.

2001). Over 50% of patients will die within 2 years of their diagnosis of ascites (Garcia & Sanyal, 2001).

EMERGENCY SITUATIONS

Emergencies in ESLD result from one or, more likely, a combination of factors: (1) bleeding, (2) mental status changes, (3) electrolyte imbalance, and/or (4) infections. The goal of palliative care is to have a plan in place that addresses what actions to take if a crisis occurs. The development of this plan should be a joint undertaking by the patient and his or her circle of caregivers. Nurses, family members, and other medical personnel must be willing to respect the wishes of the patient. What has changed in the medical community is the willingness to accept exacerbations or collateral diseases as a part of a natural process. Although, as health care professionals, we have the capability to intervene and stop the course of a collateral disease process such as pneumonia, should we? This section addresses the key emergency conditions that will likely result in the death of older patients with ESLD. The interventions outlined range from the aggressive to comfort care.

Esophageal Varices

The most immediate life-threatening emergency in liver failure is hemorrhage secondary to esophageal varices. A gradual decline in hemoglobin level or changes in stool toward a dark or tarry consistency herald a slow, low-grade hemorrhage. The differential diagnosis of these changes includes ulcerative or cancerous lesions in the upper gastrointestinal tract. A careful history that includes a thorough assessment of alcohol use focuses the clinician to evaluate the liver and esophagus. If varices are discovered on endoscopy, they can be sclerosed surgically.

An alcoholic vomiting bright red blood is always an emergency. Even when this occurs in a hospital emergency room, the bleeding may be so severe, and the patient so debilitated by the disease, that survival is doubtful. Aggressive intervention in hemorrhage includes intubation to protect the airway, the careful infusion of blood products and crystalloid, and then endoscopy to sclerose the varices. Endoscopic sclerotherapy or banding is more effective than balloon tamponade and pharmacologic treatment

to increase survival in patients with varices. The primary surgical intervention used in patient rescue at this time is a transjugular intrahepatic portosystemic shunt (TIPS), in which a metal tube is placed connecting the portal and hepatic veins, thereby reducing portal hypertension (Hegab & Luketic, 2001). Like many of the treatments for varices, TIPS does not improve survival rates.

Dementia

ESLD-induced dementia is usually a gradual process, but dramatic changes are possible. Rapid behavioral changes can be secondary to (1) resumption of heavy drinking, (2) ingestion of other hepatotoxic chemicals such as acetaminophen, (3) cerebrovascular disease, (4) electrolyte imbalance, or (5) infection. Stopping the alcohol or other drugs is the first step, and may return the patient's mental status back near baseline. If the change is due to acetaminophen overdose, the antidote (N-acetylcysteine) must be given within 10 hours if it is to be effective.

Cerebrovascular Accident

Cerebrovascular accident (stroke or transient ischemic attack) can result in the abrupt onset of dementia in ESLD patients. Family members will report that these changes occurred "overnight" or within a matter of hours. On examination, the patient may not show unilateral weakness or hemiparalysis. Unless the stroke is hemorrhagic, computed tomography of the head has little diagnostic utility. Care of the stroke patient is discussed in Chapter 12, and comorbid ESLD does not significantly change those interventions. The patient with slow-progressing liver disease, however, may be more malnourished than a healthy elder who has a stroke.

Chemical Imbalance and Infections

Assuming that someone is providing daily care directly to the elder with ESLD, infections and electrolyte changes lead to a gradual change in behavior rather than the more abrupt changes of a stroke. Because the patient may not be able to reliably relate pain or other symptoms, aggressive evaluation of the patient includes (1) complete blood count with differential, (2) blood cultures, (3) urinalysis, (4) blood chemistries, and (5) chest radiography. Chemical imbalances in ESLD often result from low serum albumin levels caused by malnutrition or fluid shifts. Aggressive intervention for electrolyte imbalances includes parenteral nutrition and hydration.

The site of the infection in a patient with ESLD is most likely to be the lungs, bladder, or perineum, as in any other older person. Peritonitis associated with ascites is a risk factor only in the ESLD patient. Spontaneous bacterial peritonitis (SBP) is common in patients with ascites and presents with fever, chills, and generalized abdominal pain (rarely, rebound tenderness). However, symptoms may be vague in the confused and debilitated patient. Intravenous cefotaxime coupled with an aminoglycoside is initiated while waiting for the results of the ascites culture. Left untreated, the elder with SBP will quickly slip into septic shock (Garcia & Sanyal, 2001).

COMMON SYMPTOMS—EARLY TO LATE

Fatigue, itching, decreased appetite, and abdominal bloating singly or in combination may be the presenting symptoms of an elder with ESLD. The patient will usually complain of fatigue with activity, or lack of stamina. He or she will feel best early in the morning and later will need periods of rest between activities of daily living. Chronic nausea may be accompanied by alterations in taste and aversion to food and food preparation smells.

The itch of liver failure is not localized and is not associated with a rash. In some instances, the patient may have open superficial wounds on the sun-exposed areas of the skin that are slow to heal and may reoccur. The patient may report increasing right upper quadrant abdominal pain as the sack enclosing the liver expands with the increase in the size of the liver.

Darkening of the urine as bilirubin is excreted occurs before the development of jaundice. Jaundice, or the accumulation of bilirubin in the skin, is usually a sign of advanced disease and may only present as death approaches. The development of jaundice may be so slow that family members do not recognize the change.

Ascites may be distinguished from gas by having the patient lie flat. In ascites, the abdomen is round or distended and is dull to percussion. Gas bloating has a tympanic sound to percussion, and the abdomen may not be uniform in its contour. With ascites, a fluid wave can be balotted by placing one's hands on both sides of the patient's abdomen and pushing one side in quickly. A ripple in the skin of the abdomen, rolling toward the other hand, will be seen as abdominal fluid moves in response to the push.

Because of the resilient nature of the liver, blood tests may be normal despite advanced disease. Likewise, measurements of liver function may be elevated for problems that do not have their origin in this organ. Laboratory testing is fivefold. First, liver damage is assessed through liver function tests (LFTs). Second, blood work is used to determine if the patient is malnourished and, if so, the degree of malnutrition. Regardless of age, any patient with a blood albumin level of less than 4 g/L should be considered malnourished. If the albumin drops below 2.1 g/L, the patient is extremely malnourished. Third, a complete blood count is used to determine the fluid and electrolyte balance of the patient. High mineral concentrations indicate dehydration. Approximately half of patients with chronic liver disease have macrocytosis and thrombocytopenia, but the rest will have no significant change to their complete blood count.

The fourth lab test in patients in liver failure is determination of the ammonia level. Samples for an ammonia level require special handling and are best drawn at the lab running the test. In the hospital, the nurse should check the protocol for this test. An elevated ammonia level indicates PSE. Finally, a hepatitis panel is used to determine if there is an infectious cause to the liver disease. Muscle wasting can also result in an elevated serum ammonia level, so the ammonia level cannot be taken alone as a measure of PSE.

LFTs are measurements of serum bilirubin, albumin, and prothrombin time. The serum bilirubin level is a measure of hepatic conjugation and excretion, and the serum albumin level and prothrombin time are measures of protein synthesis. Abnormalities of bilirubin, albumin, and prothrombin time are typical of hepatic dysfunction. Decreased intake and absorption of vitamin K is common in alcohol cirrhosis, and prolonged bleeding times can make the rupture of varices deadly. Bilirubin found in the urine is conjugated bilirubin, and its presence implies liver disease. A urine dipstick test can give the same information as the serum bilirubin and is almost 100% accurate.

Although a thorough history, physical examination, and the testing just described will provide enough information to make a diagnosis, liver biopsy is the gold standard for grading and staging of the disease.

COMPLICATIONS OF END-STAGE LIVER DISEASE

The onset of ascites or esophageal varices coupled with low albumin or any gastrointestinal bleeding should be sentinel events in the decision to initiate palliative care in advanced liver disease (McGrew, 2001). Because continued alcohol consumption will hasten the progress of dementia, and result in adverse interactions with many medications, essential to any palliative treatment is abstinence from alcohol.

Ascites

The patient, the family, and even the clinician may misidentify ascites as the bloating of simple fluid retention or weight gain. This "bloating" may be attributed to excess sodium in the diet or congestive heart failure. Without a thorough physical examination, the first reaction to a patient presenting with fluid "bloating" is to prescribe a diuretic. Diuretics can cause hypovolemia, thereby concentrating ammonia; the elder may then quickly become disoriented, demented, and then comatose. Other causes of ascites besides liver failure include cancer, tuberculosis, renal failure, and pancreatic disease.

Progressive ascites pushes up on the diaphragm, making it difficult for patients to take a deep breath, exert themselves, or sleep lying down. As the ascites increases, the patient will feel increasing shortness of breath. All these factors raise the risk of pneumonia. Changes in the patient's center of gravity may also affect his or her ability to walk.

Bed rest is the first, nonaggressive treatment for ascites, as is keeping the elder patient reclined for a few days, which reduces the activation of the renin-angiotensin system. However, this is impractical for long-term treatment. Dietary sodium restriction is the mainstay of ascites treatment. The addition of the diuretic spironolactone (Aldactone, 100 mg per day), which reduces aldosterone-dependent sodium reabsorption, is very effective in reducing ascites if used in conjunction with dietary sodium restriction. Care must be taken because rapid diuresis can result in hyponatremia, azotemia, potassium imbalance, and onset of or increased encephalopathy.

Another treatment for ascites is paracentesis, or the drainage of excess fluid from the abdominal cavity. The primary purpose of paracentesis is decompression of chest and abdominal cavity organs. The patient will be able to breathe with less strain and will feel less bloated and therefore able to eat. The gait may be improved. Paracentesis is not without risk of secondary infection and potential puncture of an abdominal organ. Overly aggressive paracentesis can result in extracellular fluid shifts and orthostatic hypotension. A sample of the fluid is examined for infection, blood, and tumor. One kilogram of fluid can be removed in an outpatient setting if the ascites is coupled with peripheral edema. Without comorbid peripheral edema, no more than 0.5 kg should be drained. More aggressive or "large-volume" paracentesis of up to 5 L of fluid requires hospitalization and parenteral albumin supplementation (Garcia & Sanyal, 2001).

Portal-Systemic Encephalopathy

Ammonia is a by-product of protein metabolism. Restricting protein in the diet is controversial. On one side of the issue are those who recommend initiation of a low-protein diet once PSE has been confirmed by an elevated ammonia level in the arterial blood and mental status changes (McGrew, 2001). Alternatively, pharmacologic management includes 15 to 30 mL of lactulose given three times a day to reduce protein absorption in the gut. If lactulose alone is effective at reducing symptoms of encephalopathy, this regimen is continued. If encephalopathy continues, neomycin can be added to reduce bacterial activity in the gut (Abiy-Assi & Vlahcevic, 2001). Patients have difficulty staying on a regimen of neomycin and lactulose because of stomach upset, cramping, and diarrhea. Ascites will likely return, requiring multiple procedures.

Other specialists in ESLD believe that long-term protein restriction is counterproductive because of the advanced malnourished state that accompanies ESLD (Bashir & Lipman, 2001). Vitamin and mineral supplementation is a special need with alcoholic cirrhosis. Dietary restriction of sodium to no more than 800 mg, or 2 g of table salt, per day may be helpful in reducing fluid retention. Diet modifications for the elder with ESLD should employ a team approach including the patient, family, health care provider, and dietitian.

Esophageal Varices

Treatment of esophageal varices is limited because the surgical interventions are invasive and have not been shown to improve the overall survival rate. A noninvasive approach is to reduce portal hypertension using nonselective beta-blockers such as propranolol (Inderal) or nadolol (Corgard). Higher doses than are normally used to treat hypertension will be required, and dosage is adjusted upward until the resting heart rate is reduced by 25%, but not below 55 beats/min. The advantage of nadolol is that it can be given in a single daily dose of 40 to 320 mg. Propranolol, at a dose between 10 and 480 mg, may be divided over the course of the day. Use of beta-blockers has been shown to reduce the risk of bleeding by 45% and bleeding-related death by 50%. Surgical intervention using a laser to cauterize the varices is a recent innovation, but can result in fatal hemorrhage. Endoscopic sclerotherapy and banding are presently the first-line treatments for bleeding varices (Hegab & Luketic, 2001).

Pain Management

Pain control and comfort are the primary patient and family concerns for terminal diseases in the older adult (Bailes, 1997; Cleary & Carbone, 1997). Pain in the later stages of ESLD can be equivalent to that of late-stage lung or colon cancer (Roth et al., 2000). Without appropriate medical pain control, the patient may turn to over-the-counter medications that may be hepatotoxic or resort to alcohol. Codeine or codeine analogues without acetaminophen, and later morphine, are the initial choices. If the elder has difficulty swallowing or retaining oral medications, transdermal fentanyl or a morphine pump may be used. Family members will likely be concerned that their loved one will become "addicted" to these pain medications or become "doped up." The patient and family need to be repeatedly reassured that comfort is the priority and that addiction is extremely rare.

Diphenhydramine (Benadryl), hydroxyzine (Vistaril), and promethazine (Phenergan) often act synergistically with pain medications in addition to reducing nausea, decreasing the severity of itching skin, and promoting rest. Often with progressing ascites and shortness of breath, the patient becomes increasingly restless and anxious even though pain is adequately controlled. Family members may become frightened when a loved one is struggling to breathe or is confused. In these cases, they are more likely to call paramedics or take the patient to the emergency room. Antianxiety agents such as lorazepam (Ativan), alprazolam (Xanax), or diazepam (Valium) are essential in reducing these symptoms. Diazepam has the advantages of being inexpensive and coming in intravenous or intramuscular injectable forms. Although finding the appropriate combination of medications to control pain, anxiety, urticaria, and nausea may require some trial and error, no patient should suffer in pain (Tremblay & Breitbart, 2001).

Hospice and palliative care services can be an effective source of information, family counseling, and pain control if this resource is initiated early in ESLD. As mentioned before, prediction of life expectancy is problematic, and clinicians often wait until death is certain and imminent before making a hospice referral. Effective pain control is therefore inconsistent, and pain appraisal is made difficult as the patient's level of consciousness diminishes. If hospice is not involved, problems with pain control are confounded by withdrawal of contact with the health care community as the patient deteriorates. In a study of people who died at home, Desbiens and Wu (2000) found that half were conscious in the last 3 days of life and, of the conscious patients, 40% reported severe uncontrolled pain.

The final days of a patient with ESLD may take several courses. Those with primarily PSE involvement will become increasingly demented, become obtunded, and eventually lapse into a coma. Without paracentesis, third-space abdominal fluid will accumulate, pushing the diaphragm upward and causing increased difficulty breathing. If conscious and without sedation, the patient will become increasingly anxious as he or she struggles to breathe. Shortly before death, the patient with bleeding esophageal varices will become increasingly weak. If the ruptured varices are large, death may occur within a matter of minutes.

CONCERNS AND IMPLICATIONS FOR NURSING PRACTICE

The goals of professional nursing care for the patient with ESLD are outlined in Box 16-4.

Elder patients with ESLD may first seek care as a result of fatigue. This sense of fatigue will increase as the disease progresses. Community health nurses need to assess the patient's capabilities and the home environment to determine what support resources are needed. The patient must learn to pace his or her activities, take frequent breaks, and build naps into the day.

Nurses are in a pivotal position to assess the family for their capacity to give care (Groen, 1999). There may be unresolved issues of guilt and recrimination surrounding the patient's alcohol abuse. The spouse and children may need counseling to deal with these issues. The circle of caregivers must be willing to help the patient avoid alcohol. Likewise, the family needs to be informed of the natural course of the disease process and what changes should be expected. There should be a written plan of the steps to be taken in the event of an emergency or rapid deterioration so that the patient's wishes are addressed. At a minimum, every family member should read and discuss this advance directive.

The first step to alcohol abstinence may be detoxification in a specialized facility. With advanced disease, the patient may be hemodynamically unstable with severe nutritional and mineral deficits. These will need to be stabilized before the patient can return to family or long-term care. Most detoxification facilities interface with Alcoholics Anonymous (AA), and arrangements for follow-up with AA should be established before the patient is discharged. Older patients may have more severe alcohol withdrawal symptoms with increased hallucinations, sleep disturbance, and confusion.

Older alcoholics are often malnourished because alcohol has been a significant source of calories. A dietitian is an essential member of the caregiver circle, especially if the decision is made to restrict protein. Vitamin and mineral supplementation is specialized to avoid chemicals that are hepatotoxic. Extra vitamin K may be needed to correct bleeding irregularities. Aspirin should be avoided and salt intake reduced. Organizations such as Meals on Wheels can deliver food to home-bound patients that conforms to a specialized diet.

Older alcoholic patients are at an increased risk of falls. Because of an increased prothrombin time, bleeding precautions such as the use of soft toothbrushes are a part of the lifestyle changes. The patient needs to be weighed daily on the same scale and to report any sudden gain of over 2 kg in a day. The patient also needs to be assessed daily for pain, itching, fever, edema, increased shortness of breath, and mental status changes (Martin, 1992).

FAMILY CONCERNS AND CONSIDERATIONS—CAREGIVER FEARS

The progression to death from liver disease is often a slow and tedious process. Roth et al. (2000) studied 575 patients with ESLD. Two thirds of these patients died within 2 years. Eighty-nine percent of the patients rated their quality of life as fair to poor, with the inability to perform activities of daily living as the major source of dissatisfaction. Eighty-eight percent of the study's patients had a family caregiver in the home, and two thirds required professional home health services. One third of these families had had their savings devastated by the costs of health care for the dying patient.

Pain control and comfort measures are universal goals in the care of patients with ESLD. African Americans, Hispanics, and recent immigrants are less likely to utilize advance directives (Huff & Kline, 1999; Waters, 2001). This is primarily due to distrust of or lack of familiarity

---

Box 16-4 **Goals for Caring for the Patient with ESLD**

- Maintain activities of daily living.
- Prepare the family and circle of caregivers for their roles in patient care interventions.
- Encourage and help the patient to avoid alcohol and other hepatotoxic chemicals.
- Maintain nutrition and hydration.
- Provide management of symptoms such as pain and itching.

EVIDENCE-BASED PRACTICE

Reference: Phillips, R., Hamel, M. B., Teno, J. M., Soukup, J., Lynn, J., Califf, R., et al. (2000). Patient race and decisions to withhold or withdraw life-sustaining treatments for seriously ill hospitalized adults. *American Journal of Medicine, 108*, 14–19.

Research Problem: The extent to which race or ethnicity plays a role in the withdrawal of treatment for terminally ill patients has been the source of much debate and research. Can the difference in resource use be attributed to more frequent or earlier decisions to withhold life-sustaining therapies.

Design: Retrospective chart review.

Sample and Setting: Review of over 9000 charts of patients in five teaching hospitals who had illnesses for which the 6-month mortality was 50%. The mean age of the patients was 63. African Americans accounted for 16% of the sample, and 44% were women. Can the difference in resource use be attributed to more frequent or earlier decisions to withhold or withdraw life-sustaining therapies.

Methods: Adults hospitalized at five geographically diverse teaching hospitals participating in the Study to Understand Prognoses and Preferences for Outcomes and Risks of Treatments (SUPPORT) were included in the sample. Examined the presence and timing of decisions to withhold or withdraw ventilator support and dialysis, and decisions to withhold surgery. Analyses were adjusted for demographic characteristics, prognosis, severity of illness, function, and patients' preferences for life-extending care.

Results: Slightly more than half of the patients who had been diagnosed with a disease for which there was a 6-month life expectancy were alive after 6 months. The researchers found no significant difference in the percentage of African Americans who chose to withdraw or withhold life support in comparison to their counterparts in other races. Likewise, there was no significant difference in the timing of the decision to withdraw or withhold life support. Also of interest is the proportion of people who chose life support by disease state. Of those patients diagnosed with acute respiratory or multiorgan system failure with sepsis, only 25% chose to withdraw support. Those with lung cancer, cirrhosis, or congestive heart failure were more likely to stop treatment than to continue.

Implications for Nursing Practice: African Americans may not be as reluctant to discuss withdrawal of life support as has been reported in other studies. Patient and family counseling provided by nurses should therefore be a part of the nursing assessment and care plan.

Conclusion: Patient race does not appear to be associated with decisions to withhold or withdraw ventilator support or dialysis, or to withhold major surgery, in seriously ill hospitalized adults.

---

with the medical system in the United States. However, in a study of palliative care choices, Phillips et al. (2000) found no differences between races with regard to decisions to withdraw or withhold life support for dying patients. Clergy should be included as a part of the caregiving circle early in the disease process, while the patient is oriented and can have meaningful interaction. In many ethnic, national, and religious groups, clergy can act as a bridge between the family and health care providers.

Although hepatitis will likely result in the death of many older adults in the future, alcoholic cirrhosis is the more common origin of ESLD today. Alcohol cirrhosis and hepatitis from drug use or sexual contact will likely create issues of guilt and blame that will be difficult to resolve as the patient deteriorates rapidly. The caring circle, including health professionals and family members, needs to be rallied around the patient in the present, rather than dwelling on the patient's past actions.

Support of the family members by health professionals is extremely important, particularly in certain cultures. Children and spouses of a dying alcoholic parent will likely harbor memories of neglect or even abuse. The codependent model may be exceeding difficult to maintain if the codependent partner is frail and unable to provide the increasingly demanding day-to-day care of the alcoholic spouse. Family members also need to be informed of the mental status changes that take place when death is imminent. In Roth's study, less than 10% of the patients showed confusion 6 months before death; however, within the last month of life, one third displayed serious mental status changes.

Case Study Conclusion

In the night, Rachel heard her mother vomiting and rushed in to find her lying on the bathroom floor and the toilet water tinted with bright red blood. She managed to help her mother to the car and drove her 30 miles to the nearest emergency room. When she arrived at the emergency room, Mrs. M. could be aroused, but quickly fell back asleep. She knew her name but was otherwise disoriented. In the emergency room, an intravenous infusion was started and blood was drawn. Mrs. M.'s blood alcohol level was 0.32 and her liver enzymes were six times normal values. Her hemoglobin was 9.8 g/dL and she had an elevated serum ammonia level. She had significant ascites and a hard liver margin. The sun-exposed areas of her skin had numerous half-centimeter sores in various stages of healing.

Mrs. M.'s daughter was counseled that her mother likely had advanced cirrhosis of the liver and that a biopsy would be scheduled for the next day to confirm it. Rachel was told that the alcohol and the elevated ammonia level were the likely source of her mother's confusion.

Prior to transfer to a general medicine floor, Mrs. M. began coughing and gagging. She rolled to one side of the gurney. Over and over, she vomited bright red blood onto the floor before losing consciousness. Within 5 minutes she went into cardiac arrest. Several attempts at intubation were obscured by massive hemorrhaging from the esophagus. Despite cardiopulmonary resuscitation and transfusions, Mrs. M. was pronounced dead within 3 hours of arriving at the emergency room.

Mrs. M.'s liver disease had been developing for many years. She would have been reluctant to discuss her drinking unless a health care provider or family member could have recognized early signs of alcoholism. Although ESLD affects three men for every woman, health care providers should not assume that a widowed woman does not drink excessively.

CONCLUSION

As with Mrs. M., more than 30% of America's older adults, predominantly women, live alone (Cleary & Carbone, 1997). Although people often prefer to die at home, lack of an in-home caregiver makes this goal difficult. The problems faced by Mrs. M. and her daughter in the case study are shared by many older adults. These issues include

1. Social isolation as a result of the dispersion of the American extended family and economic changes that dictate a dual-income family. These changes have resulted in the rise of the nursing home industry. There is a need for family-centered care provided in a supportive and caring homelike setting.
2. Loss of spouse and immediate family, which often results in depression and social isolation. Older Americans often self-medicate their depression with alcohol. Lack of social interaction does not provide a system of behavioral checks and balances. By only seeing her mother once or twice a year, Mrs. M.'s daughter could not observe her drinking habits or the subtle clues to her depression.
3. Inconsistent distribution of health care results to medically underserved rural and inner city elders. Demographic changes have resulted in a depopulation of the inner city as well as rural America as working-age adults seeking employment and housing move into suburban neighborhoods in between these two regions. Often left behind are older adults.

In addition, access to and utilization of Alcoholics Anonymous (AA) is not uniform. Seeking help from AA may not be considered necessary if the older adult's drinking is an integral part of his or her lifestyle. Without co-worker, family, or peer pressure to intervene, obtain help, and shape behavior, the amount of alcohol consumed increases with tolerance.

The etiology of ESLD in America will remain predominantly alcoholic cirrhosis and will predominantly affect those above the age of 50. Liver cancer and failure caused by viral hepatitis will be increasing and affecting younger age groups.

REFERENCES

Abiy-Assi, S., & Vlahcevic, Z. R. (2001). Hepatic encephalopathy: Metabolic consequence of cirrhosis often is reversible. *Postgraduate Medicine, 109*, 52-70.

Anderson, R. N. (2001). Deaths: Leading causes for 1999. *National Vital Statistics Reports, 49*(11).

Bailes, J. S. (1997). Health care economics of cancer in the elderly. *Cancer, 80*, 1348-1350.

Bashir, S., & Lipman, T. O. (2001). Nutrition in gastroenterology and hepatology. *Primary Care: Clinics in Office Practice, 28*, 629-645.

Butterworth, R. F. (1995). The role of liver disease in alcohol-induced cognitive defects. *Alcohol and Health Research World, 19*, 122-129.

Cleary, J. F., & Carbone, P. P. (1997). Palliative medicine in the elderly. *Cancer, 80*, 1335-1347.

Davis, Turner, & Young (2000).

Desbiens, N. A., & Wu, A. W. (2000). Perspectives and reviews of support findings: Pain and suffering in seriously ill hospitalized patients. *Journal of the American Geriatrics Society, 48*(Suppl. 5), S176-S182.

El-Serag, H. B. (2001). Liver tumors. *Clinics in Liver Disease, 5*, 87-107.

Fingerhood, M. (2000). Progress in geriatrics: Substance abuse in older people. *Journal of the American Geriatrics Society, 48*, 985-995.

Fox, E., Landrum-McNiff, K., Zhong, Z., Dawson, N. V., Wu, A. W., & Lynn, J. (1999). Evaluation of prognostic criteria for determining hospice eligibility in patients with advanced lung, heart, or liver disease. *Journal of the American Medical Association, 282*, 1638-1645.

Gambert (1997). Alcohol abuse: medical effects of heavy drinking in late life. *Geriatrics, 52*(6), 30-34, 36-37.

Garcia, N., & Sanyal, A. J. (2001). Minimizing ascites: Complications of cirrhosis signals clinical deterioration. *Postgraduate Medicine, 109*, 91-96, 101-103.

Ghany, M., & Hoofnagle, J. H. (2001). Liver and biliary tract disease. In E. Braunwald, S. L. Hauser, A. S. Fauci, D. L. Longo, D. L. Kasper, & J. L. Jameson (Eds.), *Harrison's principles of internal medicine* (pp. 1707-1711). New York: McGraw-Hill.

Groen, K. A. (1999). Primary and metastatic liver cancer. *Seminars on Oncology Nursing, 15*, 48-57.

Hegab, A. M., & Luketic, V. A. (2001). Bleeding esophageal varices: How to treat this dreaded complication of portal hypertension. *Postgraduate Medicine, 109*(2), 75-76, 81-86, 89.

Hoyert, D. L., Arias, E., Smith, B. L., Murphy, S. L., & Kochanek, K. D. (2001). Deaths: Final data for 1999. *National Vital Statistics Reports, 49*(8).

Huff, R. M., & Kline, M. V. (1999). *Promoting health in multicultural populations: A handbook for clinicians*. Thousand Oaks, CA: Sage Publications.

Jemal, A., Thomas, A., Murray, T., & Thun, M. (2002). Cancer statistics, 2002. *CA: A Cancer Journal for Clinicians, 52*, 23-47.

Keith, J. S. (1985). Hepatic failure: Etiologies, manifestations, and management. *Critical Care Nurse, 5*(1), 60-86.

Lau, W. Y. (2000). Primary liver tumors. *Seminars in Surgical Oncology, 19*, 135-144.

Malik, A. H., & Lee, W. M. (2000). Chronic hepatitis-B infection: Treatment strategies for the next millennium. *Annals of Internal Medicine, 132*, 723-731.

Marchesini, G., Brizi, M., Bianchi, G., Tomassetti, S., Bugianesi, E., Lenzi, M., et al. (2001). Nonalcoholic fatty liver disease: A feature of the metabolic syndrome. *Diabetes, 50*, 1844-1850.

Martin, F. L. (1992). When the liver breaks down. *RN, 55*(8), 52-57.

McGlynn, K. A., Tsao, L., Hsing, A. W., Devesa, S. S., & Fraumeni, J. F. (2001). International trends and patterns of primary liver disease. *International Journal of Cancer, 94*, 290-296.

McGrew, D. M. (2001). Chronic illness and the end of life. *Primary Care: Clinics in Office Practice, 28*, 339-347.

National Hospice Organization. (1996). *Medical guidelines for determining prognosis in selected non-cancer diseases* (2nd ed.). Arlington, VA: Author.

Phillips, R., Hamel, M. B., Teno, J. M., Soukup, J., Lynn, J., Califf, R., et al. (2000). Patient race and decisions to withhold or withdraw life-sustaining treatments for seriously ill hospitalized adults. *American Journal of Medicine, 108*, 14-19.

Rigler, S. K. (2000). Alcoholism in the elderly. *American Family Physician, 61*, 1710-1716.

Roth, K., Lynn, J., Zhong, Z., Borum, M., & Dawson, N. V. (2000). Dying with end stage liver disease with cirrhosis: Insights from SUPPORT. *Journal of the American Geriatric Society, 48*(Suppl.), S122-S130.

Singh, G., & Hoyert, D. I. (2000). Social epidemiology of chronic liver disease and cirrhosis mortality in the United States, 1935-1997: Trends and differential by ethnicity, socioeconomic status, and alcohol consumption. *Human Biology, 72*, 801-820.

Stuart, K. E., Anand, A. J., & Jenkins, R. L. (1996). Hepatocellular carcinoma in the United States: Prognostic features, treatment outcome and survival. *Cancer, 77*, 2217-2222.

Tremblay, A., & Breitbart, W. (2001). Psychiatric dimensions of palliative care. *Neurologic Clinics, 19*, 949-967.

Trotto, N. E. (2000). Meeting the challenge of alcoholic liver disease. *Patient Care, 34*(11), 110-113, 116-123.

Waters, C. M. (2001). Understanding and supporting African Americans' perspectives of end-of-life care planning and decision making. *Qualitative Health Research, 11*, 385-398.

III SYMPTOM MANAGEMENT AND RELATED ISSUES

Susan A. Derby

Palliative care for the older adult at the end of life consists of a comprehensive assessment of symptoms and planned interventions, involving an interdisciplinary team skilled in the needs of older adults. The urgent need for nurses skilled in providing palliative care to older adults is clear; the projected growth of the older adult population is staggering. By the year 2030, the U. S. population age 65 and over is projected to be 20% (U.S. Bureau of the Census, 1996). A primary goal of care for the older adult at the end of life includes maintenance of function and quality of life. The most common co-morbid conditions experienced by older adults—arthritis, hypertension, heart diseases, sensory impairments, diabetes, cerebrovascular disease, emphysema, cancer, and dementia—all contribute to an added symptom burden. In addition, the added disabilities resulting from chronic illness renders them more susceptible to new illnesses and treatment.

The overall goals of care for the older adult at the end of their life should be based on the palliative care needs that have been identified. Quality symptom management at the end of life care for older adults provides positive outcomes for both the patient and the family. Provision for a peaceful death should be a main concern to nurses and doctors.

However, the provision of symptom management may be limited by the uncertain prognoses of many chronic illnesses and lack of clear goals of care. When the goals of care lack clarity, coupled with uncertainty identifying terminal stages of illness, there may be overzealous interventions and over utilization of resources in the acute, as well as the long term, care setting. Numerous studies have documented the most common symptoms at the end of life and indicate that many patients experience a high degree of suffering. The most prevalent and distressing symptoms at the end of life in older adults are dyspnea, pain, and confused states, as well as gastrointestinal symptoms and fatigue (Coyle, Adelhardt, Foley, & Portenoy, 1990; Fainsinger, Miller, & Bruera, 1991; Seale, & Cartwright, 1994). Relief of dyspnea is aimed at treatment of the underlying disease process. However when death is imminent, symptom relief is paramount (Ripamonti & Bruera, 1997; Dudgeon & Lertzman, 1998) through the pharmacologic use of benzodiazepines, opioids, and corticosteroids. The use of morphine to control dyspnea at the end of life is advocated by palliative care clinicians, but often there is reluctance among staff due to lack of familiarity with dosing and titration, low priority given to this symptom, and fear of hastening death.

Pain is also a common symptom which is not adequately assessed and treated in the older adult. Pharmacologic intervention is the mainstay of treatment for the management of pain in the older adult at the end of life. Knowledge of age-related pharmacokinetics, including absorption, distribution, metabolism, and excretion will aid the advanced practice nurse in determining which opioids to use, the most appropriate route of administration, and how to titrate these drugs. Generally, older adults have more complex health problems and are more likely to experience pain, and less likely to complain of pain, especially if cognitively impaired. In this population, untreated or undertreated pain may drain energy, decrease functional status and mobility, decrease interaction, and cognition, as well as lead to depression.

In all settings, delirium is a common symptom in the older adult at the end of life (Breitbart & Strout, 2000). Delirium contributes significantly to increased morbidity and mortality. In elder hospitalized patients, delirium prevalence ranges from 10% to 40% and up to 80% at the end of life (Breitbart & Strout, 2000). Factors that predispose the older adult to delirium include age-related changes in the brain, brain damage, sensory changes, infection, impaired pharmacokinetics, malnutrition, co-morbid disease, and polypharmacy. Adequate assessment and management of delirium in the older adult requires the expertise of nurses.

Often gastrointestinal symptoms are related to bowel obstruction. Bowel obstruction at the end of life in elderly patients is a particularly difficult and painful symptom to manage, often requiring hospitalization for care. Bowel obstruction may be caused by advanced intraabdominal and pelvic disease, or may be a feature of recurrent disease. Scopolamine butylbromide and octreotide have been used successfully when the aim is to reduce gastrointestinal symptoms, thus avoiding the use of a nasogastric tube (Ripamonti et al, 2000).

Fatigue is also a symptom that is poorly understood and may overlap with other symptoms including dyspnea, pain, and depression especially at the end of life. Generally, it is thought to be multidimensional with a variety of causes. Prevalence in the dying population may be as high as 90% but often its cause may be idiopathic (Clarke & Lacasse, 1998; Curt et al, 2000).

In the palliative setting, elderly patients often have more than one co-morbid condition, necessitating treatment with multiple medications, and thereby placing them at risk for adverse drug reactions. When multiple drugs are used, the side effect profile may increase, potentially limiting the use of one or more drugs. For example, at the end of life, it is not uncommon to treat dyspnea and pain with a benzodiazepine and an opioid. In the older adult, excessive sedation may occur. However, it may be the wish of both the dying elder and their family that he or she be as alert as possible for as long as possible. Polypharmacy therefore further complicates symptom management in this population.

A key principle of palliative care is the commitment to involving a interdisciplinary team, which allows for aggressive comfort and symptom management. The interdisciplinary team further promotes quality of life and dying throughout the illness trajectory. The role of the advanced practice nurse within this framework has been well supported. Nurses, including advanced practice nurses, can enhance the quality of life for the older adult across the illness trajectory by a comprehensive assessment of the symptoms related to advanced illness and knowledge of pharmacologic and complementary therapies that relieve associated suffering.

REFERENCES

Breitbart, W., & Strout, D. (2000). Delirium in the terminally ill. *Clinical Geriatric Medicine, 16*(2), 357-372.

Clarke, P.M., & Lacasse, C. (1998). Cancer-related fatigue: Clinical practice issues. *Clinical Journal of Oncology Nursing, 2*(2), 45-53.

Coyle, N., Adelhardt, J., Foley, K., & Portenoy, R. (1990). Character of terminal illness in the advanced cancer patient: pain and other symptoms during the last four weeks of life. *Journal of Pain and Symptom Management, 5*(2), 83-93.

Curt, G.A., Breitbart, W., Cella, D., Groopman, J.E., Horning, S.J., & Itri, L.M., et al. (2000). *Oncologist, 5*(5),353-360.

Fainsinger, R., Miller, M.J., & Bruera, E. (1991). Symptom control during the last week of life on a palliative care unit. *Journal of Palliative Care, 7*(1), 5-11.

Ripamonti, C., Mercadante, S., Groff, L., Zecca, E., De Conno, F., & Casuccio, A. (2000). Role of octreotide, scopolamine butylbromide, and hydration in symptom control of patients with inoperable bowel obstruction and nasogastric tubes: a prospective randomized trial. *Journal of Pain and Symptom Management, 19*(1), 23-34.

Ripamonti, C., & Bruera, E. (1997). Dyspnea: Pathophysiology and assessment. *Journal of Pain and Symptom Management, 13*(4), 220-232.

Seale, C., & Cartwright, A. (1994). *The year before death.* Brookfield VT: Ashgate Publishing Company.

U.S. Bureau of the Census. (1996). *Current population reports: Special studies P23-190, 65+ in the United States.* Washington, DC: U.S. Government Printing Office.

17 DYSPNEA

Cindy R. Balkstra

Case Study

Mr. S., a patient on the subacute unit, was 68 years old and retired from the military. He struggled with the symptoms of emphysema, a result of smoking 2 packs of cigarettes per day for nearly 50 years, although he had been smoke-free for the last 7 years. He also had severe rheumatoid arthritis that crippled his extremities and caused a condition known as rheumatoid lung that resulted in his having both restrictive and obstructive lung disorders simultaneously. It was not surprising that Mr. S. was huffing and puffing at rest. Initially, the nurse assessed his level of understanding of his disease. He was fairly knowledgeable, but admitted he often denied the severity of his illness, causing him to avoid follow-up physician visits and to ignore his symptoms.

Finally, when he couldn't deny them any longer, Mr. S. sought assistance; this hospitalization was the result of such action. He spoke of how scary it was for him; he had been in intensive care for 2 weeks without much improvement. His poor condition upon arrival set the stage for a long uphill climb to recovery. He agreed that, in the future, early recognition and acknowledgment of his symptoms would be necessary to maintain his health. The nurse reviewed with him the signs and symptoms of worsening chronic obstructive pulmonary disease (COPD) that would be a reason to consult with the doctor.

Over the weeks that the nurse continued to work with Mr. S. and his wife, a positive relationship developed. Mr. S. typically welcomed the nurse with a play-by-play account of his day. However, he grew depressed at his lack of progress on the subacute unit. He easily tired and remained extremely short of breath, rating his dyspnea an 8 on a scale of 10 with even slight activity. It varied between 6 at rest and 10 with physical exertion. Muscle atrophy of his lower extremities caused weakness that made it even more difficult for him to comply with the demands of physical therapy. Pursed-lip breathing helped, but this was sometimes not enough. Energy conservation measures became essential; an occupational therapist worked with him daily to teach various techniques that allowed him to breathe more easily while performing activities of daily living. Anxiolytic agents and an antidepressant were added to combat the psychological effects of his illness. On the weekends, pet therapy was ordered to help lift his spirits. His wife, the primary support for him at home, was encouraged to make frequent visits.

INTRODUCTION

According to an American Thoracic Society (ATS, 1999) consensus statement, dyspnea is "a subjective experience of breathing discomfort that consists of qualitatively distinct sensations that vary in intensity. The experience derives from interactions among multiple physiological, psychological, social and environmental factors, and may induce secondary physiological and behavioral responses" (p. 1). In general, the definition of dyspnea is the perception of difficult breathing, including the person's reaction to that perception. Dyspnea can be acute, chronic, or terminal (Spector & Klein, 2002).

Acute dyspnea consists of high-intensity, time-limited shortness of breath that occurs as an immediate response to an acute physiologic or psychological event, seen in such conditions as myocardial infarction or pulmonary emboli, or with hyperventilation from an excitatory state.

Chronic dyspnea is persistent shortness of breath of variable intensity, usually seen in chronic conditions such as COPD or congestive heart failure (CHF). Terminal dyspnea occurs in people with end-stage diseases and may also be described as air hunger. Common descriptions of dyspnea include choking, congestion, tightness, and strangling as well as emotional responses such as panic, fear, worry, and frustration (Schwartzstein, 1999).

INCIDENCE OF DYSPNEA

Dyspnea is a frequent and devastating symptom that occurs in 55% to 70% of patients with advanced diseases, primarily those with cancer and end-stage heart or lung disease (Bruera, Schmitz, Pither, Neuman, and Hanson, 2000; Reuben & Mor, 1986). However, 24% of terminal patients participating in the National Hospice Study reported dyspnea despite the absence of pulmonary or cardiac disease. Moreover, 41% of patients in palliative care experience dyspnea and 46% of those describe the severity as moderate to severe (Cleary & Carbone, 1997). Dyspnea can seriously affect quality of life in those who experience it and may limit activity to the extent that even the slightest exertion may precipitate breathlessness (Dudgeon and Rosenthal, 1996). For example, eating may cause significant respiratory distress, which will impact the nutritional state as well as the mobility and functional status of older adults.

In the terminal phase of the elder's illness, fear of suffocation may be experienced (Dudgeon and Rosenthal, 1996). The frequency and severity of dyspnea often increase with the progression of disease and/or when death is approaching. In advanced cancer patients, dyspnea is considered a prognostic indicator of decreased survival time, whether alone or in association with other symptoms and/or reduced performance status (Maltoni et al., 1995). Mercadante, Casuccio, and Fulfaro (2000) reported that advanced cancer patients treated at home experienced worsening dyspnea with advancing disease, peaking in the last week of life. This correlated with a reduction in performance status and a survival range of 4 to 6 days.

MECHANISMS OF DYSPNEA

Although the mechanisms of dyspnea are complex and not well understood, it may help to review the control of respiration. The respiratory center in the medulla activates the muscles that expand the chest wall, inflate the lungs, and produce ventilation. The process of breathing regulates the oxygen and carbon dioxide balance and hydrogen ion concentration in the blood and body tissues. The automatic regulation of breathing is controlled by chemoreceptors in the blood and brain. Changes in the partial pressures of carbon dioxide and oxygen are sensed by central chemoreceptors in the medulla and peripheral chemoreceptors in the carotid and aortic bodies that send feedback to the brainstem respiratory centers to adjust breathing to maintain blood gas and acid–base homeostasis (ATS, 1999). All the input returned to the brain from body sensors contributes in some fashion to the individual's perception of dyspnea.

Although several physiologic mechanisms remain under investigation, three are recognized as dominant in the creation of the dyspneic sensation:

1. A conscious awareness of the neuromotor command to the respiratory muscles (e.g., an increased sense of effort experienced with aging, malnutrition, deconditioning, and hypoxemia)
2. Stimulation of the receptors in the airways, lungs, and chest wall, which detect changes in lung volume, stretch, and pressure (e.g., the sensation of respiratory muscle abnormalities, such as those found in neuromuscular conditions and respiratory muscle fatigue, as well as diseases that inhibit normal airflow and ventilation, such as COPD, asthma, and pulmonary fibrosis)
3. Stimulation of the chemoreceptors (e.g., the sensation of blood gas abnormalities, such as hypoxia and hypercapnia, that indirectly trigger ventilation, thereby causing dyspnea)

These mechanisms support the idea that dyspnea is caused by a "mismatch" between central respiratory motor activity and feedback from receptors in the airways, lungs, and chest wall. However, psychological, social, spiritual, and environmental factors interact with the physiologic ones to produce the subjective sensation of dyspnea. Without recognizing all of the components contributing to the total suffering of dyspnea, successful management is difficult to achieve (Zepetella, 1998).

ASSESSMENT

Dyspnea is a personal experience that accounts for a high proportion of disability, impaired quality of life, and suffering for the older adult. Thorough interdisciplinary assessment includes a careful, comprehensive history to obtain a complete understanding of the elder patient's experience with dyspnea. Specific information about dyspnea, including its timing, precipitating factors, associated symptoms, alleviating factors, and quality of the symptoms, should be obtained.

History

Timing

The sudden onset of dyspnea may reflect bronchoconstriction, pulmonary embolism, cardiac ischemia, or sudden airway occlusion. Chronic dyspnea occurs gradually and is likely to be manifested in slowly progressive disorders such as COPD, interstitial lung disease, or a slow-growing tumor. If the dyspnea occurs more at night, then it may be secondary to the redistribution of fluid in the supine position occurring in diseases such as CHF. Dyspnea can also result from an exacerbation of gastroesophageal reflux disease (GERD) that triggers bronchoconstriction. Assessing whether dyspnea is present with activity and/or at rest offers insight into the severity of the condition.

Precipitating Factors

Identification of precipitating factors assists in determining the underlying cause of the dyspnea. Exercise or overexertion commonly precipitates dyspnea in most chronic cardiopulmonary conditions. Anticipation of stressful events is another typical precipitant. Inhalation of allergens (pollen, grass, and weeds), smoke, fumes, and other aerosolized substances may trigger bronchospasm in patients with COPD and asthma. Respiratory infections usually cause an exacerbation of symptoms. The latter two factors are more likely to occur in older adults because aging increases susceptibility to both infections and allergens as a result of a diminished immune system (Sheahan & Musialowski, 2001).

Other effects of aging include a prevalence of silent GERD and sleep apnea secondary to discoordinated activity of the upper airway muscles and the diaphragm. Neurologically, age reduces chemoreceptor functioning, causing an inade-

quate ventilatory response to hypercapnia and acute hypoxia (Thompson, 1996). This makes older adults more sensitive and vulnerable to adverse outcomes from conditions that produce lower oxygen levels, such as pneumonia and COPD.

Associated Symptoms

Dyspnea is rarely an isolated problem. Concurrent symptoms can help clinicians identify the underlying pathophysiology. Clutching sternal chest pain is most likely indicative of myocardial ischemia, while brief, sharp lateral chest pain suggests pulmonary embolism, pneumothorax, or pleurisy. Wheezing is usually a sign of asthma, COPD, or CHF. Coughing, if productive, may indicate the presence of an infection. Nonproductive coughing occurs with rhinitis, reactive airway disease, interstitial fibrosis, GERD, and other diseases. Hemoptysis is most common with tuberculosis, lung cancer, and pulmonary embolism.

Alleviating Factors

Pharmacologic and nonpharmacologic strategies are necessary to relieve dyspnea and associated discomfort. Medications should be prescribed based on the identified etiology of dyspnea, such as cardiac or pulmonary problems. Bronchodilators relax bronchial smooth muscle and work well in diseases such as COPD and asthma. Nitroglycerin is the initial drug of choice for myocardial ischemia, which may cause dyspnea. Benzodiazepines often provide relaxation by decreasing the anxiety that frequently accompanies shortness of breath. Position changes can also offer clues as to etiology. Sitting up in a high Fowler's position or standing may relieve shortness of breath by allowing for better diaphragmatic expansion in the case of pulmonary disease or promoting redistribution of fluid in CHF.

Quality of Dyspnea

Schwartzstein (1999) has demonstrated that dyspnea is composed of many distinct sensations that are distinguishable by the patients who experience them; patients' descriptive language regarding dyspnea can lead to a better understanding of its etiology and management. It is important to carefully question the older adult about the quality of the dyspnea experienced. For example, elders with more severe dyspnea may say they have an "urge to breathe," or they "need more air," or may report a "sense of suffocation." Those older adults with neuromuscular or chest wall disease may describe it as "heavy breathing."

The assessment should include a thorough review of the patient's past medical history, including all current and recent medications. Some medications become problematic in relation to drug–drug interactions that can occur secondary to multiple prescribers. Beta-blockers, for example, antagonize beta$_2$-receptors and inhibit their potential bronchodilating effect.

An adequate nutritional history is valuable because malnutrition contributes to respiratory muscle fatigue and thus promotes dyspnea. Information about exposure to chemicals, smoke, fumes, and other environmental pollutants adds to the data obtained from the history.

Physical Examination

A focused physical examination of the head, neck, and chest will yield specific information about the older adult's condition and assist with identification of treatment options. Inspection should include the color of skin, nails, and lips; nutritional state; sternal/spinal deformities and chest shape and movement; breathing rate and rhythm; capillary refill; the presence or absence of nasal flaring, tracheal deviation, jugular venous distention, costal retractions, accessory muscle use; and clubbing. Other clues include facial and/or oral expression and the inspiration:expiration ratio. Palpation can yield information about tenderness, fremitus, masses, nodes, and crepitus. Percussion of the chest will indicate the degree of resonance; dullness indicates consolidation of tissue and tympanic resonance indicates the presence of air. Auscultation of the lungs will detect adventitious or diminished breath sounds, voice sounds, and pleural friction rubs.

Diagnostic Tests

Based on the need to determine the underlying cause(s) of dyspnea, several diagnostic tests may be of value. These include chest radiography, pulmonary function tests, pulse oximetry (preferred) or arterial blood gas analysis, electrocardiography, an electrolyte profile, and a complete blood count. Performance of any test should take into consideration the risk:benefit ratio, the elder's and his or her family's wishes, the prognosis, and goals of care.

Utilizing data obtained from the physical examination and diagnostic testing requires taking note of the physiologic effects of aging on the pulmonary system (Table 17-1). Three major factors contribute to these effects: an increase in chest wall stiffness, a decline in respiratory muscle strength, and a decrease in lung elasticity (Mahler, Rosiello, & Loke, 1986).

Measurement of Dyspnea

Because shortness of breath is a subjective symptom, it is important that instruments used to measure dyspnea take the patient's perception into account. Frequently, a visual analogue scale is recommended because of its ease of use and availability. On a 100-mm either horizontal or vertical line, the anchors "not at all breathless" on the low end and "severely breathless" at the high end represent the extremes of dyspnea (Gift, 1989). Another commonly used tool is the modified Borg Scale (see Chapter 15), which has the numbers 0 to 10 listed horizontally with descriptors along the line. On both, the elder is asked only to rate the shortness of breath; no other dimensions are measured. While nonverbal older adults can simply point to a number or position, some may find it difficult and need assistance to rate their symptom. Nevertheless, each tool is reliable and valid and can be helpful when assessing dyspnea in a variety of settings.

Other tools for measuring dyspnea have been developed and tested, but few are appropriate for older adults in palliative care. One exception, the Cancer Dyspnea Scale, has recently been piloted with patients who are at the end of life. This is a 12-question self-report of shortness of breath that includes the multidimensional aspects of dyspnea, such as the sense of effort, anxiety, and discomfort caused by the symptom. Validity scores have been reported as adequate, but reliability is still being determined (Tanaka, Akechi, Okuyama, Nishiwaki, & Uchitomi, 2000).

Whichever instrument is used, the elder and family should feel comfortable with it and be encouraged to utilize it to evaluate current therapeutic interventions. Consistency over time will maximize the relevance and usefulness of the

Table 17-1 **Effects of Aging Process on Pulmonary System**	
Changes with Aging	Result

STRUCTURAL CHANGES

Upper airways
   Nasal cartilage weakens, causing obstruction — Difficulty breathing through the nose
   Nasal blood flow decreases — Drying of secretions; nasal congestion
   Nasal turbinates shrink — Drying of secretions; nasal congestion
   Mucus increases in viscosity — Lodges in nasopharynx and stimulates coughing
Large airways
   Trachea and large bronchi stiffen — Decreases air exchange
Small airways
   Diameter decreases
   Alveolar ducts dilate
   Alveolar surface area decreases
     Combined changes — Increase residual volume
Thoracic cage
   Ribs decalcify — Affects posture
   Costal cartilages calcify — Affects posture
   Costal-vertebral joints stiffen (arthritic changes) — Decreases height
   Dorsal kyphosis occurs — Increases anterior-posterior diameter (barrel shape)
     Combined changes — Decrease vital capacity, increase residual volume
Pulmonary vasculature
   Arteries enlarge and thicken (lose distensibility) — Decreases cardiac output during exercise/exertion

MECHANICAL CHANGES

Small airways
   Premature closure — Air trapping/hyperinflation; impairs gas exchange and mucociliary clearance

Respiratory musculature
   Strength decreases; oxygen needs increase — Muscle fatigue; less reserve
Lung volumes, capacities, flow rates
   Forced expiratory volume in 1 second decreases — Increases residual volume
   Forced vital capacity decreases — Increases residual volume
   Functional residual capacity increases — Increases work of breathing
   Diffusing capacity decreases — Impairs gas exchange

Data from Sheahan, S.L., & Musialowski, R. (2001). Clinical implications of respiratory system changes in aging. *Journal of Gerontological Nursing, 27*(5), 26-34; Thompson, L.F. (1996). Failure to wean: Exploring the influence of age-related pulmonary changes. *Critical Care Nursing Clinics of North America, 8*(1), 7-16.

measurement. It is important to reemphasize that physiologic parameters may not always correlate with the degree of dyspnea reported. The elder must remain the singular authority on the symptom; if the older adult is unable to communicate, objective indicators of dyspnea can be used, such as tachypnea, gasping, use of accessory muscles, anxiety, restlessness, agitation, grimacing, and tachycardia.

Evaluation of Dyspnea and Functional Capacity

Although it is unusual to physically stress patients in palliative care, Booth and Adams

(2001) recently validated the effectiveness of the shuttle walking test (SWT) in evaluating interventions aimed at improving dyspnea in cancer patients. The SWT had previously been validated in patients with COPD, heart failure, and pacemakers; unsolicited comments from the study participants demonstrated a surprising positive effect. Patients realized better than expected physical capability, which improved their self-confidence as well as the confidence of their relatives. It is often difficult to evaluate the outcome of interventions in patients who are breathless solely on exertion. Booth and Adams (2001) recommended the SWT as an ideal test in the ambulatory patient with dyspnea to evaluate the impact of breathlessness on functional capacity.

MANAGEMENT
Nonpharmacologic Treatment and Interventions

Cooling and Vibration

When stimulated, temperature and mechanical receptors of the trigeminal nerve in the cheek and nasopharynx alter feedback to the brain and modify the perception of dyspnea. The use of a fan, set on low speed and directed toward the elder's face, will stimulate this response (Rousseau, 1997). Cooling the body may have a beneficial effect as well. Simple techniques include applying cool, damp cloths to the forehead or chest, offering a cool-water sponge bath, or providing a clean, fresh pillow. Altering the environment by circulating cool air either with an air-conditioning unit or a ceiling fan or by placing the older adult by an open window may add an element of comfort.

Stimulation of the mechanical receptors in the respiratory muscles can alter the sensation of dyspnea too. This accounts for why chest wall vibration is helpful in some elders (ATS, 1999). An electric massager, which also helps with relaxation and relief of pain, can be purchased for this use.

Breathing Retraining

Diaphragmatic and pursed-lip breathing have been advocated to relieve dyspnea, especially in elders with COPD; however, relief is highly variable among patients. Moreover, patients often resort to rapid, shallow breathing when unobserved. Despite these inconsistencies, these techniques offer an option that has no associated cost, is readily available, and can be easily learned. Families can play an active role in the care of the older adult by learning these techniques and coaching the elder during daily interactions.

Positioning

Patients should be assisted to find a position of comfort. The forward-leaning position has been reported to improve overall inspiratory muscle strength, increase diaphragm recruitment, and decrease abdominal paradoxical breathing as well as reduce dyspnea in patients with COPD (ATS, 1999). While reducing participation of the chest wall and neck muscles overall, sitting and leaning forward with arms supported on a table facilitates a more focused effort on respiration rather than on maintenance of body posture and/or arm movement (Campbell, 1996).

Optimal comfort as well as ventilation and perfusion may be accomplished by placing the patient's good lung in a dependent position in which gravity may assist in perfusing the healthiest area of lung tissue. In some patients, terminal dyspnea may be relieved only by an upright position, in which vital capacity is increased because of the lowered diaphragm. The clinician should accept the patient's position of choice, even if it belies traditional thinking.

Energy Conservation

Activities of daily living strain the dyspneic elder, even if he or she is passive during the activity. Oxygen consumption is increased with any activity, so it is important to allow for an adequate recovery period. All care should be evaluated with regard to what the patient can tolerate and what is desired. In some cases, the activity or intervention can be modified to accommodate the elder's decreased tolerance. For example, a bath and linen change could be stretched out over the course of several hours, focused on face and hands only, or eliminated entirely. As noted earlier, a position of comfort is not only helpful, but also critical to accommodating the elder's wants/needs with any required activities. However, if the care is more burdensome than beneficial, it should be reevaluated regarding the value of continuing it.

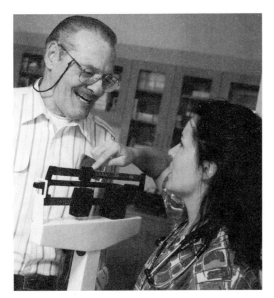

Focusing on health promotion along the illness trajectory. (Courtesy Mathy Mezey.)

Cognitive-Behavioral Approaches and Complementary Therapies

Distraction and relaxation strategies are important and useful adjuncts in the treatment of dyspnea. Distraction helps to focus the patient on something other than breathing. Relaxation eases muscular tension, thereby allowing breathing to be less strenuous and more effective. One method, guided imagery, uses mental images to promote relaxation. Other therapeutic activities include massage, music therapy, Reiki, therapeutic touch, and aromatherapy.

A number of essential oils (highly concentrated plant constituents) are thought to enhance respiration (Cooksley, 1996). These oils possess certain qualities such as expectorant, mucolytic, antiallergic, or immune-stimulant effects; some also have antiviral and antibacterial benefits. Most of the essential oils useful in respiratory conditions come from the bark, leaves, berries, and branches of certain trees. Once properly diluted, essential oils can be applied directly to the skin (check for sensitivity first) or in the form of massage, placed on pulse points, or inhaled through the use of a diffuser, aroma lamp, vaporizer, humidifier, or an absorbent material such as a cotton ball. Oils are non–habit forming and

excreted via the kidneys, skin, or lungs. Some recommended essential oils that can be used for dyspnea include eucalyptus, peppermint, ginger, hyssop, lavender, bergamot, basil, pine, sandalwood, and cypress. Blends of various oils are commonly used to achieve the maximum effect.

Education of the elder and family on management techniques and the basic rationale for each empowers them to take an active role in the treatment plan. Coaching both the older adult and the family reinforces these interventions. Active listening and emotional support by the nurse encourages expression of thoughts and feelings and also helps with early identification of potential problems. Benefits have been achieved using a rehabilitative approach that combined breathing retraining, psychosocial support, and help to develop adaptive strategies for breathlessness (Corner, Plant, A'Hern, & Bailey, 1996).

Transfusion Therapy

For elders with advanced cancer, blood transfusions are commonly used to alleviate symptoms such as dyspnea, fatigue, weakness, and tachycardia (Ripamonti, 1999). There are few data documenting symptom relief and improvement of the subjective sense of well-being after blood transfusions in anemic elders. With the potential risks of a transfusion reaction and adverse responses to blood transfusions, a safer, effective nontransfusion form of therapy might be considered, such as recombinant human erythropoietin. Disadvantages to this therapy include cost and the significant length of time required for an improvement in hemoglobin concentration, which is normally 4 to 6 weeks.

Noninvasive Positive Pressure Ventilation

Noninvasive positive-pressure ventilation (NIPPV) represents an alternative method to treat dyspnea. Although it can also be used as a curative intervention, it has found a place in palliative care for some patients with respiratory failure to either relieve symptoms or allow time for completion of life-closure tasks (Benditt, 2000). Advantages include a lack of adverse effects when compared to medications, continued patient participation, and maintenance of communication, as well as relief of dyspnea and other symptoms related to hypoxia or hypercarbia.

Disadvantages include the cost of equipment, hospice restrictions, lack of hypercarbic effect at the end of life (potential for increased suffering), the potential for decreasing the use of analgesics and anxiolytics prematurely, and the question of when and how to discontinue therapy. No studies have yet been done on NIPPV at the end of life. Studies that have been done on neuromuscular disease patients without palliative intent demonstrate improvement of dyspnea and other symptoms, quality of life, and cognitive function (Cazzoli & Oppenheimer, 1996; Hill, Eveloff, Carlisle, & Goff, 1992; Lyall et al., 2000; Meduri et al., 1991).

Adverse effects include facial irritation or discomfort, gastric distention, nasal/oral dryness or congestion, air leaks, failure to ventilate effectively, failure to tolerate, and, rarely, aspiration. As yet, many questions remain about the role of NIPPV at the end of life. However, if used in conjunction with traditional therapies, it may evolve into an effective tool for relieving dyspnea and improving quality of life in terminally ill elders. Other technological advances that may be of value for the dyspneic elder include laser therapy and the placement of endobronchial or tracheal stents to facilitate airway dilation, especially with tumor encroachment.

Pharmacologic Therapies

Oxygen

Supplemental oxygen depresses the hypoxic drive, thereby reducing ventilation and subsequently relieving dyspnea. This physiologic response occurs at rest and during exertion in elders with a variety of lung diseases. Oxygen should be titrated to the elder's comfort level using the least restrictive device possible (e.g., a nasal cannula does not interfere with eating and communication). Booth, Kelly, Cox, Adams, & Guz (1996) suggest a trial of 15 minutes of therapy at 4 L/min as a means of identifying those elders more likely to benefit from oxygen. Although at or above this liter flow, humidification is recommended for comfort and to prevent drying of mucous membranes. Continuous oxygen has been proven to be beneficial, although some older adults may prefer to use oxygen intermittently; however, assurance of the immediate availability of oxygen may be of greater importance.

High concentrations of oxygen can be problematic for elders with COPD who are carbon dioxide retainers (i.e., their only drive to breathe is the hypoxic drive), but this should not be a major concern in the final hours of life because hypercarbia produces a sedating effect. It should be noted that the benefit of oxygen therapy for elders without hypoxemia remains controversial (Rousseau, 1997; Zepetella, 1998).

Opioids

Opioids reduce dyspnea through a number of mechanisms. They act on the respiratory center by decreasing the ventilatory response to hypercapnia and hypoxia, reducing metabolic rate and oxygen consumption, and altering the perception of breathlessness. Furthermore, the cardiovascular effects of vasodilation and decreased peripheral resistance help to improve oxygen supply and reduce lung congestion.

Despite concerns regarding the use of opioids in dyspneic elders, morphine therapy forms the basis for treatment of dyspnea at the end of life. Opioids are very beneficial for many cardiopulmonary conditions, including lung cancer, CHF, COPD, and interstitial lung disease, as well as neuromuscular problems and others.

There is no ceiling dose with opioids, so it is appropriate to titrate the morphine to the desired effect; limited only by intolerable side effects. Commonly seen side effects include constipation, urinary retention, altered mental status, and drowsiness; tolerance to all of these side effects, except constipation, usually occurs within a week. A bowel regimen should always be established when opioids are prescribed to prevent constipation.

The oral route of morphine is preferred for elders at the end of life because it is better tolerated, least invasive, and less costly. Other routes can be utilized, such as sublingual, rectal, intravenous, subcutaneous, or aerosolized. Opioid-naive older adults are started with the morphine equivalent of 2.5 to 10 mg orally every 4 hours; the dose is increased by 30% to 50% daily or more frequently until dyspnea is relieved or sedation or other adverse effects become problematic (Rousseau, 1997). For elders already receiving morphine and experiencing dyspnea as a new symptom, the dose should be increased by 30% to 50% daily (or more frequently) and titrated according to symptoms (Rousseau, 1997).

EVIDENCE-BASED PRACTICE

Reference: Quigley, C., Joel, S., Patel, N., Bakash, A., & Slevin, M. (2002). A Phase I/II study of nebulized morphine-6-glucuronide. *Journal of Pain and Symptom Management, 23,* 7-9.

Research Problem: Determine the clinical efficacy, toxicity, and pharmacokinetics of nebulized morphine 6-glucuronide (M6G), the active metabolite of morphine, at different doses in patients with cancer-related breathlessness.

Design: Experimental Phase I/II study.

Sample and Setting: 9 patients from the department of oncology at a hospital. The age range was 45 to 77 years; median age was 51 years. Six patients were already receiving morphine.

Methods: Subjects were placed into three treatment groups in which each patient received a single dose of M6G at one of three dose levels (5 mg [3 patients], 10 mg [3 patients], or 20 mg [3 patients]) inhaled via nebulizer over 15 minutes. Breathlessness, anxiety, and effort of breathing were measured pretreatment and 15, 30, and 60 minutes after the treatment using a 100-mm visual analogue scale (VAS) and a modified Borg Scale. VAS and verbal rating scales (VRS) were used to assess nausea, drowsiness, and other adverse effects. Plasma samples were analyzed to determine pharmacokinetics.

Results: Although all patients reported subjective improvement in breathlessness, the change in value from baseline measurements was not significant. However, a significant difference was observed in dyspnea scores on the VAS with time. Furthermore, when the pretreatment value was excluded from the analysis, there was no longer a difference in the post-treatment VAS dyspnea scores. The researchers determined that this indicated an effect of treatment. However, there was no significant difference between the three treatment groups across all time points and when the pretreatment value was excluded, suggesting no difference between the three doses of M6G. Similar analyses were done for Borg scores, VAS anxiety scores, and VAS effort of breathing scores.

Implications for Nursing Practice: Cancer-related dyspnea remains a difficult symptom to control. Consider all available alternatives when traditional therapies do not achieve the desired results.

Conclusion: M6G may represent a safe, possibly therapeutic alternative to nebulized morphine for dyspnea in cancer patients. A randomized controlled study is planned comparing nebulized M6G and nebulized saline in patients with cancer-related breathlessness.

Because opioid receptors have been demonstrated to exist in the airways, nebulized morphine can be given in addition to systemic opioids or alone. Some patients experience relief of dyspnea with fewer side effects as a result of the lack of systemic concentration achieved by inhalation. This method of delivery remains controversial because studies have been conflicting, with most demonstrating no symptomatic improvement. However, a starting dose of 15 to 20 mg every 4 hours, possibly up to 100 mg, has been suggested (Zepetella, 1998).

One protocol recommends nebulized morphine only when intolerable side effects have occurred from systemic administration (Specter,

Klein, & Rice-Wylie, 2000). This protocol begins at a very conservative dose of 5 mg and titrates up to a maximum of 40 mg every 4 hours; the protocol includes frequent reevaluation of the dyspnea. Dyspnea refractory to other routes of administration may justify a trial of nebulized morphine. However, further research is needed to determine which patients may achieve maximum benefit. A recent exploratory study utilized the active metabolite of morphine (morphine 6-glucuronide) in a nebulized form for treatment of cancer-related breathlessness (Quigley, Joel, Patel, Baksh, & Slevin, 2002); nine patients reported subjective improvement in dyspnea. A randomized controlled trial is planned.

Anxiolytics

Anxiety is often one of the dimensions of dyspnea; therefore, when morphine is not completely effective, an anxiolytic may help relieve dyspnea. Benzodiazepines are the category of anxiolytics most commonly used in the management of dyspnea. These drugs have hypnotic, sedative, anxiolytic, anticonvulsant, and muscle-relaxant actions, therefore achieving control of dyspnea via multiple mechanisms of action. Benzodiazepines depress the hypoxic/hypercapnic ventilatory response, as well as alter the emotional response to dyspnea. Specifically, they bind to a site on the gamma-aminobutyric acid (GABA) receptor and potentiate the action of GABA, which acts as an inhibitory neurotransmitter in the central nervous system.

Unfortunately, studies have demonstrated a lack of consistent therapeutic benefit and poor tolerance to some benzodiazepine side effects (primarily sedation and cognitive impairment) (Rousseau, 1997). Nevertheless, lorazepam, 0.5 to 1.0 mg sublingually/orally every 6 to 8 hours as needed or around the clock, is frequently used. Side effects include drowsiness, ataxia, reduced psychomotor performance, loss of appetite, and perceptual disturbances. Diazepam or phenothiazines (e.g., chlorpromazine or haloperidol [Haldol]) are considered alternative medications. The use of Haldol increases the risk of extrapyramidal side effects, although it has been used successfully in intractable dyspnea unresponsive to opioids, corticosteroids, and benzodiazepines. Haldol reduces air hunger and anxiety with minimal side effects, and is particularly efficacious during the final days of life (Rousseau, 1997).

Corticosteroids

Corticosteroids are of value in the treatment of dyspnea because they reduce inflammation by suppressing the migration of polymorphonuclear leukocytes and reversing the increase in capillary permeability. Euphoria occurs in the form of an overall feeling of well-being, and an increase in appetite is exhibited as a secondary response. In the lungs, corticosteroids decrease airway inflammation that may be experienced with COPD and radiation pneumonitis, reduce edema associated with tracheal or lung tumors, and increase vital capacity in interstitial disease.

Corticosteroids can improve airway obstruction in cases of lymphangitis carcinomatosa or superior vena cava syndrome. The standard dose of dexamethasone is 8 mg orally per day; that of prednisone is 10 to 20 mg orally per day, but can increase to as much as 60 mg/day. Starting doses are usually high, then reduced to a lower maintenance dose. Adverse reactions (e.g., insomnia, nervousness, indigestion, and hyperglycemia) are dose and duration dependent; the nurse should monitor the elder closely for any untoward outcomes. Benefits are generally felt within 48 hours in most patients, but may take a couple of weeks. Corticosteroids can be given orally, subcutaneously, intramuscularly, intravenously, or by inhalation.

For many terminally ill elders, opioids, corticosteroids, and benzodiazepines remain the mainstays of therapy and frequently obviate the need for more aggressive evaluation and intercession (Rousseau, 1997).

Bronchodilators

A trial of bronchodilator therapy is warranted to relieve dyspnea, especially with COPD, asthma, and other problems associated with reactive airways. Beta$_2$-agonists and anticholinergics cause smooth muscle dilation of the airways, thus removing any impedance to airflow. Specifically, bronchodilators exert synergistic action on cyclic adenosine 3′,5′-monophosphate. They also stabilize mast cells and stimulate the respiratory tract cilia to expel mucus. The preferred route is inhaled, either by metered-dose inhaler or nebulizer, but these drugs are also available in oral preparations. Side effects, such as tremors, agitation, and anxiety that may heighten the dyspnea, are due to sympathetic stimulation. These potential systemic effects, however, are greater with the oral route. The elder's response should dictate the use of bronchodilators.

Diuretics

Dyspnea may be associated with fluid volume excess, which can be treated with diuretics such as furosemide to mobilize edema, normalize blood volume, reduce vascular congestion, and reduce the workload of the heart. Furosemide inhibits reabsorption of sodium and chloride in the ascending loop of Henle and distal renal tubule, interfering with the chloride-binding cotransport system, thus causing increased excretion of water and electrolytes. Normal doses can be administered orally, subcutaneously, intramuscularly, intravenously, and by inhalation. For conditions in which diuresis is needed urgently (e.g., CHF, pulmonary edema), the intravenous form may be preferred. Other disease states in which diuretics may be helpful to relieve dyspnea include pulmonary hypertension and abdominal ascites. For control of dyspnea refractory to standard treatments, Shimoyama and Shimoyama (2002) reported on the use of inhaled furosemide. Three terminal cancer patients with severe dyspnea were treated with nebulized furosemide. Twenty milligrams of furosemide was nebulized and inhaled four times daily. Dyspnea improved dramatically without adverse reactions. The effect was sustained throughout the final weeks of life (approximately 3 weeks).

Antibiotics

Antibiotics may be indicated when dyspnea occurs secondary to a respiratory infection. Rather than pursue a traditional work-up for infection, an empirical trial of antibiotics is appropriate when an elder is near death. Antibiotics can provide symptom relief and facilitate comfort in the presence of a respiratory infection characterized by an elevated temperature, abnormal breath sounds, acute cough, and nasal/chest congestion.

Anticholinergics

The lack of ability to protect one's airway in the final hours of life contributes to the buildup of secretions that leads to what is commonly referred to as the "death rattle" (i.e., noisy breathing). This is an extremely disturbing symptom to families, loved ones, and caregivers of the

---

EVIDENCE-BASED PRACTICE

Reference: Shimoyama, N., & Shimoyama, M. (2002). Nebulized furosemide as a novel treatment for dyspnea in terminal cancer patients. *Journal of Pain and Symptom Management, 23,* 73-76.

Research Problem: Investigate an alternative treatment for severe cancer-related dyspnea unrelieved with traditional therapy (morphine, oxygen, and bronchodilator).

Design: Experimental case reports.

Sample and Setting: 3 terminal cancer patients (bladder cancer with lung metastasis, esophageal cancer with tracheal metastasis, malignant lymphoma) with intractable dyspnea in a hospital setting. All were male, with an age range of 49 to 53 years.

Methods: Each patient was given 20 mg furosemide in 2 mL saline via nebulizer four times daily. Dyspnea was measured by a 10-cm visual analogue scale (VAS) anchored by no breathlessness (0) and worst possible breathlessness (10) before and after initiation of furosemide inhalation.

Results: Dyspnea improved and was controlled for as long as 3 weeks. Dyspnea VAS scores ranged from 7 to 10 before furosemide to 1 to 3 after furosemide. Peak effect occurred within 20 to 30 minutes of the nebulizer treatment and was sustained throughout the course. No side effects were noted, nor were observable systemic effects (urine output before and after intervention was relatively unchanged).

Implications for Nursing Practice: Cancer-related dyspnea can be intractable to standard therapies. Consider alternatives to manage this difficult symptom. Tailor therapy to the individual and think beyond traditional modes. Utilize available pharmacologic agents, but combine these with comfort measures both known and unusual.

Conclusion: Furosemide may be a reasonable alternative for the treatment of severe dyspnea; a randomized controlled trial is planned.

patient. It occurs in 56% to 92% of dying patients (Bennett, 1996). The "death rattle" is caused by the collection of secretions in the posterior oropharynx, an absent cough reflex, and, in severe cases of cardiopulmonary failure, pulmonary edema (Picella, 1997).

Transdermal hyoscine (scopolamine) or oral or sublingual hyoscyamine can be used to manage excessive secretions in the upper respiratory tract. The mechanism of action is the blockade of acetylcholine at parasympathetic sites in smooth muscle, secretory glands, and central nervous system, with the primary clinical effect of inhibition of salivary secretions. The dosage is one to three patches every 3 days or 0.8 to 3.2 mg subcutaneously every day. However, not all patients will respond to hyoscine; the exact reasons are unknown (Bennett, 1996). In these cases, an antispasmodic agent such as oxybutynin, 5 to 10 mg orally three times per day, should be considered (Storey, 1994). Anecdotal reports from hospice nurses suggest the use of atropine eyedrops sublingually as a reasonable alternative, as long as side effects (bradycardia) are monitored.

Anesthetics

Recent reports in the literature suggest that ketamine may have a place in treating intractable symptoms, specifically pain, during a patient's final hours (Fine, 1999). Ketamine, a neuromuscular depolarizing agent, has strong analgesic, anxiolytic, and amnestic properties that make it attractive as a treatment for uncontrollable dyspnea (R. Witte, personal communication, December 13, 2002). Anecdotal reports on a small number of patients with severe dyspnea unresponsive to usual therapy suggest that a conservative induction of ketamine can be successful (Witte, 2002). Using trial and error, the following regimen has safely facilitated control of severe dyspnea: give an initial intravenous bolus dose of 0.15 mg/kg; repeat every 10 to 15 minutes twice as needed (Witte, 2002). If no effect is noted at this time, other options should be explored. If symptom(s) subside, a ketamine infusion can be started at a rate determined by dividing the relief-duration time into the total induction dose (Witte, 2002). (For example, in a 50-kg person, 0.15 mg/kg = a 7.5-mg intravenous bolus. Duration of relief is 3 hours; thus 7.5 mg

divided by 3 hours = a 2.5-mg/hr infusion.) The patient may need to receive a second bolus at the start of the infusion. Side effects are rare because the dose is subtherapeutic for anesthesia (Fine, 1999). There is no interaction with opioids; however, opioids can usually be tapered without increasing symptoms (Witte, 2002). Although the benefit to the patient is relief of symptoms without drowsiness and other untoward effects, tolerance rapidly develops (R. Witte, personal communication, December 13, 2002). There may be difficulty accessing this drug in palliative care, as well as issues regarding starting an intravenous infusion at the end of life. Based on these preliminary reports, however, further investigation into using ketamine to treat extreme dyspnea and other severe symptoms seen at the very end of life is warranted.

Case Study Conclusion

Despite all efforts to restore his health, Mr. S. again developed pneumonia with respiratory failure that required mechanical ventilation. Acting as his health care proxy, his wife, within a few days, came to terms with the fact that he was not going to come home and made the decision to forego further life-sustaining therapies. He was moved to a room that offered more privacy and space. Mr. S. was given intravenous morphine prior to extubation, and then as needed for relief of breathlessness. Because of the severity of his pulmonary condition combined with the inflammatory effects of his rheumatoid arthritis, Mr. S. required frequent morphine administration that was difficult for the nursing staff to handle and did not effectively manage his symptoms. However, with the addition of intravenous lorazepam, Mr. S. became less dyspneic, less agitated, and more alert, and less frequent doses of morphine were needed. He was able to focus on his family for a few moments at a time.

Intravenous corticosteroids helped reduce the painful effects of the inflammation. During the course of his illness, Mr. S. had become reassured by oxygen therapy, so it was offered by nasal cannula, the least restrictive device. A scopolamine patch was placed when his secretions became excessive. His family and a few close friends gathered at his bedside. They played his favorite country-western music, expressed their love for him, reminisced about the good times they had had together, and told a few jokes. His priest came and offered the Sacrament of the Anointing of the Sick. His wife and son were encouraged to stay at the bedside as much as they wanted and were supported in their grief by friends, hospital staff, clergy, and the physicians involved in his care. Mr. S. drifted in and out of consciousness until the last few hours of his life. He died peacefully with his family at his side.

CONCLUSION

Dyspnea has long been recognized as a prevalent symptom near the end of life (Fainsinger, Miller, & Bruera, 1991; Lichter & Hunt, 1990; Nauck, Klaschik, & Ostgathe, 2000; Ventafridda, Ripamonti, DeConno, Tamburini, & Cassileth, 1990). Similarly, noisy breathing (death rattle) is frequently observed in the last hours and days of life. Morita, Ichiki, and Tsunoda (1998) reported a mean of 57 hours till death once noisy breathing began. A retrospective chart review of 185 residents who died in a long-term care facility indicated that dyspnea was the most commonly recorded symptom (62%) and noisy breathing was the third (39%). However, in nearly a quarter of the patients with dyspnea, symptoms were not treated. Of those who did receive treatment, oxygen was the therapy most often utilized. Opioids accounted for 27% of the treatment and nonpharmacologic measures for 6%. About half of the cases with "noisy breathing" went untreated; those who did receive therapy were either suctioned or given hyoscine. The nurse was the only health care professional involved 40% of the time (Hall, Schroder, & Weaver, 2002).

Although the authors conducted only a chart review and used a convenience sample, which are study limitations, the findings nonetheless point to the tremendous need for end-of-life education and research, especially for dyspnea management. As the population ages and the symptoms of chronic diseases become even more prevalent, more people will suffer unnecessarily unless nurses advocate for quality end-of-life care.

REFERENCES

American Thoracic Society. (1999). Dyspnea mechanisms, assessment, and management: A consensus statement. *American Journal of Respiratory and Critical Care Medicine, 159,* 321-340.

Benditt, J. O. (2000). Noninvasive ventilation at the end of life. *Respiratory Care, 45,* 1376-1381.

Bennett, M. I. (1996). Death rattle: An audit of hyoscine (scopolamine) use and review of management. *Journal of Pain and Symptom Management, 12,* 229-233.

Booth, S., & Adams, L. (2001). The shuttle walking test: A reproducible method for evaluating the impact of shortness of breath on functional capacity in patients with advanced cancer. *Thorax, 56,* 146-150.

Booth, S., Kelly, M. J., Cox, N. P., Adams, L., & Guz, A. (1996). Does oxygen help dyspnea in patients with cancer? *American Journal of Respiratory and Critical Care Medicine, 153,* 1515-1518.

Bruera, E., Schmitz, B., Pither, J., Neumann, C. M., & Hanson, J. (2000). The frequency and correlates of dyspnea in patients with advanced cancer. *Journal of Pain & Symptom Management, 19,* 357-362.

Campbell, M. (1996). Managing terminal dyspnea: Caring for the patient who refuses intubation or ventilation. *Dimensions in Critical Care Nursing, 15,* 4-13.

Cazzoli, P. A., & Oppenheimer, E. A. (1996). Home mechanical ventilation for amyotrophic lateral sclerosis: Nasal compared to tracheal intermittent positive pressure ventilation. *Journal of Neurological Science, 139* (Suppl.), 123-128.

Cleary, J. F., & Carbone, P. P. (1997). Palliative medicine in the elderly. *Cancer, 80,* 1335-1347.

Cooksley, V. G. (1996). Aromatherapy treatments for the respiratory system. In *Aromatherapy: A lifetime guide to healing with essential oils* (pp. 92-112). Paramus, NJ: Prentice Hall.

Corner, J., Plant, H., A'Hern, R., & Bailey, C. (1996). Nonpharmacological intervention for breathlessness in lung cancer. *Palliative Medicine, 10,* 299-305.

Dudgeon, D. J., & Rosenthal, S. (1996). Management of dyspnea and cough in patients with cancer. *Hematology/Oncology Clinics of North America, 10,* 157-171.

Fainsinger, R., Miller, M., Bruera, E., Hanson, J., & Maceachern, T. (1991). Symptom control during the last week of life on a palliative care unit. *Journal of Palliative Care, 7* (1), 5-11.

Fine, P. G. (1999). Low-dose ketamine in the management of opioid nonresponsive, terminal cancer pain. *Journal of Pain and Symptom Management, 17,* 296-300.

Gift, A. G. (1989). Clinical measurement of dyspnea. *Dimensions of Critical Care Nursing, 8,* 210-216.

Hall, P., Schroder, C., & Weaver, L. (2002). The last 48 hours of life in long-term care: A focused chart audit. *Journal of the American Geriatrics Society, 50,* 501-506.

Hill, N. S., Eveloff, S. E., Carlisle, C. C., & Goff, S. G. (1992). Efficacy of nocturnal nasal ventilation in patients with restrictive thoracic disease. *American Review of Respiratory Diseases, 145,* 365-371.

Lichter, I., & Hunt, E. (1990). The last 48 hours of life. *Journal of Palliative Care, 6* (4), 7-15.

Lyall, R. A., Fleming, T. A., Newsome-Davis, I., Wood, C., Leigh, P. N., & Moxham, J. (2000). A prospective controlled study of the effect of NIPPV on quality of life in amyotrophic lateral sclerosis. *American Journal of Respiratory and Critical Care Medicine, 161,* A358.

Mahler, D. A., Rosiello, R. A., & Loke, J. (1986). The aging lung. *Geriatric Clinics of North America, 2,* 215-225.

Maltoni, M., Pirovan, M., Scarpi, E., Marinari, M., Indelli, M., Arnoldi, E., et al. (1995). Prediction of survival of patients terminally ill with cancer. *Cancer, 75,* 2613-2622.

Meduri, G. U., Abou-Shala, N., Fox, R. C., Jones, C. B., Leeper, K. V., & Wunderink, R. G. (1991). Noninvasive face mask mechanical ventilation in patients with acute hypercapnic respiratory failure. *Chest, 100,* 445-454.

Mercadante, S., Casuccio, A., & Fulfaro, F. (2000). The course of symptom frequency and intensity in advanced cancer patients followed at home. *Journal of Pain and Symptom Management, 20,* 104-112.

Morita, T., Ichiki, T., & Tsunoda, J. (1998). A prospective study on the dying process in terminally ill cancer patients. *American Journal of Hospice & Palliative Care, 15,* 217-222.

Nauck, F., Klaschik, E., & Ostgathe, C. (2000). Symptom control during the last three days of life. *European Journal of Palliative Care, 7,* 81-84.

Picella, D. V. (1997). Palliative care for the patient with end stage respiratory illness. *Perspectives in Respiratory Nursing, 8* (4), 1-10.

Quigley, C., Joel, S., Patel, N., Baksh, A., & Slevin, M. (2002). A Phase I/II study of nebulized morphine-6-glucuronide in patients with cancer-related breathlessness. *Journal of Pain and Symptom Management, 23,* 7-9.

Reuben, D. B., & Mor, V. (1986). Dyspnea in terminally ill cancer patients. *Chest, 89,* 234-236.

Ripamonti, C. (1999). Management of dyspnea in advanced cancer patients. *Supportive Care for Cancer, 7,* 233-243.

Rousseau, P. (1996). Nonpain symptom management in terminal care. *Clinics in Geriatric Medicine, 12,* 313-327.

Rousseau, P. (1997). Management of dyspnea in the dying elderly. *Clinical Geriatrics, 5* (6), 42-48.

Schwartzstein, R. M. (1999). The language of dyspnea: Using verbal clues to the diagnosis. *Journal of Critical Illness, 14,* 435-441.

Sheahan, S. L., & Musialowski, R. (2001). Clinical implications of respiratory system changes in aging. *Journal of Gerontological Nursing, 27* (5), 26-34.

Shimoyama, N., & Shimoyama, M. (2002). Nebulized furosemide as a novel treatment for dyspnea in terminal cancer patients. *Journal of Pain and Symptom Management, 23,* 73-76.

Spector, N., & Klein, D. (2002, March). Assessing and managing dyspnea. *Nursing Profile,* pp. 20-24.

Spector, N., Klein, D., & Rice-Wiley, L. (2000, December). Terminally ill patients breathe easier with nebulized morphine. *Nursing Spectrum,* pp. 1-6.

Storey, P. (1994). Symptom control in advanced cancer. *Seminars in Oncology, 21,* 748.

Tanaka, K., Akechi, T., Okuyama, T., Nishiwaki, Y., & Uchitomi, Y. (2000). Development and validation of the Cancer Dyspnoea Scale: A multidimensional, brief, self-rating scale. *British Journal of Cancer, 82,* 800-805.

Thompson, L. F. (1996). Failure to wean: Exploring the influence of age-related pulmonary changes. *Critical Care Nursing Clinics of North America, 8,* 7-16.

Ventafridda, V., Ripamonti, C., DeConno, F., Tamburini, M., & Cassileth, B. R. (1990). Symptom prevention and control during cancer patients' last days of life. *Journal of Palliative Care, 6* (3), 7-11.

Witte, R. (2002, July). *Terminal agitation and sedation.* Presented at the HOPE regional meeting, Tomah, WI.

Zepetella, G. (1998). The palliation of dyspnea in terminal disease. *American Journal of Hospice & Palliative Care,* Nov-Dec, 322-330.

18 ANXIETY, DEPRESSION, AND DELIRIUM

Constance M. Dahlin

Case Study

Mrs. M. is an 85-year-old retired school principal who has atrial fibrillation and coronary artery disease, additionally suffering from anxiety and depression in her later years. She had lived alone in the house she and her husband had shared for 55 years, even after he died of cancer 10 years ago. His death was a peaceful experience for the family; they used the services of a local hospice to care for him at home. Mrs. M.'s two daughters live nearby, but she insisted she didn't need much help. Mrs. M. had been fiercely independent as she attended to her own shopping, errands, and church activities.

Everything changed 2 years ago when she began to have more trouble caring for herself. She became more fatigued, lost interest in her personal appearance, and had trouble managing her home. After much discussion, she moved into an assisted living facility, and did fairly well at the residence the first year. She was able to participate in activities and walk to the dining room for meals.

She then developed several bouts of pneumonia within a 6-month period, requiring multiple hospital admissions. After four admissions, Mrs. M. was much weaker and unable to care for herself. She was admitted to the nursing home affiliated with the assisted living residence because she needed skilled care.

She also was experiencing more physical symptoms, pain, occasional delirium, and extreme shortness of breath. A cardiac work-up revealed an ejection fraction of 15%, an oxygen saturation of approximately 89%, and a functional status so poor that she needed help with all activities of daily living. She was subsequently diagnosed with end-stage heart failure and chronic anxiety. Both of these conditions impacted her breathing; in addition, she experienced delirium from carbon dioxide retention and exacerbation of depression for which she had a previous history, and was worsened because of her loss of independence.

INTRODUCTION

The developmental tasks of late adulthood include role changes related to retirement, widowhood, or caring for a spouse. In addition, there are normal biologic changes in physical appearance and function that may result in loss of health and independence. Indeed, the older adult may have a keen sense of his or her mortality and limited life span (Buckwalter & Piven, 1999). In response to such events, individuals cope in many ways. Sometimes they develop psychiatric symptoms, including anxiety, depression, and delirium. However, the diagnoses of anxiety, depression, and delirium are strongly correlated with life-limiting illness (Shuster & Jones, 1998).

As transient events, anxiety, depression, and delirium may not cause long-term issues. However, in severe forms, they inhibit the ability to have meaningful communication with family and friends as part of life closure. They may cause suffering in and of themselves, thereby greatly affecting quality of life.

Anxiety, depression, and delirium are common symptoms during the dying process. In older adults, these symptoms may be the first sign of a medical problem, making it difficult to differentiate between these three disorders and other medical conditions (Reichel & Gallo, 1999). Because these disorders may occur concurrently, diagnosis and treatment are even more challenging. In some cases, anxiety may precede depression in the diagnosis of certain medical conditions such as myocardial infarction or dementia. Often anxiety and depression are seen together, for example, with the shock of the diagnosis of a terminal illness. Delirium may cause anxiety stemming from the ensuing alteration of consciousness. This is particularly true if the delirium waxes and wanes and the patient has a sense of his or her loss of cognitive faculties. Depression may result if an elder patient understands his or her cognitive deficits (Lovejoy, Tabor, & Deloney, 2000; Reichel & Gallo, 1999).

Because the initial presentation of a medical condition may manifest as a psychiatric symptom, misdiagnosis of anxiety, depression, and delirium is common in the older adult. With the additional overlay of a life-threatening illness, diagnosis may be much more difficult and more complex. Cardinal signs of a disease may be hidden or diminished, such as decreased pain in a myocardial infarction, or minimal fever in an infection. Other examples include the presentation of delirium in a patient with a neurologic process, depression in a patient who has underlying pancreatic cancer, and anxiety in a patient with underlying cardiac ailments (Reichel & Gallo, 1999).

Once a diagnosis is made, treatment issues related to the older adult must be considered. In particular, the health care practitioner must take into account the older adult's more pronounced therapeutic and adverse effects from medications as a result of potential diminishing functional and physiologic processes, as well as the possible lack of social supports (Reichel & Gallo, 1999). Because successful treatment of the older adult includes pharmacologic therapy, complementary therapy, and mobilization of social support of the patient and family, this chapter addresses the holistic care necessary in effective diagnosis, assessment, and treatment of anxiety, depression, and delirium in the palliative care older adult population.

ANXIETY
Definition
Anxiety is defined as feelings of distress and tension that lack a known stimulus (Lehmann & Rabins, 1999). Generalized anxiety disorder is described as chronic uncontrollable nervousness,

fearfulness, and sense of worry that lasts for 6 months or longer (Carmin et al., 1999; Lantz, 2002; Lehmann & Rabins, 1999). Patients may describe this as a sense of worry, fear, concern, or even foreboding. Although anxiety is a very subjective experience, it is often accompanied by somatic complaints such as tachycardia, fatigue, restlessness, difficulty concentrating, muscle tension, headaches, palpitations, sweating, abdominal discomfort, dizziness, urinary frequency, and sleep disturbances. For a diagnosis of generalized anxiety disorder, symptoms must be present for at least 6 months and cause impairment in social or occupational functioning. In older adults, there may be a sense of phobia that causes them to stay at home because they are fearful to leave. They may also stop activities and become more isolated (Lantz, 2002).

Incidence
Generalized anxiety is the most common anxiety disorder found in late life. It occurs at a rate of 10% to 20%, with a prevalence of 7% in adults older than age 55 (Reichel & Gallo, 1999). Anxiety has been associated with female gender, young age, and low socioeconomic status. However, as a life-threatening disease progresses and a person's physical status declines, anxiety may increase (Tremblay & Breitbart, 2001). Anxiety symptoms may develop in any individual diagnosed with a life-limiting illness. In one study, over half of cancer patients fit the International Classification of Diseases criteria for anxiety (Stark, Kiely, Smith, Velikova, & Selby, 2002). This anxiety is a natural response to the crisis precipitated by such a diagnosis, including the threat to life and the future (Payne & Massie, 2000). Treatment issues arise when the anxiety symptoms persist.

Etiology
Anxiety in older patients with a life-limiting illness is common and has numerous causes; it may be an element of adjustment to the disease process or an agitated depression (Breitbart, Chochinov, & Passik, 1998). The etiology of anxiety includes a multitude of medical conditions such as poorly managed pain; endocrine disorders, including hypo- and hyperglycemia, hypo- and hyperthyroidism, and Cushing's disease; and carcinoid syndrome (Table 18-1). Cardiovascular conditions that cause anxiety

Table 18-1 **Medical Conditions Associated with Anxiety**	
Category/Basis	**Examples**
Cardiovascular conditions	Angina, congestive heart failure, hypovolemia, mitral valve prolapse, myocardial infarction, paroxysmal atrial tachycardia
Endocrine disorders	Carcinoid syndrome, Cushing's disease, hyperglycemia, hypoglycemia, hyperthyroidism/hypothyroidism
Immune conditions	AIDS, infections
Metabolic conditions	Anemia, hyperkalemia, hyperthermia, hypoglycemia, hyponatremia
Respiratory conditions	Asthma, chronic obstructive pulmonary disease, hypoxia, pneumonia, pulmonary edema, pulmonary embolus
Neurologic conditions	Akathisia, encephalopathy, brain lesion, seizure disorders, postconcussion syndrome, vertigo, cerebrovascular accident, dementia
Cancer	Hormone-producing tumors (e.g., pheochromocytoma)
Medication and substances	Withdrawal from alcohol, benzodiazepines, or sedatives
	Use of steroids, stimulants, and neuroleptics such as metoclopramide or prochlorperazine
Uncontrolled pain	

AIDS, acquired immunodeficiency syndrome.
Sources: Breitbart, W., Chochinov, H. M., & Passik, S. (1998). Psychiatric aspect of palliative care. In D. Doyle, W. C. Hanks, & N. MacDonald, Eds. *Oxford textbook of palliative medicine*. (2nd ed.). New York: Oxford University Press; Lantz, M. (2002). Generalized anxiety in anxious times: helping older adults cope. *Clinical Geriatrics*, 10(1), 36-38; McCullough, P. K. (1992). Evaluation and management of anxiety in the older adult. *Geriatrics*, 47(4), 35-38; Pasacreta, J. V., Minarik, P. A., & Nield-Anderson, L. (2001). Anxiety and depression. In B. Ferrell, & N. Coyle. *Textbook of palliative nursing*. New York: Oxford University Press; Waller, A. & Caroline, N. L. (2000). *Handbook of palliative care in cancer*. (2nd ed.). Boston: Butterworth-Heinemann.

include myocardial infarctions, angina, congestive heart failure, mitral valve prolapse, and hypovolemia; respiratory conditions include asthma, chronic obstructive pulmonary disease (COPD), pneumonia, pulmonary edema, dyspnea, and hypoxia. Neoplasms and neurologic conditions such as akathisia, encephalopathy, seizure disorder, and postconcussion disorders can also contribute to or exacerbate anxiety disorders (Pasacreta, Minarik, & Nield-Anderson, 2001; Pollack, Smoller, & Lee, 1998).

Stimulant substances that may contribute to anxiety include caffeine, which is present in coffee, tea, chocolate, and soda; ephedrine, which is present in cold remedies; and stimulant-type drugs such as methylphenidate (*Medical Letter*, 2002). In addition, withdrawal from medications such as benzodiazepines, alcohol, and barbiturates may cause anxiety. Psychological distress, such as worries about family relationships and finances, may also cause anxiety for elders with a life-limiting illness. These may be exacerbated by concern about being a burden to other family members. Lastly, a family history may be a component of anxiety that may become more pronounced in older patients as they lose physical functioning.

Cardinal Signs

Anxiety has four manifestations: physical symptoms, affective symptoms, behavioral responses, and cognitive responses (Pollack et al., 1998) as outlined in Table 18-2. Generalized anxiety can be accompanied by symptoms of depression, panic, and phobias; however, in the elder patient, depression is the most common accompanying condition (Well-Connected, 1998a). Patients may be observed to have a tense posture and to sigh frequently. Older adults are more likely to minimize emotions and feelings and report somatic complaints (Lantz, 2002). In addition, they have many attributes of suicide vulnerability, which include pain and suffering, poor prognosis, depression, delirium, loss of control, and lack of social support (Breitbart et al., 1998). In differentiating anxiety from fear, evaluation

Table 18-2 **Four Manifestations of Anxiety**	
Classification	Manifestations
Physical symptoms	Autonomic responses such as tachycardia, tachypnea, diaphoresis, lightheadedness
Affective symptoms	Nervous behaviors such as pacing, picking, frequent movement, edginess, panic, terror
Behavioral responses	Avoidance, compulsions
Cognitive responses	Worry, apprehension, obsession, thoughts of self physical or emotional damage

From Pollack, M. H., Smoller, J. W., & Lee, D. (1998). Approach to the anxious patient. In T. A. Stern, J. B. Herman, & P. L. Slavin (Eds.) *The MGH guide to psychiatry in primary care* (pp. 23-32). New York: McGraw-Hill.

Severity

Anxiety, in its mildest form, assists any person to participate in general life activities; it serves as an impetus to perform various functions in learning, working, and adapting to the ongoing changes in life. Levels of anxiety include mild, which is normal, moderate, and severe (Lehmann & Rabins, 1999; Pasacreta et al., 2001). In its most severe form, anxiety becomes panic, which prevents an elder from doing anything. The person may become paralyzed with fear and confined to his or her immediate surroundings, such as home or a bedroom. Box 18-1 outlines the characteristics of anxiety, ranging from mild to panic.

Assessment of the Older Adult

Assessment for anxiety requires vigilance. A history and review of medical conditions for potential causes of anxiety is part of the initial evaluation. This should be followed by a thorough discussion of psychosocial situations, including living conditions, recent changes in the patient's life, and anticipated changes. This conversation is most revealing if it includes both

Box 18-1 **Mild to Severe Anxiety and Its Effects**	
Mild	Awareness
	Alert attention
Moderate	Perceptual field narrowed
	Observation decreased
	Selective attention
Severe	Reduced perceptual field
	Scattered
	Anxiety escalates
	Unable to attend
Panic	Feelings of awe, dread, fear, panic
	Inability to focus
	No perceptual field

Adapted from Pasacreta, J. V., Minarik, P. A., & Nield-Anderson, L. (2001). Anxiety and depression. In B. Ferrell & N. Coyle (Eds.), *Textbook of palliative nursing* (pp. 267-269). New York: Oxford University Press.

the patient and family or friends. Moreover, there should be an assessment of whether the anxiety is a secondary response to any of the following: an organic factor, a primary psychiatric disorder, or reactive or situationally related stress (Pollack et al., 1998).

Physical Exam

A physical exam may reveal tachycardia, tachypnea, skin changes, tongue changes, rapid speech, restlessness, and tremors. Further assessment includes ruling out associated conditions; for example, if an elder has tachycardia, a thyroid function panel can rule out hyperthyroidism. For patients feeling anxious, a glucose test can rule out hypoglycemia. If there is a sore tongue along with the anxiety, testing folate levels can rule out nutritional deficiencies. Similarly, pulmonary function tests and arterial blood gases can rule out hypoxia and pulmonary disease (McCullough, 1996).

Assessment Tools

A tool for further assessing anxiety is the Anxiety Sensitivity Index (ASI) (Box 18-2). This is a 16-item self-report index; responses are rated from 0 to 4. A mean score of 20 and below indicates no anxiety. A mean score in the 20s is common for those with generalized anxiety disorders. A mean score of 35 and above indicates

Box 18-2 **Anxiety Sensitivity Index**

1. It scares me when my heart beats rapidly.
2. It scares me when I become short of breath.
3. It scares me when I am nauseous.
4. It scares me when I feel faint.
5. When I notice my heart is beating rapidly, I worry I might have a heart attack.
6. Unusual body sensations scare me.
7. It scares me when I feel "shaky."
8. It embarrasses me when my stomach growls.
9. When my stomach is upset, I worry that I might be seriously ill.
10. When I am nervous, I worry that I might be mentally ill.
11. When I cannot keep my mind on a task, I worry that I might be going crazy.
12. It scares me when I am unable to keep my mind on a task.
13. It scares me when I am nervous.
14. Other people notice when I feel shaky.
15. It is important to me to stay in control of my emotions.
16. It is important for me not to appear nervous.

Responses are rated from 0 (not true) to 4 (extremely true). Mean score of 20 and below indicates no anxiety. Mean score in the 20s is common for those with generalized anxiety disorders. Mean score of 35 and above indicates panic disorder. From Reiss, S., Peterson, R. A., Gursky, D. M., & McNally, R. J. (1986). Anxiety sensitivity, anxiety frequency, and the prediction of fearfulness. *Behaviour Research and Therapy, 24,* 1-8.

Table 18-3 **Medications to Treat Older Adults with Anxiety**

Medication	Dosage
BENZODIAZEPINES (SHORT ACTING)	
Lorazepam (Ativan)	0.25-5 mg tid–qid
Oxazepam (Serax)	10-15 mg tid–qid
Temazepam (Restoril)	15-30 mg at bedtime
NEUROLEPTICS	
Haloperidol (Haldol)	0.5-5 mg q 2-12 h
Chlorpromazine (Thorazine)	12.5-50 q 4-6h
ANTIHISTAMINES	
Diphenhydramine (Benadryl)	25-75 mg bid
Hydroxyzine (Vistaril)	10-50 mg qid–q 6 h
AZAPIRONE	
Buspirone (BuSpar)	5-20 mg tid

Sources: Breitbart, W., Chochinov, H. M., & Passik, S. (1998). Psychiatric aspect of palliative care. In D. Doyle, W. C. Hanks, & N. MacDonald, Eds. *Oxford textbook of palliative medicine.* (2nd ed.). New York: Oxford University Press; Lavretsky, H. (2001). Choosing appropriate treatment for geriatric depression. *Clinical Geriatrics, 9*(5), 30-46; Payne, D. K., & Massie, M. J. (2000). Anxiety in palliative care. In H. M. Chochinov, & W. Breitbart, Eds. *Handbook of psychiatry in palliative medicine.* New York: Oxford University Press; Pasacreta, J. V., Minarik, P. A., & Nield-Anderson, L. (2001). Anxiety and depression. In B. Ferrell, & N. Coyle, *Textbook of palliative nursing.* New York: Oxford University Press.

panic disorder (Candilis, 1998; Reiss, Peterson, Gursky, & McNally, 1986).

Management
Pharmacologic

In a younger, healthier population, benzodiazepines, along with tricyclic antidepressants and beta-adrenergic agents, are used to treat anxiety. However, in the geriatric population, benzodiazepines are preferred because tricyclics and beta-adrenergic agents are not well tolerated. Even so, in the older adult, one should not use longer-acting benzodiazepines because they may cause more confusion; use of shorter-acting agents such as lorazepam, oxazepam, and temazepam may be more appropriate (Table 18-3). Suggested doses are 0.25 to 5 mg three times a day for lorazepam, or 10 to 15 mg three times a day for oxazepam. Selective serotonin reuptake inhibitors (SSRIs) may be worthwhile if benzodiazepines are not successful. These agents include fluoxetine, 20 to 80 mg/day, and sertraline, 50 to 200 mg/day (Pollack et al., 1998). If insomnia is also an issue, temazepam, 15 to 30 mg at bedtime, may be helpful. Drug-induced anxiety may be caused by neuroleptic medications such as haloperidol. For older adult patients with generalized anxiety and a history of substance abuse, buspirone may be useful. In patients with severe respiratory function, low-dose antihistamines may be helpful, because benzodiazepines may be too sedating and may inhibit respiratory drive (Pasacreta et al., 2001; Payne & Massie, 2000).

Nonpharmacologic

In severe anxiety and panic, medications are usually necessary; nonpharmacologic or complementary therapy may help in mild to moderate anxiety. Nonpharmacologic treatment of anxiety includes modalities such as adjustment of dietary intake, stress management, and psychotherapy. Adjusting dietary intake includes evaluating the diet for caffeine and alcohol (McCullough, 1992). Caffeine is an ingredient in tea, coffee, chocolate, and colas, as well as other products; sometimes, just decreasing the daily amount ingested is helpful. However, in many cases, the caffeine intake needs to be completely eliminated. If this is the case, weaning off the caffeine in a planned process helps avoid headache, nausea, and general malaise. High alcohol intake is common in anxious patients, although it does not actually help the anxiety and, if fact, may worsen it because it affects sleep and cognition. Alcohol may be commonly ingested as beer, wine, or hard liquors and may also be found in cough medicines. Again, reduction of alcohol intake may be helpful, or it may need to be eliminated from the diet.

Stress management can include exercise programs, breathing exercises, relaxation techniques, massage, touch, distraction, music therapy, and visualization. Many senior centers or YWCAs/YMCAs offer gentle exercise programs or special programs directed at keeping older adults healthy. Shopping malls often offer older adults the opportunity to walk in a safe, climate-friendly environment. For patients in assisted living or skilled nursing facilities, physical therapists can often help promote gentle exercise.

Massage therapy can be an effective method to help elders relax. However, as with any person, the older adult's degree of comfort with physical touch must be respected. Many older adults may not have had the experience of a formal massage and may be uncomfortable with such intimate touch. However, they may receive modified massages from health care personnel in various facilities if they do not live at home.

Distraction occurs in many forms, ranging from just having a television or radio on to participating in arts and crafts, performing hobbies, and reading. It is important to assess how the older adult spends his or her time and what activities are distracting for them and therefore helpful in reducing anxiety. Various volunteer organizations in the community can help with the provision of these sorts of activities.

Environmental manipulation may be very important. The older adult may be fearful of the place where he or she lives; therefore, manipulation of the physical environment to make it safe can ease an older adult's anxiety immensely. Physical therapists (PTs) and occupational therapists (OTs) can assist with home safety evaluations. Social workers can assist with issues of personal safety. This may include questionable situations of abuse and neglect, transportation, or nutrition. In addition, anxiety can be reduced by helping the elder maintain control of his or her daily schedule of activities. Too often, the older patient is not allowed much control over the structure of his or her day. Facilitating the elder's ability to schedule when appointments, meals, and other activities occur can help him or her feel less anxious and out of control.

Psychotherapy may include counseling, spiritual care, and cognitive behavioral therapy. Counseling should include an acknowledgment of fears and specific conversations about fears. Spiritual care should focus on existential fears regarding death and dying (Payne & Massie, 2000). Cognitive behavioral therapy focuses on restructuring the issues that are distressing to the older adult.

Dependent, Independent, and Collaborative Interventions

Treatment of anxiety in the older adult requires a collaborative approach by an interdisciplinary team. Specifically, the team needs to review the patient's history and medications, and determine symptom management together. Because treatment usually requires psychological support and medication management, clear delineation of roles should be clarified for the elder and his or her family. This provides consistent direction and support to the patient and family without provoking further anxiety. Usually a physician or an advanced practice registered nurse can diagnose and treat anxiety as well as provide medications and psychological support. A social worker can be quite effective in assessing the living conditions and family dynamics that affect anxiety, as well as offering both counseling and stress management techniques. An OT or PT can assess in-home safety. A pharmacist can examine a medication regimen for polyphar-

EVIDENCE-BASED PRACTICE

Reference: Stark, D., Kiely, A., Smith, G., Velikova, A., & Selby, P. (2002). Anxiety disorders in cancer patients: Their nature, associations, and relations to quality of life. *Journal of Clinical Oncology, 20,* 3137-3148.

Research Problem: Anxiety is a common symptom for patients with a life-threatening illness. However, there has been limited research regarding the severity of anxiety in patients at the end of their lives.

Design: Cross Sectional Observational Study using computer touch screen technology questionnaires measuring psychological symptoms, quality of life, and social support.

Sample and Setting: 178 oncology patients with lymphoma, renal cell carcinoma, malignant melanoma, or plasma cell dyscrasia at cancer center in Northeast England.

Methods: Over a 9-month period from May 1999 to January 2000, this cancer center evaluated anxiety in patients with myriad cancer diagnoses. This was done through the use of several questionnaires, including the State-Trait Anxiety Inventory (STAI), the Schedule for Clinical Assessment in Neuropsychiatry (SCAN), the European Organization for Re-

search and Treatment of Cancer Quality of Life Questionnaire (EORTC QLQC30), and the Hospital Anxiety and Depression Scale for Anxiety (HAD-A).

Results: Of the 178 patients able to complete the study, half reported symptoms that merited a diagnosis of anxiety. However, follow-up interview and survey revealed that only 30% actually had an anxiety diagnosis.

Implications for Nursing Practice: Nurses must maintain an awareness for anxiety, probably integrated as a review of palliative care symptoms, as well as look for secondary symptoms identified with anxiety to be sure one is treating the correct symptom.

Conclusion: Upon examination of the study results, the authors concluded that anxiety decreased quality of life and that insomnia secondary to anxiety was minimized. Further research as to the etiology of the anxiety (whether it is caused by the life-threatening illness or by other coexistent problems) needs to be done. This study has a high degree of power because of the access to possible subjects and the multiplicity of tools. However, it would be interesting to perform this study on patients with various forms of life-threatening illnesses to see if some illnesses have a higher anxiety component than others.

macy. However, an intervention common to all disciplines in dealing with anxious patients is to remind all team members to recognize their own anxiety and manage it so as not to transfer any anxiety to the patient and family (Payne & Massie, 2000). It is also helpful to remind colleagues how to diffuse an elder's anxiety when it begins to escalate.

Family Concerns and Considerations

Education for the family and caregivers is important. The patient and family should understand anxiety and how it manifests itself. This enables early recognition and helps the patient utilize both medications and complementary strategies to manage symptoms. The patient and family should also understand that long-term use of medications to treat anxiety might be necessary.

Moreover, these medications may cause some or all of the following side effects: daytime somnolence, confusion, unsteady stance or gait, paradoxical effects, memory disturbance, depression, withdrawal, abuse, dependence, and respiratory problems. Therefore, safety may be an issue, and how to prevent problems with medications should be discussed. The patient and family may need to discuss the risk:benefit ratio of interventions if medication side effects are debilitating and worse than the anxiety itself.

Medication information is imperative. This includes information on both prescription medications and over-the-counter medications, because the latter can also cause anxiety. A careful review of each medication, its intent, and its dosage can help decrease confusion and help with compliance. A medication box prefilled by family members or health care personnel with medications in the correct time slots can be tremendously helpful in assuring correct medication dosage and timing. Or, a patient or family member can keep a diary of when medications were taken to allow examination for correct time and dosage. In creating medication schedules, it is best to work around previous rituals such as mealtimes and activities of daily living, particularly wake time and bedtime.

Further information necessary for the family includes stress management techniques that can be utilized by both the patient and family. This can involve promotion of some control for the older adult over his or her environment, such as simple planning of daily activities, toileting, mealtimes, and visiting times. It also includes review of the symptoms (including their recognition), management, and prevention of anxiety. Education should also be provided regarding how to diffuse anxiety in the elder and techniques of management by family members so as not to escalate the patient's stress.

For the terminally ill elder patient, care should be taken to simplifying the day by not overbooking activities. Health care personnel should encourage family members or significant others to allow time for ventilation of feelings or concerns regarding the illness. In addition, preparing the elder for any treatment, change in plans, or visitation by other medical personnel can greatly help to decrease anxiety because the patient knows what to expect. Finally, all persons involved with the elder need be patient, speak calmly, and provide any direct care as gently as possible.

DEPRESSION

At the end of life, it is common for patients to experience psychological distress. For many years, it was thought that grief and depression were normal coping mechanisms in response to a terminal illness (Block, 2000; McDonald et al., 1999). Consequently, it was thought that treatment of depression was unnecessary because the treatment would interfere with the natural dying process and the emotional work of dying. In fact, the reverse is true. Not treating depression may interfere with a patient's ability to bring closure to his or her end-of-life issues and concerns.

Identifying depression in the older adult at the end of life is particularly complicated by possible numerous comorbidities. These include cardiovascular conditions, neurologic conditions, autoimmune diseases, endocrine disorders, and other conditions (Pasacreta et al., 2001). In cancer, depressive symptoms can mimic those caused by the cancer treatment regimen, including loss of appetite from chemotherapy, fatigue induced by the metabolic changes in cancer, and lack of sleep from compliance with continuous pain and symptom medication regimens (Lebowitz et al., 1997; McDonald et al., 1999).

Depression in the older adult may be masked by the normal aging process, including changes in the sleep-wake cycle, appetite changes, and changes in the ability to continue previous pursuits in life (Lebowitz et al., 1997; McDonald et al., 1999; Pasacreta et al., 2001). McDonald et al. (1999) documented that depression was overlooked because health care focuses on physiologic treatment and management of side effects rather than emotional responses to an individual's changes in health.

Specifically in the elder patient, depression may not be identified secondary to the misperception that all elders become depressed as part of the aging process. There is also a cohort characteristic to depression in that the current generation of older adults may be embarrassed to report psychological problems in general and depressive symptoms in particular because of a perceived stigma that depression represents weakness (Valente, Saunders, & Cohen, 1994).

Further complicating the diagnosis and treatment of depression in the older adult is the possibility that health care providers may feel ill equipped to treat depression. Treatment necessitates time to work on psychological issues and prescribing psychotropic agents that can cause adverse effects. Under the time constraints of various medical practices, the time required to perform a complete assessment may feel overwhelming to the novice clinician. Ageist attitudes on the part of the prescribing clinician can also affect treatment. Some clinicians express feelings that the life-limiting illness is hopeless and cannot be well treated (Block, 2000). Many clinicians, including nurses, may feel that, by asking about depression, they may add to the patient's psychological distress by further upsetting him or her (McDonald et al., 1999; Valente & Saunders, 1997). Lastly, clinicians may feel

EVIDENCE-BASED PRACTICE

Reference: Hypericum Depression Trial Study Group (2002). Effect of *Hypericum perforatum* (St John's wort) in major depressive disorder: A randomized controlled study.

Research Problem: Depression is a pervasive illness. Often, many patients use *Hypericum perforatum* (St John's wort) to avoid the adverse side effects of prescription antidepressants. In 1996, St John's wort was found to be better than placebo for mild-to-moderate depression. However, there have been questions about these studies as none addressed major depression.

Design: Double-blind, randomized, placebo-controlled trial conducted in 12 settings.

Sample and Setting: 340 Adult outpatients from academic and community psychiatric research clinics across the United States.

Methods: Patients 18 and older were screened for depression using DSM-IV criteria were randomly. They were then diagnosed with major depression after the modified Structured Clinical Interview for Axis I DSM-IV disorders (SCID-Hypericum). This group then completed the Hamilton Depression Scale (HAM-D) with a score of 17-20 and the Global Assessment of Functioning with a maximal score of 60 indicating major depression. If patients remained

in major depression after a 1-week trial of placebos, they entered the 8-week double-blind study receiving placebo, St John's wort, or sertaline. Follow up included the HAM-D and other inventories to measure improvement. Additionally, patients underwent physical evaluation including physical examination, blood testing, urine testing, and EKG.

Results: Upon outcome measures, neither sertaline nor St John's wort differed significantly from placebo. However, side effect profile did vary for St John's wort and sertaline relative to placebo.

Implications for Nursing Practice: Patients often think natural products can help a variety of illnesses. However, it is important to know which medications can help. Patients with signs and symptoms of depression must be able to assess and differentiate between mild and major depression. This will enable the nurse to offer appropriate treatment options. Although St John's wort may be useful for mild depression, major depression will not be effectively treated with this antidepressant.

Conclusion: Upon examination, the trial failed to support the efficacy of St John's wort in major depression because there was no change in the assessment scales. However, those patients who received sertaline rated much higher on the clinical global impression Scale for Improvement.

that, once they have identified depression, they must attend to all the elements of the disease at once to cure the patient, rather than understanding that treatment of depression is a process (Valente & Saunders, 1997).

Definition

Depression is defined as a mood disorder and contains both psychological and somatic symptoms that alter mood, affect, and personality. It is a compilation of signs and symptoms that are not usually a normal reaction to daily life occurrences. According to the *Diagnostic and Statistical Manual of Mental Disorders, Fourth Edition* (DSM-IV) (American Psychiatric Association [APA], 2000), depression is defined as an episode of 2

weeks or longer in which there is loss of interest or pleasure in nearly all activities. Accompanying this would be at least four additional symptoms from the following list: changes in appetite, sleep, weight, or psychomotor activity; decreased energy; feelings of worthlessness or guilt; difficulty thinking, concentrating, or making decisions; and recurrent thoughts of death, suicidal ideation, or attempts at such (APA, 2000).

Depression can be persistent and lasts months if left untreated. There may be a family history of the disease. Usually, the patient has inconsistent memory or complaints of memory loss, increased speech latency, and an irritable affect (Rosenbaum & Fava, 1998). However, there is lack of consensus on the criteria to define depression in older adults with cancer because their disease and treatment side effects alone result in many of the criteria in the depression profile (NIH Consensus Development Program, 2002).

Incidence

In patients over age 65, depression is a major health problem and the most common psychiatric disorder secondary to the events that occur later in life (Buckwalter & Piven, 1999; Edelstein, Kalish, Drozdick, & McKee, 1999). However, it may be overlooked and/or mistaken for dementia (Costa, et al., 1996). Most studies on depression look at prevalence rather than incidence. At the recent National Institutes of Health (NIH) State-of-the-Science Conference on Symptom Management in Cancer: Pain, Depression and Fatigue, the consensus was that there were no reliable incidence studies on depression in cancer patients (NIH Consensus Development Program, 2002). Recent geriatric studies report a 1% to 2% prevalence of major depression. Estimates are that about 25% of patients with cancer and over 50% of patients with life-threatening diseases suffer from depression (Lebowitz et al., 1997).

Etiology

The etiology of depression is multifactorial and falls into four categories: physical, psychological, social, and biologic (Kane, Ouslander, & Abrass, 1999) (Table 18-4). Physical factors encompass medical conditions (Table 18-5), specific diseases, medication effects, and sensory deprivation from loss of vision or hearing (Kane et al., 1999). Medical conditions include cardiovascular conditions (e.g., congestive heart failure, myocardial infarction, cardiac arrhythmias); neurologic conditions (e.g., cerebrovascular accidents and cerebral anoxia; Huntington's, Parkinson's, and Alzheimer's diseases; dementia; epilepsy; multiple sclerosis; postconcussion syndrome; myasthenia gravis; narcolepsy; subarachnoid hemorrhage); autoimmune diseases (e.g., human immuno-deficiency virus infection, rheumatoid arthritis, polyarteritis nodosa); endocrine disorders (e.g., hypothyroidism, hyperparathyroidism, diabetes mellitus, folate deficiency, hypoadrenalism, Cushing's and Addison's diseases); and other conditions such as anemia, alcoholism, systemic lupus erythematosus, infection with Epstein-Barr virus, hepatitis, malignancies, malnutrition, sex-

Table 18-4 Etiology of Depression

Category	Examples
Physical	Medical conditions, specific diseases, medication effects, sensory deprivation
Psychological	Unresolved conflict, memory loss, loss of independence, change in living situation, financial consequences from illness
Social	Loss of family and friends, isolation, loss of employment, previous conflicted relationships
Biologic	Family history, previous episodes of depression, neurotransmission deficiencies, central nervous system effects of cytokine

Data from Edelstein, B., Kalish, K. D., Drozdick, L. W., & McKee, D. R. (1999). Assessment of depression and bereavement in older adults. In P. A. Lichtenberg (Ed.), *Handbook of assessment in clinical gerontology* (pp. 22-25). New York: Wiley; and Kane, R. L., Ouslander, J. G., & Abrass, I. B. (1999). *Essentials of clinical geriatrics.* New York: McGraw-Hill.

ually transmitted diseases (STDs), and encephalitis. Medications that may trigger depression include propranolol, reserpine, and metoclopramide (Rosenbaum & Fava, 1998).

Psychological issues may include unresolved conflicts, memory loss, loss of independence, change in living situations, and the possible financial consequences incurred from a life-limiting illness. Coping with the debilitating physical aspects of having a life-limiting illness may also cause depression. These include the inability to participate in daily functioning and changes in body image caused by treating the disease.

Social issues include loss of family or friends, isolation, loss of job, and previous conflicted relationships (Edelstein et al., 1999; Kane et al., 1999). Even without dealing with terminal illness, older adults face much loss in living. Close friends and family of similar age may predecease them. Retirement may wreak havoc by producing multiple losses, including loss of social position as a working person, change in socioeconomic status, loss of friends and acquaintances, loss of routine, and a loss of purpose.

Table 18-5 **Medical Conditions Associated with Depression**	
Category/Basis	Examples
Endocrine disorders	Hypothyroidism, hyperparathyroidism, diabetes, Cushing's and Addison's diseases
Cardiovascular conditions	Congestive heart failure, myocardial infarction, cardiac arrhythmias
Neurologic conditions	Cerebrovascular accident, anoxia, Huntington's chorea, Alzheimer's disease, dementia, multiple sclerosis, postconcussion syndrome, myasthenia gravis, narcolepsy, subarachnoid hemorrhage
Immune disorders	AIDS, rheumatoid arthritis, polyarteritis nodosa
Cancer	Pancreatic
Other	Pain, alcoholism, anemia, lupus

AIDS, acquired immunodeficiency syndrome.
Sources: Well-Connected. (1998b). *Depression* (Report # 8). Atlanta: A.D.A.M., Inc.; Pasacreta, J. V., Minarik, P. A., & Nield-Anderson, L. (2001). Anxiety and depression. In B. Ferrell, & N. Coyle, *Textbook of palliative nursing.* New York: Oxford University Press; Rosenbaum J. F., & Fava, M. (1998). Approach to the patient with depression. In T. A. Stern, J. B. Herman, & P. L. Slavin. *The MGH guide to psychiatry in primary care.* New York: McGraw-Hill.

Biologic factors include family history, prior episodes of depression, neurotransmission deficiencies, and central nervous system effects of cytokines (Kane et al., 1999). Data suggest that deficiencies in serotonin, norepinephrine, and prolactin, as well as abnormal cortisol and dopamine levels, cause depressive symptoms (Lovejoy et al., 2000).

Cardinal Signs

Buckwalter and Piven (1999) described a triad of depressive symptoms: 1) changes in mood; 2)

perceptual disturbances of oneself, the environment, and the future; and 3) vegetative and behavioral signs. Depression may affect all aspects of an older person's life because of the possible elements of depression involved in other conditions, such as aches and pains, confusion, agitation, anxiety, or irritability. Depression is not a symptom of normal aging; rather, it has a relatively discrete onset. Indeed, the older adult may develop more physical symptoms than changes in emotional affect (Buckwalter & Piven, 1999).

Patients may present with a dysphoric mood, or lack of pleasure. Other signs in the older adult include poor personal hygiene and grooming; slow thought processes and speech; sadness, tearfulness, hopelessness, helplessness, worthlessness, and social withdrawal; changes in sleep patterns and appetite; fatigue; behavioral slowing; and complaints of diminished ability to think (Costa et al., 1996; Kane et al., 1999).

In the elder with dementia, depression is not expressed in the same way as it is in the person whose cognitive function is intact. For these patients, there may be more peripheral symptoms, such as agitation, repetitive vocalization, apathy, insomnia, food refusal, or resisting care (Volicer, 2001). Depression in this population leads to increased dependence in activities of daily living and decreased ability to engage in meaningful activities.

Most patients with a life-threatening illness fulfill several of the criteria for depression listed in the DSM-IV. The challenge lies in differentiating depression from grief (Block, 2000). Grief is a normal response to a loss, injury, insult, illness, deprivation, or disenfranchisement usually proportionate to the disruption caused by the loss (Weissman, 1998). To differentiate between grief and depression in the patient with a terminal illness, one must perform a more thorough interview that examines how the patient has coped with past crises to assess resiliency. Evaluation of the somatic distress the patient is experiencing includes whether there is a sense of hopelessness or helplessness, whether he or she still has the capacity for joy, and whether he or she looks to the future. If he or she still has joy and can look forward to the future, and the symptoms come in wavelike fashion, the patient probably has grief rather than depression (Block, 2000).

Severity

Depression in its most severe form puts a person at risk for suicide. Among older adults, suicide is the third leading cause of death (Lehmann & Rabins, 1999; Well-Connected, 1998b). One of five suicides involves a person age 65 years or older (Edelstein et al., 1999). Suicidal behavior in the older adult differs from that in younger people in that older people are less likely to express suicidal ideation and more likely to utilize lethal methods. Older single males are at a higher risk for suicide than older single females (Edelstein et al., 1999).

Suicidal ideation should be considered a psychiatric emergency and assessed on an urgent basis. It is essential to assess for depression in any patient who verbalizes suicidal ideation because it plays a significant role. Lack of a previous suicide attempt may not be significant in assessing suicide risk because the majority of older patients who commit suicide have no prior suicidal behaviors. Many elders who commit suicide have been found to have the most treatable types of depression; however, they have not received appropriate interventions (Depression Guideline Panel, 1993; Edelstein et al., 1999).

Risk for suicide in the general population includes prior psychiatric diagnosis (including previous depression), increasing age, family history of suicide, poor social support, delirium, disfiguring disease or surgery, substance abuse, and poorly controlled pain (Depression Guideline Panel, 1993). The following issues are specific to the evaluation of the older adult's potential for suicide: strong character, refusal of assistance/fear of becoming a burden, fear of dependence/fear of loss of control, fear of financial issues (retired or unemployed), severe pain that is unrelieved, poor functional status, poor health, poor/bad relationships with family, isolation, and previous psychiatric distress (Filiberti et al., 2001; Kane et al., 1999). Other factors include retirement, recent changes (such as a move), changes in health, history of poor interpersonal relationships, and a terminal diagnosis (Kane et al., 1999).

Assessment

Assessment of depression includes both cognitive and physical assessment. The Depression Guideline Panel (1993) outlined the steps in detecting and treating depression: 1) be vigilant for depression and evaluate risk factors, 2) perform a clinical interview, and 3) consider any mood disorders using clinical history, interview, and report by family, and evaluate other potential factors that may cause depression, such as medications, medical conditions, previous psychiatric disorders, and substance abuse. In addition, the racial and ethnic culture of the older adult should be considered in assessment. This is particularly important because most of the depression literature, including that related to description, presentation, and experience of depression, focuses on that of the white culture (Edelstein et al., 1999). However, in many other cultures, depression may be expressed in somatic complaints and certain affects. Therefore, it may be necessary to use interpreters when English is not the patient's first language, as well as consult religious elders and community-specific experts to assist with examining common practices within another culture.

Assessment focuses on the cognitive processes of the patient, including a mental status examination. Other assessment areas include the following: the ability of patient to engage in life (boredom vs. inability to be active); a patient's interest in the world around him or her (lack of interest vs. delight in shock, humor, etc.); engagement in hobbies (joy vs. lack of interest); presence of anhedonia (inability to anticipate anything with pleasure); the patient's view of life (feelings of hopelessness vs. optimism and plans for the future); the patient's sense of self-worth (worthfulness vs. worthlessness); any expressions of guilt or self-recrimination; and, lastly, expression of suicidal ideation (Block, 2000; Buckwalter & Piven, 1999; Lloyd-Williams, 2001) (Box 18-3).

Suicidal ideation should be evaluated for its severity. There should be an examination of any suicide plan, specifically looking at the risk:rescue ratio and the level of planning. The patient's level of hopelessness should be examined. Further assessment of the possible precipitants, as well as social supports, should be determined. Finally, the issue of suicidal ideation should be discussed with family and friends (Lagomasino & Stern, 1998).

In further assessment of the elder patient with depression, laboratory and/or diagnostic tests should be ordered to rule out other conditions

Box 18-3 **Depression Assessment Areas**

AREAS OF PSYCHOSOCIAL ASSESSMENT FOR THE PATIENT

- Ability to engage in life
- Interest in world around him/her
- Engagement in hobbies
- Presence of anhedonia (inability to anticipate anything with pleasure)
- View of life
- Self-worth
- Any expressions of guilt or self-recrimination
- Expression of suicidal ideation
- Boredom vs. inability to be active
- Lack of interest vs. delight in shock, humor, etc.
- Joy vs. lack of interest
- Feelings of hopelessness vs. optimism and plans for the future
- Worthfulness vs. worthlessness

Sources: Block, S. D. (2000). Assessing and managing depression in the terminally ill patient. *Annals of Internal Medicine, 132*(2), 209-213; Buckwalter, K. C., & Piven, ML. S. (1999). Depression. In J. T. Stone, J. F. Wyman, & S. A. Salisbury. *Clinical gerontological nursing—a guide to advanced practice.* Philadelphia: Saunders; Lloyd-Williams, M. (2001). Screening for depression in palliative care patients: a review. *European Journal of Cancer Care, 10,* 31-35.

(see Table 18-5) as long as, in doing so, an undue burden is not placed on the older adult and if there are plans to treat whatever deficiencies are found. These tests would include determination of serum electrolytes to rule out dehydration, a complete blood count and hematocrit to rule out anemia, a thyroid profile to rule out hypothyroidism, a Venereal Disease Research Laboratory screen to rule out an STD, determination of vitamin B_{12} and folate levels to rule out vitamin deficiencies, liver function tests (LFTs) to rule out liver failure, renal function tests to rule out renal failure, a urinalysis to rule out infections, and an electrocardiogram to rule out cardiac problems (Kane et al., 1999).

Patients with preexisting neurovegetative conditions such as Alzheimer's or Parkinson's disease are usually unable to respond to questioning. Performing a cognitive assessment may be impossible or may yield little helpful information. Volicer (1999) described the high incidence of depression in this population and stressed the importance of surveillance for behaviors that may indicate depression. These behaviors include food refusal, angry affect, labile mood, agitation, repetitive movements, or increased withdrawal. Treatment of possible depression with medications serves as a diagnostic tool (Volicer, 1999). The current standard is to initiate treatment and see if there is a response. Even without any outward clues to the presence of depression, medications may improve behavior. Volicer (1999) stated that it is important, however, to continue treatment for a least a year because this population is vulnerable to relapse.

Physical assessment includes general examination of the following areas: cardiopulmonary, gastrointestinal, genitourinary, and neurologic (Kane et al., 1999). If an older adult develops pain, radiologic and gastrointestinal studies are indicated to rule out fractures, ulcers, and neoplasms. Complaints of chest pain should be evaluated with an electrocardiogram, and noninvasive cardiovascular studies should be done to rule out myocardial infarction, congestive heart failure, and arrhythmias. Shortness of breath justifies chest radiographs, a pulmonary function test, pulse oximetry, and determination of blood gases to rule out COPD, lung neoplasms, and other pulmonary conditions. The presence of constipation indicates the need for a fecal occult blood test, a barium enema, and a thyroid function test to rule out neoplasms and ineffective thyroid. Neurologic changes warrant an electroencephalogram with computed tomography or magnetic resonance imaging to rule out cerebrovascular accidents, tumors, or other brain conditions (Kane et al., 1999).

All too often the symptom complaints of older adults are not taken seriously. The symptoms of depression can signal a medical condition, and a physical work-up may be necessary to find the cause of problems. However, if the older adult is already known to have a terminal illness, the extent of a work-up will depend on quality-of-life issues and how much a further work-up would change an inevitable outcome. If a condition is suspected that is reversible and treatment can have a positive effect on a patient, then at least a preliminary work-up may be appropriate. Thus evaluation of appropriate treatments needs to occur on an individualized basis wherein the health care team can examine the totality of the patient's health condition and weigh the risks and benefit of work-up and treatment.

Assessment Tools

Assessment tools specific to screening for depression in the geriatric population include the Beck Depression Inventory (BDI) and the Geriatric Depression Scale (GDS) (Box 18-4). The BDI consists of 21 items with a 4-point scale, although there is a shorter 13-item version (Candilis, 1998). This self-report inventory investigates neurovegetative, cognitive, and mood symptoms. This scale is useful in examining psychological symptoms to differentiate those patients who are depressed and those who are not (Lloyd-Williams, 2001). Candilis (1998) explained that a cutoff score of 10 indicates mild depression, a score of 16 indicates mild to moderate depression, a score of 20 indicates moderate to severe depression, and a score of 30 indicates severe depression. The GDS (Fig. 18-1) was specifically developed for use with older adults. It is a 30-item questionnaire that takes approximately 10 minutes to complete. A score of 11 or more indicates depression (Yesavage, Brink, & Rose, 1983). Additionally, there is a briefer 15-item GDS (Costa et al., 1996; Edelstein et al., 1999).

Asking the key question "Are you depressed?" as suggested by Block (2000) may not be as appropriate in the older adult population as in younger adults because elders do not have the same culture and support to express such emotions or to answer a question so direct. However, another measure of depression is the mood of the health care provider after an encounter. If a health care provider feels down, hopeless, or negative after an encounter, or has a desire to avoid the patient, there should be a high index of suspicion for depression in the patient and a rapid follow-up depression assessment (Lee, Back, Block, & Stewart, 2002). Of note, the U. S. Preventive Services Task Force (2000) found little evidence to recommend one assessment tool as more effective than another. Instead, they stated that a simple assessment may be just as effective as a formal assessment tool. They offered two simple screening questions that relate to mood and anhedonia:

1. Over the past 2 weeks, have you felt down, depressed, or hopeless?
2. Over the past 2 weeks, have you felt little interest or pleasure in doing things?

Box 18-4 Depression Scales

BECK DEPRESSION INVENTORY (BDI)
- 21-item questionnaire
- Multiple choice
- Scale of 11 or higher indicates depression
  11-19: mild depression
  20-30: moderate depression
  31 or higher: severe depression

GERIATRIC DEPRESSION SCALE (GDS)
- 30-item scale
- Yes/no format
- Scale of 11 or more is positive for depression

Data from Edelstein, B., Kalish, K. D., Drozdick, L. W., & McKee, D. R. (1999). Assessment of depression and bereavement in older adults. In P. A. Lichtenberg (Ed.), *Handbook of assessment in clinical gerontology* (pp. 22-25). New York: Wiley.

Suicide assessment includes some specific questioning. One tool is the Suicidal Ideation Screening Questionnaire (SIS-Q), a four-item screening tool that examines sleep disturbances, mood disturbances, guilt, and hopelessness with the following questions:

1. Have you ever had a period of 2 weeks or more when you had trouble falling asleep, staying asleep, waking up too early, or sleeping too much?
2. Have you ever had 2 weeks or more during which you felt sad, blue, depressed, or when you lost interest and pleasure in things that you usually cared about or enjoyed?
3. Has there ever been a period of 2 weeks or more when you felt worthless, sinful, or guilty?
4. Has there been a period of time when you felt that life was hopeless?

A single positive response to a question correlates with suicidal ideation in 84% of patients and necessitates further assessment (Candilis, 1998).

Kane et al. (1999) and Buckwalter and Piven (1999) suggested the following questions:

1. Do you feel life is not worth living?
2. Have you thought about harming yourself?
3. Are you thinking about suicide or taking your own life?
4. Do you have a plan? What is it?
5. Have you ever attempted suicide?

A positive or "yes" answer to any question warrants further questioning, assessment, and intervention with the patient and family.

Choose the best answer for how you felt over the past week.

1.	Are you basically satisfied with your life?	YES	NO
2.	Have you dropped many of your activities and interests?	YES	NO
3.	Do you feel that your life is empty?	YES	NO
4.	Do you often get bored?	YES	NO
5.	Are you hopeful about the future?	YES	NO
6.	Are you bothered by thoughts you can't get out of your head?	YES	NO
7.	Are you in good spirits most of the time?	YES	NO
8.	Are you afraid that something bad is going to happen to you?	YES	NO
*9.	Do you feel happy most of the time?	YES	NO
10.	Do you often feel helpless?	YES	NO
11.	Do you often get restless and fidgety?	YES	NO
12.	Do you prefer to stay at home rather than going out and doing things?	YES	NO
13.	Do you frequently worry about the future?	YES	NO
14.	Do you feel you have more problems with memory than most?	YES	NO
*15.	Do you think it is wonderful to be alive now?	YES	NO
16.	Do you often feel downhearted and blue?	YES	NO
17.	Do you feel pretty worthless the way you are now?	YES	NO
18.	Do you worry a lot about the past?	YES	NO
*19.	Do you find life very exciting?	YES	NO
20.	Is it hard for you to get started on new projects?	YES	NO
*21.	Do you feel full of energy?	YES	NO
22.	Do you feel that your situation is helpless?	YES	NO
23.	Do you think that most people are better off than you are?	YES	NO
24.	Do you frequently get upset over little things?	YES	NO
25.	Do you frequently feel like crying?	YES	NO
26.	Do you have trouble concentrating?	YES	NO
*27.	Do you enjoy getting up in the morning?	YES	NO
28.	Do you prefer to avoid social gatherings?	YES	NO
*29.	Is it easy for you to make decisions?	YES	NO
*30.	Is your mind as clear as it used to be?	YES	NO

Score: ☐

Norms

Normal	5 ± 4
Mildly depressed	15 ± 6
Very depressed	13 ±

*Non-depressed answers = yes, all others = no

Fig. 18-1 Geriatric Depression Scale (GDS). (From Yesavage, J., Brink, T. L., & Rose, T. L. [1983]. Development and validation of a geriatric screening scale: A preliminary report. *Journal of Psychiatric Research, 17,* 37-49.)

Management

Pharmacologic

Because physical pain and discomfort increase depression, treatment of depression first involves management of pain and other unpleasant symptoms (Block, 2000), which will ensure that optimal comfort is achieved. Treatment of some of the major types of pain and discomfort includes the use of medications such as antiemetics for nausea and vomiting; opioids for cancer pain, chest pain, and dyspnea; nonsteroidal medications for bone pain, arthritis-type pain, and various aches; and even low-dose antidepressant medications for nerve pain. By treating any of these types of pain, the patient's mood may improve. However, in the last category of treating nerve pain, the use of low-dose tricyclic antidepressants (TCAs) may simultaneously treat the depression and the pain.

For the older adult, it is judicious to use the lowest dose possible for any medication (Well-Connected, 1996b). This dose range may particularly vary in elders who have had a stroke, have Parkinson's or Alzheimer's disease, or have other comorbidities. Furthermore, the older patient may need longer treatment (Lavretsky, 2001). The underlying principle of medication management is to "start low and go slow." Practitioners should be careful not to stop therapy with a specific medication too soon because older patients may need a longer time to respond (Lavretsky, 2001).

For patients with a prognosis of 1 month or less, a psychostimulant, such as methylphenidate, may be very helpful. Psychostimulants typically work within 1 to 2 days. If the prognosis is longer than 1 month, one can start a psychostimulant to get an immediate effect and also start a longer-acting antidepressant medication. The effect a patient gets from the psychostimulant can help with predicting how he or she will respond to a longer-term medication; after a week on the psychostimulant, the dose can be decreased as the longer-acting antidepressant dose is increased (Rozans, Dreisbach, Lertora, & Kahn, 2002).

In elder patients, TCAs and SSRIs are roughly equivalent in efficacy (Lebowitz et al., 1997). However, the older adult tends to tolerate SSRIs better than TCAs. Side effects of TCAs include sedation, confusion, orthostatic hypotension, cardiac arrhythmias, dry mouth, constipation, ataxia, and confusion (Lavretsky, 2001; Lebowitz et al., 1997). SSRIs have fewer anticholinergic effects (Lebowitz et al., 1997), with other side effects of SSRIs including nausea, anorexia, diarrhea, and insomnia (Lavretsky, 2001). Data are limited on newer agents known as selective norepinephrine reuptake inhibitors relative to an elder's tolerance. In severe depression, TCAs may be more efficacious (Well-Connected, 1998b). Of note is that the use of herbal medications for treatment has shown no benefit over standard antidepressant therapy. More important is that these herbs (St. John's wort, kava, and valerian) may interfere with other medications and foods or may have serious adverse interactions (Payne & Massie, 2002). Table 18-6 reviews the medications commonly used in treating depression.

Nonpharmacologic

The mainstay of nonpharmacologic interventions for depression is psychotherapy. Psychological counseling may be even more important in older patients because they may not physically

Table 18-6 **Medications to Treat Depressed Older Adults**		
Medication	Starting Dose (mg)	Daily Dose (mg)
PSYCHOSTIMULANTS		
Dextroamphetamine	2.5-5	10-20 8:00 AM/noon
Methylphenidate	2.5-5	5-10 8:00 AM/noon
SSRIS (LESS SIDE EFFECTS)		
Sertraline	12.5-25	50-100
Fluoxetine	5-10	20-40
Paroxetine	5-10	20-40
Nefazodone	100-500	
Fluvoxamine	50-300	
SNRI		
Venlafaxine	37.5	37.5-225
TRICYCLICS		
Amitriptyline	25-50	25-125
Imipramine	25-50	25-125
Desipramine	25-50	25-125
Nortriptyline	25-50	25-125
AZAPIRONE		
Bupropion		200-450

SNRI, selective norepinephrine reuptake inhibitor; *SSRIs*, selective serotonin reuptake inhibitor.
Sources: Lavretsky, H. (2001). Choosing appropriate treatment for geriatric depression. *Clinical Geriatrics*, 9(5), 30-46; Wilson, K. G., Chochinov, H. M., de Faye, B. J., & Breitbart, W. (2000). Diagnosis and management of depression in palliative care. In H. M. Chochinov, & W. Breitbart. Eds. *Handbook of psychiatry in palliative medicine*. New York: Oxford University Press; Block, S. D. (2000). Assessing and managing depression is the terminally ill patient. *Annals of Internal Medicine*, 132(2), 209-213; Breitbart, W., Chochinov, H. M., & Passik, S. (1998). Psychiatric aspect of palliative care. In D. Doyle, W. C. Hanks, & N. MacDonald. Eds. *Oxford textbook of palliative medicine*. (2nd ed.). New York: Oxford University Press.

tolerate medications (Cremens & Harari, 1998; Lavretsky, 2001). The ability to express emotions and feelings may be a novel process to the older adult and may take some adjustment. Nonetheless, psychotherapy allows the reduction of emotional distress and the improvement of morale and coping (Payne & Massie, 2002). Psychotherapy may focus on issues surrounding death and dying, including reminiscence and life review. In therapy sessions, clinicians can help patients set realistic goals, provide compassionate listening, and validate the patient's feelings. Cognitive behavioral therapy focuses on reframing and restructuring events. Clinicians can help patients develop structure for their day and activities (Pasacreta et al., 2001). This may allow the patient to identify accomplishments, improve interactions, and reduce fears of death, as well as provide a sense of making amends.

Music therapy and movement therapy may be helpful in stimulating interaction, providing sensory input, and increasing circulation. Music therapy allows a person to access his or her inner feelings because music can tap into emotions that words are unable to access. Other therapies may include pet therapy, group activities, and sensory stimulation. Pet therapy enhances self-worth and fulfills a need to love and be loved in a safe environment while allowing tactile stimulation. Group activities and sensory stimulation increase contact and response to surroundings, stimulate thought and communication, and encourage interaction with other people (Buckwalter & Piven, 1999).

Dependent, Independent, and Collaborative Interventions

The effective management of depression in the older adult requires a team approach. A team participating in a case conference can identify vulnerable patients with factors predisposing to depression. Reviewing specific patients in case conferences also can reveal subtle changes in behavior assessed by different team members that may indicate depression. The various team members may interact with the older adult in different ways. Sometimes certain behaviors are difficult for a single team member to evaluate; review of these behaviors by the whole team may help to identify problems. Moreover, the team approach is helpful because team members have different functions and interactions with the patient. Physicians and advanced practice nurses may prescribe antidepressant medications. The social worker can provide counseling and assessment of social supports. In particular, family caregivers should be assessed for stress and finances should be reviewed for potential burden. The pastoral care worker can provide spiritual support

(Block, 2000). Volunteers can add to the web of social support. If a patient has home care, a psychiatric clinical nurse specialist can help with continuing care needs. Seeing the patient across the continuum and working within a collaborative approach may increase response to treatment.

Family Concerns and Considerations

Education is very important in depression; often the family and patient do not understand depression and think that social withdrawal and slowing of activities is part of the aging process. Families should understand that depression is neither a necessity of life nor a sign of weakness or failure; rather, it is a medical illness caused by medical conditions or polypharmacy. Families should receive information on the factors that make patients vulnerable, such as multiple health problems, untreated pain and discomfort, and multiple losses. A review of depressive symptoms can help family members recognize depression and may help the older adult to receive treatment sooner, thereby alleviating suffering. For those patients with severe depression, clinicians can assist the family in reviewing patient safety issues with regard to potential suicide, including access to weapons and leftover medications, ability to drive, and extreme isolation.

Medical information is paramount. Family members and the patient should understand that concurrent use of medications may cause depression or interfere with response to antidepressant medications. Discussion of treatment options should include a discussion of side effects of antidepressant medication. These side effects include blurred vision, constipation, dry mouth, urinary retention, excessive perspiration, orthostatic hypotension, fatigue, weakness, drowsiness, tremors, twitching, and hallucinations. Family members should understand that the side effects in themselves cause further depressed affect. With regard to medications and dosages, the family needs to understand that, in the older adult population, lower medication doses are prescribed because of lower metabolism (Buckwalter & Piven, 1999; Depression Guideline Panel, 1993). The patient and family also need to be reminded that it takes several weeks before the full effect of the medication is reached. The family and patient need encouragement to continue the medication for at least 6 weeks to receive the maximal effect, even if the patient feels no specific changes, and to continue the medication even when the patient feels better and thinks that he or she can stop taking it.

Most important, the family and patient should be reassured that, the majority of the time, symptoms of depression may be effectively treated (Waller & Caroline, 2000). They should be reassured that the patient will not be abandoned, and that a thoughtful treatment plan will be developed to improve quality of life. In the meantime, education about severe depression should include information about support and obtaining emergency care if the depression worsens.

DELIRIUM

Delirium is defined as an acute confusional state resulting from a more global impairment in mental function (Ingham & Caraceni, 2002; Waller & Caroline, 2000), and may also be referred to as confusion or agitation. This inconsistency in terminology makes management difficult. In the older adult population, this confusion is even more prevalent. The aging process makes the elder more susceptible to delirium because of decreased kidney function causing inability to rid the body of toxic substances, decreased ability to metabolize medications, and decreased fluid balance mechanisms. Alterations in thought processes are very common during the last weeks of life. Historically, this confusion has been thought to be a normal part of the dying process (Langhorne, 1999).

Delirium should be considered an emergency situation (Chan & Brennan, 1999). In the elder population, delirium may be associated with higher mortality rates, longer hospital admissions, increased costs of care, greater likelihood of being placed outside the home after hospitalization, and decreased functional ability (Casarett & Inouye, 2001; Langhorne, 1999). Moreover, elder patients may be terrified of fluctuating cognitive deficits, hallucinations, misperceptions, paranoid and psychomotor agitation, and changes in sleep-wake cycles (Casarett & Inouye 2001; Lawlor, Fainsinger, & Bruera, 2000). Families may become distressed by both the unusual behaviors and the sadness they feel from the premature "loss" of their loved one. If confusion about delirium is extreme, there is sadness and/or guilt if the elder falls or is in need

of physical or chemical restraint (Casarett & Inouye, 2001; Lawlor et al., 2000). Though delirium interferes with comfort and causes distress for family members, it was previously considered a stage of dying. Now state-of-the-art palliative care includes aggressive treatment of this symptom, allowing better quality of life for older patients at the end of their lives.

Definition

According to the APA (2000), the essential feature of delirium is a disturbance of consciousness that is accompanied by a change in cognition that cannot be better accounted for by a preexisting or evolving dementia. The key elements that determine delirium, according to the DSM-IV, consist of changes in mental status in a short time; alternations in attention or consciousness; changes in cognition or memory; and a change in cognition from a direct physiologic consequence of a medical condition (APA, 2000).

Incidence

Estimates of the incidence of delirium range from 20% to 75% in cancer patients up to 90% in all terminally ill patients (Casarett & Inouye, 2001; Tremblay & Breitbart, 2001). This symptom occurs frequently during peri-death, particularly in the last days or hours, when estimates rise to 90% to 95% (Waller & Caroline, 2000). In hospitalized patients over age 70, delirium is very common, and its treatment adds costly hospital days (Chan & Brennan, 1999).

Etiology

The precise pathophysiology of delirium is not well understood; however, it is thought to involve increases in the levels of neurotransmitters in the cortical and subcortical areas of the brain. Several neurotransmitters are involved, including dopamine, serotonin, gamma-aminobutyric acid, beta-endorphins, and acetylcholine; acetylcholine is thought to play the most important role (Casarett & Inouye, 2001; Chan & Brennan, 1999). The etiology of delirium is multifactorial (Table 18-7). Causes include medications, polypharmacy, brain metastases, hypoxia, sepsis, hypercalcemia, hepatic and renal dysfunction, electrolyte imbalances, bowel obstruction, urinary tract infection, past psychiatric history, and medication withdrawal. Possible medications contributing to delirium include opioids, TCAs, diphenhydramine, antihistamines (histamine$_2$ blockers), analgesics, sedatives, and cardiovascular drugs (Chan & Brennan, 1999; Langhorne, 1999).

Brain involvement may be secondary to metastases, primary cerebral disease, cancer, or cardiovascular accident. Systemic causes include organ failure, metabolic disturbances, infection, and toxic effects of an agonist substance (Lawlor et al., 2000). Other factors specific to the older adult include preexisting dementia, a fracture, systemic infections, malnutrition, drug regimens including three or more medications, simultaneous use of neuroleptics and opioids, use of restraints, bladder catheters, and iatrogenic events (Chan & Brennan, 1999; Kane et al., 1999). Unfortunately, delirium may be misdiagnosed as dementia.

Cardinal Signs

The cardinal signs of delirium include an acute onset, fluctuating course, presence of underlying organic cause, reduced sensorium, attention deficit, and cognitive or perceptual disturbances (Chan & Brennan, 1999; Costa et al., 1996; Lawlor et al., 2000). Specific symptoms include insomnia during the night and somnolence during the day, nightmares, restlessness, hypersensitivity to light or noise, and emotional lability (Breitbart & Cohen, 2000). Early signs of delirium specific to the older adult include sundowning, withdrawal, irritability, new forgetfulness or befuddlement, and new onset of incontinence. Later signs include outbursts of anger, hostility, or abusive behavior (Waller & Caroline, 2000). Confusion, agitation, or restlessness is usually worse at night and when the older adult becomes disoriented as to person, place, date, and time.

Either increased activity (hyperactive delirium) or increased passivity (hypoactive delirium) may delineate delirium. Hyperactive or agitated delirium is characterized by agitation and hallucinations, and the delirium or confusion is readily apparent and more easily recognized. Hypoactive delirium often goes unrecognized because the patient may be quiet and lethargic and the delirium may be mistaken for sedation from opioids or for an obtunded state in the last days of life, or be viewed as a state of comfort if symptom management has been difficult (Breitbart & Cohen, 2000; Casarett & Inouye, 2001; McElhaney, 2002). There may also be times when a patient experiences a mixed delirium, which means he or she alternates between a hypoactive and a hyperactive state.

Severity

Delirium usually becomes more severe in the hyperactive form. If an elder becomes more agitated and delusional, then he or she may become a safety risk. There may be very aggressive and combative behavior that can be physically threatening to others as well as increasing the risk of harm to the patient. This can result in a tendency to want to place the patient in physical restraints to avoid injury to caregivers and to keep the patient from injuring him- or herself. However, it is best to avoid restraints because this can further exacerbate the problem when the patient cannot move and feels frustrated by the inability to move, or if he or she falls while attempting to escape the restraints. Additionally, the delirium may include delusions and hallucinations such that patients do not understand where they are. Finally, the more delusional a patient, the greater the risk of suicide (Chan & Brennan, 1999; Costa et al., 1996; Langhorne, 1999).

The result of hypoactive delirium may be premature death. If pain and symptoms have been difficult to manage, the hypoactive patient will look sedated. In particular, the elder patient may be lethargic and unable to communicate his or her confusion. The health care team may feel that they have finally managed the symptoms because the patient is very quiet. Medications will continue and the vital functioning will be depressed. The result is premature death by perhaps weeks to months (Breitbart & Cohen, 2000; Casarett & Inouye, 2001; McElhaney, 2002).

Assessment

Evaluation of delirium includes several components: history, cognitive assessment, physical exam, and laboratory studies. The first step in diagnosing delirium is awareness of it as a potential symptom. Challenges of assessment include absence of uniform classification (as seen by its several names), lack of knowledge regarding early signs, staff tolerance of confused behavior, and the assumption that, with age, most people inevitably become confused (Boyle, Abernathy, Baker, & Wall, 1998).

Assessment may be by criteria such as those in the DSM-IV defining characteristics of delirium.

Table 18-7 **Causes of Delirium**

Category/Basis	Examples
Disease process	Primary brain tumor or secondary brain metastasis
Side effects of treatment	Chemotherapy
	Radiation to the brain
Pain and symptom medications	Corticosteroids
	Opioids
	Tricyclic antidepressants
	H_2 blockers (e.g., cimetidine, ranitidine)
	Anticholinergics
	Antiemetics (e.g., thioridazine, amitryptyline, diphenhydramine)
	OTC antihistamines
	Benzodiazepines
	Sedatives (e.g., triazolam)
	Acyclovir
	Cardiovascular drugs (e.g., digitalis, nifedipine, quinidine)
	Beta-blockers
Medication withdrawal	Opioids
	Benzodiazepines
	Alcohol
Pain	Uncontrolled pain syndrome
	Urinary retention
	Constipation/impaction
	Obstruction
Metabolic fluctuations	Glucose (hypoglycemia)
	Sodium (hyponatremia)
	Potassium
	Calcium
Organ failure	Brain (e.g., stroke, seizure, CVA)
	Kidney (uremia)
	Lungs (hypoxia)
	Heart (e.g., hypoxia, CO_2 retention, MI)
	Thyroid or adrenal
Infection	CNS (meningitis)
	Urinary tract
	Respiratory tract (pneumonia)
	Generalized sepsis
	Steroid-induced immunocompromise
Nutritional deficiencies	Thiamine
	Vitamin B_{12}/folate
Miscellaneous	Sleep deprivation
	Urinary retention
	Sensory deprivation
	Change in environment
	Immobilization
Past psychiatric history	Depression

CNS, central nervous system; CVA, cerebrovascular accident; H_2, histamine$_2$; MI, myocardial infarction; OTC, over the counter.
Sources: Casarett, D. J., & Inouye, S. K. (2001). Diagnosis and delirium near the end of life. *Annals of Internal Medicine, 135,* 32-40; Chan, D., & Brennan, N. (1999). Delirium: making the diagnosis, improving the prognosis. *Geriatrics, 54*(3), 28-42; Langhorne, M. (1999). Confusion or delirium: determining the difference. *Developments in Supportive Cancer Care, 3*(3), 82-87; Waller, A. & Caroline, N. L. (2000). *Handbook of palliative care in cancer.* (2nd ed.). Boston: Butterworth-Heinemann.

These include disturbance in consciousness with impaired ability to focus or shift attention; changes in cognition or the development of perceptual disturbance that is not better accounted for by a preexisting established or evolving dementia; fluctuation of the disturbance over a short period of time; and evidence from the history, physical exam, or lab findings that the disturbance is caused by psychological consequences of a general medical condition. Specific assessment tools to screen for delirium in the older adult are described below.

Assessment should first include a history and review of current conditions. This review should note the presence of disease side effects, such as those caused by a tumor; side effects of treatment, such as chemotherapy or radiation to the head; medications used to treat symptoms, including corticosteroids, opioids, cimetidine, anticholinergics, antiemetics, benzodiazepines, and acyclovir; withdrawal of medications such as opioids, benzodiazepines, or alcohol; discomfort from uncontrolled pain, urinary retention, or fecal impaction; metabolic fluctuations in glucose, sodium, potassium, or calcium; organ failure, including the kidneys, liver, lungs, heart, brain, thyroid, or adrenal glands; infection of the central nervous system, urinary tract, or respiratory tract, or generalized sepsis; and finally nutritional deficiencies such as thiamine or folate/vitamin B_{12} (Waller & Caroline, 2000). There should then be a review of the patient's behavior and sleep cycles as noted in the chart, followed by a review of the medication regimen.

A critical assessment element is an evaluation of mental status. This helps to develop a multidimensional clinical picture, including functional performance status and signs/symptoms. A mental status exam provides a baseline for monitoring the course of cognition and is a source of documentation for reference and repeat evaluations. The key aspects of mental status assessment include general state and appearance, orientation, state of consciousness, short- and long-term memory, language, visuospatial functions, cognitive functions (e.g., calculations, spelling), insight and judgment, thought control, and mood and affect (Costa et al., 1996; Kane et al., 1999).

Physical exam is important to rule out possible treatable causes (Table 18-8). Vital signs can give information regarding infection, hypoxemia,

and hypoglycemia. Integument inspection reveals sepsis or cardiac failure (cold, clammy skin) or anticholinergic reactions (hot, red skin). Examination of the head, eye, ears, nose, and throat may reveal signs of scleral icterus from liver failure, constricted pupils from opioids or dilated pupils from anticholinergic toxicity, or smooth, shiny tongue from nutritional deficiencies. The chest can be examined for rales of heart failure on auscultation or dullness to percussion from pneumonia. The abdominal exam may reveal urinary retention or fecal impaction, and examination of the extremities may reveal evidence of hypocalcemia, thiamine deficiency, and liver failure (Waller & Caroline, 2000). Helpful lab data may include levels of glucose, electrolytes, bilirubin, and lactate dehydrogenase; LFTs; urine culture results; and oxygen saturation level.

Assessment Tools

Several tools are available to assess mental status; the most frequently used is the Mini-Mental State Examination (MMSE) (Folstein, Folstein, & McHugh, 1975) (Box 18-5). The MMSE is a brief tool that measures cognitive impairment, specifically examining immediate memory, short-term memory, aphasia, apraxia, agnosia, and construction ability along with concentration and spatial ability (Costa et al., 1996). The 30-item exam requires only about 10 minutes to complete. Out of a possible 30 points, scores below 20 indicate a possible organic brain disorder. A score of 23 is sensitive to thought disorders and mood (Candilis, 1998).

Three primary tools are used to assess confusion or delirium in patients with life-limiting illnesses. These are the Confusion Assessment Method (CAM) diagnostic algorithm, the Delirium Rating Scale (DRS), and the Memorial Delirium Assessment Scale (MDAS). All have been used with the older adult and are outlined in Box 18-6.

The CAM assesses nine domains of cognitive functioning, including perceptual disturbances (e.g., hallucinations), disorganized thinking (e.g., rambling, incoherent speech), altered level of consciousness (e.g., sleepy, stuporous, hypervigilant), inattention (e.g., incorrect responses to digit span or months backward test), and acute changes in mental status with fluctuating course

Table 18-8 Physical Examination for Delirium

System	Sign	Implications
General	Cold, clammy skin	Cardiac failure, sepsis, hypoglycemia, hypocalcemia
	Warm, hot, red skin	Anticholinergic reaction
Head, ears, eyes, nose, throat		
Head (face)	Chostek's sign	Hypocalcemia
Eyes	Papilledema	Intracranial pressure
	Scleral icterus	Liver failure
	Constricted pupils	Opioid toxicity
	Dilated pupils	Anticholinergic toxicity
Mouth	Smooth, shiny tongue	Folate deficiency
Chest		
Lungs	Rales	Heart failure
	Dullness	Pneumonia
Heart	S_1 gallop	Heart failure
Abdomen	Palpable feces	Constipation or impaction
	Palpable bladder	Urinary retention
Extremities	Trousseau's sign	Hypocalcemia
	Tender, swollen calves	Thiamine deficiency
	Asterixis	Liver failure
Nervous system	Mental status exam	Evaluation of cognitive functioning
	Hemiplegia/hemiparesis	Stroke
	Proximal myopathy	Corticosteroid toxicity
	Ataxia, loss of vibration sense, loss of position sense	Thiamine or B_{12} deficiency

Data from Chan, D., & Brennan, N. (1999). Delirium: Making the diagnosis, improving the prognosis. *Geriatrics, 54*(3), 28-42; and Waller, A., & Caroline, N. L. (2000). *Handbook of palliative care in cancer* (2nd ed.). Boston: Butterworth-Heinemann.

(Chan & Brennan, 1999). The presence of at least the first three elements suggests a diagnosis of delirium (Flacker & Marcantonio, 1998).

The DRS (Box 18-7) is a 10-item structured interview in which each answer is rated on a 0 to 3 scale. It is the most widely used assessment of delirium with the longest history of use in the psychiatric setting. It measures such factors as mood, onset of perceptual disturbances (including hallucinations and delusions), and behavior (Kuebler, English, & Heidrich, 2001).

The MDAS (Box 18-8) is a 10-item assessment tool measuring awareness and cognitive impairment, with attention to memory and psychomotor responses. Each response is rated from 0 to 3, with a score of 13 or higher being diagnostic of delirium (Breitbart et al., 1997; Breitbart & Cohen, 2000).

Management

To treat delirium, it is first necessary to decide on goals of care. Specifically, it must be determined if the elder is close to death and whether the delirium is reversible. A stepwise approach is taken regarding treatment (Boyle et al., 1998). Constipation and urinary retention should be treated, and any potential contributing factors should be removed. For example, the clinician may initiate the discontinuation of problematic medications one by one to determine the causative drug. If complete discontinuation of the offending medication is not appropriate, then decreasing the dose may be helpful. Elders may be sensitive to medications needed for pain and symptom management; therefore, discussion regarding the benefits and burdens of pain and

Text continued on p. 346

Box 18-5 **Mini-Mental State Examination**

ORIENTATION

	Maximum Score	Score
What is the _____ _____ _____ _____ _____ ? year season date day month	5	( )
Where are we _____ _____ _____ _____ _____ ? state county town hospital floor	5	( )

REGISTRATION

Name 3 objects: 1 second to name each. Then ask the patient to repeat all 3 objects after you have said them. Give 1 point for each correct answer. Then repeat. Count trials and record.	3	( )

TRIALS:
ATTENTION AND CALCULATION

Serial 7s. 1 point for each correct. Stop after 5 answers. Alternatively, spell "world" backward.	5	( )

RECALL

Ask for the 3 objects repeated above. Give 1 point for each correct.	3	( )

LANGUAGE

Name a pencil and watch (2 points).
Repeat the following: "No ifs, ands, or buts." (1 point)
Follow a 3-stage command: "Takes a paper in your right hand, fold it in half, and put it on the floor." (3 points)
Read and obey the following:
    Close your eyes. (1 point)
    Write a sentence. (1 point)
    Copy design. (1 point)
	9	( )

Total score _____ (A score of less than 24 indicates cognitive disorder).
Assess level of consciousness along a continuum:

|_____|_____|_____|
    Alert   Drowsy   Stupor   Coma

Place "X" at appropriate point on continuum.

Instructions for Administration of Mini-Mental State Examination

1. Ask for the date. Then ask specifically for part omitted (e.g., "Can you also tell me what season it is?"). 1 point for each correct answer.

2. Ask, "Can you tell me the name of this hospital?" (town, county, etc.). 1 point for each correct.

Registration

Ask the patient if you may test his or her memory. Then say the name of 3 unrelated objects, clearly and slowly, about 1 second for each. After having said all 3, ask the patient to repeat them. This first repetition determines his or her score (0-3), but keep saying them until the patient can repeat all 3, up to 6 trials. If he or she does not eventually learn all 3, recall cannot be meaningfully tested.

Attention and Calculation

1. Ask the patient to begin with 100 and count backward by 7. Stop after subtractions (93, 86, 79, 72, 65). Score the total number of correct answers.

2. If the patient cannot or will not perform this task, ask him or her to spell the word "world" backward. The score is the number of letters in correct order (e.g., DLROW = 5; DLORW = 3).

From Folstein, M. F., Folstein, S., & McHugh, P. R. [1975]. Mini-mental state: A practical method for grading the cognitive state of patients for the clinician. *Journal of Psychiatric Research, 12,* 189-198.

Continued

Box 18-5 **Mini-Mental State Examination—cont'd**

Language

1. Naming: Show the patient a wrist watch and ask him or her what it is. Repeat for pencil. Score 0-2.

2. Repetition: Ask the patient to repeat the sentence after you. Allow only one trial. Score 0 or 1.

3. Three-stage command: Give the patient a plain blank paper and repeat the command. Score 1 point for each part correctly executed.

4. Reading: On a blank piece of paper print the sentence, "Close your eyes," in letters large enough for the patient to see clearly. Ask him or her to read it and do what it says. Score 1 point only if the patient actually closes his or her eyes.

5. Writing: Give the patient a blank piece of paper and ask him or her to write a sentence for you. Do not dictate a sentence; it is to be written spontaneously. It must contain a subject and a verb and be sensible. Correct grammar and punctuation are not necessary.

6. Copying: On a clean piece of paper, draw intersecting pentagons, each side about 1 inch, and ask the patient to copy it exactly as it is. All 10 angles must be present, and 2 must intersect to score 1 point. Tremor and rotation are ignored.

Scoring

Add the scores from each of the areas. This is the total score.

Box 18-6 **Delirium Assessment Scales**

DELIRIUM RATING SCALES
DELIRIUM RATING SCALE (DRS) (APPENDIX 3)

- 10-item scale
- 4-point clinician-rated scale
- Assesses
  - Temporal onset
  - Perceptual disturbance
  - Hallucinations
  - Delusions
  - Psychomotor behavior
  - Cognitive status
  - Physical disorder
  - Sleep-wake disturbance
  - Mood lability
  - Symptom variability
- Score of 12 or above from range of 0-32 indicates presence of delirium

MEMORIAL DELIRIUM ASSESSMENT SCALE (MDAS) (APPENDIX 4)

- 10-item scale
- 4-point clinician-rated scale
- Assesses
  - Level of consciousness
  - Disorientation
  - Memory
  - Repetition
  - Attention
  - Thought clarity
  - Perceptual disturbances
  - Delusions
  - Psychomotor activity
  - Sleep-wake disturbance
- Score of 13 or above from range of 0-30 indicates presence of delirium

DIAGNOSTIC INSTRUMENTS
CONFUSION ASSESSMENT METHOD (CAM)

- 10-item scale
- Clinician-rated scale
- Assesses 9 domains from DSM-III-R
  - Level of consciousness
  - Thought clarity
  - Perceptual disturbances
  - Psychomotor activity
  - Attention
  - Sleep-wake disturbance
  - Disorientation
  - Memory
  - Temporal onset and fluctuation
- Presence of first 3-4 items indicates presence of delirium

DSM-III-R, *Diagnostic and Statistical Manual of Mental Disorders (Third Edition, Revised)* (American Psychiatric Association, 1987). Sources: Breitbart, W., & Cohen, K. (2000). Delirium in the terminally ill. In H. M. Chochinov, & W. Breitbart. Eds. *Handbook of psychiatry in palliative medicine*. New York: Oxford University Press; Casarett, D. J., & Inouye, S. K. (2001). Diagnosis and delirium near the end of life. *Annals of Internal Medicine, 135,* 32-40; Kuebler, K. K., English, N., & Heidrich, D. (2001). Delirium, confusion, agitation, and restlessness. In B. Ferrell, & N. Coyle. *Textbook of palliative nursing*. New York: Oxford University Press.

Box 18-7 **The Delirium Rating Scale (DRS)**

ITEM 1: TEMPORAL ONSET OF SYMPTOMS

This item addresses the time course over which symptoms appear; the maximum rating is for the most abrupt onset of symptoms—a common pattern for delirium. Dementia is usually more gradual in onset. Other psychiatric disorders, such as affective disorders, might be scored with 1 or 2 points on this item. Sometimes delirium can be chronic (e.g., in geriatric nursing home patients), and unfortunately only 1 or 2 points would be assessed in that situation.

0   No significant change from long-standing behavior; essentially a chronic or chronic-recurrent disorder
1   Gradual onset of symptoms, occurring within a 6-month period
2   Acute change in behavior or personality occurring over a month
3   Abrupt change in behavior, usually occuring over a 1- to 3-day period

ITEM 2: PERCEPTUAL DISTURBANCES

This item rates most highly the extreme inability to perceive differences between internal and external reality, while intermittent misperceptions such as illusions are given 2 points. Depersonalization and derealization can be seen in other organic mental disorders like temporal lobe epilepsy, in severe depression, and in borderline personality disorder and thus are given only 1 point.

0   None evident by history or observation
1   Feelings of depersonalization or derealization
2   Visual illusions or misperceptions including macropsia, micropsia; e.g., may urinate in wastebasket or mistake bedclothes for something else
3   Evidence that the patient is markedly confused about external reality; e.g., not discriminating between dreams and reality

ITEM 3: HALLUCINATION TYPE

The presence of any type of hallucination is rated. Auditory hallucinations alone are rated with less weight because of their common occurrence in primary psychiatric disorders. Visual hallucinations are generally associated with organic mental syndromes, although not exclusively, and are given 2 points. Tactile hallucinations are classically described in delirium, particularly due to anticholinergic toxicity, and are given the most points.

0   Hallucinations not present
1   Auditory hallucinations only
2   Visual hallucinations present by patient's history or inferred by observation, with or without auditory hallucinations
3   Tactile, olfactory, or gustatory hallucinations present with or without visual or auditory hallucinations

ITEM 4: DELUSIONS

Delusions can be present in many different psychiatric disorders, but tend to be better organized and more fixed in nondelirious disorders and thus are given less weight. Chronic fixed delusions are probably most prevalent in schizophrenic disorders. New delusions may indicate affective and schizophrenic disorders, dementia, or substance intoxication but should also alert the clinician to possible delirium and are given 2 points. Poorly formed delusions, often of a paranoid nature, are typical of delirium.

0   Not present
1   Delusions are systematized, i.e., well organized and persistent
2   Delusions are new and not part of a preexisting primary psychiatric disorder
3   Delusions are not well circumscribed; are transient, poorly organized, and mostly in response to misperceived environmental cues; e.g., are paranoid and involve persons who are in reality caregivers, loved ones, hospital staff, etc.

ITEM 5: PSYCHOMOTOR BEHAVIOR

This item describes degrees of severity of altered psychomotor behavior. Maximum points can be given for severe agitation or severe withdrawal to reflect either the hyperactive or the hypoactive variant in delirium.

0   No significant retardation or agitation
1   Mild restlessness, tremulousness, or anxiety evident by observation and a change from patient's usual behavior

Continued

Box 18-7 The Delirium Rating Scale (DRS)—cont'd

ITEM 5—cont'd

2   Moderate agitation with pacing, removing IVs, etc.

3   Severe agitation, needs to be restrained, may be combative; or has significant withdrawal from the environment, but not due to major depression or schizophrenic catatonia

ITEM 6: COGNITIVE STATUS DURING FORMAL TESTING

Information from the cognitive portion of a routine mental status examination is needed to rate this item. The maximum rating of 4 points is given for severe cognitive deficits while only 1 point is given for mild inattention, which could be attributed to pain and fatigue seen in medically ill persons. Two points are given for a relatively isolated cognitive deficit, such as memory impairment, which could be due to dementia or organic amnestic syndrome as well as to early delirium.

0   No cognitive deficits, or deficits which can be alternatively explained by lack of education or prior mental retardation

1   Very mild cognitive deficits which might be attributed to inattention due to acute pain, fatigue, depression, or anxiety associated with having a medical illness

2   Cognitive deficit largely in one major area tested, e.g., memory, but otherwise intact

3   Significant cognitive deficits which are diffuse, i.e., affecting many different areas tested; most include periods of disorientation to time or place at least once each 24-hr period; registration and/or recall are abnormal; concentration is reduced.

4   Severe cognitive deficits, including motor or verbal perseveration, confabulations, disorientation to person, remote and recent memory deficits, and inability to cooperate with formal mental status testing

ITEM 7: PHYSICAL DISORDER

Maximum points are given when a specific lesion or physiological disturbance can be temporally associated with the altered behavior. Dementias are often not found to have a specific underlying medical cause, while delirium usually has at least one identifiable physical cause. . . .

0   None present or active

1   Presence of any physical disorder which might affect mental state

2   Specific drug, infection, metabolic, central nervous system lesion, or other medical problem which can be temporally implicated in causing the altered behavior or mental status

ITEM 8: SLEEP-WAKE CYCLE DISTURBANCE

Disruption of the sleep-wake cycle is typical in delirium, with demented persons generally having significant sleep disturbances much later in their course. Severe delirium is on a continuum with stupor and coma, and persons with a resolving coma are likely to be delirious temporarily.

0   Not present; awake and alert during the day, and sleeps without significant disruption at night

1   Occasional drowsiness during day and mild sleep continuity disturbance at night; may have nightmares, but can readily distinguish from reality

2   Frequent napping and unable to sleep at night, constituting a significant disruption of or a reversal of the usual sleep-wake cycle

3   Drowsiness prominent, difficulty staying alert during interview, loss of self-control over alertness and somnolence

4   Drifts into stuporous or comatose periods

ITEM 9: LABILITY OF MOOD

Rapid shifts in mood can occur in various organic mental syndromes, perhaps due to a disinhibition of one's normal control. The patient may be aware of this lack of emotional control and may behave inappropriately relative to the situation or to his/her thinking state, e.g., crying for no apparent reason. Delirious patients may score points on any of these items depending upon the severity of the delirium and upon how their underlying psychological state "colors" their delirious presentation. Patients with borderline personality disorder might score 1 or 2 points on this item.

Box 18-7 **The Delirium Rating Scale (DRS)—cont'd**

0   Not present; mood stable

1   Affect/mood somewhat altered and changes over the course of hours; patient states that mood changes are not under self-control

2   Significant mood changes which are inappropriate to situation, including fear, anger, or tearfulness; rapid shifts of emotion, even over several minutes

3   Severe disinhibition of emotions, including temper outbursts, uncontrolled inappropriate laughter, or crying

ITEM 10: VARIABILITY OF SYMPTOMS

The hallmark of delirium is the waxing and waning of symptoms, which is given 4 points on this item. Demented as well as delirious patients, who become more confused at night when environmental cues have decreased, could score 2 points.

0   Symptoms stable and mostly present during daytime

2   Symptoms worsen at night

4   Fluctuating intensity of symptoms, such that they wax and wane during a 24-hr period

From Trzepacz, P. T., Baker, R. W., & Greenhouse, J. (1988). A symptom rating scale for delirium. *Psychiatry Research, 23*, 89-97.

Box 18-8 **Memorial Delirium Assessment Scale (MDAS)**

INSTRUCTIONS

Rate the severity of the following symptoms of delirium based on current interaction with subject or assessment of his/her behavior or experience over past several hours (as indicated in each time).

ITEM 1–REDUCED LEVEL OF CONSCIOUSNESS (AWARENESS)

Rate the patient's current awareness of an interaction with the environment (interviewer, other people/objects in the room, for example, ask patients to describe the surroundings)

0: none   Patient spontaneously fully aware of environment and interacts appropriately

1: mild   Patient is unaware of some elements in the environment, or not spontaneously interacting appropriately with the interviewer; becomes fully aware and appropriately interactive when prodded strongly; interview is prolonged but not seriously disrupted

2: moderate   Patient is unaware of some or all elements in the environment, or not spontaneously interacting with the interviewer; becomes incompletely aware and inappropriately interactive when prodded strongly; interview is prolonged but not seriously disrupted

3: severe   Patient is unaware of all elements in the environment with no spontaneous interaction or awareness of the interviewer, so that the interview is difficult to impossible, even with maximal prodding

ITEM 2–DISORIENTATION

Rate current state by asking the following 10 orientation items: date, month, day, year, season, floor, name of hospital, city, state, and country.

0: none   Patient knows 9-10 items
1: mild   Patient knows 7-8 items
2: moderate   Patient knows 5-6 items
3: severe   Patient knows no more than 4 items

ITEM 3–SHORT-TERM MEMORY IMPAIRMENT

Rate current state by using repetition and delayed recall of 3 words (patient must immediately repeat and recall words 5 minutes later after an intervening task). Use alternate sets of 3 words for successive

Continued

Box 18-8 Memorial Delirium Assessment Scale (MDAS)—cont'd

evaluation (e.g., apple, table, tomorrow, sky, cigar, justice).

0: none   All 3 words repeated and recalled
1: mild   All 3 repeated, patient fails to recall 1
2: moderate All 3 repeated, patient fails to recall 2
3: severe   Patient fails to repeat 1 or more words

ITEM 4—IMPAIRED DIGIT SPAN

Rate current performance by asking subjects to repeat first 3, 4, then 5 digits forward and then 3, then 4 backward; continue to the next step only if patient succeeds at the previous one.

0: none   Patient can do at least 5 numbers forward and 4 backward
1: mild   Patient can do at least 5 numbers forward, 3 backward
2: moderate Patient can do 4-5 numbers forward, cannot do 3 backward
3: severe   Patient can do no more than 3 numbers forward

ITEM 5—REDUCED ABILITY TO MAINTAIN AND SHIFT ATTENTION

As indicated during the interview by questions needing to be rephrased and/or repeated because patient's attention wanders, patient loses track, patient is distracted by outside stimuli or over-absorbed in a task

0: none   None of the above; patient maintains and shifts attention normally
1: mild   Above attention problems occur once or twice without prolonging the interview
2: moderate Above attention problems occur often, prolonging the interview without seriously disrupting it
3: severe   Above attention problems occur constantly, disrupting and making the interview difficult to impossible

ITEM 6—DISORGANIZED THINKING

As indicated during the interview by rambling, irrelevant, or incoherent speech, or by tangential, circumstantial, or faulty reasoning. Ask patient a somewhat complex question (e.g., "Describe your current medical condition.").

0: none   Patient's speech is coherent and goal-directed
1: mild   Patient's speech is slightly difficult to follow; responses to questions are slightly off target but not so much as to prolong the interview
2: moderate Disorganized thoughts or speech are clearly present, such that interview is prolonged but not disrupted
3: severe   Examination is very difficult or impossible due to disorganized thinking or speech

ITEM 7—PERCEPTUAL DISTURBANCE

Misperceptions, illusions, hallucinations inferred from inappropriate behavior during the interview or admitted by subject as well as those elicited from nurse/family/chart accounts of the past several hours or of the time since last examination

0: none   No misperceptions, illusions, or hallucinations
1: mild   Misperceptions or illusions related to sleep, fleeting hallucinations on 1-2 occasions without inappropriate behavior
2: moderate Hallucinations or frequent illusions on several occasions with minimal inappropriate behavior that does not disrupt the interview
3: severe   Frequent or intense illusions or hallucinations with persistent inappropriate behavior that disrupts the interview or interferes with medical care

ITEM 8—DELUSIONS

Rate delusions inferred from inappropriate behavior during the interview or admitted by the patient as well as delusions elicited from nurse/family/chart accounts of the past several hours or of the time since the previous examination.

Box 18-8 **Memorial Delirium Assessment Scale (MDAS)—cont'd**

0: none	No evidence of misinterpretations or delusions
1: mild	Misinterpretations or suspiciousness without clear delusional ideas or inappropriate behavior
2: moderate	Delusions admitted by the patient or evidenced by his/her behavior that do not or only marginally disrupt the interview or interfere with medical care
3: Severe	Persistent and/or intense delusions resulting in inappropriate behavior, disrupting the interview or seriously interfering with medical care

ITEM 9—DECREASED OR INCREASED PSYCHOMOTOR ACTIVITY

Rate activity over past several hours as well as activity during interview by circling (a) hypoactive, (b) hyperactive, or (c) elements of both present

0: none			Normal psychomotor activity
a	b	c	
1: mild			Hypoactivity is barely noticeable, expressed as slightly slowing of movement
a	b	c	Hyperactivity is barely noticeable or appears as simple restlessness
2: moderate			Hypoactivity is undeniable with marked reduction in the number of movements or marked slowness of movement; subject rarely spontaneously moves or speaks
a	b	c	Hyperactivity is undeniable, subject moves almost constantly In both cases, exam is prolonged as a consequence
3: severe			Hypoactivity is severe, patient does not move or speak without prodding or is catatonic

a	b	c	Hyperactivity is severe; patient is constantly moving, overreacts to stimuli, and requires surveillance and/or restraint Getting through the exam is difficult or impossible

ITEM 10—SLEEP-WAKE CYCLE DISTURBANCE (DISORDER OF AROUSAL)

Rate patient's ability to either sleep or stay awake at the appropriate times. Utilize direct observation during the interview as well as reports from nurses, family, patient, or charts describing sleep-wake cycle disturbance over the past several hours or since last examination. Use observations of the previous night for morning evaluations only.

0: none	At night, sleeps well; during the day, has no trouble staying awake
1: mild	Mild deviation from appropriate sleepfulness and wakefulness states; at night difficulty falling asleep or transient night awakenings, needs medication to sleep well; during the day, reports periods of drowsiness or, during the interview, is drowsy but can easily fully awaken him/herself
2: moderate	Moderate deviations from appropriate sleepfulness and wakefulness states at night, repeated and prolonged night awakening; during the day, reports of frequent and prolonged napping or, during the interview, can only be roused to complete wakefulness by strong stimuli
3: severe	Severe deviations from appropriate sleepfulness and wakefulness states at night, sleeplessness; during the day, patient spends most of the time sleeping, or, during the interview, cannot be roused to full wakefulness by any stimuli

From Breitbart, W., Rosenfeld, B., Roth, A., Smith, M. J., Cohen, K., & Passik, S. (1997). The Memorial Delirium Assessment Scale. *Journal of Pain and Symptom Management, 13,* 128-137. Copyright 1997 by the U.S. Cancer Pain Relief Committee.

Table 18-9 Comparison of Depression, Delirium, and Dementia

Depression	Delirium	Dementia	
Onset	Coincides w/ major life changes	Acute/abrupt	Insidious, chronic
Course	Diurnal effects—worse in AM usually	Short diurnal fluctuations	Long, no diurnal effects
	Situational fluctuations	Worse at night	Progressive
Progression	Variable—rapid or slow	Abrupt	Slow—uneven
Duration	Persistent—at least 2 weeks	Days to hours—less than 1 month	Months to years
Awareness	Clear	Clear	Reduced
Alertness	Normal	Fluctuates	Generally normal
Attention	Minimal impairment	Impaired	Generally normal
Orientation	Selective	Generally impaired	Possibly impaired
Memory	Selective or patchy impairment	Recent and immediate impairment	Recent memory worse, remote impairment
Thinking	Intact w/ hopelessness, helplessness	Disorganized, distorted, fragmented, incoherent	Difficulty w/abstraction, word finding
Perception	Intact except severe cases	Distorted, illusions, hallucinations	Misperceptions usually absent
Psychomotor behavior	Variable—retardation or agitation	Variable—hypokinetic or hyperkinetic	Normal with apraxia
Sleep/wake cycle	Disturbed, early AM waking	Cycle reversed	Fragmented
Affect	Depressed/irritable	Labile	Variable
Family history	May be positive	Noncontributory	May be positive for dementia of Alzheimer's type

Sources: Breitbart, W., & Cohen, K. (2000). Delirium in the terminally ill. In H. M. Chochinov, & W. Breitbart. Eds. *Handbook of psychiatry in palliative medicine*. New York: Oxford University Press; Chan, D., & Brennan, N. (1999). Delirium: making the diagnosis, improving the prognosis. *Geriatrics, 54*(3), 28-42; Falk, W. (1998). Approach to the patient with memory problems or dementia. In T. A. Stern, J. B. Herman, & P. L. Slavin. *The MGH guide to psychiatry in primary care*. New York: McGraw-Hill; Langhorne, M. (1999). Confusion or delirium: determining the difference. *Developments in Supportive Cancer Care*, 3(3), 82-87.

symptom management is critical. Alcohol or benzodiazepine withdrawal should be considered (Chan & Brennan, 1999). Any treatments provided should include promotion of appropriate pacing and time for rest and sleep. Metabolic fluctuations should be corrected, including hydration, if appropriate within the elder's entire clinical picture. The patient should be assessed for infection, and treated if it is present. Last, it may be appropriate to do further work-up with particular emphasis on differentiating delirium from dementia or possible depression. Table 18-9 compares the differences between depression, delirium, and dementia.

Bruera and Neumann (1998) suggested an algorithm approach in the patient with advanced disease and delirium. Their algorithm begins by determining whether it is a hypoactive or hyperactive delirium. If the delirium is hypoactive, then reversible causes should be ruled out. Assessment includes evaluating for causative factors by checking for abnormal lab exams, metastatic processes, sepsis, and use of opioid medications. Hydration and a change in opioid may be necessary. The patient should be reassessed following treatment to determine if the delirium is reversing. If the delirium is hyperactive, then the patient should be started on haloperidol. If delirium continues in spite of high doses of haloperidol, then the older patient could receive a trial of methotrimeprazine. If this medication had no effect, a benzodiazepine drip may be appropriate. Either midazolam, diazepam, or lorazepam may be appropriate. Throughout the

Table 18-10 **Treatment of Delirium**	
Medications	**Dosage (mg)**
NEUROLEPTICS	
Haloperidol	0.5-5 q 2-12h
Thioridazine	10-75 q 4-8h
Chlorpromazine	12.5-50 q 4-12h
Methotrimeprazine	12.5-50 q 4-8h
BENZODIAZEPINES	
Lorazepam	0.5-2.0 q 1-4h
Midazolam	1.0-4.0 q 1-4h
ANESTHETIC	
Propofol	10-mg bolus w/ 10-20mg/hr

Sources: Breitbart, W., Chochinov, H. M., & Passik, S. (1998). Psychiatric aspect of palliative care. In D. Doyle, W. C. Hanks, & N. MacDonald. Eds. *Oxford textbook of palliative medicine*. (2nd ed.). New York: Oxford University Press; Casarett, D. J., & Inouye, S. K. (2001). Diagnosis and delirium near the end of life. *Annals of Internal Medicine, 135*, 32-40; Kuebler, K. K., English, N., & Heidrich, D. (2001). Delirium, confusion, agitation, and restlessness. In B. Ferrell, & N. Coyle. *Textbook of palliative nursing*. New York: Oxford University Press.

treatment of delirium, counseling and education would be offered to the elder patient, his or her family, and support staff, with continual reassessment focusing on determining any other causes of the delirium.

Pharmacologic

Pharmacologic interventions depend on the suspected problem. For undetermined causes, neuroleptics are the drugs of first choice; haloperidol (a potent dopamine blocker) is the preferred medication (Chan & Brennan, 1999; Waller & Caroline, 2000). The initial dose is a 1-mg tablet three times a day (Waller & Caroline, 2000). Historically, chlorpromazine has been used, but it is much more sedating. Risperidone has been suggested, but older adults tend to experience more side effects (Zarate et al., 1997). Benzodiazepines may be helpful, particularly during medication withdrawal (Conn & Lieff, 2001); short-acting ones are better tolerated, making lorazepam the preferred drug. Doses can range from 0.5 to 1 mg every 4 hours. For brain metastases, a trial of steroids may help; the dose for dexamethasone ranges from 16 to 36 mg

every morning (Waller & Caroline, 2000). In patients with Parkinson's disease, risperidone may be helpful (Chan & Brennan, 1999). If delirium is intractable and no treatment is successful, palliative sedation may be necessary (Wein, 2000). This may best be achieved through the use of propofol or midazolam (Casarett & Inouye, 2001; Waller & Caroline, 2000; Wein 2000). Table 18-10 offers suggestions for medications and dosages in the treatment of delirium.

Nonpharmacologic

Nonpharmacologic treatments focus on management of the environment, which includes creating a safe environment, reducing stimuli, and providing reassurance. A basic, but often ignored, intervention is to make sure elders have access to their hearing aids and glasses, which facilitate communication and promote reassurance. Other strategies focus on the patient's room and climate; for example, soft lighting that does not cause harsh images or shadows can prevent hallucinations. Cognitive assist devices (e.g., calendars or clocks) can cue orientation to time and date. Familiar sounds, smells, and touch may help promote calmness (Boyle et al., 1998; Simon, Jeuel, & Brokel, 1997). Personal effects (e.g., lotions, perfumes, foods) and family and friends provide reorientation and reassurance.

Having a consistent roster of nurses caring for the patient may also be of benefit. In order to avoid using restraints, family or health care providers may need to provide "sitters." Confused elders may unintentionally harm themselves trying to slip out of restraints (Conn & Lieff, 2001). Sitters can help with reorientation, respond to patient fear, and watch the elder to prevent falls.

Sleep deprivation may cause further confusion, so the elimination of both visual and sensory stimuli is paramount. Scheduling medications without constant interruption of sleep during the night can decrease sleep loss. Reduction or elimination of noise pollution, such as radios, television, or overhead intercom announcements, can also increase rest and promote sleep.

Family Concerns and Considerations

Education of the family is a cornerstone of management of the prevention and treatment of delirium. Families need to understand predisposing risk factors that can lead to delirium, includ-

EVIDENCE-BASED PRACTICE°

Reference: Gagnon, P., Allard, P., Masse, B., & DeSerres, M. (2000). Delirium in terminal cancer: A prospective study using daily screening, early diagnosis, and continuous monitoring. *Journal of Pain and Symptom Management, 19,* 412-426.

Research Problem: Delirium is common in palliative care patients. The purpose of this study was to evaluate delirium frequency and outcome in more terminal cancer patients.

Design: Prospective pilot cohort study.

Sample and Setting: 89 cancer patients, fairly equally represented in terms of gender, with a median age of 66, studied over 4 months in a 15-bed hospice unit.

Methods: Patients underwent screening and re-screening with the Confusion Rating Scale. If this screen was positive, the patient was then assessed with the Confusion Assessment Method tool.

Results: Thirty-four patients (38%) remained negative for delirium screening throughout their hospice stay. The other 55 patients (62%) had positive results at some point during their hospice stay. The prevalence of delirium symptoms within the first 24 hours of admission was 20%. Although the prevalence of confirmed delirium was 13%, the remaining 87% experienced delirium at some point during their stay. For the patients with delirium, the common characteristic was opioid intake that was only minimally higher than that in the patients without the diagnosis of delirium.

Implications for Nursing Practice: Nurses should institute the useful practice of initial and ongoing screening for delirium in the setting of opioid use. They also should gain familiarity with the various delirium scales so as to gain facility in their usage.

Conclusion: Because these patients had metastatic cancer, opioid metabolism could be altered just enough to increase its effects, which could result in delirium. This study is limited in that its population was only cancer patients in a hospice setting, where clinicians are attuned to the presence of delirium. It is also limited in not covering the aspects of terminal care that take place outside a hospice setting, where a patient may be taking more medications.

ing pressure sores, poor nutrition, incontinence, sleep disturbances, and decreased functional ability, including vision and hearing (Casarett & Inouye, 2001; Flacker & Marcantonio, 1998). Helping to prevent these conditions and providing education about the issues may help prevent delirium and the necessity for treatment. Teaching should be multifaceted; instructions regarding the use of cognitive assist devices such as glasses and hearing aids can help maintain safety for the older adult. Assessment of the home environment can be quite revealing, particularly in regard to whether the patient has the basic necessities of food, finances, and medications. Family members should understand the importance of skin care, as well as the importance of a well-balanced diet and hydration, to the extent that the older adult does not see these interventions as a burden or source of distress.

The elder patient, family, and friends should be offered information on all treatment choices to prevent delirium. The primary role of the nurse is advocacy for appropriate care. Preventative measures include judicious use of Foley catheters or removal of unnecessary tubes; no restraints for confusion; prevention of skin ulcers; and maximal social support to the family caregivers (McElhaney, 2002).

When an elder patient becomes delirious at the end of life, ongoing support of the family is important. Delirium may be irreversible because of the various medical conditions the elder is experiencing as well as the dying process. In deciding on treatment, an informed discussion of the realistic options should occur in the context of life expectancy and the risk versus benefit of any treatment. Families often welcome this clear discussion of all the current issues, including possible dying scenarios and what to expect. This information prepares them for the anticipated events.

Health care providers should model the art of "presence," or being with a patient. The patient's family should be encouraged to provide ongoing, soothing communication, reassuring the elder patient that he or she is safe, while not confronting the patient about what she or he sees or hears. Gentle reorientation should be provided.

Often, in the search to find an explanation for delirium, the very fact that an elder is actively dying is overlooked. Therefore, families may need education that delirium may be a signal that their loved one is nearing the end of his or her life. The other signs and symptoms of the dying process should be reviewed in the larger context of the terminal illness (see Chapter 25). Family members should be encouraged to talk to the older adult even when death is imminent. They should also be reassured that pain and symptom management will continue.

Case Study Conclusion

Mrs. M. was a perfect candidate for palliative care. She began receiving 5 to 6 L/min of oxygen via nasal cannula and was placed on a scheduled dose of a short-acting benzodiazepine (lorazepam, 0.5 mg every 6 hours). This smaller dose was chosen because Mrs. M. weighed only about 60 pounds. The lorazepam helped decrease her anxiety, which in turn assisted her breathing. She was also given morphine elixir, 0.5 to 1.0 mg every 6 hours, to ease any additional chest pain and labored breathing. Although she had been on long-term antidepressants, those were reexamined and she was started on sertraline, 12.5 mg/day. In addition, Mrs. M. clarified her wishes not to be returned to the hospital and was subsequently referred to hospice care. They provided expert pain and symptom management in the nursing home as well as more pastoral support.

Mrs. M. was much more comfortable with the additional medications, and less anxious. In fact, she felt so much better that she thought she should stop her medications. However, with coaxing, she was made to understand the importance of the scheduled doses of these medications. She remained comfortable and died very peacefully at the nursing home.

CONCLUSION

The older adult has many experiences in late adulthood that affect coping ability in crisis. Psychiatric symptoms may develop in the event of a life-threatening illness. Anxiety, depression, and delirium may be the first sign of an illness, or may be the response to an illness. Biologic issues such as diminished functional and slower physiologic processes affect treatment considerations. These issues include a slower metabolism, a higher side effect profile for many medications, and a lower threshold for any imbalances.

Social issues such as isolation and lack of family supports may also have negative effects on treatment. The family effort may be the most challenging because of the increased mobility of families, with members often spread across the country. Elders may be living alone in one town with their adult children living in cities a long distance away. The very issue of the basics of living may be affected by distance between aging parents and adult children. Aging adults may not want to burden their children with their daily struggle (Reichel & Gallo, 1999).

Effective treatment of anxiety, depression, and delirium for the older patient necessitates a collaborative effort between the patient, family, and health care team. The patient may perceive that something is wrong but cannot articulate the problem; family members may perceive that something is wrong but feel that it is part of the aging process. The health care provider may not account for the biologic differences in older adults when evaluating the problem. These factors make communication and vigilance necessary components of care.

Anxiety, depression, and delirium can be difficult disorders to recognize and treat in the older adult population. These conditions cause suffering by reducing both daily functioning and quality of life. The result may be unnecessary placement in an institution outside the home and increased stress for family caregivers. Anxiety, depression, and delirium can be effectively treated; however, evaluation and treatment of older adults requires skill, time, and patience. The goal of palliative care is a holistic approach that improves physical, psychological, spiritual, and emotional well-being. It is incumbent upon clinicians to be vigilant and have a high index of suspicion for the presence of these disorders. A collaborative approach can provide a partnership in caring for the older adult that supports his or her independence and dignity as long as possible.

REFERENCES

American Psychiatric Association. (2000). *Diagnostic and statistical manual of mental disorders* (4th ed., text revision). Washington, DC: Author.

Barsevik, A. M., Sweeney, C., Haney, E., & Chung, E. (2002). A systemic qualitative analysis of psychoeducational interventions for depression in patients with cancer. *Oncology Nursing Forum, 29*, 73–87.

Block, S. D. (2000). Assessing and managing depression in the terminally ill patient. *Annals of Internal Medicine, 132*, 209-213.

Boyle, D. M., Abernathy, G., Baker, L., & Wall, A. C. (1998). End of life confusion in patients with cancer. *Oncology Nursing Forum, 25*, 1335-1343.

Breitbart, W., Chochinov, H. M., & Passik, S. (1998). Psychiatric aspect of palliative care. In D. Doyle, W. C. Hanks, & N. MacDonald (Eds.), *Oxford textbook of palliative medicine* (pp. 933-959). (2nd ed.). New York: Oxford University Press.

Breitbart, W., & Cohen, K. (2000). Delirium in the terminally ill. In H. M. Chochinov, & W. Breitbart (Eds.), *Handbook of psychiatry in palliative medicine* (pp. 75-90). New York: Oxford University Press.

Bruera, E. D., & Neumann, C. M. (1998). The uses of psychotropics in symptom management of advanced cancer. *Psycho-Oncology, 7*, 346-358.

Buckwalter, K. C., & Piven, M. L. S. (1999). Depression. In J. T. Stone, J. F. Wyman, & S. A. Salisbury (Eds.), *Clinical gerontological nursing—a guide to advanced practice* (pp. 587-412). Philadelphia: Saunders.

Candilis, P. (1998). The use of screening tests for detection of psychiatric disorders. In T. A. Stern, J. B. Herman, & P. L. Slavin (Eds.), *The MGH guide to psychiatry in primary care* (pp. 643-650). New York: McGraw-Hill.

Carmin, C. N., Pollard, C. A., & Gillock, K. L. (1999). Assessment of anxiety disorders in the elderly. In P. A. Lichtenberg (Ed.), *Handbook of assessment in clinical gerontology* (pp. 59-90). New York: Wiley.

Casarett, D. J., & Inouye, S. K. (2001). Diagnosis and delirium near the end of life. *Annals of Internal Medicine, 135*, 32-40.

Chan, D., & Brennan, N. (1999). Delirium: Making the diagnosis, improving the prognosis. *Geriatrics, 54*(3), 28-42.

Conn, D. K., & Lieff, S. (2001). Diagnosing and managing delirium in the elderly. *Canadian Family Physician, 47*, 101-108.

Costa, P. T., Williams, T. F., Somerfield, M. S., et al. (1996). *Recognition and initial assessment of Alzheimer's disease and related dementias* (Clinical Practice Guideline 19). Rockville, MD: Agency for Health Care Policy and Research.

Cremens, M. C., & Harari, D. (1998). Approach to the geriatric patient. In T. A. Stern, J. B. Herman, & P. L. Slavin (Eds.), *The MGH guide to psychiatry in primary care* (pp. 131-138). New York: McGraw-Hill.

Depression Guideline Panel. (1993). *Depression in primary care: Vol. 1. Detection and diagnosis* (Clinical Practice Guideline 5). Rockville, MD: Agency for Health Care Policy and Research.

Drugs that may cause psychiatric symptoms. (2002). *Medical Letter on Drugs and Therapeutics, 44*, 59-62.

Edelstein, B., Kalish, K. D., Drozdick, L. W., & McKee, D. R. (1999). Assessment of depression and bereavement in older adults. In P. A. Lichtenberg (Ed.), *Handbook of assessment in clinical gerontology* (pp. 11-58). New York: Wiley.

Falk, W. (1998). Approach to the patient with memory problems or dementia. In T. A. Stern, J. B. Herman, & P. L. Slavin (Eds.), *The MGH guide to psychiatry in primary care* (pp. 207-219). New York: McGraw-Hill.

Filiberti, A., Ripamonti, C., Totis, A., Ventafridda, V., De Conno, F., Contiero, P., et al. (2001). Characteristics of terminal cancer patients who committed suicide during a home palliative care program. *Journal of Pain and Symptom Management, 22*, 544-553.

Flacker, J. M., & Marcantonio, E. R. (1998). Delirium in the elderly—optimal management. *Drugs and Aging, 13*, 119-130.

Folstein, M., Folstein, S., & McHugh, P. (1975). Mini-mental state: A practical method for grading the cognitive state of patients for the clinician. *Journal of Psychiatric Research, 12*, 189-198.

Ingham, J., & Caraceni, A. (2002). Delirium. In A. Berger, R. Portenoy, & D. Weissman (Eds.), *Principles and practice of palliative and supportive oncology* (pp. 555-576). Philadelphia: Lippincott Williams & Wilkins.

Kane, R. L., Ouslander, J. G., & Abrass, I. B. (1999). *Essentials of clinical geriatrics*. New York: McGraw-Hill.

Kuebler, K. K., English, N., & Heidrich, D. (2001). Delirium, confusion, agitation, and restlessness. In B. Ferrell, & N. Coyle (Eds.), *Textbook of palliative nursing* (pp. 290-308). New York: Oxford University Press.

Lagomasino, I. L., & Stern, T. (1998). Approach to the suicidal patient. In T. A. Stern, J. B. Herman, & P. L. Slavin (Eds.), *The MGH guide to psychiatry in primary care* (pp. 15-22). New York: McGraw-Hill.

Langhorne, M. (1999). Confusion or delirium: Determining the difference. *Developments in Supportive Cancer Care, 3*(3), 82-87.

Lantz, M. (2002). Generalized anxiety in anxious times: Helping older adults cope. *Clinical Geriatrics, 10*(1), 36-38.

Lavretsky, H. (2001). Choosing appropriate treatment for geriatric depression. *Clinical Geriatrics, 9*(5), 30-46.

Lawlor, P. G., Fainsinger, R. L., & Bruera, E. D. (2000). Delirium at the end of life—critical issues in clinical practice and research. *Journal of the American Medical Association, 284*, 2427-2429.

Lebowitz, B. D., Pearson, J. L., Schneider, L. S., Reynolds, C. F. 3rd, Alexopoulos, G. S., Bruce, M. L., et al. (1997). Diagnosis and treatment of depression in late life—consensus statement update. *Journal of the American Medical Association, 248*, 1186-1190.

Lee, S., Back, A., Block, S., & Stewart, S. (2002). Enhancing physician-patient communication. *Hematology, 1*, 464-478.

Lehmann, S. W., & Rabins, P. V. (1999). Clinical geropsychiatry. In J. J. Gallo, J. Busby-Whitehead, P. V. Rabins, R. A. Silliman & J. B. Murphy (Eds.), *Reichels's care of the elderly—clinical aspects of aging* (pp. 179-189). Philadelphia: Lippincott Williams & Wilkins.

Lloyd-Williams, M. (2001). Screening for depression in palliative care patients: A review. *European Journal of Cancer Care, 10*, 31-35.

Lovejoy, N. C., Tabor, D., & Deloney, P. (2000). Cancer-related depression: Part ii—neurologic alterations and evolving approaches to psychopharmacology. *Oncology Nursing Forum, 27*, 795-808.

McCullough, P. K. (1992). Evaluation and management of anxiety in the older adult. *Geriatrics, 47*(4), 35-38.

McDonald, M. V., Passik, S. D., Dugan, W., Rosenfeld, B., Theobald, D. E., & Edgerton, S. (1999). Nurses' recognition of depression in their patients with cancer. *Oncology Nursing Forum, 26*, 593-599.

McElhaney, J. E. (2002, April 1). Delirium in elderly patients: How you can help. *Consultant*, pp 484-490.

Meagher, D. J. (2001). Delirium: Optimizing management. *BMJ, 322*, 144-149.

NIH Consensus Development Program. (2002, October 26). *NIH State-of-the-Science Conference on Symptom Management in Cancer: Pain, Depression and Fatigue—Final statement.* Retrieved from consensus.nih.gov/ta/022/022_statement.html

Pasacreta, J. V., Minarik, P. A., & Nield-Anderson, L. (2001). Anxiety and depression. In B. Ferrell, & N. Coyle (Eds.), *Textbook of palliative nursing* (pp. 269-289). New York: Oxford University Press.

Payne, D. K., & Massie, M. J. (2000). Anxiety in palliative care. In H. M. Chochinov, & W. Breitbart (Eds.), *Handbook of psychiatry in palliative medicine* (pp. 577-592). New York: Oxford University Press.

Payne, D. K., & Massie, M. J. (2002). Depression and anxiety. In A. Berger, R. Portenoy, & D. Weissman (Eds.), *Principles and practice of palliative and supportive oncology.* Philadelphia: Lippincott Williams & Wilkins.

Pollack, M. H., Smoller, J. W., & Lee, D. (1998). Approach to the anxious patient. In T. A. Stern, J. B. Herman, & P. L. Slavin (Eds.), *The MGH guide to psychiatry in primary care* (pp. 23-37). New York: McGraw-Hill.

Reichel, W., & Gallo, J. J. (1999). Essential principles in the care of the elderly. In J. J. Gallo, J. Busby-Whitehead, P. V. Rabins, R. A. Silliman & J. B. Murphy (Eds.), *Reichels's care of the elderly—clinical aspects of aging* (pp. 3-19). Philadelphia: Lippincott Williams & Wilkins.

Reiss, S., Peterson, R. A., Gursky, D. M., & McNally, R. J. (1986). Anxiety sensitivity, anxiety frequency, and the prediction of fearfulness. *Behaviour Research and Therapy, 24*, 1-8.

Rosenbaum, J. F., & Fava, M. (1998). Approach to the patient with depression. In T. A. Stern, J. B. Herman, & P. L.

Slavin (Eds.), *The MGH guide to psychiatry in primary care* (pp. 1-14). New York: McGraw-Hill.

Rozans, M., Dreisbach, A., Lertora, J., & Kahn, M. (2002). Palliative uses of methylphenidate in patients with cancer: A review. *Journal of Clinical Oncology, 20*, 335-339.

Shuster, J. L., & Jones, G. R. (1998). Approach to the patient receiving palliative care. In T. A. Stern, J. B. Herman, & P. L. Slavin (Eds.), *The MGH guide to psychiatry in primary care* (pp. 147-157). New York: McGraw-Hill.

Simon, L., Jewell, N., & Brokel, J. (1997). Management of acute delirium in hospitalized elderly: A process improvement project. *Geriatric Nursing, 18*, 150-154.

Stark, D., Kiely, A., Smith, G., Velikova, A., & Selby, P. (2002). Anxiety disorders in cancer patients: Their nature, associations, and relations to quality of life. *Journal of Clinical Oncology, 20*, 3137-3148.

Tremblay, A., & Breitbart, W. (2001). Psychiatric dimensions of palliative care. *Neurology Clinics, 19*, 949-967.

U. S. Preventive Services Task Forces. (2000). *Screening for depression: Recommendations and rationale.* Rockville, MD: Agency for Healthcare Research and Quality.

Valente, S. M., & Saunders, J. M. (1997). Diagnosis and treatment of major depression among patients with cancer. *Cancer Nursing, 10*, 168-177.

Valente, S. M., Saunders, J. M., & Cohen, M. Z. (1994). Evaluating depression among patients with cancer. *Cancer Practice, 2*(1), 65-71.

Volicer, L. (1999, May). Clinical guidelines for the treatment of Alzheimer's disease and other progressive dementias. *Federal Practitioner, 16*(Suppl.), 16-25.

Volicer, L. (2001). Management of severe Alzheimer's disease and end of life issues. *Clinics in Geriatric Medicine, 17*, 377-391.

Waller, A., & Caroline, N. L. (2000). *Handbook of palliative care in cancer* (2nd ed.). Boston: Butterworth-Heinemann.

Wein, S. (2000). Sedation in the imminently dying patient. *Oncology, 14*, 585-592.

Weissman, A. (1998). The patient with acute grief. In T. A. Stern, J. B. Herman, & P. L. Slavin (Eds.), *The MGH guide to psychiatry in primary care.* New York: McGraw-Hill.

Well-Connected. (1998a). *Anxiety* (Report # 28). Atlanta: A.D.A.M., Inc. URL: www.well-connected.com.

Well-Connected. (1998b). *Depression* (Report # 8). Atlanta: A.D.A.M., Inc. URL: www.well-connected.com.

Wilson, K. G., Chochinov, H. M., de Faye, B. J., & Breitbart, W. (2000). Diagnosis and management of depression in palliative care. In H. M. Chochinov, & W. Breitbart (Eds.), *Handbook of psychiatry in palliative medicine* (pp. 25-50). New York: Oxford University Press.

Yesavage, J., Brink, T. L., & Rose, T. L. (1983). Development and validation of a geriatric screening scale: A preliminary report. *Journal of Psychiatric Research, 17*, 37-49.

Zarate, C. A., Baldessarini, R. J., Siegel, A. J., Nakamura, A., McDonald, J., Muir-Hutchinson, L. A., et al. (1997). Risperidone in the elderly: A pharmacoepidemiologic study. *Journal of Clinical Psychiatry, 58*, 311-317.

19

GASTROINTESTINAL SYMPTOMS

Pamala D. Larsen and Nichole M. Irish

Case Study

Mr. S., 68, has been admitted to the palliative care unit. Three months ago he was diagnosed with gallbladder cancer and metastases to the liver. He has been nonambulatory for 3 weeks because of advancing weakness, disease progression, and a decreasing level of consciousness. He lives at home with his wife. Mr. S.'s daughter has also recently moved in, providing care and added support. His current medications include oxycodone (OxyContin, 40 mg twice a day, and OxyIR, 5 to 10 mg every 3 to 4 hours as needed for breakthrough pain), and senna (Senokot), 15 mg given as one tablet in the morning and two tablets at night.

His wife reports that Mr. S. has been having bowel movements every 2 to 3 days with small amounts of loose stools over the past 7 to 10 days. She is unable to remember when his last formed, normal bowel movement occurred, but estimates it to be over 2 weeks ago. She has noticed his abdomen becoming larger and more distended. His appetite has decreased significantly in the past few days, with nausea and vomiting preventing him from tolerating anything other than sips of water.

Physical assessment reveals a thin, white patient with jaundiced skin and sclera and a large, distended abdomen. Bowel sounds are hypoactive. There is no evidence of a fecal impaction on digital rectal exam. Radiography reveals a small bowel obstruction related to metastatic disease (abdominal carcinomatosis). Labs reveal elevated coagulopathy studies and increased ammonia level.

Palliative care staff and the physician met with the family to discuss the plan of care and code status. The decision was made to change the code status of Mr. S. to do not resuscitate, secondary to a poor prognosis. Referrals were made to an oncology counselor and chaplain.

INTRODUCTION

In most countries of the world, sharing meals with others is a social activity. The primary purpose of the meal may be consumption of food, but the enjoyment and stimulation of another's company may be even more important. Communities, organizations, and churches often have potluck suppers where individuals gather to share a meal and socialize.

For the older adult at the end of life with gastrointestinal (GI) symptomatology, the physical problems may be burdensome, but they also affect the individual's ability to participate in social activities, such as sharing a meal with others. The effect on the emotional health of the individual at the end of life from being socially isolated and unable to participate in such activities may outweigh the physical effects of the symptoms.

From an anecdotal perspective, patients at the end of life suffer from GI symptoms, although there are few data available to indicate the extent to which this is true. For some patients, GI symptoms may be present but limited in scope. However, for those patients suffering from continuous nausea, vomiting, and diarrhea that preclude them from leaving their care setting, whether it be home, assisted living, or a long-term care facility, GI symptoms affect their quality of life and the ability to function normally. D'Olimpio (2001) stated that, although much progress has been made in the area of pain control in advanced illness, similar results have not yet been seen with regard to GI symptomatology. Nausea, vomiting, retching, reflux dysphagia, hiccup, constipation, and diarrhea are among the most difficult symptoms to be controlled in palliative care, and all can become intractable (D'Olimpio, 2001, p. 419).

This chapter addresses GI symptoms that are commonly seen in older adults at the end of life. Some symptoms may be the result of the disease process itself, and others may be complications of the disease, concurrent disorders, iatrogenic in nature, or due to an unidentified cause.

NAUSEA AND VOMITING

Nausea and vomiting (N&V) are unpleasant GI symptoms and have been described by some patients as worse than pain and more disabling (Fallon & Welsh, 1998). Although nausea may occur without vomiting on rare occasions, they most commonly occur together and are discussed together in this chapter.

Nausea is a nonobservable subjective symptom involving an unpleasant sensation experienced in the back of the throat and the epigastrium that may or may not result in vomiting (Rhodes & McDaniel, 2001). Vomiting is the forceful expulsion of gastric contents through the oral or nasal cavity (Rhodes & McDaniel, 2001).

Although N&V are typically associated with malignant disease and its treatment, they may affect patients with other advanced illnesses. N&V occur in approximately 40% of individuals at the end of life (Waller & Caroline, 1996). Patients with acquired immunodeficiency syndrome (AIDS), hepatic failure, and liver failure often have nausea during the disease process and at the end of life (Mannix, 1998). A National Hospice Study by Reuben and Mor (1986) demonstrated that 62% of terminally ill cancer patients experienced N&V at some time in their last 6 to 8 weeks of life. This study also noted that patients with stomach and breast cancer, and female patients in general, have higher rates of N&V than patients with other terminal cancers (Reuben & Mor, 1986).

Most of the literature is derived from studying chemotherapy-induced N&V. The literature is sparse about the incidence and treatment of non–chemotherapy-related N&V in patients with advanced cancer (Bruera & Neumann, 1998; Enck, 2002b) or in nonmalignant terminal illness in general. Thus our ability to understand the mechanism and determine optimal treatment of multicausal N&V or non–chemotherapy-related N&V remains limited.

Etiology

N&V involve both afferent and efferent activity at multiple levels of the nervous system, all of which is coordinated in the vomiting center in the medulla (Portenoy, 1994). These afferent and efferent impulses come from one or more of the areas outlined in Box 19-1. Box 19-2 lists potential causes and conditions associated with N&V that may occur in the older adult with terminal illness. It must be emphasized that, if the older adult has several comorbidities, the etiology of N&V may be difficult to ascertain. Without a clear indication of cause, successful treatment becomes even more difficult.

Signs and Symptoms

A sign is the objective evidence of what is occurring with the patient; the presence of vomitus in any amount is definitive objective evidence. Nausea, however, is a subjective symptom that the patient experiences, and it is not measurable by the caregiver. Although it is not objective, nausea may produce significant distress for the patient, and affect activities of daily living and quality of life.

Box 19-1 Afferent and Efferent Impulse Sources of Nausea and Vomiting

- Chemoreceptor trigger zone, which is stimulated by metabolic products produced by uremia, ketoacidosis, and hypercalcemia; tumor-generated toxins and chemotherapeutic agents; radiation; and opioids
- Cerebral cortex, which is stimulated by anxiety and thoughts; sights, smells and taste; and increased intracranial pressure
- Vestibular system (the source of motion or positional nausea)
- Upper gastrointestinal tract, which is stimulated by pressure, distention, stasis, obstruction, or irritation

From Kemp, C. (1999). *Terminal illness: A guide to nursing care* (2nd ed.). Philadelphia: Lippincott.

Box 19-2 **Causes of Nausea and Vomiting at End of Life**

METABOLIC
- Ketoacidosis
- Uremia
- Hypercalcemia
- Tumor-generated toxins
- Fluid and electrolyte imbalances

INCREASED INTRACRANIAL PRESSURE
- Cerebral edema
- Tumor or metastasis
- Intracranial bleed

GASTROINTESTINAL
- Pharyngeal irritation
- Gastritis
- Ascites
- Gastric stasis/paresis
- Stretch/distortion of gastrointestinal tract as a result of:
  - Constipation/impaction
  - Intestinal obstruction
  - Tumor enlargement/metastasis

OTHER
- Fear and anxiety
- Drug induced (NSAIDs, digoxin, anticoagulants, anticholinergics, opioids, antibiotics, chemotherapy, theophylline)
- Movement/position
- Comorbidities
- Radiation
- Sepsis

NSAIDs, nonsteroidal anti-inflammatory drugs.

Sources: Fallon, M., & Welsh, J. (1998). The management of gastrointestinal symptoms. In C. Faull, Y. Carter, & R. Woof (eds.) *Handbook of palliative care.* (pp. 134-156). Oxford: Blackwell Science; Kazanowski, M. (2001). Symptom management in palliative care. In M. Matzo, & D. Sherman (eds.) *Palliative care nursing: Quality care to the end of life.* (pp. 327-361). New York: Springer; Kemp, C. (1999). *Terminal illness: A guide to nursing care* (2nd ed.). New York: J.B. Lippincott; King, C. (2001). Nausea and vomiting. In B. Ferrell, & N. Coyle (eds.) *Textbook of palliative nursing.* (pp. 107-121). New York: Oxford University Press; Mannix, K. (1998). Palliation of nausea and vomiting. In D. Doyle, G. Hanks, & MacDonald (Eds.) *Oxford textbook of palliative medicine* (2nd ed.) (pp. 489-499). New York: Oxford University Press.

N&V may have accompanying signs and symptoms as well. With nausea, there may be accompanying signs of increased salivation and swallowing, perspiration, and tachycardia. In patients with N&V triggered by GI tract stasis, there may be accompanying epigastric pain, fullness, early satiety, flatulence, acid reflux, hiccup, and large-volume vomitus (possibly projectile). In patients with N&V associated with increased intracranial pressure (ICP), headache and nausea, both diurnal in nature, may occur. Other neurologic signs may or may not be present with increased ICP.

Assessment

A number of factors must be considered when the older patient has N&V. Some of the data will be obtained from self-report or report from family caregivers, and some will be objective. Assessment includes frequency and duration; color; amount and consistency of vomitus; contributing factors to the N&V; pattern of the N&V; presence of pain; presence of other abdominal symptoms; and disruption to the patient (e.g., can the patient continue activities of daily living and other "normal" activities with the N&V present?) Lastly, does the elder consider the N&V to affect his or her quality of life or see it merely as a nuisance? To have a clearer picture of the patient's N&V, an instrument with known reliability and validity should be used.

Instruments

Accurate assessment of signs and symptoms can better determine the pattern of occurrence, if there is one, and the effect of interventions. The MANE instrument is a self-report Likert scale that measures post-treatment and anticipatory aspects of N&V separately. Anticipatory nausea is measured on a 5-point scale, and severity of N&V is rated on a 6-point scale (Rhodes & McDaniel, 1997). This instrument's Index of Nausea, Vomiting, and Retching (INVR) measures nausea, vomiting, retching, and the associated distress. The INVR is an 8-item, 5-point Likert self-report tool. Although it was originally developed for the adult oncology population, it has been demonstrated to have use with other populations (Rhodes & McDaniel, 1997).

Other instruments include the Duke Descriptive Scale (DDS), a visual analogue scale (VAS),

Reference: Bentley, A., & Boyd, K. (2001). Use of clinical pictures in the management of nausea and vomiting: A prospective audit. *Palliative Medicine, 15,* 247-253.

Research Problem: This study evaluated the effectiveness of an established protocol, the Fairmile guide, being used in the management of nausea and vomiting (N&V) in palliative care inpatients. The Fairmile guide is one that bases treatment on the clinical picture of the patient as opposed to the more common approach based on the site receptors. It uses a clinical composite of patient activity (i.e., cranial disease, bowel obstruction, regurgitation) to treat N&V rather than making the decision based on the site receptors for N&V. This N&V treatment guideline was used to measure whether the number of episodes of N&V could be reduced and the N&V more effectively controlled.

Design: Prospective audit of charts using a standardized tool.

Sample and Setting: 37 patients in a palliative care unit.

Methods: Chart review of 40 patient episodes of N&V over a 3-month period was done. All inpatient episodes of nausea and/or vomiting were entered. The audit consisted of a 4-page questionnaire completed by the doctor responsible for the patient.

Results: Over the 3-month period, 8 patients died within a day of the study, and 3 patients were reentered because their symptoms changed. The mean number of days for complete resolution of symptoms was 3.4, with a median of 2.0 days and a range of 1 to 24 days.

Implications for Nursing Practice: This study evaluated the results of an ongoing protocol to relieve N&V in palliative care patients. Nurses in all settings need to recognize the importance of evaluating what is considered standard practice or protocol in an effort to better care for patients in all settings.

Conclusion: Adequate symptom control was obtained using the Fairmile guide in the treatment of N&V. Patients who did not respond died shortly after being admitted to the study, indicating a very advanced state of disease. As a result of this small prospective study, a larger study to include patients in all of the United Kingdom hospices is being developed.

and the Functional Living Index–Emesis (FLIE) (Rhodes & McDaniel, 1997). The use of reliable and valid instruments is necessary in developing evidence-based interventions to better assist older adult patients with these symptoms.

Management

Interventions should take into account the symptoms and the central emetogenic pathways involved (Mannix, 1998). In the older adult who is at the end of life, there may be multiple causes of N&V.

Pharmacologic Interventions

Although progress has been made in identifying antiemetic agents that alleviate chem-otherapy-induced N&V, little work has been accomplished in establishing drugs that alleviate the N&V experienced at the end of life. Different antiemetics act on different parts of the N&V process; therefore, when antiemetics are not prescribed correctly, optimal results will not occur. Drugs should be prescribed according to the etiology. For example, drugs that act on the chemoreceptor trigger zone would be given to patients with N&V stemming from uremia-, chemotherapy-, radiation-, or opioid-induced nausea.

Mannix (1998) recommended seven steps in choosing the appropriate antiemetic. These are (1) identify the cause; (2) identify the pathway triggering the vomiting reflex; (3) identify the neurotransmitter receptor involved; (4) select those medications that are the most potent antagonists to the receptors identified; (5) choose the route of administration that ensures optimal action; (6) titrate the dosage; and (7) if symptoms persist, review the cause (p. 490).

Currently, there are nine classifications of antiemetics that are used in palliative care for N&V (King, 2001) (Box 19-3). Table 19-1 lists the drug categories, examples of those drugs, indications of their usage, and comments.

Nonpharmacologic and Complementary Interventions

Often there are adjunct interventions to accompany medications. Establishing a research basis for those interventions is more difficult, although much has been written using anecdotal data versus research data. Research that is present in the literature is based on patients with chemotherapy-induced N&V and not patients with N&V at the end of life.

Simple self-care strategies, which may consist of dietary and environmental changes, may be instituted to control N&V (Box 19-4). Encourage the elder to use interventions that have relieved N&V at other times in his or her life, such as during pregnancy, illness, or times of stress. A particular food associated with a positive past experience can be suggested (Enck, 2002b). Dietary changes such as drinking clear liquids and eating bland foods may be helpful. Minimizing or even eliminating liquids prior to or during a meal may decrease nausea (Kemp, 1999).

The older adult and family should be encouraged to keep a self-care log of symptoms, interventions, and responses. The log reinforces interventions that work for the patient and may demonstrate "good days" when the N&V was less. The log can also help the patient feel more in control of his or her life in addition to providing the caregiver with information on which to base interventions.

Music therapy has shown some benefits as an adjunct therapy. Ezzone, Baker, Rosselet, and Terepka (1998) demonstrated that music therapy was a statistically significant adjunct treatment during high-dose chemotherapy to reduce N&V. Relaxation techniques and guided imagery are other adjuvant therapies that can be used to decrease N&V and reduce anxiety. However, the research basis of these nonpharmacologic interventions (Table 19-2) needs to be established to support evidence-based practice.

Box 19-4 Self-Care Activities for Nausea and Vomiting (N&V)

- Oral hygiene after each emesis
- Cool, damp washcloth to the forehead, neck, and wrists
- Eat bland, cool foods
- Have fresh air with a fan or open window
- Limit environmental stimuli that precipitate N&V
- Lie flat for 2 hours after eating
- Eat small meals
- Practice relaxation techniques and/or guided imagery
- Provide distraction

Sources: Enck, R. C. (2002). *The medical care of terminally ill patients.* (2nd ed.) Baltimore: Johns Hopkins University Press; Kemp, C. (1999). *Terminal illness: A guide to nursing care* (2nd ed.). New York: J.B. Lippincott; King, C. (2001). Nausea and vomiting. In B. Ferrell, & N. Coyle (eds.) *Textbook of palliative nursing.* (pp. 107-121). New York: Oxford University Press; Rhodes, V., & McDaniel, R. (1997). Measuring nausea, vomiting and retching. In M. Frank-Stromberg, & S. Olsen (eds.) *Instruments for clinical health-care research* (2nd ed.) (pp. 509-517). Sudbury, MA: Jones & Bartlett.

Box 19-3 Classifications of Antiemetics

- Antihistamines
- 5-HT$_3$ receptor antagonists
- Steroids
- Cannabinoids
- Benzodiazepines
- Butyrophenones
- Prokinetic agents
- Phenothiazides
- Anticholinergics

5-HT$_3$, 5-hydroxytryptamine$_3$ (serotonin).
From King, C. (2001). Nausea and vomiting. In B. Ferrell & N. Coyne (Eds.), *Textbook of palliative nursing* (pp. 107-121). New York: Oxford University Press.

Table 19-1 **Antiemetic Drugs in Palliative Care**

Drug Category	Indication	Comments
Butyrophenones (haloperidol, droperidol)	Opioid-induced nausea, chemical & mechanical nausea	Use when anxiety symptoms aggravate N&V; may have additive effects with other CNS depressants
Prokinetic agents (metoclopramide, domperidone)	Gastric stasis, ileus	Use diphenhydramine to decrease extrapyramidal symptoms; rectal route for domperidone
Cannabinoids (dronabinol)	2nd- or 3rd-line antiemetic	More effective in young adults
Phenothiazines (prochlorperazine, chlorpromazine)	General N&V	Not recommended for routine use in palliative care
Antihistamines (cyclizine, diphenhydramine)	Intestinal obstruction, increased ICP, vestibular causes, peritoneal irritation	Cyclizine is the least sedative
Anticholinergics (scopolamine)	Intestinal obstruction, increased ICP, peritoneal irritation	Useful if N&V exist with colic
Steroids (dexamethasone)	May be used with other agents	Compatible with 5-HT$_3$ receptor antagonists; may increase efficacy when used with other antiemetics
5-HT$_3$ receptor antagonists (ondansetron, granisetron)	Chemotherapy, abdominal radiation, postoperative N&V	Use in moderate to highly emetogenic chemotherapies; ideal for elderly patients
Benzodiazepines (lorazepam)	Used with anxiety as well	Caution with use in patients with hepatic or renal dysfunction

CNS, central nervous system; 5-HT$_3$, 5-hydroxytryptarninc$_3$ (serotonin); ICP, intracranial pressure; N&V, nausea and vomiting.
Sources: King, C. (2001). Nausea and vomiting. In B. Ferrell, & N. Coyle (eds.) *Textbook of palliative nursing*. (pp. 107-121). New York: Oxford University Press; Enck, R. C. (2002). *The medical care of terminally ill patients*. (2nd ed.) Baltimore: Johns Hopkins University Press; Mannix, K. (1998). Palliation of nausea and vomiting. In D. Doyle, G. Hanks, & MacDonald (Eds.) *Oxford textbook of palliative medicine* (2nd ed.) (pp. 489-499). New York: Oxford University Press; Wickham, R. (1999). Nausea and vomiting. In C. Yarbro, M. Frogge, & M. Goodman (Eds.) *Cancer symptom management* (2nd ed.). (pp. 228-253). Sudbury, MA: Jones & Bartlett.

Acupuncture and ginger are two common complementary interventions used to manage nausea and vomiting (Fallon & Welsh, 1998). Acupuncture is an ancient healing art using fine-gauge needles to palliate symptoms. The needles are inserted into carefully chosen acupuncture points and left in place for up to 20 minutes. Vickers (1996), in his review of acupuncture studies, found 11 high-quality, randomized, placebo-controlled trials that demonstrated positive results using acupuncture as an anti-emetic intervention. Ginger has been used for centuries in folk medicine to decrease nausea (Langmead & Rampton, 2001; Wickham, 1999). Langmead and Rampton (2001) reported that, of four research studies that have been conducted using ginger in postoperative N&V, two demonstrated statistically significant results.

Family Concerns and Considerations

N&V are visible signs of an unhealthy state, and therefore family caregivers can be distressed and

Table 19-2 Nonpharmacologic Interventions for Nausea and Vomiting

Techniques	Description	Comments
BEHAVIORAL INTERVENTIONS		
Self-hypnosis	Evocation of physiologic state of altered consciousness and total body relaxation. This technique involves a state of intensified attention and receptiveness to an idea.	Used to control anticipatory nausea and vomiting Limited studies, mostly children and adolescents Easily learned No side effects Decreases intensity and duration of nausea Decreases frequency, severity, amount, and duration of vomiting
Relaxation	Progressive contraction and relaxation of various muscle groups.	Often used with imagery Can use for other stressful situations Easily learned No side effects Decreases nausea during and after chemotherapy Decreases duration and severity of vomiting Not as effective with anticipatory nausea and vomiting
Biofeedback	Control of specific physiologic responses by receiving information about changes in response to induced state of relaxation.	Two types: electromyographic and skin temperature Used alone or with relaxation Easily learned No side effects Decreases nausea during and after chemotherapy More effective with progressive muscle relaxation
Imagery	Mentally take self away by focusing mind on images of a relaxing place.	Most effective when combined with another technique Increases self-control Decreases duration of nausea Decreases perceptions of degree of vomiting Feel more in control, relaxed, and powerful
Distraction	Learn to divert attention from a threatening situation and to relaxing sensations.	Can use videos, games, and puzzles No side effects Decreases anticipatory nausea and vomiting Decreases postchemotherapy distress
Desensitization	Three-step process involving relaxation and visualization to decrease sensitization to aversive situations.	Inexpensive Easily learned No side effects Decreases anticipatory nausea and vomiting
OTHER INTERVENTIONS		
Acupressure	Form of massage using meridians to increase energy flow and affect emotions.	Inconclusive literature support Acupressure wrist bands may be helpful to decrease nausea and vomiting
Music therapy	Use of music to influence physiologic, psychological, and emotional functioning during threatening situations.	Often used with other techniques No side effects Decreases nausea during and after chemotherapy Decreases perceptions of degree of vomiting

From King, C. (1997). Nonpharmacologic management of chemotherapy-induced nausea and vomiting. *Oncology Nursing Forum*, 24 (Suppl.), 41-48.

anxious about their loved one. It is important that the nurse address the family's anxiety associated with N&V. Family education is key to facilitating their functioning as care team members and helping the loved one experience an optimal quality of life.

Families should be taught to systematically assess the patient's N&V. Use of a simple log of what activity the patient is engaging in when the episode of N&V occurs provides evidence to the family and patient as to when the nausea increased or decreased, and how and when the vomiting occurred as well. The family and health care provider can then assess the situation by viewing the log and determine what pharmacologic and/or nonpharmacologic interventions work best for the patient.

DYSPHAGIA

Dysphagia is defined as difficulty in swallowing food or liquid; pain may or may not be associated. Best estimates of the prevalence of dysphagia in the older adult population in long-term care settings are that one third of the residents have some degree of dysphagia (Curless & James, 1992). Outside of the long-term care setting, most of the data on incidence of dysphagia come from patients affected by head and neck cancer. These patients may suffer from dysphagia in the early, middle, and terminal stages of the disease. One source indicates that 79% of those patients have significant eating problems (Barbour, 1999).

Dysphagia is a primary symptom of esophageal malignancies, which occur in 3 to 4 per 100,000 patients (Murray, Rao, & Schulze-Delrieu, 1997). In the late stages of multiple sclerosis (MS), dysphagia is reported in 10% to 33% of patients (Dahlin & Goldsmith, 2001). In amyotrophic lateral sclerosis (ALS), 25% of patients present with dysphagia as their initial complaint at diagnosis (Dahlin & Goldsmith, 2001).

Etiology

Swallowing is a complex activity that requires intact anatomy; normal mucosa; normal functioning of six cranial nerves and the brainstem; and the coordination of the cortex, limbic system, basal ganglia, cerebellum, brainstem centers involved in respiration and salivation, and motor function of 34 skeletal muscles (Twycross & Regnard, 1998). Dysphagia may

occur as a result of a disruption in any of the four phases of swallowing: oral preparatory phase; oral phase; pharyngeal phase; and esophageal phase.

Both the oral preparatory and oral phases of swallowing are voluntary actions. In the oral preparatory phase, food is taken into the mouth and saliva helps form a paste bolus. During the oral phase, the bolus is centered and moved to the posterior oropharynx. The pharyngeal phase is not voluntary, but rather reflexive, with the swallowing reflex carrying the food bolus through the pharynx. Peristaltic waves carry the food bolus to the stomach during the esophageal phase.

Each of the phases of swallowing is affected by aging, and dysphagia is a common complaint of the older adult. The skeletal muscles involved with swallowing may undergo the age-related changes of atrophy and weakness that can occur in all skeletal muscles (Timiras, 1994). Each of the phases of swallowing is a precisely timed contraction-relaxation sequence and can be affected by the aging process. The sequence may become desynchronized and the entire process of swallowing may become ineffective (Timiras, 1994).

Dahlin and Goldsmith (2001) listed five causes of dysphagia commonly seen in palliative care: neoplasms, to include brain tumors, head and neck cancer, and esophageal tumors; progressive neuromuscular diseases such as ALS, Parkinson's disease, and MS; dementia; systemic dysphagia as a result of inflammatory and infectious factors; and general deconditioning, which may include multisystem disease and multisystem organ failure and the side effects of medications and/or polypharmacy.

Each cause of dysphagia may occur for a different reason. For example, in Parkinson's disease there is disruption in the oral phase of swallowing because of rigidity of the lingual musculature. As a result of this rigidity, pharyngeal swallow responses are delayed and aspiration may occur before or during the swallow (Dahlin & Goldsmith, 2001). In head and neck cancers, dysphagia may occur because of the pressure and size of the tumor, or as a result of chemotherapy, radiation, or the surgery itself. Two common side effects of radiation, mucositis and xerostomia, may further exacerbate dysphagia (Rudd &

Table 19-3 **Signs and Symptoms of Dysphagia**

ORAL PHASE

Drooling

Pocketing of food

Excessive chewing

Facial asymmetry or weakness

Tongue weakness

Inability to close lips tightly or move lips

Weakness or absence of gag reflex

Weakness or absence of swallowing reflex

Nasal drainage as a result of nasal regurgitation

Loss of internal or external sensation of the oral cavity or face

PHARYNGEAL PHASE

Delayed or absence of swallowing

Coughing while drinking or eating fluids

History of aspiration pneumonia

Wet, gurgling, moist, or nasal voice

Frequent clearing of throat

Complaints of burning

ESOPHAGEAL PHASE

Burping or substernal distress caused by esophageal reflux

Coughing or wheezing

From Hickey, J. (1997). Rehabilitation of neuroscience patients. In J. Hickey (Ed.), *The clinical practice of neurological and neurosurgical nursing* (4th ed., p. 255). Philadelphia: Lippincott.

Box 19-5 **Goals of Assessment of Dysphagia**

1. Identify the underlying physiological nature of the disorder.
2. Determine whether any short-range interventions can alleviate the dysphagia.
3. Together with the patient, family, and caregivers, decide on the safest and most efficient method of providing nutrition and hydration.

From Dahlin, C. M., & Goldsmith, T. (2001). Dysphagia, dry mouth, and hiccups. In B. R. Ferrell & N. Coyle (Eds.), *Textbook of palliative nursing* (pp. 122-138). New York: Oxford University Press.

that he or she will be unable to breathe as a result of food "going down the wrong pipe."

Some older adults exhibit no signs of choking, although food or liquids may be entering the trachea and lung; these patients are known as "silent aspirators." Noting the quality of the patient's voice and whether or not any expressive aphasia or dysphasia is present may provide cues to the nurse that the patient is aspirating (Easton, 1999).

Depending on the phase of swallowing that is affected, the signs of dysphagia may differ. Table 19-3 delineates characteristics of dysphagia associated with the oral, pharyngeal, and esophageal phases. Each characteristic may have varying degrees of seriousness.

Assessment

In the terminal stages of illness, it is likely that dysphagia is not a new symptom, but rather one that has been present for some time and is worsening. In a swallowing assessment of the older adult at the end of life, the goals of assessment should be clear (Dahlin & Goldsmith, 2001) (Box 19-5).

Difficulty with specific food consistencies provides the nurse with some assessment data, but may be misleading. Lesions and/or tumors that produce an obstruction generally produce dysphagia for solids first as opposed to liquids. However, patients with neuromuscular disorders may have dysphagia for both solids and liquids (Twycross & Regnard, 1998).

The prognosis of the patient will determine whether a professional swallowing evaluation

Worlding, 1998), as may pain on swallowing, anorexia, or anxiety (Baines, 1992).

Dysphagia may not be a part of the terminal illness itself but rather a result or symptom of a comorbidity. An example would be an older adult who is terminally ill with cancer and also has advanced Parkinson's disease or has suffered from a previous cerebrovascular accident and is hemiplegic and dysphagic.

Cardinal Signs and Symptoms

An initial indication of dysphagia is choking or coughing when eating or drinking. A patient may complain of having the feeling that something is caught in his or her throat. These signs of dysphagia are often accompanied by fear and anxiety on the part of the elder: fear that food may actually be trapped in his or her lungs, and the anxiety

---

Box 19-6 **Management of Dysphagia**

1. Rate of decline of the patient
2. Patient's opinion
3. Opinions of significant other and/or family
4. Opinions of formal caregivers
5. Feasibility/advantages/disadvantages of alternative feeding routes

---

From Twycross, R., & Regnard, C. (1998). Dysphagia, dyspepsia, and hiccup. In D. Doyle, G. W. Hanks, & N. MacDonald (Eds.), *Oxford textbook of palliative medicine* (2nd ed., pp. 499-512). New York: Oxford University Press.

merits consideration. If the patient's life expectancy is reasonably long and the patient is clearly in distress, an evaluation performed by a speech therapist with expertise in swallowing disorders may be indicated. A modified barium swallow is used to radiologically determine the phase of swallowing in which the disturbance is occurring and thus identify potential interventions, as well as evaluate the compensatory mechanisms of the patient (Dahlin & Goldsmith, 2001).

Management

If the patient clearly has a very short prognosis (days), it may be determined by the patient, family, and caregivers that hydration and/or feeding are not warranted. If the patient has a longer prognosis, medically assisted feeding and hydration may be attempted. Twycross and Regnard (1998) listed factors to help determine the appropriateness of such interventions (Box 19-6).

Transnasal intubation, percutaneous endoscopic gastrostomy or jejunostomy, or surgical gastrostomy or jejunostomy may be considered if the prognosis of the patient determines that these interventions will provide optimal palliation. Any surgical intervention is clearly undertaken with significant input from the patient and family and is determined by the goals of care.

Pharmacologic Interventions

If dry mouth and/or oral lesions are present and are exacerbating the dysphagia, pharmacologic treatment is appropriate. The most common mucosal infection causing oral lesions is candidiasis. Antifungal medication such as nystatin, ketoconazole, miconazole, and fluconazole may be used in treatment (Dahlin & Goldsmith, 2001; Twycross & Regnard, 1998).

Dry mouth (xerostomia) could be a result of prescribed medications, particularly anticholinergics and opiates. These medications may need to be continued if there are limited alternatives to treat other symptoms, making the dry mouth unavoidable. In that case, artificial saliva, such as Salogen or porcine mucin, may be used. Glycerin and lemon should be avoided because glycerin dehydrates the mucosa and lemon affects the salivary glands (Twycross & Regnard, 1998).

Nonpharmacologic Interventions

After a thorough evaluation of the patient has determined that oral intake is safe, the guiding principle of management is that a maximum amount of calories should be ingested for the least amount of effort (Dahlin & Goldsmith, 2001). If the degree of dysphagia is limited, simple positioning may be the primary intervention. Patients should be positioned upright with the head tilted slightly forward and the chin tucked in to prevent food from moving to the posterior oropharynx before it is properly chewed. If the patient is unable to hold his or her head independently, the caregiver can assist the patient in maintaining this position. If the older adult has had a past stroke, pocketing of food on the affected side of the mouth is a common problem. Either the patient, family, or caregiver can sweep the mouth with a finger after each bite to alleviate this problem.

Simple dietary changes such as providing pureed or blenderized food may be appropriate. Patients with oropharyngeal dysphagia may require thickened liquids. There are a number of commercial products that are used in rehabilitation facilities (e.g., Thick-it) to address these issues; however, simple food starch can be used as effectively.

Family Concerns and Considerations

Positioning techniques that allow the patient to continue oral feeding can be easily explained and taught to the older adult and/or the family. Dietary changes, such as using thickening agents, if appropriate, should be suggested to the family. Any interventions that can be taught to the family will increase their feeling of being able to help the elder.

As described previously, eating is considered a social activity as much as it is a necessity of life. Society has conditioned us to believe that eating wholesome, healthy food will keep us well. As family members sitting by the bedside of their loved one see that oral intake is impossible because of dysphagia and potential aspiration, feelings of helplessness and anxiety may occur. Family may feel that they are neglecting their obligation to the older adult. For both the elder and the family, the act of eating is viewed as compatible with life; the inability to eat is a harbinger of death. Such factors influence decisions regarding feeding at the end of life.

The decision to discontinue oral feeding and initiate alternate feeding methods is not easy. It is clearly difficult to make the initial decision to feed a patient or loved one "artificially," and more difficult if a decision is made to discontinue feedings. The patient and family must be fully aware of the risks and benefits of artificial nutrition and hydration. During this period of time, the support of the nurse to the elder and family is paramount. In addition to explaining what is occurring, the nurse must verbally support the decision of the patient and family even if he or she disagrees with it.

BOWEL DYSFUNCTION

Older adults with terminal illness commonly have alterations in bowel function. The most frequently encountered types of bowel dysfunctions include diarrhea, constipation, and bowel obstruction. The impact on quality of life for the older adult caused by bowel dysfunction may be overlooked because of the focus on disease management. Along with having a profound impact on activities of daily living, nutritional intake, socialization, and comfort, alterations in bowel function may potentially result in serious complications such as severe pain, dehydration, fluid and electrolyte imbalance, and bleeding (Bisanz, 1997).

Primary control processes in normal bowel function include activity of the small intestine, colonic motility, and defecation. The principle activity of the small intestine is the mixing of contents and absorption of nutrients. Stimulation of this activity occurs when there is food in the stomach, and concludes upon gastric emptying. The normal time of small intestine transit

is 9 hours, in contrast to the extended length of time of transit occurring in the large intestine, which ranges from 1 to 48 hours. Any change in colonic transit time results in bowel dysfunction.

Colonic propulsion occurs through mass peristalsis. Relaxations and contractions are required for bowel motility. Strong motor contractions are estimated to occur six times per day. The strongest burst is upon awakening, and the afternoon meal triggers a second, less intense burst. The process of defecation is initiated by rectal distention. This action involves the involuntary and voluntary relaxation of the anal sphincters. The coordinated effect of all of these processes maintains normal bowel function (Economou, 2001).

Constipation

One of the most common symptoms in advanced illness is constipation, and it is often one of the easiest symptoms to manage (Kemp, 1999). It occurs in 10% of the general population and in up to 78% of patients with terminal cancer (Levy, 1991); for some patients constipation is a lifelong pattern. Constipation is defined as fewer than three bowel movements per week, reduced fecal volume, harder fecal consistency, straining on more than 25% of occasions, and the presence of excess feces on rectal or radiographic examination (Woodward, 1999a). Essentially, constipation is a result of decreased motility of the large intestine.

Alternative definitions for constipation are numerous. The Rome criteria for diagnosing chronic constipation indicate that patients with functional constipation have an average of fewer than two bowel movements per week for at least 12 months, or have two or more symptoms for at least 12 months without laxative use (Box 19-7).

Constipation can also be divided into two subtypes: functional constipation (criteria defined above), and rectal outlet delay. Rectal outlet delay, also referred to as rectal dyschezia, is a result of impaired rectal sensation, reduced rectal tone, and a variation in rectal dilation (Woodward, 1999a). It occurs when there is anal blockage 25% of the time, and prolonged defecation with manual disimpaction is necessary at times (Schaefer & Cheskin, 1998).

Box 19-7 **Symptoms of Constipation**

1. Less than three bowel movements per week
2. Excessive straining at defecation for at least 25% of bowel movements
3. A sensation of incomplete evacuation for at least 25% of bowel movements
4. The passage of hard, pellet-like stool for at least 25% of bowel movements

From Whitehead, W. E., Chaussade, S., Corazziari, E., et al. (1991). Report of an international workshop on management of constipation. *Gastroenterology International, 4,* 99–113.

Etiology

Constipation can be caused by a number of factors, occurring independently or in combination with each other. There is some debate as to whether normal GI changes that occur with aging include slowed bowel motility. According to Woodward (1999a), colonic transit time is prolonged in older individuals as a result of factors other than age, such as reduced oral intake, immobility, or medications. Others indicate that the cause of constipation in older adults is related to bowel motility changes, in contrast to spastic causes (i.e., irritable bowel syndrome), which occur more frequently in younger persons (Cheskin & Schuster, 1994).

Among the most common direct causes (Box 19-8) of constipation in elder patients at the end of life are medications, advanced disease states, dietary inadequacies, metabolic conditions, and mechanical obstruction (Kemp, 1999). The most frequent nonobstructive factor attributed to chronic constipation is medication side effects (Schaefer & Cheskin, 1998). Medications known for causing slowed bowel motility include opioids, anticholinergics (antipsychotics, tricyclic antidepressants, antiparkinsonian drugs, and antispasmodics), aluminum-containing antacids, anticonvulsants, iron supplements, calcium channel blockers, phenothiazines, nonsteroidal anti-inflammatory agents, antiemetics, and chemotherapeutic agents. Prolongation in colonic transit time results in increased absorption of fluids and electrolytes, causing dryer, more rigid stools.

Tolerance to the constipating effects of opioids is often absent or slow to develop (Bisanz, 1997;

Box 19-8 **Causes of Constipation in Terminal Illness**

DIRECT CAUSES
MEDICATION SIDE EFFECTS
- Opioids
- Anticholinergics
- Aluminum-containing antacids
- Iron supplements
- Calcium channel blockers
- Phenothiazines
- Nonsteroidal anti-inflammatory drugs
- Antiemetics
- Chemotherapeutics

ADVANCED DISEASE STATES
- Weakness
- Immobility
- Decreased activity
- Depression
- Confusion/dementia
- Sedation

DIETARY INADEQUACIES
- Appetite changes
- Decreased fiber intake
- Decreased fluid intake
- Increased fiber intake with decreased fluid intake
- Nausea and vomiting

METABOLIC DYSFUNCTIONS
- Hypercalcemia
- Hypokalemia
- Hypothyroidism

MECHANICAL OBSTRUCTION
- Tumor growth
- Bowel obstruction

INDIRECT CAUSES
- Privacy issues
- Unfamiliar toileting facility

Adapted from Kemp, C. (1999). *Terminal illness: A guide to nursing care* (2nd ed.). New York: J.B. Lippincott; Schaefer, D. C., & Cheskin, L. J. (1998). Constipation in the elderly. *American Family Physician.* Retrieved April 1, 2002, http://www.aafp.org/afp/98091/schaefer.html; Woodward, M. C. (1999a). Constipation: Aetiology and diagnosis. In R. N. Ratnaike (Ed.), *Diarrhoea and constipation in geriatric practice* (pp. 187-193). Cambridge, UK: Cambridge University Press.

Enck, 2002b; Ross & Alexander, 2001). Narcotic bowel syndrome occurs with extended use of opioid analgesics. The symptoms include abdominal pain, distention, nausea, vomiting, and constipation and may subside with the discontinuation of opioid therapy (Enck, 2002b).

Older adults with terminal illness may also have other conditions that contribute to slowed bowel motility, such as weakness, immobility or decreased activity, depression, confusion, and sedation. Changes in appetite and intake are not uncommon with chronic illness. Inadequate fiber or fluid intake decreases frequency of bowel movements, and a high-fiber diet in combination with low fluid intake results in hard stool formation and an increased potential for fecal impactions.

Metabolic dysfunctions, more specifically alterations in calcium and potassium, have a role in bowel dysfunction as well. Hypercalcemia causes a conduction delay in terms of innervation to the colon. Hypokalemia decreases GI smooth muscle stimulation by neuronal dysfunction of acetylcholine. Hypothyroidism may cause GI mucosal edema and an increase in water absorption, leading to constipation (Woodward, 1999a). Abdominal, pelvic, or bowel tumor growth and invasion can result in neurologic dysfunction or bowel compression. Indirect causes such as privacy issues and unfamiliarity with toileting facilities can be unrelated to the terminal illness but contribute to constipation.

Cardinal Signs and Symptoms

Classic signs and symptoms accompanying constipation are abdominal pain, cramping, flatus, bloating, nausea, poor appetite, and weight loss. Diarrhea from bacterial breakdown of fecal material higher in the colon may be present with obstruction or severe impaction. Colicky abdominal pain occurs as the colonic muscle attempts to propel hardened fecal matter (Sykes, 1998).

Assessment

The process of symptom assessment in constipation is highly subjective, which suggests that a patient-based constipation assessment tool is helpful (Frank, Kleinman, Farup, Taylor, & Miner, 1999). Normal frequency of bowel movements ranges from three times a day to three times per week. Patients may define constipation relative to the consistency of stool or straining effort associated with defecation (Schaefer & Cheskin, 1998). The Patient Assessment of Constipation (PAC) was developed to measure constipation over time as experienced by the patient. This instrument is divided into two separate questionnaires and is used to address symptom components independently, or to evaluate the effects of symptoms on quality of life. Tested by Frank et al. (1999), the PAC was successful at detecting changes over time, and has been found to be a reliable and valid assessment of constipation in adult patients.

Although history of past and current bowel activity (i.e., size, character, and frequency) is important, it is also necessary to assess for other factors that contribute to constipation. These include questioning the use of medications known to cause constipation, new medications or changes to a specific regimen, dietary fiber and fluid intake, and history of bowel dysfunction. Polypharmacy is an issue to be addressed with all elder patients. Particularly when providing palliative care, attention should be given to discontinuing all unnecessary medications. The Constipation Assessment Scale (Fig. 19-1) is a good indicator of bowel function and can be used as an initial evaluation tool or for ongoing management. Requiring just a few minutes to complete, it consists of eight questions about the occurrence of constipation symptoms for the previous 3 days (McMillan & Williams, 1989). Scores are added to show the severity of constipation. Total scores range from 0 (no constipation) to 16 (the most severe constipation).

When individuals are confused, sedated, or exhibiting signs of dementia, obtaining a complete history may involve acquiring assessment data not only from the elder, but also from the family or caregivers. A complete history is essential to determine the severity and location of discomfort and may indicate specific factors leading to constipation. For instance, if there is lack of a bowel movement for longer than 5 days or a history of inadequate fluid and food intake, a high impaction in the ascending, transverse, or descending colon should be ruled out (Bisanz, 1997).

Constipation, although often thought of as benign, may predispose the older adult to further complications. Fecal impaction may cause bowel obstruction, potentially leading to intestinal perforation and infection that could be fatal.

Directions: Circle the appropriate number to indicate whether, during the past three days, you have had NO PROBLEM, SOME PROBLEM, or a SEVERE PROBLEM with each of the items listed below

Item	No Problem	Some Problem	Severe Problem
1. Abdominal distention or bloating	0	1	2
2. Change in amount of gas passed rectally	0	1	2
3. Less frequent bowel movements	0	1	2
4. Oozing liquid stool	0	1	2
5. Rectal fullness or pressure	0	1	2
6. Rectal pain with bowel movement	0	1	2
7. Small stool size	0	1	2
8. Urge but inability to pass stool	0	1	2

Fig. 19-1 Constipation Assessment Scale. (From McMillan, S., & Williams, F. [1989]. Validity and reliability of the Constipation Assessment Scale. *Cancer Nursing, 12,* 183-188.)

Urinary incontinence may occur as a result of bladder outlet irritation. Anorectal disorders that result from constipation include prolapse, hemorrhoids, and fissures; hemorrhoids are of particular concern because of the risk of anemia if bleeding occurs. Decreased appetite and N&V often accompany constipation, and are poorly tolerated by elders with a terminal condition (Woodward, 1999a). It is for those reasons that constipation should be identified and managed promptly in the older adult.

Physical exam may reveal abdominal distention, diminished or hypoactive bowel sounds, and palpation of stool in the large intestine. Rebound tenderness occurs with inflammation, and may signify peritonitis. Percussion of tympany over the abdomen indicates gas in the bowel, and dullness is related to a solid mass, which could be intestinal fluid, tumor, or feces (Economou, 2001). A digital rectal exam may reveal impaction, impaired sphincter tone, anal fissures, or hemorrhoids.

Diagnostic tests are used to confirm or determine the extent of bowel dysfunction caused by constipation. The need for an extensive work-up in palliative care is rare, and one should only be done when necessary to continue with comfort measures. If indicated, testing may include upright and flat plate radiographs of the abdomen to check for air–fluid levels indicative of a partial or complete intestinal obstruction that is either due to tumor or secondary to fecal impaction. Magnetic resonance imaging or computed tomography may also be appropriate to assess the abdomen. Laboratory data used to evaluate constipation may include blood urea nitrogen, elevations of which signify dehydration, and blood glucose, elevated levels of which may indicate a diversion of fluids from the GI tract to the kidneys with excess renal fluid loss (Bisanz, 1997).

Management

Pharmacologic Interventions. Prophylactic management of constipation is a primary consideration in older adults with terminal illness, especially those receiving medications that slow bowel motility, such as opioids (Box 19-9). Management of chronic constipation should be continuous (Sykes, 1998). Stool softeners, stimulant laxatives, and increased dietary fiber and fluids are among the most common prophylactic measures prescribed. With the exception of bulk-forming agents, long-term use of laxatives for chronic constipation is normally discouraged (Wong & Kadakia, 1999), except when the goal is comfort and symptom relief. For the elder patient receiving palliative care, correction of metabolic dysfunction using potassium supplements can aid in restoration of bowel motility. If fecal impaction occurs, digital rectal disimpaction may be required. It is often necessary to precede disimpaction attempts with an olive oil (120 mL) retention enema. Following disimpaction, a high milk and molasses or saline enema may be used to clear remaining stool. Sodium biphosphate (Fleet) enemas are effective, but a milk and molasses enema (Box 19-10) is recom-

Box 19-9 Management of Constipation

INDEPENDENT INTERVENTIONS

- Encourage fluids
- Offer fluids a patient likes
- Diet education—high fiber
- Increase activity if possible—assistance with mobility
- Facilitate toileting to provide adequate time, comfort, and privacy
- Provide toileting access after breakfast
- Bowel retraining
- Ongoing assessment to help with prevention of complications/impactions

DEPENDENT INTERVENTIONS

- Administration of laxatives and enemas as prescribed
- Use of nonsedative pain medications during the day
- Antidepressants
- Constipation prophylaxis
- Correction of metabolic dysfunction

COLLABORATIVE INTERVENTIONS

- Measures to counteract depression—referral to counseling
- Dietary consult for fiber intake calculation
- Physical therapy for strengthening and range of motion

Box 19-10 Milk and Molasses Enema

1. Mix 8 oz warm water and 3 oz powdered milk.
2. Add 4.5 oz of molasses and shake until completely mixed.
3. Add to enema bag for administration.

May be given every 6 hours (a total of 3 times) until results are achieved.

Adapted from Bisanz, A. (1997). Managing bowel elimination problems in patients with cancer. *Oncology Nursing Forum, 24,* 679–686.

mended because it is less irritating to the GI mucosal lining (Bisanz, 1997).

A multitude of specific bowel programs have been recommended, primarily for cancer-related constipation (Derby & Portenoy, 1997; Levy, 1991; Robinson et al., 2000). Combined use of fecal softeners and laxatives works best to manage persistent constipation in terminal illness (Baines, 1992). Bulk-forming agents may be contraindicated if there is poor fluid intake because of the risk for developing an impaction (Woodward, 1999b). Additional pharmacologic measures, along with dosages and side effects, are listed in Table 19-4.

Two categories of medications are used to treat constipation: softening agents and stimulating agents. Laxatives that function as softeners include lubricant, osmotic, surfactant, saline, and bulk-forming agents. Anthracene and polyphenolic laxatives act as stimulants to increase intestinal motility.

SOFTENING PREPARATIONS. Lubricant laxatives such as mineral oil aid in elimination by lubricating and penetrating the stool to cause softening. They are more effective for management of intermittent or acute episodes and fecal impaction than for chronic constipation. Chronic use may lead to malabsorption of fat-soluble vitamins (A, D, E, and K).

Osmotic laxatives cause the intestinal lumen to retain water, primarily in the small intestine. Residual effects are minimal in the colon because of bacterial degradation and production of short-chain organic acids that stimulate peristalsis (Sykes, 1998). Osmotic cathartics are especially effective in treating opioid-induced constipation, but are contraindicated if bowel obstruction is suspected. Examples include lactulose (Duphalac), mannitol, polyethylene glycol (MiraLax), and sorbitol. Sorbitol is reported to be less expensive than and as effective as lactulose (Lederle, Busch, Mattox, West, & Aske, 1990).

Surfactant laxatives, also called detergent laxatives, increase absorption of water and fats into dry stools by decreasing surface tension of intestinal mucosa. At higher doses, peristalsis may be induced. Examples of surfactant laxatives include docusate sodium, poloxalene, and calcium salt.

Saline laxatives increase water in the bowel lumen, similar to osmotic laxatives, thereby decreasing transit time throughout the small and large intestines. Two types of saline laxatives are

Table 19-4 Pharmacologic Agents for Constipation Management

	Softening Agents	Dose	(Time to) Results	Side Effects
Lubricant laxatives (intermittent or acute episodes of constipation)	Mineral oil	10-30 mL PO qd or 100 mL PR as an enema	1-3 days	Seepage from the rectum. Not recommended if risk for aspiration
Osmotic laxatives (opioid-induced constipation)	Lactulose (Duphalac) Polyethylene glycol (MiraLax) Sorbitol	15-60 mL qd–tid Dissolve 17 g in 8 oz water qd; may use up to 2 wk 15-60 mL qd–bid	1-2 days 2-4 days 2-6 hr	Contraindicated if bowel obstruction. Electrolyte imbalance. Flatulence Dehydration
Surfactant (detergent) laxatives	Docusate sodium Calcium salt (Surfak)	300 mg PO qd 240 mg qd or bid	1-3 days 1-3 days	Bitter taste Nausea
Saline laxatives Magnesium salts	Magnesium hydroxide (Milk of Magnesia) Magnesium Sulfate (Epsom Salts) Magnesium Citrate	30-60 mL 5-15 g ½ to 1 bottle	30 min-6 hr 3-6 hr 30 min-6 hr 1-6 hr	Do not use with renal or cardiac disorders
Sodium salts	Sodium phosphate (Fleet Phosphot-Soda)	20-30 mL qd-bid with 12 oz water		Strong purging properties Cramping
Bulk-forming agents (mild to moderate constipation)	Methyl cellulose (Citrucel) Psyllium Ispaghula Metamucil	3-4 g qd 3-4 g qd 7 g tid	2-4 days 2-4 days 2-4 days	Flatulence Abdominal distention/pain Large amounts of water prevents viscous mass and obstruction Not to be used if obstruction suspected
Anthracene (anthraquinone)	Senna (Senokot)	15 mg qd 50 mg qd	6-12 hr 6-12 hr	Danthron causes pink discoloration of urine
Laxatives (continuous treatment of opioid-induced constipation)	Danthron Cascara	325 mg hs	6-12 hr	May cause perianal rash
Polyphenic laxatives	Bisacodyl (Dulcolax)	10 mg qd	15-60 min rectal 6-12 hr oral	Dermatitis Electrolyte imbalance

Sources: Schaefer, D. C., & Cheskin, L. J. (1998). Constipation in the elderly. *American Family Physician.* Retrieved April 1, 2002, http://www.aafp.org/afp/98091/schaefer.html; Wong, P. W., & Kadakia, S. (1999). How to deal with chronic constipation: A stepwise method of establishing and treating the source of the problem. *Postgraduate Medicine, 106,* 6. Retrieved April 1, 2002, http://www.postgradmed.com/issues/1999/11_99/wong.htm; Bisanz, A. (1997). Managing bowel elimination problems in patients with cancer. *Oncology Nursing Forum, 24*(4), 679-686; Sykes, N. P. (1998). Constipation and diarrhoea. In D. Doyle, G. W. Hanks, & N. MacDonald (Eds.), *Oxford textbook of palliative medicine* (2nd ed.), (pp. 513-526). New York: Oxford University Press.

Box 19-11 Decreased Effectiveness of Bulk-Forming Agents in Palliative Medicine

1. Increased water intake (200-300 mL) is required, and these agents are of a thick consistency that is not well tolerated by terminal care patients.
2. If not taken with adequate amounts of water, a viscous mass may occur, resulting in obstruction, especially if prior mass or malignancy is present.
3. They are minimally effective against severe constipation.

From Sykes, N. P. (1998). Constipation and diarrhoea. In D. Doyle, G. W. Hanks, & N. MacDonald (Eds.), *Oxford textbook of palliative medicine* (2nd ed., pp. 513-526). New York: Oxford University Press.

Box 19-12 Types of Enemas

SMALL VOLUME
Fleet Enema
- Stimulation of lower bowel
- Softens hard or impacted stool

Fleet Mineral Oil retention enema
- Best given prior to large-volume enema
- Stimulation of lower bowel

Milk and molasses enema
- Softens hard or impacted stool
- Causes peristalsis, pressure, and evacuation

LARGE VOLUME
Tap water enema
- Stimulates peristalsis

Soap suds enema
- Stimulates lower bowel
- Promotes evacuation
- Can be irritating

Saline enema
- Stimulates lower bowel
- Promotes evacuation

Adapted from Derby, S., & Portenoy, R. K. (1997). Assessment and management of opioid-induced constipation. In R. K. Portenoy & E. Bruera (Eds.), *Topics in palliative care*, *Vol. 1* (pp. 95-112). New York: Oxford University Press.

magnesium salts and sodium salts. Magnesium salts consist of magnesium hydroxide (Milk of Magnesia), magnesium sulfate, and magnesium citrate. The most commonly used sodium salt, sodium phosphate (Fleet Phospho-Soda), should be used as a last resort because of its strong purging properties (Sykes, 1998). Magnesium preparations are usually more potent than sodium preparations. Magnesium and sodium salts are not recommended in patients with cardiac heart failure or renal disorder because of systemic absorption of the ions (Enck, 2002b).

Bulk-forming agents are resistant to bacterial breakdown and provide material to remain in the lumen to shorten transit time. There is a balance between the mechanisms of softening hard stool and making loose stools firmer. Examples of these agents include methyl cellulose (Citrucel) and psyllium (Ispaghula, Metamucil). Sykes (1998) provided three reasons why bulk-forming agents are less effective in palliative medicine (Box 19-11).

PERISTALSIS-STIMULATING PREPARATIONS. Anthracene laxatives (anthraquinones) primarily affect the large intestine and induce peristalsis by direct stimulation of the myenteric plexus. Anthracenes have been found helpful in the prevention of constipation, especially in cases of medications causing decreased bowel transit time (Enck, 2002b). Examples include senna, danthron, and cascara. Anthracenes are commonly used as a continuous treatment for opioid-induced constipation, but may also be used intermittently as needed (Derby & Portenoy, 1997).

Polyphenolic laxatives have the same action as anthracene: myenteric plexus stimulation and induction of peristalsis. Bisacodyl (Dulcolax) and sodium picosulfate are examples of polyphenolics. Bisacodyl given orally may take longer to act and cause uncomfortable cramping as compared to suppository administration, in which results typically occur within 15 to 60 minutes (Economou, 2001).

OTHER RECTAL PREPARATIONS. Enemas and suppositories are most helpful in the management of fecal impaction and acute constipation. Rectal administration is contraindicated in thrombocytopenic patients (Derby & Portenoy, 1997). Box 19-12 lists the specific types of enemas.

Lubricant rectal laxatives are enemas that are retained to aid with evacuation or manual disimpaction of feces in the rectum. The older adult's ability to retain the enema determines the efficacy. This type of rectal laxative includes arachis oil and olive oil, which may be used one to three times per week. Osmotic rectal laxatives include glycerine suppositories and sorbitol enemas. Surfactant rectal laxatives include sodium docusate, sodium lauryl sulfacetate, and sodium alkyl sulfacetate enemas. These agents work by promoting water penetration of the fecal mass and softening stool. Saline rectal laxatives stimulate rectal or colonic peristalsis and increase water availability within the lumen. These include sodium phosphate suppositories (Carbalax) and enemas such as sodium phosphate and sodium citrate.

PROKINETIC AGENTS. One of the most commonly used prokinetic agents is metoclopramide (Reglan). Although the indication for direct management of constipation has not been clearly defined, these medications are regularly used for gastroesophageal reflux disease. Subsequent treatment of constipation by these agents comes as a result of their cholinergic and dopaminergic antagonist properties and the ability to accelerate gastric emptying time.

Naloxone (Narcan), an opioid antagonist, has been successful in treating patients who develop opioid analgesic–induced constipation (Sykes, 1996). Because of its first-pass hepatic metabolism, naloxone provides a laxative effect by increasing transit time in the transverse and rectosigmoid colon, without reversing the actual analgesic effects (Economou, 2001).

Nonpharmacologic and Complementary Interventions. Preventing dehydration is of primary concern in the management of constipation. Palliative care measures and overall patient comfort are always the focus; therefore, constipation is not sufficient justification for parenteral fluid supplementation. A more reasonable alternative is continued encouragement of oral fluid intake, with attention given to drinks that the patient likes (Sykes, 1998). Warmed liquids may aid in the stimulation of defecation (Bisanz, 1997).

A high-fiber diet is useful in both the prevention and treatment of constipation. It is important to distinguish between the two types of dietary fiber. Soluble fiber has no significant effect on constipation (Woodward, 1999b). Foods with

Table 19-5 **Sources of Dietary Fiber**		
	Source	Benefit
Soluble dietary fiber	Prunes Oats, oat bran, oatmeal Rice bran Barley Rye Legumes (dried beans & peas) Apples Oranges Grapefruit Pears Peaches Grapes Strawberries Broccoli Potatoes	Minimal benefit in constipation prevention
Insoluble dietary fiber	Whole-wheat breads Whole-grain pasta or rice Brown rice Wheat cereals Wheat bran Nuts Weeds Dried beans Green beans Cabbage Beets Carrots Brussels sprouts Turnips Cauliflower Apple skin	Helpful to prevent constipation

soluble fiber include, peas, lentils, oats, pears, and apples. Insoluble dietary fibers such as wheat, bran, and barley are more helpful in increasing intestinal motility and stool bulk. Insoluble fibers should be avoided if fecal impaction or obstruction is suspected (Woodward, 1999b). A list of foods (Table 19-5) containing insoluble fiber, along with other foods that contribute to constipation, should be provided to the patient, family, or caregivers.

Activity should be increased if possible. Patients should have assistance with mobility when needed and be encouraged to use the lavatory or bedside commode, rather than a bedpan. Adequate time, comfort, and privacy should be provided to facilitate improved toileting habits, along with providing access to toileting following breakfast, when the gastrocolic reflex is active (Woodward, 1999b).

Herbal supplements with laxative properties may be used in management of constipation. Mulberry and rhubarb are similar to senna, but should be used with caution because drug interactions are not well known and have not been thoroughly researched (Economou, 2001). The Food and Drug Administration does not regulate herbal products, and therefore the content of different brands of herbs varies.

Family Concerns and Considerations

Family concerns regarding constipation can be addressed through education about the causes of constipation, methods of prevention, and complications. Special attention should be given to patient or family preferences with regard to treatment modalities. Comfort level with routes of medication administration should be assessed, and, if it is determined that rectal administration is not something the family is able to do, caregiver assistance should be provided.

Diarrhea

When compared to the occurrence of constipation, diarrhea is less common in palliative care (Sykes, 1998); the incidence is estimated at less than 10% (Fallon & O'Neill, 1997). The exception are patients diagnosed with human immunodeficiency virus (HIV) infection, among whom 80% experience diarrhea (Ratnaike, 1999). Diarrhea is described as frequent passage of loose stools, and more specifically defined as three or more stools within 24 hours (Sykes, 1998). Chronic diarrhea persisting longer than 3 weeks may become profuse, and may cause incontinence.

Etiology

Diarrhea may result from decreased absorption or increased secretion of fluid within the intestinal lumen. Classifications of diarrhea are large and small volume. Large-volume diarrhea occurs with increased water or oversecretion; small-volume diarrhea is the result of increased intestinal motility (Kemp, 1999).

There are four mechanisms of diarrhea: secretory, osmotic, hypermotile, and exudative. Secretory diarrhea persists with fasting and may be difficult to control (Economou, 2001). It occurs as a result of hypersecretion tumors and endogenous mediators affecting electrolyte and water transport (Ratnaike, 1999). Enteral feedings, bleeding in the bowel, and lactose intolerance are all related to osmotic diarrhea (Economou, 2001). Increased intestinal motility in hypermotile diarrhea may result from overgrowth of bacteria, incomplete digestion of fat in the small intestine causing it to be expelled in stool (steatorrhea), or chemotherapeutic agents (Economou, 2001). Prostaglandins are released secondary to inflammation of the intestinal mucosa in exudative diarrhea (Economou, 2001). This type of diarrhea is commonly associated with radiation therapy.

The use of high-dose laxatives to relieve constipation is the most common cause of diarrhea in older adult patients (Fallon & O'Neill, 1997). In terminal illness, diarrhea may be attributable to a number of causes occurring independently or concurrently. Malignancy is the second most common cause (Sykes, 1998). Partial bowel obstruction often presents with alternating diarrhea and constipation, while complete obstruction may lead to intractable diarrhea (Sykes, 1998). Subsequent to malabsorption processes or gastrectomy or other bowel-shortening procedures, many patients experience dumping syndrome, causing diarrhea after eating secondary to osmotic and hypermotile mechanisms (Levy, 1991). Diarrhea caused by constipation occurs when liquid stool is expelled around fecal impactions.

In addition to laxatives, other medications associated with the risk of diarrhea include antacids, antibiotics, iron preparations, and nonsteroidal anti-inflammatory drugs (Sykes, 1998). Chemotherapy and radiation directly affect intestinal mucosa, causing bacteria overgrowth, which may contribute to diarrhea (Economou, 2001). Patients receiving eternal feedings are particularly at risk for diarrhea as a result of the use of sorbitol as a sweetener in the majority of these mixtures (Edes, Walk, & Austin, 1990).

Assessment

Initial assessment includes identification of the underlying cause of diarrhea. Specific description of previous bowel habits, along with current symptoms, may help to identify the etiology and appropriate management approaches. Fatty, pale yellow stool that is difficult to control may indicate an etiology of malabsorption. If diarrhea occurs after a period of constipation, fecal impaction should be suspected (Sykes, 1998). Diarrhea that persists beyond 2 to 3 days of fasting may be attributable to osmotic or secretory mechanisms (Economou, 2001).

Varying bowel habits make it difficult to assess diarrhea from the history alone. Typically, the complaint of loose, watery, or frequent stool is indicative of diarrhea. However, some patients describe diarrhea as frequent bowel movements even if consistency remains normal. Although the most accurate account of diarrhea is obtained from a 24- to 48-hour collection and measurement (Wadler, 2001), in clinical practice this is rarely a reasonable method of assessment. Moreover, there is little need for this type of investigation in the palliative care setting. A more logical and objective approach to assessment would be the criteria for grading severity of diarrhea developed by the National Cancer Institute (Table 19-6).

It is also important to review all past, current, and new medications or treatment modalities. Metabolizing capabilities vary in older adults, but generally this population is more susceptible to medication side effects. Use of laxatives in conjunction with fiber intake should be explored. If antibiotics are in use, stool culture for *Clostridium difficile* toxin or other intestinal infectious processes should be performed (Economou, 2001). Additionally, abdominal or pelvic radiation may cause diarrhea up to 2 to 3 weeks after completion (Sykes, 1998).

Psychosocial effects of diarrhea, whether acute or chronic in onset, must be evaluated. Physical activity may be limited as a result of dehydration and weakness if diarrhea has been an ongoing problem. The inability to control bowel movements can cause depression (Economou, 2001) and insecurity for the older adult. Diarrhea may prevent elders from completing their activities of daily living and cause social isolation.

Table 19-6 **National Cancer Institute Common Toxicity Criteria for Grading Severity of Diarrhea**

	Grade 1	Grade 2	Grade 3	Grade 4
Patients without a colostomy	Increase of <4 stools/day over pretreatment	Increase of 4-6 stools/day or nocturnal stools	Increase of ≥7 stools/day or incontinence or need for parenteral support for dehydration	Physiologic consequences requiring intensive care, or hemodynamic collapse
Patients with a colostomy	Mild increase in loose, watery colostomy output compared with pretreatment	Moderate increase in loose, watery colostomy output compared with pretreatment, but not interfering with normal activity	Severe increase in loose, watery colostomy output compared to pretreatment and interfering with daily activity	Physiologic consequences requiring intensive care, or hemodynamic collapse

From Cancer Therapy Evaluation Program. (2003, June 10). Common terminology criteria for adverse events v3.0 (CTCAE). Bethesda, MD: National Cancer Institute. Retrieved from http://ctep.cancer.gov/forms/CTCAEv3.pdf

Management (Box 19-13)

Pharmacologic Interventions. The antidiarrheal therapy of choice in palliative medicine is opioids, specifically loperamide (Imodium) (Sykes, 1998). Initially 4 mg is given, followed by 2 mg after each loose stool up to a maximum of 16 mg/day. Codeine phosphate is also effective at a dose of 10 to 60 mg every 4 hours, and has the added benefit of being relatively inexpensive (Sykes, 1998). Diphenoxylate (Lomotil), 2.5 mg, may be given after each loose stool up to a maximum of eight doses per day (Levy, 1991).

Secretory diarrhea, specifically in HIV patients, is often treated with octreotide (Sandostatin), 50 to 200 mg subcutaneously two to three times daily (Levy, 1991). Although costly, the somatostatin analogue octreotide has the ability to control even the most severe, intractable diarrhea (Doyle, 1994). Reduction of peristalsis and gastric secretions can also be accomplished using anticholinergics such as atropine and scopolamine (Economou, 2001).

Nonpharmacologic Interventions. It is important to prevent dehydration and associated complica-

tions for older adults who are at the end of their lives. Sykes (1998) recommended supportive care and rehydration by encouraging oral liquids rather than the parenteral route. A minimum of 2 quarts/day of un-carbonated fluids is suggested (Bisanz, 1997). Glucose and electrolyte concentrations (flat ginger ale; Pedialyte) are most helpful in rehydration (Sykes, 1998).

Dietary modifications include clear liquids and only simple or light carbohydrates, such as toast or crackers, which should be offered frequently in small amounts (Kemp, 1999). As diarrhea resolves, proteins and fats should be gradually reintroduced (Sykes, 1998). Additional dietary changes with diarrhea include avoidance of greasy, spicy, and raw foods, as well as very hot or cold liquids, caffeine, fruit juices, and alcohol (Kemp, 1999; Ratnaike, 1999).

Family Concerns and Considerations

Incontinence of stool can be a disturbing problem for the older adult and the caregiver. Frequent checks and toileting should be done in cases in which patients are confused or unable to express when they need to have a bowel movement. Nurses play a significant role in educating caregivers and family members regarding these issues. Care should be taken to prevent skin breakdown, perineal pain, and other complications with infection. Protective ointments and anesthetics can be applied for comfort measures, and should be initiated prior to skin problems developing (Kemp, 1999). It is also helpful to avoid toilet tissue after a few days of diarrhea; a spray bottle for warm water washes, or mild skin cleansers, may be less painful.

If the etiology of diarrhea is infectious, appropriate contact precautions should be instituted. Patients, family members, and caregivers should be instructed on proper hand-washing techniques to prevent the spread of infection. Disposable briefs should be discarded and tied in plastic bags to prevent contamination.

Bowel Obstruction

Bowel obstruction occurs when intraluminal or extraluminal etiologies prevent normal GI propulsion. It occurs throughout the course of disease, but most often in advanced states (Mercadante, 1997). Obstruction is more commonly the result of extrinsic pressure of tumor

---

Box 19-13 Management of Diarrhea

INDEPENDENT INTERVENTIONS
- Encourage fluids—clear liquids
- Offer fluids a patient likes
- Dietary modifications—simple carbohydrates, progress to proteins and fats
- Avoid caffeine, juices, spicy foods, greasy foods, and alcohol
- Disimpaction
- Prevention of skin breakdown
- Client/family/caregiver education—contact precautions, hand washing, etc.
- Promote comfort
- Ongoing assessment and evaluation

DEPENDENT INTERVENTIONS
- Discontinuation of laxatives
- Antidiarrheal agents
- Stool cultures
- Antimicrobial agents

COLLABORATIVE INTERVENTIONS
- Dietary modifications

Table 19-7 Symptoms and Signs of Intestinal Obstruction

Site	Pain	Vomiting	Distention	Bowel Sounds
Duodenum	None	Severe; large amounts with undigested food	None	Succussion splash may be present
Small bowel	Upper to central abdominal colic	Moderate to severe	Moderate	Usually hyperactive with borborygmi
Large bowel	Central to lower abdominal colic	Develops late	Great	Borborygmi

From Baines, M. J. (1998). The pathophysiology and management of malignant intestinal obstruction. In D. Doyle, G. W. Hanks, & N. MacDonald (Eds.), *Oxford textbook of palliative medicine* (2nd ed., pp. 526-534). New York: Oxford University Press.

growth, rather than tumor reoccurrence within the lumen (Enck, 2002b), and any location within the bowel can be affected (Baines, 1998). Although the general incidence of malignant bowel obstruction is unknown, studies of advanced cancer patients at St. Christopher's Hospice in London estimated that obstruction was experienced by 3% of patients with terminal illness and 10% of patients with colorectal cancer (Baines, Oliver, & Carter, 1985).

Etiology

Bowel obstruction can occur anywhere along the GI tract, including the gastric outlet, duodenum, small or large bowel, and rectosigmoid junction. Bowel obstructions attributed to causes within the lumen are termed *intraluminal* and may arise from a primary or metastatic process. Intramural obstruction results from lateral tumor growth within the musculature of the bowel, and extramural causes are abdominal adhesions and mesenteric or omental masses (Baines, 1998). Pseudo-obstruction occurs when a segment of bowel has impaired or absent motility. Motility disorders involving multiple sites of the bowel are common with advanced cancer states, especially in ovarian carcinomas (Baines, 1998). Mechanical bowel obstruction can be attributed to complications of constipation, impaction, ascites, fibrosis, and intestinal muscle fatigue (Baines, 1998).

Cardinal Signs and Symptoms

Bowel obstruction is characterized by a gradual onset of symptoms that include abdominal pain or distention, vomiting, and constipation.

Malignant obstruction may present more suddenly (Baines, 1998). Specific presentation of symptoms depends on the location of obstruction (Table 19-7).

Assessment

Assessment regarding the elder's history of bowel patterns is needed, but may not distinguish the diagnosis of bowel obstruction from constipation. Physical examination includes assessment of bowel sounds throughout all abdominal quadrants and gentle palpation for masses, dilated bowel segments, or distention. Rectosigmoid impaction or obstruction may be identified by digital rectal exam.

The most helpful diagnostic procedure to confirm obstruction is abdominal radiography (Economou, 2001), which will also help to locate the specific area of bowel where the obstructive problem is occurring. To prevent unnecessary procedures, it is important to clearly define the goals of care. If the prognosis for survival is greater than 3 months or palliative surgery is a consideration, a more extensive work-up to determine etiology may be performed (Sykes, 1998).

Management (Box 19-14)

Pharmacologic Interventions. A variety of medications can be used to provide symptomatic relief in elder patients with intestinal bowel obstruction. Antiemetics, analgesics, antispasmodics, and antisecretory agents are commonly used to relieve N&V, abdominal pain, and distention. Oral administration should be avoided because of the unknown amount of drug absorption (Mercadante, 1997).

Box 19-14 Management of Bowel Obstruction

INDEPENDENT INTERVENTIONS
- Encourage oral intake
- Small, frequent meals
- Control of nausea and vomiting

DEPENDENT INTERVENTIONS
- Nasogastric tube suction
- Venting gastrostomy or jejunostomy
- Symptomatic relief with medications
  - Antiemetics
  - Analgesics
  - Antispasmodics

COLLABORATIVE INTERVENTIONS
- Palliative surgery—ostomy formation or bowel resection

The antiemetic agent of choice in terminally ill patients is haloperidol (Haldol), 0.5 to 2 mg orally, intravenously, or subcutaneously every 6 hours initially, then titrated (Fainsinger, Spachynski, Hanson, & Bruera, 1994). Metoclopramide is generally avoided, particularly if complete obstruction is suspected, because of its prokinetic effects of increased abdominal cramping and pain (Baines, 1998). However, metoclopramide, 10 to 20 mg orally every 6 hours, may be used as an antiemetic in partial obstruction.

Morphine is effective in relieving abdominal pain associated with bowel obstruction and may be titrated until relief is achieved. Subcutaneous morphine is the most common analgesic used (Fainsinger et al., 1994). The antispasmodic hyoscine butylbromide (scopolamine), 10 to 20 mg subcutaneously, intramuscularly, or intravenously, may be used up to four times per day, and is effective in relieving spasms that contribute to pain with bowel obstruction (Baines, 1998). It is also available orally in the form of hyoscine hydrobromide at the same dosages, or rectally at 10 mg three to four times per day.

Nonpharmacologic Interventions. Older adults with bowel obstruction may be encouraged to continue oral intake as tolerated (Baines, 1998). If intake is limited, crushed ice may be given to prevent dry mouth. High intestinal obstruction may cause profuse emesis and the inability to tolerate any oral intake. In these cases, nasogastric tube insertion or venting gastrostomy should be considered to relieve symptoms. Nasogastric tube suctioning decompresses the stomach, removing air and fluids that would be vomited, and has been found beneficial in high intestinal obstruction and gastric outlet obstructions (Mercadante, 1997). Oral intake is halted, and intravenous fluids may be given to allow time for determining a continued plan of care or whether to proceed with palliative surgery (Baines, 1998). It is important to determine if the nasogastric tube is a burden or a benefit; resolution of obstruction may occur for some, while others are unable to tolerate the discomfort (Mercadante, 1997). Venting gastrostomy or jejunostomy can be performed at the bedside under local anesthesia. A full liquid diet is encouraged, and the tube may be clamped for meals for as long as tolerated. Venting is considered more effective than nasogastric suctioning in relieving N&V in cases of inoperable obstruction (Baines, 1998).

A more invasive method of treating bowel obstruction is palliative surgery. In the evaluation of individual cases, prognosis and the ability to tolerate the procedure must be seriously considered. A conservative approach with medications or one of the modalities mentioned previously should be attempted prior to surgery. Surgical techniques vary from resections to ostomy formations, depending on the type and location of obstruction. Reoccurrence of obstruction and other complications are common after surgery (Gallick, Weaver, Sachs, & Bouwman, 1986).

OTHER CONDITIONS
Hiccups
Hiccups, also referred to as singultus, are typically an intermittent phenomenon that is annoying but benign. The exception is those hiccups termed *persistent* or *protracted*, lasting longer than 48 hours (Kolodzik & Eilers, 1991). Chronic reoccurring hiccups can negatively impact advanced conditions by causing dehydration, insomnia, or abdominal muscle pain (Kemp, 1999). Hiccups lasting longer than 1 month are considered intractable (Kolodzik & Eilers, 1991), and can produce exhaustion if sleep is disturbed for an extended period of time (Dahlin &

Reference: Espinel, J., Vivas, S., Munoz, F., Jorquera, F., & Olcoz, J. L. (2001). Palliative treatment of malignant obstruction of gastric outlet using an endoscopically placed enteral wallstent. *Digestive Diseases and Sciences, 46,* 2322-2324.

Research Problem: The standard treatment for malignant gastric outlet obstruction is surgical gastro-jejunostomy, a procedure associated with high morbidity and mortality. The study was designed to evaluate the efficacy and safety of a new self-expandable metal stent to be used for palliation in malignant gastrointestinal obstruction. The new procedure is performed using endoscopy rather than surgery.

Design: Outcomes analysis determined the median survival time and symptom reoccurrence following the procedure. The data were used to show the safety and effectiveness of the stents.

Sample and Setting: 6 patients with malignant bowel obstruction (5 female and 1 male) who were determined to be inappropriate for surgery because of advanced age and progressive illness.

Methods: The patients underwent self-expanding stent placement under conscious sedation using endoscopy with fluoroscopic guidance. Following the procedure, the patients were observed for complications and reoccurrence of symptoms. Specific factors assessed included the ability to eat a regular diet, length of hospital stay postprocedure, and median survival time.

Results: The mean hospital stay was 2.5 days, with none of the patients experiencing complications from the procedure. All six patients were able to tolerate pureed or regular diet within 24 hours after the procedure, with no reoccurrence of obstructive symptoms. The median survival time was 9 weeks, with a 95% confidence interval of 3 to 15 weeks.

Implications for Nursing Practice: Nurses are continuously providing highly specialized care to patients at the end of life. Managing the symptoms of bowel obstruction is one of the frequently encountered nursing challenges with this population. This procedure can be used for symptom relief and decreased length of hospitalization for patients with malignant bowel obstruction. Nursing care pre- and postprocedure includes continuous monitoring for recurrent obstruction, complications, and maintenance of comfort.

Conclusion: The self-expandable metal stents were shown to have no complications and to provide quick symptom relief with short hospitalization time. During the survival time, the stents allowed good quality of life without recurrent obstruction. In all of the cases the cause of death was disease progression.

Goldsmith, 2001). Intractable or persistent hiccups are more likely to be associated with anatomic or organic disorders, and may have complications including oxygen desaturation, ventilatory disturbances, and cardiac arrhythmias (Rousseau, 1995).

The characteristic sound of a hiccup is the result of a sudden, involuntary contraction of one or both sides of the diaphragm, causing a sudden inspiratory response and closure of the glottis (Twycross & Regnard, 1998). The incidence of hiccup in terminal cancer is unknown; however, protracted hiccups are 82% more common in men than women (Rousseau, 1995).

Etiology
Although the exact pathophysiology is unknown, common causes of hiccups include esophagitis, gastric distention, diaphragmatic irritation, phrenic nerve irritation, uremia, infection, brain tumor, and possibly psychogenic origin (Lewis, 1985). The numerous causes for hiccups are described with relationship to the type: benign, persistent, or intractable. Some of the most common causes of benign hiccups are alcohol intake, emotional stress, sudden excitement, smoking, laughter, and gastric distention from carbonated beverages, eating too fast, overeating, and indigestion. Gastric distention is

thought to be the most common cause of hiccups in older adult patients with terminal cancer (Twycross & Regnard, 1998).

Persistent and intractable hiccups can be classified as resulting from central nervous system causes, diaphragmatic (phrenic nerve) irritation, or vagal nerve irritation, or as drug or toxin induced, postoperative, infectious, metabolic, psychogenic, and idiopathic. Central nervous system causes of hiccups include structural lesions, neoplasms, hydrocephalus, encephalitis, epilepsy, vascular lesions, and head trauma (Kolodzik & Eilers, 1991). Diaphragmatic irritation may result from a hernia, organomegaly, esophageal neoplasms, pericarditis, intra-abdominal abscess, and gastroesophageal reflux disease. Irritation of any of the branches of the vagus nerve (auricular, meningeal, pharyngeal, laryngeal, thoracic, and abdominal) may cause intractable or persistent hiccups.

The etiology of medication- or toxin-induced hiccups is not completely understood. Barbiturates, diazepam, general anesthetics, morphine, and nicotine are among the most common drugs that may induce hiccups. Postoperative procedures linked to hiccups include any that involve manipulation of the diaphragm or adjacent organs, craniotomy, laparotomy, and thoracotomy. Cholera, herpes zoster, influenza, meningitis, and rheumatic fever are infectious causes of hiccups. Metabolic disorders resulting in hiccups include uremia, diabetes, hypocalcemia, hypokalemia, hyponatremia, gout, and hypocarbia. Among the psychogenic causes of prolonged hiccups are grief reactions, sudden emotional shock, hysterical neurosis, personality disorders, and anorexia (Kolodzik & Eilers, 1991).

Assessment

In obtaining a thorough assessment of symptoms, it is necessary to inquire about duration, prior episodes, and the impact on activities of daily living. Interference with resting and sleeping may cause a patient to present with symptoms of exhaustion and fatigue. If the hiccups are so severe that eating habits are affected and appetite is diminished, the patient may be dehydrated, thin, and weak, and may even appear cachectic. The already predisposed terminally ill elder may exhibit signs of sepsis or metabolic dysfunction secondary to immunocompromised states. It may be necessary to perform lab work to determine if metabolic dysfunction is the underlying cause of the hiccups (Dahlin & Goldsmith, 2001). These causes are often easily treated and may resolve persistent hiccups.

In palliative care, a comprehensive work-up to determine the etiology of persistent hiccups is appropriate only if the result assists in identifying an intervention. A chest radiograph may be necessary if mediastinal or pulmonary processes are suspected (Dahlin & Goldsmith, 2001).

Management (Box 19-15)

Pharmacologic   Interventions. Pharmacologic interventions are selected based on the presumed etiology of hiccups. Hiccups are generally preventable or manageable by decreasing gastric distention and resolving esophageal irritation.

Gastric distention is likely to be the focus of an initial treatment approach in palliative care. Among the most effective medications for gastric distention are simethicone and metoclopramide (Reglan). Simethicone, 15 to 30 mL, is recommended before and after meals and at bedtime. Metoclopramide, 10 to 20 mg orally or intra-

---

Box 19-15 Management of Hiccups

INDEPENDENT INTERVENTIONS
- Drinking liquids quickly
- Drinking a cold liquid
- Swallowing dry bread or granulated sugar
- Breathing into a paper bag
- Hyperventilation
- Vagal stimulation
- Behavioral therapy

DEPENDENT INTERVENTIONS
- Pharmacological approaches
  - Simethicone
  - Metoclopramide
  - Chlorpromazine
  - Haloperidol
  - Anticonvulsants
  - Lidocaine
  - Baclofen
- Nasogastric tube

venously up to four times a day, can be used alone or in combination with simethicone. Metoclopramide works to decrease gastric distention by increasing overall gastric motility. This medication should be used with caution in elder patients. Metoclopramide should not be used concurrently with peppermint water, another treatment, because of opposing effects on the lower esophageal sphincter (Twycross & Regnard, 1998). Esophageal disorders or irritation can be treated with peppermint water, which decreases gastric distention that sometimes leads to esophageal irritation.

Chlorpromazine (Thorazine), 25 to 50 mg orally, works by reticular formation and hiccup reflex suppression, and may be taken up to three times per day (Kolodzik & Eilers, 1991). It is an option for prophylactic treatment of intractable hiccups. However, because of its side effects of central nervous system depression and postural hypotension, caution should be exercised with older adult patients (Twycross & Regnard, 1998).

Haloperidol (Haldol), 5 mg orally or intravenously for acute treatment followed by regular dosing at bedtime for prophylactic management, is successful for resistant cases of hiccups, and is suggested to be a convenient regimen (Twycross & Regnard, 1998). Anticonvulsants such as carbamazepine (Tegretol), phenytoin (Dilantin), and valproic acid (Depakote, Depakene) are most effective when the cause of hiccups is of central origin (Kolodzik & Eilers, 1991). The skeletal muscle relaxant baclofen, 5 to 10 mg orally three times per day, is also effective for treatment of hiccups (Ramirez & Graham, 1992; Piper et al., 1989; Walker, Watanabe, & Bruera, 1998).

In severe cases, surgical intervention in the form of phrenic nerve interruption may be necessary to improve the patient's quality of life. Another alternative that has been used when all other methods fail is intravenous infusion of lidocaine (Twycross & Regnard, 1998).

Nonpharmacologic   Interventions. Determining the underlying cause of hiccups is the primary factor to consider when selecting treatment. This is not always possible, and therefore the health care provider should be most concerned with assessing the overall effect of persistent hiccups on the elder's quality of life. The aggressiveness of treatment depends on how bothersome the hiccups are to the older adult.

Patients and family members often attempt nonpharmacologic measures before they report this symptom to their health care practitioners. Pharyngeal stimulation by drinking a cold liquid or swallowing sugar granules or dry bread has been effective with acute attacks of hiccups (Baines, 1992). Increasing retention of carbon dioxide by re-breathing into a paper bag has also been suggested to be helpful in relieving an acute attack (Baines, 1992).

Digital rectal massage and carotid massage can be used for vagal stimulation (Dahlin & Goldsmith, 2001). Gastric distention can be relieved by nasogastric tube insertion for decompression or lavage, along with induction of vomiting (Lewis, 1985). Collaborative and complementary therapies that may be useful in the management of hiccups include chest physiotherapy to disrupt diaphragmatic spasms (Twycross & Regnard, 1998).

Family Concerns and Considerations

It is necessary to discuss treatment options with the older adult patient, his or her family, and caregivers. All methods and alternatives should be clearly outlined. Various treatment benefits, along with medication side effects, are necessary to make an informed decision regarding regimens they would like to pursue. When hiccups become overly disruptive to daily life, the patient may be willing to explore more aggressive therapies to obtain relief.

Ascites

Ascites refers to the presence of excess fluid in the peritoneal cavity. It is a common manifestation of many disorders, but is most frequently found in chronic liver disease. Malignancy is the cause of ascites in 10% of all patients with ascites (Runyon, Hoefs, & Morgan, 1988). Estimated survival at 1 year is 40%, and less than 10% of patients live 3 years (Bain, 1998). The exception to the poor prognostic implications associated with ascites is ovarian cancer, in which the survival rate may be improved with surgical intervention (Mercadante, LaRosa, Nicolosi, & Garofalo, 1998). Bain (1998) described four subtypes and the pathogenesis of malignant ascites (Table 19-8). Both central and peripheral malignant ascites result in compression of the lymphatic and portal venous systems. Central

Table 19-8 **Subtypes of Malignant Ascites**	
Type	**Etiology**
Central malignant ascites	Tumor invasion of hepatic parenchyma
Peripheral malignant ascites	Tumor cells located on the parietal or visceral peritoneal surface
Mixed malignant ascites	Tumor invasion in the liver and on the peritoneal surface
Chylous malignant ascites	Obstruction of lymphatic flow as a result of tumor invasion of the retroperitoneal space

Adapted from Bain, V. G. (1998). Jaundice, ascites, and hepatic encephalopathy. In D. Doyle, G. W. Hanks, & N. MacDonald (Eds.), *Oxford textbook of palliative medicine* (2nd ed., pp. 557-571). New York: Oxford University Press.

malignant ascites involves tumor invasion of hepatic parenchyma, as opposed to peripheral malignant ascites, in which tumor cells located on the parietal or visceral peritoneal surface lead to blockage at the level of the peritoneal space. Peripheral is the most common type of malignant ascites. Mixed-type malignant ascites has features of both central and peripheral types. Tumor invasion occurs in the liver parenchyma and on the peritoneal surface. Chylous malignant ascites occurs with obstructed lymphatic flow secondary to tumor invasion of the retroperitoneal space.

Etiology

In chronic liver disease, ascites initially begins with portal hypertension that leads to increased levels of nitric oxide, vasodilation, sodium retention, and decreased renal function (Runyon, 1998). Other disorders associated with the development of ascites resulting from increased hydrostatic pressure include congestive heart failure, constrictive pericarditis, and hepatic vein occlusion (Runyon et al., 1992). According to Runyon et al. (1992), tuberculosis, bacterial peritonitis, and malignant disease of the peritoneum may cause ascites, along with the decreased colloid osmotic pressure seen in malnutrition, nephritic syndrome with protein loss, and end-stage liver disease.

Cardinal Signs and Symptoms

Patients often complain of abdominal bloating and that their clothes no longer fit across their abdomen. Pain is often associated with the bloating and increase in abdominal girth. Some patients may have heartburn, nausea, and a

decreased appetite. If the ascites is pronounced, dyspnea may be apparent.

Assessment

The most distressing physical symptom associated with ascites may be abdominal discomfort or pain caused by the distention. Additional complications, such as dehydration and electrolyte imbalances, should be assessed in the older adult. Depending on the extent of fluid present, scrotal edema may occur along with weakened hernial orifices (Heneghan & O'Grady, 2001). Physical mobility may be difficult, especially for patients who are weakened or fatigued secondary to the excess weight and pressure that occurs with ascites.

The most obvious sign of ascites is increased abdominal girth. Patients may complain of bloating, nausea, and decreased appetite. Secondary to increased abdominal pressure, there may be worsening of gastroesophageal reflux or heartburn (Economou, 2001), as well as dyspnea or orthopnea (Bain, 1998). In the supine position, physical exam may reveal dullness on abdominal percussion in the dependent flank areas because ascitic fluid typically follows gravity. Tympany may be present toward the center of the abdomen. Shifting dullness can be assessed by turning the patient onto one side and noting that the dullness on percussion shifts to the dependent side while tympany shifts to the top (Bates, Bickley, & Hoekelman, 1995). Approximately 1500 mL of fluid must be present before dullness occurs with percussion of fluid alone (Cattau, Benjamin, Knuff, & Castell, 1982). A fluid wave test is performed by asking an assistant to press down firmly on the midline of the abdomen (to stop transmission of a wave through fat) while tapping on one flank of the abdomen. This causes an impulse to be transmitted through ascitic fluid that is felt on the other flank; if the impulse is easily palpable, it suggests the presence of ascites (Bates et al., 1995). Liver enlargement, tumor, or mass may also be palpable.

Management (Box 19-16)

Pharmacologic Interventions. The use of diuretics to decrease sodium reabsorption and urinary retention, along with increasing urinary excretion, is the primary intervention for ascites. As helpful as diuretic therapy may be, approximately 10% to 20% of patients will not respond to this intervention (Heneghan & O'Grady, 2001). Loop diuretics and aldosterone-inhibiting diuretics are typically not effective because malignant ascites is related to sodium retention; however, central malignant ascites may be more responsive to these therapies (Enck, 2002a. The potassium-

---

Box 19-16 Management of Ascites

INDEPENDENT INTERVENTIONS
- Symptomatic relief
- Medication administration
- Patient and family education
- Positioning to promote comfort and prevent dyspnea
- Ongoing physical assessment to identify progression of ascites
- Identifying complications
  - Infection
  - Difficulty breathing
  - Gastroesophageal reflux

DEPENDENT INTERVENTIONS
- Therapeutic paracentesis—serial paracentesis
- Peritoneovenous shunting
- Prevention of electrolyte imbalances
- Diuretic therapy
- Antibiotic therapy
- Albumin replacement

COLLABORATIVE INTERVENTIONS
- Dietary consultation regarding sodium and fluid restrictions

---

sparing agent spironolactone (100 to 400 mg/day) is the diuretic of choice for ascites, but it may be necessary to initiate diuresis with a loop diuretic such as furosemide (40 to 80 mg/day) (Bain, 1998). Supplementation of potassium (10 to 20 mEq/day) is necessary when using loop diuretics, especially in older adults, who are sensitive to mild electrolyte imbalances. Additional complications that may occur with diuretics include hepatic encephalopathy and prerenal failure.

Ascitic fluid may be analyzed to determine if albumin replacement is necessary, as well as for bacterial infection of the fluid, which may require antibiotic therapy. Practitioner discretion and family requests will determine if antibiotic therapy is appropriate, given the goals of care of elder patients who are at the end of their lives. However, confusion and delirium are common when older adults experience infection, and may influence decisions regarding antibiotic therapy.

Administration of medications to help with diuresis and pain control is a primary intervention with ascites. Treatment for infection or albumin and potassium replacement may also be warranted. Paracentesis or shunt placement and the prevention of infection may be important components of management. Nursing interventions include monitoring the older adult to promote symptomatic relief, and educating the elder and his or her family about ascites and the interventions being performed.

If diuresis is accomplished with diuretic therapy, it is necessary to make elimination as easy as possible for the patient and caregivers. This may include urinary catheterization if needed to prevent injury if the patient has difficulty getting out of bed or in elders who are confused and become agitated from urinary distention. Although it is important to monitor for signs and symptoms of urinary tract infection with catheterization, this intervention is usually considered a safe and effective treatment for older adults at the end of life.

Nonpharmacologic Interventions. The goal of providing palliative care to a patient with ascites is to relieve discomfort. The poor prognosis related to ascites lends itself to palliation of symptoms without the expectation of altering patient survival rates. Management of ascites includes sodium restriction to prevent additional fluid retention. Ascites will be decreased from restriction of dietary sodium to 40 to 60 μg/day, or 1 to 1.5 g of salt, without the need for any further interventions (Heneghan & O'Grady, 2001). When there is marked sodium retention, restriction of sodium must be to less than 20 μg/day, a goal that not only is difficult to achieve but may impair nutritional status (Heneghan & O'Grady, 2001).

Severe ascites requires therapeutic paracentesis alone or in combination with dietary sodium restriction. Symptomatic relief of malignant ascites may be accomplished with the removal of 5 to 10 L of fluid with each paracentesis (Bain, 1998). Complete drainage of peritoneal fluid may actually cause an increase in pain (Doyle, 1994). Following removal of the ascitic fluid, diuretic therapy is often initiated to prevent reaccumulation. Heneghan and O'Grady (2001) cited conflicting data regarding albumin replacement to prevent electrolyte imbalance when large amounts of fluid are withdrawn. According to Doyle (1994), albumin replacement is rarely justified in palliative care and should be discussed with the older adult and his or her family.

Refractory ascites occurs when repeated attempts to restrict sodium and diuretic therapy are both unable to prevent reoccurrence of ascitic fluid. If drainage is frequently required or there is increased discomfort for the patient, placement of a shunt may be warranted. Peritoneovenous shunting provides benefit for 3 to 4 weeks; however, insertion has high mortality rates (Doyle, 1994). Candidates for shunting include those with abdominal scars preventing serial paracentesis, and limited access to or distance from a physician able or willing to perform serial paracentesis (Heneghan & O'Grady, 2001).

Comprehensive nursing assessment is essential to identify any complications that may occur with ascitic fluid accumulation. The nurse should observe for signs and symptoms of infection or peritonitis. The elder must be monitored for increased shortness of breath or dyspnea; the physician should be notified if positioning does not relieve dyspnea. With diuresis, older patients are also at increased risk of dehydration leading to poor nutritional status and skin breakdown. Frequent repositioning is necessary not only for comfort, but also for prevention of pressure ulcers.

Collaborative care may include dietary consultation to aid with planning meals for sodium restriction, and it may also involve frequent discussions with the physician or palliative care team to accomplish symptom relief from refractory ascites. The nurse must act as the advocate for the older adult and discuss assessment findings to inform the physician of any problems the elder may be experiencing.

Family Concerns and Considerations

The older adult and his or her caregivers will need instruction on positioning. It may be difficult to achieve a comfortable position in which the pressure of ascitic fluid does not inhibit breathing or make breathing more strenuous. The nurse should explain the importance of sodium restriction and provide education regarding how this may help to prevent fluid retention and the associated discomfort. If refractory ascites is present, the risks and benefits of paracentesis should be clearly discussed to ensure that informed decisions about management can be made. It is important that patients and caregivers understand the risks associated with reaccumulation of fluid.

Xerostomia

Xerostomia (dry mouth) can be the result of three primary factors: reduced salivary secretion, buccal mucosa erosion, and dehydration (Ventafridda, Ripamonti, Sbanotto, & De Conno, 1998). Xerostomia is indicated when there is an unstimulated salivary flow rate of less than 0.1 mL/min (Sreebny & Valdini, 1987). Despite popular belief, xerostomia is not a normal occurrence of aging, and should be considered an indication of a disorder or a side effect of a treatment (Baum & Ship, 1994). Prevalence in the general population is 29% (Sreebny & Valdini, 1988), and greater than 50% in cancer patients (Conill et al., 1997).

Etiology

A reduction in salivary production by the parotid and submandibular glands occurs as a result of radiotherapy, oral surgery, medication side effects, gland obstruction, brain neoplasms, and hypothyroidism. Saliva functions as a protective mechanism against infection, dental caries, and extreme temperatures in food. It is also contains water, mucus, and enzymes that facilitate nutrition (Cooke, Admedzel, & Mayberry, 1996).

Clinical practice suggests that it is common for elder patients with cancer who are receiving morphine to experience xerostomia (White, Hoskin, Hanks, & Bliss, 1989). A greater incidence of dry mouth was observed by Ventafridda, Ripamonti, Bianchi, Sbanotto, and De Conno (1986) following the administration of oral liquid morphine than with other tablet forms of morphine.

Medications may contribute to xerostomia both indirectly and directly. These may include anticholinergics, anticonvulsants, antidepressants, antihistamines, corticosteroids, opioid analgesics, nonsteroidal anti-inflammatory agents, calcium channel blockers, beta-blockers, and diuretics. Antidepressants directly interfere with nerve supply to the salivary glands to decrease saliva production, and diuretics inhibit actual production of saliva (Davies, Broadley, & Beighton, 2001). Indirect effects involve impairment of taste sensation, leading to a decreased secretion of saliva. Some polypharmacy is common for older adults, especially those who are terminally ill. It is likely that combinations of these drugs increase the incidence of xerostomia. A study by Davies et al. (2001) revealed a positive correlation between the total number of drugs taken and the presence of xerostomia in elders with cancer.

Oral cancer, chemotherapy or radiation therapy, stomatitis, and oral infections may cause actual erosion of buccal mucosa. Local causes of dehydration, such as oxygen therapy or mouth breathing, may contribute to xerostomia, along with the systemic causes of diarrhea, vomiting, anorexia, and polyuria (Dahlin & Goldsmith, 2001).

Cardinal Signs and Symptoms

Xerostomia is generally considered a subjective sensation; the severity is related to the amount of discomfort or pain that the elder experiences. Symptoms that are most frequently voiced in relation to dry mouth include diminished taste (dysgeusia), difficulty chewing foods without fluids (dysmasesis), dysphagia, needing fluids during the night, and a burning sensation on the tongue (Ventafridda et al., 1998).

Assessment

When assessing the oral cavity of the older adult, the nurse should inspect the oral mucosa for dryness, cracking, fissures, pale color, ulcerations, and gingivitis (Cooke et al., 1996). Dentures should be removed to inspect for problems that may otherwise be hidden. Structures that should be evaluated on routine examination are the hard and soft palate, pharynx, buccal areas, floor of the mouth, gum and tooth or denture condition, and top, bottom, and sides of the tongue. The nurse should also evaluate the lips for dry, cracked areas or lesions, along with the degree of mouth opening.

Xerostomia can be determined at the bedside utilizing a quick and easy test. Following inspection of the oral cavity, an attempt is made to stick the tongue blade on the top surface of the tongue. If it remains in place, xerostomia is present (Cooke et al., 1996). Another test that can be attempted is the cracker/biscuit test. This involves asking the patient to eat a dry cracker or biscuit; if he or she is unable to do so, xerostomia is present (Sreebny & Valdini, 1987). It may be difficult to perform this second test if patients are limited in their ability to tolerate oral intake. Caution should be used to prevent aspiration.

The Oncology Nursing Society has introduced a standardized documentation tool for xerostomia and nursing care. A zero is recorded for no evidence of dry mouth; 1 for mild dryness, slightly thickened saliva, and minimal taste change; 2 for moderate dryness, thick and sticky saliva, and marked altered taste change; 3 for complete mouth dryness; and 4 for actual salivary necrosis (Oncology Nursing Society, 1994).

Management (Box 19-17)

Pharmacologic Interventions. Interventions in managing xerostomia can be accomplished by a stepped approach (Dahlin & Goldsmith, 2001). Identification and treatment of underlying infection or disease is the first step. This involves using a nystatin swish and swallow or a one-time dose of fluconazole (Diflucan), 150 mg orally. Second, it should be determined if the cause is related to medications. If so, interventions may include decreasing dosages or adjusting medication schedules when possible. Stimulation of salivary secretion using both pharmacologic and nonpharmacologic measures is the third and final step

---

Box 19-17 Management of Xerostomia

INDEPENDENT INTERVENTIONS
• Good oral hygiene
• Frequent mouth care
• Humidification of air
• Gustatory stimulation—chewing gum
• Provide cool liquid drinks as needed
• Provide bland diet
• Monitoring for signs of infection

DEPENDENT INTERVENTIONS
• Treatment of underlying infection
• Medication adjustments

COLLABORATIVE INTERVENTIONS
• Dietary consult to maintain adequate nutrition

---

in the approach to managing xerostomia (Cooke et al., 1996).

Pilocarpine hydrochloride (Salagen), 5 to 10 mg orally three times per day, improves saliva production but can take up to 12 weeks for results if xerostomia is radiation induced (Johnson et al., 1993). Cholinergic side effects such as dizziness, headache, hypertension, tachycardia, watery eyes, sweating, and urinary frequency may occur secondary to parasympathetic stimulation of pilocarpine. Sweating is the most common side effect, usually leading to discontinuation (Johnson et al., 1993).

Nonpharmacologic Interventions. Implications for reversing symptoms accompanying xerostomia include discontinuing or changing medication regimens when possible. In palliative care, this is rarely a viable option when the medications are utilized for pain and symptom management.

Independent interventions for prevention of xerostomia include maintenance of good oral hygiene as frequently as every 2 hours and humidifying the air, especially when oxygen is being administered (Ventafridda et al., 1998). Gustatory stimulation can be enhanced using peppermint water or sugarless gum. Unfortunately, the results from these interventions tend to be short lived (Cooke et al., 1996). Vitamin C and citric acids may be helpful, but have been found to cause a burning sensation, and are not

recommended if oral lesions are present (Davies, 1997). Acupuncture has been suggested to be effective in management of various types of xerostomia (Blom, Dawidson, & Angmar-Manson, 1992), but the evidence to support this claim is limited.

Case Study Conclusion

A gastrostomy tube was placed for comfort to relieve Mr. S.'s gastric distention and nausea. Patient-controlled analgesia using subcutaneous morphine, with a continuous basal rate, was added for additional pain control. Prochlorperazine (Compazine), 10 mg every 6 to 8 hours as needed by mouth, or 25 mg per rectum every 8 hours, was ordered for nausea and vomiting.

Mr. S. was discharged from the hospital to continue with palliative care from the local hospice agency. He was kept comfortable with adjustments to the morphine and had no further nausea or vomiting. The gastrostomy tube was also successful in relieving abdominal distention and discomfort. Mr. S. died 2 weeks later with his wife and family by his side.

Mr. S. had a rapid decline from initial diagnosis. Disease progression contributed to the small bowel obstruction, and changes in level of consciousness were directly related to increasing ammonia levels. Ongoing nursing assessment and maintaining comfort through pain management for Mr. S. was the priority. Palliation to relieve gastric distention, rather than aggressive surgery, was an appropriate treatment choice. A need for aggressive family intervention to provide support for death and grief issues was identified, playing an important role in the rapid development of a plan of care for Mr. S.

CONCLUSION

Gastrointestinal symptoms are common in terminal illness. Many patients have described the constant nausea, vomiting, and diarrhea as more disabling and disturbing than pain (Fallon & Welsh, 1998). Gastrointestinal symptoms affect patients' activities of daily living and influence their quality of life.

As in all palliative care, ongoing assessment of the older adult patient is necessary to determine what interventions are working and which ones need modification. Interventions include pharmacologic, nonpharmacologic, and complementary therapies. Patient and family input remains the most important data to be considered in the assessment, planning, implementation, and evaluation of interventions.

REFERENCES

Bain, V. G. (1998). Jaundice, ascites, and hepatic encephalopathy. In D. Doyle, G. W. Hanks, & N. MacDonald (Eds.), *Oxford textbook of palliative medicine* (2nd ed., pp. 557-571). New York: Oxford University Press.

Baines, M. J. (1992). Symptom management and palliative care. In J. G. Evans & T. F. Williams (Eds.), *Oxford textbook of geriatric medicine* (pp. 685-696). New York: Oxford University Press.

Baines, M. J. (1998). The pathophysiology and management of malignant intestinal obstruction. In D. Doyle, G. W. Hanks, & N. MacDonald (Eds.), *Oxford textbook of palliative medicine* (2nd ed., pp. 526-534). New York: Oxford University Press.

Baines, M., Oliver, D. J., & Carter, R. L. (1985). Medical management of intestinal obstruction in patients with advanced malignant disease: A clinical and pathological study. *Lancet, 2,* 990-993.

Barbour, L. (1999). Dysphagia. In C. Yarbro, M. Frogge, & M. Goodman (Eds.), *Cancer symptom management* (2nd ed., pp. 209-227). Sudbury, MA: Jones & Bartlett.

Bates, B., Bickley, L. S., & Hoekelman, R. A. (1995). *A guide to physical examination and history taking* (6th ed., pp. 331-360). Philadelphia: Lippincott.

Baum, B. J., & Ship, J. A. (1994). The oral cavity. In W. R. Hazzard, E. L. Bierman, J. P. Blass, W. H. Ettinger Jr., & J. B. Halter (Eds.), *Principles of geriatric medicine and gerontology* (3rd ed., pp. 431-439). New York: McGraw-Hill.

Bisanz, A. (1997). Managing bowel elimination problems in patients with cancer. *Oncology Nursing Forum, 24,* 679-686.

Blom, M., Dawidson, I., & Angmar-Manson, B. (1992). The effect of acupuncture on buccal blood flow assessed by laser Doppler flowmeter: A pilot study. *Caries Research, 24,* 428.

Bruera, E., & Neumann, C. (1998). Management of specific symptom complexes in patients receiving palliative care. *Canadian Medical Association Journal, 158,* 1717-1726.

Cattau, E. L., Benjamin, S. B., Knuff, T. E., & Castell, D.O. (1982). The accuracy of the physical exam in the diagnosis of suspected ascites. *Journal of the American Medical Association, 247,* 1164-1167.

Cheskin, L. J., & Schuster, M. M. (1994). Constipation. In W. R. Hazzard, E. L. Bierman, J. P. Blass, W. H. Ettinger, Jr., & J. R. Halter (Eds.), *Principles of geriatric medicine and gerontology* (3rd ed., pp. 1267-1273). New York: McGraw-Hill.

Conill, C., Verger, E., Henriquez, I., Saiz, N., Espier, M., & Lugo, F. (1997). Symptom prevalence in the last week of life. *Journal of Pain and Symptom Management, 14,* 328-331.

Cooke, C., Admedzel, S., & Mayberry, J. (1996). Xerostomia—a review. *Palliative Medicine, 10,* 284-292.

Curless, R., & James, O. F. W. (1992). The oesophagus. In J. G. Evans & T. F. Williams (Eds.), *Oxford textbook of geriatric medicine* (pp. 196-211). New York: Oxford University Press.

Dahlin, C. M., & Goldsmith, T. (2001). Dysphagia, dry mouth, and hiccups. In B. R. Ferrell & N. Coyle (Eds.), *Textbook of palliative nursing* (pp. 122-138). New York: Oxford University Press.

Davies, A. (1997). The management of xerostomia: A review. *European Journal of Cancer Care, 6,* 209-214.

Davies, A. N., Broadley, K., & Beighton, D. (2001). Xerostomia in patients with advanced cancer. *Journal of Pain and Symptom Management, 22,* 820-825.

Derby, S., & Portenoy, R. K. (1997). Assessment and management of opioid-induced constipation. In R. K. Portenoy & E. Bruera (Eds.), *Topics in palliative care, Vol. 1* (pp. 95-112). New York: Oxford University Press.

D'Olimpio, J. (2001). Contemporary drug therapy in palliative care: New directions. *Cancer Investigation, 19,* 413-423.

Doyle, D. (1994). *Domiciliary palliative care: A handbook for family doctors and community nurses* (Oxford General Practice Series 27). New York: Oxford University Press.

Easton, K. (1999). *Gerontological rehabilitation nursing.* Philadelphia: Saunders.

Economou, D. C. (2001). Bowel management: Constipation, diarrhea, obstruction, and ascites. In B. R. Ferrell & N. Coyle (Eds.), *Textbook of palliative nursing* (pp. 139-155). New York: Oxford University Press.

Edes, T. D., Walk, B. E., & Austin, J. L. (1990). Diarrhea in tube-fed patients: Feeding formula not necessarily the cause. *American Journal of Medicine, 88,* 91-93.

Enck, R. (2002a). Malignant ascites [Editorial]. *American Journal of Hospice and Palliative Care, 19,* 7-8.

Enck, R. C. (2002b). *The medical care of terminally ill patients* (2nd ed.). Baltimore: Johns Hopkins University Press.

Ezzone, S., Baker, C., Rosselet, R., & Terepka, E. (1998). Music as an adjunct to antiemetic therapy. *Oncology Nursing Forum, 10,* 27-35.

Fainsinger, R. L., Spachynski, K., Hanson, J., & Bruera, E. (1994). Symptom control in terminally ill patients with malignant bowel obstruction. *Journal of Pain and Symptom Management, 9,* 12-18.

Fallon, M., & O'Neill, B. (1997). ABC of palliative care: Constipation and diarrhea. *British Medical Journal, 315,* 1293-1296.

Fallon, M., & Welsh, J. (1998). The management of gastrointestinal symptoms. In C. Faull, Y. Carter, & R. Woof (Eds.), *Handbook of palliative care* (pp. 134-156). Oxford: Blackwell Science.

Frank, L., Kleinman, L., Farup, C., Taylor, L., & Miner, P. (1999). Psychometric validation of a constipation symptom assessment questionnaire. *Scandinavian Journal of Gastroenterology, 9*, 870-877.

Gallick, H. L., Weaver, D. W., Sachs, R. J., & Bouwman, D. L. (1986). Intestinal obstruction in cancer patients: An assessment of risk factors and outcome. *American Surgeon, 52*, 434-437.

Heneghan, M. A., & O'Grady, J. G. (2001). Palliative care in liver disease. In J. M. Addington-Hall & I. J. Higginson (Eds.), *Palliative care for non-cancer patients* (pp. 82-103). New York: Oxford University Press.

Hickey, J. (1997). Rehabilitation of neuroscience patients. In J. Hickey (Ed.), *The clinical practice of neurological and neurosurgical nursing* (4th ed., p. 255). Philadelphia: Lippincott.

Johnson, J. T., Ferretti, G. A., Nethery, W. J., Valdez, I. H., Fox, P. C., Ng, D., et al. (1993). Oral pilocarpine for post-irradiation xerostomia in patients with head and neck cancer. *New England Journal of Medicine, 329*, 390-395.

Kazanowski, M. (2001). Symptom management in palliative care. In M. Matzo & D. Sherman (Eds.), *Palliative care nursing: Quality care to the end of life* (pp. 327-361). New York: Springer.

Kemp, C. (1999). *Terminal illness: A guide to nursing care* (2nd ed.). Philadelphia: Lippincott.

King, C. (2001). Nausea and vomiting. In B. Ferrell & N. Coyle (Eds.), *Textbook of palliative nursing* (pp. 107-121). New York: Oxford University Press.

Kolodzik, P. W., & Eilers, M. A. (1991). Hiccups (singultus): Review and approach to management. *Annals of Emergency Medicine, 20*, 565-573.

Langmead, L., & Rampton, D. S. (2001). Review article: Herbal treatment in gastrointestinal and liver disease—benefits and dangers. *Alimentary Pharmacology Therapy, 15*, 1239-1252.

Lederle, F. A., Busch, D. L., Mattox, K. M., West, M. J., & Aske, D. M. (1990). Cost-effective treatment of constipation in the elderly: A randomized double-blind comparison of sorbitol and lactulose. *American Journal of Medicine, 89*, 597-601.

Levy, M. H. (1991). Constipation and diarrhea in cancer patients. *Cancer Bulletin, 43*, 412-422.

Lewis, J. H. (1985). Hiccups: Causes and cures. *Journal of Clinical Gastroenterology, 12*, 539-552.

Mannix, K. (1998). Palliation of nausea and vomiting. In D. Doyle, G. Hanks, & N. MacDonald (Eds.), *Oxford textbook of palliative medicine* (2nd ed., pp. 489-499). New York: Oxford University Press.

McMillan, S. C., & Williams, F. A. (1989). Validity and reliability of the Constipation Assessment Scale. *Cancer Nursing, 12*, 183-188.

Mercadante, S. (1997). Assessment and management of mechanical bowel obstruction. In R. K. Portenoy & E. Bruera (Eds.), *Topics in palliative care, Vol. 1* (pp. 113-130). New York: Oxford University Press.

Mercadante, S., LaRosa, S., Nicolosi, G., & Garofalo, S. L. (1998). Temporary drainage of symptomatic malignant ascites by a catheter inserted under computerized tomography. *Journal of Pain and Symptom Management, 15*, 374-378.

Murray, J., Rao S., & Schulze-Delrieu, K. (1997). Esophageal diseases. In A. Perlman & K. Schulze-Delrieu (Eds.), *Deglutition and its disorders: Anatomy, physiology, clinical diagnosis and management* (pp. 383-418). San Diego: Singular Publishing.

Oncology Nursing Society. (1994). *Radiation therapy patient care record: A tool for documenting nursing care*. Pittsburgh: Oncology Nursing Society Press.

Piper, B. F., Lindsey, A. M., Dodd, M. J., Ferketich, S., Paul, S. M., & Weller, S. (1989). The development of an instrument to measure the subjective dimension of fatigue. In S. G. Funk, E. M. Tornquist, M. T. Champangen, L. A. Copp., & Weise, R. A. (Eds.). Key aspects of comfort: *Management of pain, fatigue and nausea* (pp. 199-208). New York: Springer Publishers.

Portenoy, R. (1994). Management of common opioid side effects during long term therapy of cancer pain. *Annals of the Academy of Medicine of Singapore, 23*, 160-170.

Ramirez F. C., & Graham D. Y. (1992). Treatment of intractable hiccup with baclofen: results of a double-blind randomized, controlled, cross-over study. *American Journal of Gastroenterology, 87*, 1789-1791.

Ratnaike, R. N. (1999). *Diarrhoea and constipation in geriatric practice*. New York: Cambridge University Press.

Reuben, D., & Mor, V. (1986). Nausea and vomiting in terminal cancer patients. *Archives of Internal Medicine, 146*, 2021-2023.

Rhodes, V., & McDaniel, R. (1997). Measuring nausea, vomiting and retching. In M. Frank-Stromberg & S. Olsen (Eds.), *Instruments for clinical health-care research* (2nd ed., pp. 509-517). Sudbury, MA: Jones and Bartlett.

Rhodes, V., & McDaniel, R. (2001). Nausea, vomiting and retching: Complex problems in palliative care. *CA: A Cancer Journal for Clinicians, 51*, 232-248.

Robinson, C. B., Fritch, M., Hullett, L., Petterson, M. A., Sikkema, S., & Theuninck, L. (2000). Development of a protocol to prevent opioid-induced constipation in patients with cancer: A research utilization project. *Clinical Journal of Oncology Nursing, 4*(2), 79-84.

Ross, D. D., & Alexander, C. S. (2001). Management of common symptoms in terminally ill patients: Part II. Constipation, delirium, and dyspnea. *American Family Physician, 64*, 1019-1026.

Rousseau, P. (1995). Hiccups. [Review Article]. *Southern Medical Journal, 88*, 175-181.

Rudd, N., & Worlding, J. (1998). The management of people with head and neck cancers. In C. Faull, Y. Carter, & R. Woof (Eds.), *Handbook of palliative care* (pp. 240-255). Malden, MA: Blackwell Science.

Runyon, B. A. (1998). Ascites and spontaneous bacterial peritonitis. In M. Feldman, B. F. Scharschmidt, & M. H.

Sleisenger (Eds.), *Sleisenger and Fordtran's gastrointestinal and liver disease: Pathophysiology, diagnosis, management, Vol. 2.* (6th ed., pp. 1310-1333). Philadelphia: Saunders.

Runyon, B. A., Hoefs, J. C., & Morgan, T. R. (1988). Ascitic fluid analysis in malignancy-related ascites. *Hepatology, 8,* 1104-1109.

Runyon, B. A., Montano, A. A., Akrivadis, E. A., Antillon, M. R., Irving, M. A., & McHutchison, J. G. (1992). The serum-ascites gradient is superior to the exudate-transudate concept in the differential diagnosis of ascites. *Annals of Internal Medicine, 117,* 215.

Schaefer, D. C., & Cheskin, L. J. (1998). Constipation in the elderly. *American Family Physician, 58,* 907-919. Retrieved April 1, 2002, from http://www.aafp.org/afp/980915ap/schaefer.html

Sreebny, L. M., & Valdini, A. (1987). Xerostomia: A neglected symptom. *Archives of Internal Medicine, 147,* 1333-1337.

Sreebny, L. M., & Valdini, A. (1988). Xerostomia. Part I: Relationship to other oral symptoms and salivary gland hypofunction. *Oral Pathology, 66,* 451-458.

Sykes, N. P. (1996). An investigation of the ability of oral naloxone to correct opioid-related constipation in patients with advanced cancer. *Palliative Medicine, 10,* 135-144.

Sykes, N. P. (1998). Constipation and diarrhoea. In D. Doyle, G. W. Hanks, & N. MacDonald (Eds.), *Oxford textbook of palliative medicine* (2nd ed., pp. 513-526). New York: Oxford University Press.

Timiras, P. (1994). Aging of the gastrointestinal tract and liver. In P. Timiras (Ed.), *Physiological basis of aging and geriatrics* (pp. 247-257). Boca Raton, FL: CRC Press.

Twycross, R., & Regnard, C. (1998). Dysphagia, dyspepsia, and hiccup. In D. Doyle, G. W. Hanks, & N. MacDonald (Eds.), *Oxford textbook of palliative medicine* (2nd ed., pp. 499-512). New York: Oxford University Press.

Ventafridda, V., Ripamonti, C., Bianchi, M., Sbanotto, A., & De Conno, F. (1986). A randomized study on oral morphine and methadone in the treatment of cancer pain. *Journal of Pain and Symptom Management, 1,* 203-207.

Ventafridda, V. Ripamonti, C., Sbanotto, A., & De Conno, F. (1998). Mouth care. In D. Doyle, G. W. Hanks, & N. MacDonald (Eds.), *Oxford textbook of palliative medicine* (2nd ed., pp. 691-707). New York: Oxford University Press.

Vickers, A. J. (1996). Can acupuncture have specific effects on health? A systematic literature review of acupuncture anti-emesis trials. *Journal of the Royal Society of Medicine, 89,* 303-311.

Wadler, S. (2001). Treatment guidelines for chemotherapy-induced diarrhea. *Oncology Special Edition, 4,* 81-84.

Walker, P., Watanabe, S., & Bruera, E. (1998). Baclofen, a treatment for chronic hiccup. *Journal of Pain and Symptom Management, 16,* 125-132.

Waller, A., & Caroline, N. (1996). *Handbook of palliative care in cancer.* Newton, MA: Butterworth-Heinemann.

White, I. D., Hoskin, P. J., Hanks, G. W., & Bliss, J. M. (1989). Morphine and dryness of the mouth. *BMJ, 298,* 1222-1223.

Whitehead, W. E., Chaussade, S., Corazziari, E., et al. (1991). Report of an international workshop on management of constipation. *Gastroenterology International, 4,* 99-113.

Wickham, R. (1999). Nausea and vomiting. In C. Yarbro, M. Frogge, & M. Goodman (Eds.), *Cancer symptom management* (2nd ed., pp. 228-253). Sudbury, MA: Jones and Bartlett.

Wong, P. W., & Kadakia, S. (1999). How to deal with chronic constipation: A stepwise method of establishing and treating the source of the problem. *Postgraduate Medicine, 106,* 6. Retrieved April 1, 2002, from http://www.post-gradmed.com/issues/1999/11_99/wong.htm

Woodward, M. C. (1999a). Constipation: Aetiology and diagnosis. In R. N. Ratnaike (Ed.), *Diarrhoea and constipation in geriatric practice* (pp. 187-193). Cambridge, UK: Cambridge University Press.

Woodward, M. C. (1999b). Constipation: Issues and management. In R. N. Ratnaike (Ed.), *Diarrhoea and constipation in geriatric practice* (pp. 194-200). Cambridge, UK: Cambridge University Press.

20 FATIGUE AND WEAKNESS

Marianne LaPorte Matzo and Deborah Witt Sherman

Case Study

Ms. L. is a 68-year-old woman diagnosed with metastatic breast cancer. Following a lumpectomy, she began a four-cycle course of chemotherapy with doxorubicin (Adriamycin) and cyclophosphamide (Cytoxan), which was followed by paclitaxel (Taxol). She is now receiving adjuvant radiation. She realizes that the intent of treatment is not cure, but rather to prevent further disease progression and promote her quality of life. Members of the palliative care team have followed Ms. L. from the cancer center. Concerned with her physical, emotional, social, and spiritual health, the palliative care nurse practitioner assesses her symptoms, including fatigue. Ms. L. reports "feeling exhausted with little or no physical or emotional energy for work." As a single woman who owns an advertising agency, she feels the pressures of maintaining her business, and emphasizes the emotional investment she has in her work. She begins to cry as she expresses her sense of "overwhelming tiredness, yet an inability to sleep through the night." Her comment is "I can't seem to keep it together. I am even having trouble concentrating, and everything I do takes twice as long. I am very irritable and feel down. My friends do help me, but it is very difficult since I have really no family to rely on."

The palliative care nurse recognizes the cumulative effects of surgery, chemotherapy, and radiation, as well as the emotional and existential burdens of diagnosis with a life-threatening illness. In order to identify the underlying, multidimensional aspects of fatigue, a complete history, review of systems, physical examination, and laboratory data are warranted, as well as an assessment of Ms. L.'s emotional well-being. It is recognized that depression and fatigue can be correlated.

Ms. L. has experienced the physical and emotional trauma of surgery, anesthesia, and anesthetics, as well as fatigue induced by chemotherapy. She became neutropenic and anemic during the chemotherapy regimen and was treated with epoetin alfa (Procrit) and pegfilgrastim (Neulasta). The radiation therapy now exacerbates her fatigue, which nearly 100% of patients experience toward the end of the treatment cycle. Given the various etiologies of fatigue, the palliative care team, in accordance with Ms. L.'s goals and preferences, extent of disease, and coexisting symptoms, must develop a comprehensive plan of care. The goals of care will be to focus on treating symptoms that exacerbate fatigue, preventing fatigue, identifying activities that increase fatigue, and restoring energy.

INTRODUCTION

Fatigue is one of the most common symptoms experienced by older adults with cancer and other incurable, progressive illnesses that negatively influence the quality of their lives (Ferrell, Grant, Dean, Funk, Ly, 1996; Richardson & Ream, 1996). Fatigue affects patients' relationships with others, self-perception, ability to function, and sense of hope. It can also compound the suffering associated with life-threatening illness. As an invisible wound that can be extremely debilitating, fatigue can begin to shape the life

Adapted from Morrison, R. S., Meier, D. E. (Eds.). (2003). *Geriatric palliative care*. New York: Oxford University Press.

of the older adult and pose great challenges (Harpham, 1999). Like pain, fatigue is what the patient says it is; it is a subjective experience that must be taken seriously by health care practitioners. In palliative care, it is of value to understand the experience of fatigue by older adults and its relevance to various disease states and associated therapies (Small & Lamb, 1999).

PREVALENCE OF FATIGUE

The symptom of fatigue has been poorly clinically defined. A study conducted by the World Health Organization, which included 1840 palliative care patients, documented that half (51%) of the patients experienced fatigue (Vainio & Auvinen, 1996). The overall prevalence of fatigue, defined as diminished energy, for patients with metastatic cancer has been reported to exceed 75% in multiple surveys (Breitbart, Esch, & Portenoy, 1997). In a study of the dimensions of symptom distress in women with advanced lung cancer, fatigue was reported as one of the most prevalent symptoms (Sarna & Brecht, 1997). Prevalence rates have been reported to be as high as 95% for patients receiving chemotherapy, radiation therapy, and immunotherapy (Irvine, Vincent, Bubela, Thompson, & Graydon, 1991).

Fatigue is also a common symptom for patients with human immunodeficiency virus (HIV) infection and acquired immunodeficiency syndrome (AIDS), with a prevalence that ranges from 20% to 60% (Adinolfi, 2001), affecting a greater percentage of women with AIDS (69%) than men (49%) (Breitbart, McDonald, Rosenfeld, Monkman, & Passik, 1998). In a study of patients with stage IV AIDS, more than half reported fatigue (Darko, McCutchan, Kripke, Gillin, & Golshan, 1992). The prevalence of fatigue has also been documented in patients with end-stage renal disease, coronary artery disease, and all gradations of rheumatoid arthritis, diseases that commonly afflict older adults (Dean & Anderson, 2001).

With regard to palliative care, a retrospective study was conducted based on the charts of 100 consecutive cancer patients who had been referred to a palliative care consult team within a tertiary acute care hospital (Jenkins, Schulz, Hanson, & Bruera, 2000). The results indicated, based on the Edmonton Symptom Assessment Scale (ESAS), that fatigue, loss of appetite, and diminished well-being were the most intense symptoms reported. The authors concluded that the assessment and management of fatigue should be a priority of the palliative care team.

FATIGUE IN THE OLDER ADULT

When treating the older adult in palliative care, the potential for confounding pathology secondary to the patient's age cannot be ignored. It is often very difficult to discern if the fatigue that the elder is experiencing is secondary to depression, various treatment modalities, congestive heart failure, anemia, hypothyroidism, diabetes, or fibromyalgia, to name a few conditions to be considered in the differential diagnosis. A study by Karlsen, Larsen, Tandberg, and Jorgensen (1999) compared the prevalence of fatigue in patients with Parkinson's disease (PD) with that in healthy older adults to determine if fatigue was an independent symptom of PD. Forty-four percent of the elders with PD and 18% of the elder control subjects reported fatigue. Fatigue was associated in this study with depression, dementia, the use of sleeping pills, disease severity and duration, and levodopa dose. It was concluded that fatigue was an independent symptom of PD that overlapped, but was not causally related to, depressive symptoms.

Often, the conventional wisdom is that, because a person is of advanced age, fatigue is a normal consequence of the aging process. Many elder patients erroneously consider fatigue to be inevitable, and therefore not a symptom to be treated. In fact, older adults may not even report symptoms of weakness and fatigue to their primary care provider. Therefore, the health care provider should include a careful assessment of fatigue for all older adult patients. Many causes of fatigue can be treated, even for the elder palliative care patient. The goal for the health care provider related to the symptom of fatigue is to improve the patient's quality of life by treating the symptom and teaching the older adult coping mechanisms and lifestyle changes.

CONCEPT OF FATIGUE

Fatigue has been characterized by patients with such descriptors as "worn out," "weary," "exhausted," "sleepiness," "low energy," "worn down," "bone-tired," and "rubber knees."

EVIDENCE-BASED PRACTICE

Reference: Studenski, S., Perera, S., Wallace, D., Chandler, J., Duncan, P. W., Rooney, E., et al. (2003). Physical performance measures in the clinical setting. *Journal of the American Geriatrics Society, 51,* 314-322.

Research Question: The study was designed to assess the ability of gait speed alone and a three-item lower extremity performance battery to predict 12-month rates of hospitalization, decline in health, and decline in function in primary care settings serving older adults.

Design: Prospective cohort study of primary care programs.

Sample and Setting: 487 persons ages 65 and older utilizing a Medicare health maintenance organization (HMO) and the Veterans Affairs (VA) system for primary health care.

Methods: Lower extremity performance was evaluated on the Established Population for Epidemiologic Studies of the Elderly (EPESE) battery, which included gait speed, chair stands, and tandem balance tests. In addition, data were collected on demographics, health care use, health status, functional status, Probability of Repeated Admission scale (Pra) scores, and primary physician's hospitalization risk estimate.

Results: Veterans had poorer health and higher health care use than HMO members did. Gait speed alone and the EPESE battery predicted hospitalization; 41% (21/51) of slow walkers (gait speed < 0.6 m/sec) were hospitalized at least once, compared with 26% (70/266) of intermediate walkers (0.6 to 1.0 m/sec) and 11% (15/136) of fast walkers (>1.0 m/sec) ($p < .0001$). The relationship was stronger in the HMO than in the VA population. Both performance measures remained independent predictors after accounting for Pra score. The EPESE battery was superior to gait speed when both Pra score and primary physician's risk estimate were included. Both performance measures predicted decline in function and health status in both health systems. Performance measures, alone or in combination with self-report measures, were more able to predict outcomes than self-report alone.

Implications for Nursing Practice: Gait speed and a physical performance battery are brief, quantitative estimates of future risk for hospitalization and decline in health and function in clinical populations of older adults.

Conclusion: Physical performance measures might serve as easily accessible "vital signs" to screen older adults in clinical settings.

Practitioners also use terms such as *listlessness, lassitude, lethargy,* and *malaise.* The historical development of the concept of fatigue has produced the following identifying criteria of fatigue: (1) a subjective perception; (2) an alteration in neuromuscular and metabolic processes; (3) a decrease in physical performance; and (4) a deterioration in mental and physical activities (Dean & Anderson, 2001). To date, there has been no clear consensus regarding the definition of fatigue or a description of the phenomenon. However, there is an appreciation of the differentiation between "normal" fatigue experienced by the majority of the population, and clinical fatigue associated with disease or its treatments (Breitbart et al., 1997). The assessment of etiol-

ogy, severity, duration, and impact of clinical fatigue will be important in developing a conceptual and operational definition of fatigue.

Currently, there are various definitions of fatigue documented in the literature. Piper, Lindsey, Dodd, et al. (1989) defined fatigue as "a subjective feeling of tiredness that is influenced by circadian rhythm; it can vary in unpleasantness, duration, and intensity; when acute it serves a protective function and when prolonged, excessive or chronic, it may lead to an aversion to activity." The North American Nursing Diagnosis Association has defined fatigue as "an overwhelming, sustained sense of exhaustion and decreased capacity for physical or emotional work" (Tiesinga, Dassen, & Halfens, 1996, p. 87).

One of the most comprehensive definitions, relevant to palliative care, is of fatigue as "the awareness of a decreased capacity for physical and/or mental activity due to an imbalance in the availability, utilization, and/or restoration of resources needed to perform activity" (Aaronson et al., 1999, p. 45).

Some practitioners differentiate fatigue from weakness, while others believe that they accompany each other and comprise a syndrome known as asthenia (Dean & Anderson, 2001). Asthenia is an unpleasant sensation experienced when an individual's physiologic resources are exceeded, particularly within the context of several clinical conditions including chronic fatigue syndrome, depression, acute or chronic infection, endocrine diseases such as diabetes, chronic heart failure, chronic pulmonary disease, AIDS, and cancer (Neuenschwander & Breura, 1998).

At various points in the course of their illness, older adults may interpret fatigue differently. For many elders newly diagnosed with a life-threatening illness, fatigue has been an indication or warning symptom of the diagnosis. As treatment ensues, fatigue may be understood as the side effects of treatment, and for older adults with recurrence or exacerbation of illness, fatigue is interpreted as the end of a very long struggle (Dean & Anderson, 2001).

In a qualitative study of the experience of fatigue in cancer patients (Magnusson, Moller, Ekman, & Wallgren, 1999), fatigue was illustrated as a process with three major categories. The first was the experience of fatigue (of loss, need, psychological stress, emotional affect, malaise, abnormal weakness, and difficulty taking initiative). The second category was the consequence of fatigue, specifically social limitation, affected self-esteem, and affected quality of life. The third category was the action, or coping with the fatigue. These authors stated that how fatigue is expressed is important in caring for patients with cancer.

Multidimensional Aspects of Fatigue

Fatigue, like pain, is a multidimensional, subjective experience of diverse etiologies (Breitbart et al., 1997). As a complex phenomenon, fatigue has physical, emotional, cognitive, and behavioral dimensions (Richardson & Ream, 1996).

The possible physical etiologies of fatigue in the medically ill elder include medical and physical conditions (specifically the underlying disease itself), associated treatment of disease (chemotherapy, radiation, surgery, and biologic response modifiers), intercurrent systemic disorders (anemia, infection, pulmonary disorders, hepatic failure, heart failure, renal failure, malnutrition, and neuromuscular disorders), sleep disorders, chronic pain, use of centrally acting drugs, and lack of mobility and lack of exercise (Chochivov & Breitbart, 2000). From a physiologic perspective, fatigue has been attributed to excessive energy consumption and the depletion of hormones, neurotransmitters, or other essential substrates (Aaronson et al., 1999).

Research indicates that the pathophysiology or mechanisms of fatigue/asthenia differ from one clinical condition to another. Within a physiologic context, fatigue can be classified according to two types: central or peripheral. In central fatigue, the motor pathways in the central nervous system fail to sustain recruitment and/or frequency of motor units or the generation of descending volleys in the motor cortex as a result of neurotransmitter depletion. Research data suggest that pharmacologically altered brain 5-hydroxytryptamine (serotonin) activity may influence dopamine concentration in the brain, altering the perception of fatigue. Central fatigue most closely correlates with chronic disease (Swain, 2000).

In peripheral fatigue, there is failure in the propagation of muscle action potential resulting in impaired excitation–contraction coupling (Neuenschwander & Breura, 1998). Peripheral fatigue is observed in chronic diseases that involve muscle wasting, inflammation, or joint abnormalities (e.g., rheumatoid arthritis, systemic lupus erythematosus) (Swain, 2000).

Thus in any specific clinical condition, the question is whether a person's failure to exert effort is caused by a failure in the neural drive, such as fatigue in the mind or central nervous system, or a failure of neurotransmission in the muscles. In the case of cancer-related fatigue (CRF)/asthenia, three associated physiologic mechanisms may affect the central nervous system or muscles (Neuenschwander & Breura, 1998):

1. Direct tumor effects (mechanically by destruction, such as metastasis, or metabolically by lipolytic factors or tumor degradation products)

2. Tumor-induced products (e.g., tumor necrosis factors [asthenin/cachectin] and other cytokines such as prostaglandin E_2, interleukins 1 and 6, and interferon)

3. Tumor-accompanying factors (e.g., cachexia, infection, anemia, hypoxia, neurologic disorders, pharmacologic side effects, paraneoplastic effects, metabolic factors, dehydration)

In cancer populations, there has been a documented relationship between asthenia and cachexia, although one may exist without the other. However, in patients with advanced cancer, both are usually present with asthenia as an epiphenomenon of the cachexia syndrome. In malignancy, changes in carbohydrate, fat, and protein metabolism, as well as the presence of tumor necrosis factors and cytokines as previously mentioned, lead to cachexia and resultant loss of muscle mass. This partially explains cachexia-related asthenia.

The concept of fatigue also encompasses emotional, cognitive, and behavioral dimensions. Psychosocial etiologic factors of fatigue in the medically ill person include anxiety or depressive disorders, stress, and related environmental reinforcers (Portenoy, 2000). In healthy individuals, overexertion may produce ordinary fatigue, which is relieved relatively quickly by rest. Fatigue may also be interpreted as a source of satisfaction given the accomplishment of hard work. However, fatigue associated with illness is perceived as more severe, and comes on after a shorter period of time and with less exertion than ordinary fatigue. It is often described as a general feeling of tiredness or "sapped" energy that occurs on a daily basis and is present intermittently throughout the day or during the evening after a day of normal activities. Fatigue also leads to a decline in mental or intellectual activities, as well as a diminished motivation or capacity to attend (Breitbart et al., 1997). With fatigue comes a decreased ability to concentrate, which impedes engagement in a variety of activities (Small & Lamb, 1999).

For many individuals, fatigue is interpreted as an exacerbation of their condition. For example, in a study by Small and Lamb (1999), patients with chronic obstructive pulmonary disease (COPD) expressed an increase in fatigue as their breathing became more labored. They believed that the cause of their fatigue was their inability to obtain sufficient oxygen, and that labored breathing was a central feature of their fatigue. With restrictions of their activities imposed by fatigue, patients with COPD also expressed a loss of strength. The less they were able to do, the more tired they became with effort. Fatigue was also exacerbated by interrupted sleep, which led to prolonged and extreme feelings of exhaustion, and by psychological stress, which affected their fatigue through its effect on their breathing.

The patients in Small and Lamb's (1999) study also described the impact of fatigue on activities of daily living. Because of fatigue, they were unable to do heavy chores around the house or spur-of-the-moment activities. For many, fatigue limited self-care abilities, such as showering, which resulted in feelings of exhaustion. Lack of energy also resulted in changes in mood, such as irritability and frustration. Patients explained that "what bothers me most is not being able to get up and do what I want to do." The psychosocial impact of fatigue also resulted in changes in family roles and interfered with family and social relationships given that patients were too tired to participate fully in related events. Furthermore, patients frequently avoided social situations that might trigger or exacerbate their fatigue.

Classification of Fatigue as Acute or Chronic

Fatigue has been classified as either acute or chronic (Swain, 2000). According to Piper (1989), acute fatigue is a protective state, identifiably linked to a single cause, in usually healthy individuals. Acute fatigue has a rapid onset and short direction, and is viewed as normal when alleviated by restorative techniques such as rest, diet, exercise, and stress management. Acute fatigue has minor effects on activities of daily living and quality of life.

In contrast, chronic fatigue has an unknown physiologic purpose, and may be experienced without any relationship to exertion or activity. Chronic fatigue is frequently experienced by patients with life-threatening illness, having an insidious onset and persisting over time, typically longer than 6 months (Swain, 2000). Chronic fatigue is viewed as abnormal or pathologic, is generally not relieved by rest, and typically is not related to exertion. As a result, chronic fatigue has a significant negative effect on activities of daily living and quality of life.

CAUSES OF FATIGUE

In a healthy individual, a biologic mechanism controlled by the parasympathetic nervous system safeguards against the exhaustion of reserves and gives the body the signal that it is fatigued, and that it needs to rest. When the body is experiencing the stress and pathology of chronic disease or cancer, the body reserves can become depleted and ultimately unable to counterbalance the physiologic insults. The elder with cancer may experience fatigue in relation to the advanced stage of the disease and concurrent anemia and cachexia. Coexisting symptoms such as nausea and vomiting, inadequate nutrient intake, pain, immobility, loss of muscle mass, infection, metabolic disturbances, shortness of breath, possible gastric obstruction, and anxiety or depression also are associated with the elder's experience of fatigue. In addition, medications such as analgesics, psychotropics, and beta-blockers, can cause fatigue, as can alcohol (Breitbart et al., 1997).

The treatment for cancer (surgery, radiation, chemotherapy, and biologic response modifiers) can cause feelings of fatigue. With surgery, there is anxiety resulting from preoperative regimens and postoperative fatigue that can result from pain, direct tissue damage, anesthesia, sedatives, analgesics, and immobility. Fatigue may continue for as long as 6 months after a surgical intervention (Groenwald, Frogge, Goodman, & Yarbo, 1993). Among patients treated with radiation therapy, nearly 100% will experience fatigue, which tends to peak toward the end of the cycle; the fatigue experienced is dose dependent. Approximately 95% of the patients who receive chemotherapy feel that fatigue is one of the worst symptoms experienced within the first 2 weeks after treatment. Biologic response modifiers (interferon and interleukins) induce dose-related fatigue in 50% to 70% of the patients treated (Breitbart et al., 1997).

Patients with chronic conditions, such as fibromyalgia, may manifest progressive symptoms of psychogenic fatigue, physiologic fatigue, and pain. Given the unknown etiology of fibromyalgia, there are limited treatment options for this disease, with relief primarily achieved by the palliation of symptoms. Older adults who have lived with conditions such as fibromyalgia, rheumatoid arthritis, or chronic fatigue syndrome are at higher risk for suicide, particularly when comorbid depression occurs. In such situations, interventions such as medication management should be initiated (Cahill, 1999).

HIV-related fatigue is typically related to many different factors. These include lack of rest or exercise, inadequate nutrition, anemia, infections, thyroid problems, side effects of medications, sleep disturbances, and fever. Psychological distress such as depression or anxiety may also compound the fatigue (Adinolfi, 2001).

CORRELATES OF FATIGUE IN VARIOUS PATIENT POPULATIONS

Fatigue has been associated anecdotally with many factors, such as sleep disorders, anemia, systemic infection, depression, or the use of centrally acting drugs, such as opioids (Breitbart et al., 1997). Fatigue has also been associated with older age, advanced disease, and combined therapies (Fobair et al., 1986).

Correlates of fatigue in older women with heart failure were examined by Friedman and King (1995), based on interviews of 80 women hospitalized in the previous 12 months for heart failure. A second interview was conducted several months later with 57 of the participants. Fatigue was the most commonly reported symptom at both measurement times, and significantly increased over time. At time 1, sleep difficulties, chest pain, and sense of weakness contributed significantly to the variance in fatigue. At time 2, dyspnea was the only physical variable that contributed to fatigue (9%). Psychological factors, such as perceived stress, satisfaction with life, and optimism, explained less than 1% of the variance in fatigue beyond the physical symptoms.

Given that fatigue is integral to the experience of heart failure, interventions are needed to assist patients to cope with the experience of fatigue, such as pacing of activities, relaxation, and restful sleep. Friedman and King (1995) suggested that exercise may reduce fatigue in patients with heart failure. However, caution was expressed regarding the safety and benefits of physical training for patients with mild to moderate heart failure, given a lack of empirical data regarding the risk:benefit ratio.

Ingles, Eskes, and Phillips (1999) studied the presence of fatigue as a symptom after having had a stroke. This study compared 181 patients admitted to a stroke service to 56 elder control subjects living independently in the community. Subjects completed the Fatigue Impact Scale and the Geriatric Depression Scale; self-reported fatigue was greater in the stroke group (68%) as compared to the control group (36%) ($p < .001$). Forty-percent of the stroke group reported that fatigue was one of their worst symptoms and that this symptom was not related to time poststroke, severity, or location of the lesion. These findings suggest that fatigue can contribute to functional impairment. Therefore, the recognition and treatment of fatigue by a palliative care provider is an important consideration.

In older populations, fatigue is a common symptom, particularly evident in the older adult in long-term care facilities. Liao and Ferrell (2000) found, based on a sample of 199 ambulatory older residents (mean age 88; 82% female) of a single residential care facility, that fatigue was experienced for a median of 44 weeks. Significant positive correlations ($p < .005$) were reported between pain ($r = .36$), number of medications ($r = .26$), depression ($r = .57$), and instrumental activities of daily living ($r = .31$) and fatigue. Fatigue was also negatively correlated with a 3-minute walk ($r = -.29$). No significant correlations were found between fatigue and age, sex, mental status, or number of medical diagnoses. Multivariate regression analysis identified pain, number of medications, depression, and a 3-minute walk as significant predictors of fatigue intensity (multiple $R = .68$, $r^2 = .46$, $p < .02$). The authors concluded that fatigue is poorly recognized and undertreated in older people.

Depression may be the causal factor if the elder reports that the fatigue is worse in the morning, particularly if accompanied by unexplained weight loss (Frazer, Leicht, & Baker, 1996). The American Psychiatric Association has identified fatigue as a symptom of depression, but often it is difficult to determine if chronic fatigue is etiologically unrelated to an affective disorder or if the symptoms of chronic fatigue precipitated the depression (Aaronson, 1999).

In a sample of 88 patients with primary biliary cirrhosis, Cauch-Dudek, Abbey, Stewart, and Heathcote (1998) studied fatigue in relation to sleep, depression, and liver disease severity. The findings indicated that 68% of the sample reported fatigue lasting greater than 6 months. The Fatigue Severity Score (FSS) was correlated with sleep quality ($p = .0001$). Furthermore, fatigued patients had more sleep disturbance and depression than nonfatigued patients did. However, the FSS was not significantly correlated with age or duration of disease.

Based on a study of 41 patients with COPD, Breslin et al. (1998) reported that fatigue was correlated with forced expiratory volume ($r = -.32$, $p < .5$), exercise tolerance ($r = -.55$, $p < .05$), depression ($r = .44$, $p < .01$), and overall quality of life ($r = .75$, $p < .01$). Among the dimensions of fatigue, depression correlated with general and mental fatigue. Physical dimensions of fatigue correlated with the increased severity of pulmonary impairment, while cognitive components of fatigue, such as reduction in motivation and mental fatigue, were not highly correlated with the physical dimension of quality of life. However, all five dimensions of fatigue—general, physical, mental, reduction of motivation, and activity—were related to the total quality-of-life score.

In a study of patients with Hodgkin's disease (ages 19 to 74 years; 56% male) (Loge, Abrahamsen, Ekeberg, & Kaasa, 2000), fatigue was also correlated with psychiatric morbidity, specifically depression and anxiety ($r = -.41$ and .44, respectively). Twenty-six percent had fatigue for 6 months or longer. A multiple logistic regression analysis revealed that advanced age, anxiety, and no self-reported psychiatric problems during treatment were predictors of fatigue.

Differences in fatigue by treatment methods in women with breast cancer was studied by Woo, Dibble, Piper, Keating, and Weiss (1998), using the Piper Fatigue Scale. The results indicated significant differences in the total fatigue scores ($p < .03$) based on type of treatment. Specifically, women who received combined chemotherapy and radiation therapy had the highest fatigue scores (mean = 4.8, standard deviation = 2.0), and those who received only radiation therapy had the lowest fatigue scores (mean = 2.7, standard deviation = 2.0). The findings suggest the need for anticipatory guidance regarding the side effects, such as fatigue, of various treatment regimens. These findings are also consistent with those of Mast (1998), who found, based on a sample of 109 women 1 to 6 years after treatment for stage I to III breast cancer, that low to moderate fatigue persisted for women and was associated with the presence of concurrent illness. When concurrent illness was taken into account, fatigue was significantly related to treatment with chemotherapy, irrespective of the length of time since treatment, age, disease stage, or tamoxifen use.

Based on a sample of 24 oncology patients receiving radiation therapy for breast cancer, Miakowski and Lee (1999) also reported a high incidence of fatigue and pain, although patients reported less morning than evening fatigue. Those

patients who completed a higher proportion of their radiation treatments also reported greater sleep disturbance, which contributed to their perceived fatigue. Fatigue was not influenced by age, stage of disease, time since surgery, weight, or length of time since diagnosis. However, fatigue was significantly related to symptom distress, psychological distress, quality of life, and self-reported fatigue relief strategies. The most frequently reported fatigue relief strategies were "sitting" and "sleeping," with sleep being the most effective strategy used. Other less frequently used strategies were socializing and handicrafts.

In a study of the patterns of exercise and fatigue in physically active cancer survivors ($N = 219$), Schwartz (1998) reported that 69% of the participants experienced problems with CRF during treatment, with 52% describing CRF as

---

EVIDENCE-BASED PRACTICE

Reference: Hwang, S. S., Chang, V. T., Cogswell, J., & Kasimis, B. S. (2002). Clinical relevance of fatigue levels in cancer patients at a Veterans Administration Medical Center. *Cancer, 94,* 2481-2489.

Research Problem: Is there a correlation between fatigue levels with functional interference, symptom distress, and quality of life? Can this be used to determine clinically significant fatigue levels?

Design: Administered standard fatigue and performance scales.

Sample and Setting: 180 consecutive patients with cancer in a Veteran's Medical Center.

Methods: Patients completed the Functional Assessment of Cancer Therapy General and Fatigue subscales, the Memorial Symptom Assessment Scale–Short Form, the Zung Depression Scale, and the Brief Fatigue Inventory. The Karnofsky performance status (KPS) was determined for each patient. Multivariate analyses of variance were performed to compare fatigue models with different cut-off points to categorize fatigue levels. Cox proportional hazards

analysis was performed to assess the association between fatigue severity and survival.

Results: Increased fatigue levels were associated with greater symptom distress and decreased quality of life. A model with usual fatigue cut-off points of 0 (no fatigue), 1 to 2 (mild fatigue), 3 to 6 (moderate fatigue), and 7 to 10 (severe fatigue) was optimal in relation to functional interference items (Wilks multivariate criterion, 0.36; $F = 11.61$; $p < .0001$), symptom distress scores (Wilks, 0.52; $F = 10.41$; $p < .0001$), and quality-of-life scores (Wilks, 0.50; $F = 0.50$; $p < .0001$). Fatigue severity predicted survival in univariate analysis (chi-square test, 25.42; $p < .0001$). The KPS, stage of disease, and number of symptoms independently predicted survival in patients with fatigue.

Implications for Nursing Practice: Clinically relevant fatigue levels are correlated with symptom and quality-of-life measurements.

Conclusion: Patients with a *usual* fatigue severity greater than 3 or a *worst* fatigue severity greater than 4 on a 1 to 10 scale may require further assessment.

affecting their whole body. Although 26% of the participants felt most fatigued before exercise, exercise and rest were the most commonly used strategies for managing their symptoms. Patients with non-Hodgkin's lymphoma experienced significantly different CRF than patients with breast or prostate cancer and reported fewer benefits of exercise. The majority of participants, however, believed that regular exercise would make them less likely to have health problems.

Berger and Farr (1999) identified indicators involving circadian activity-rest cycles associated with higher levels of CRF during the first three chemotherapy cycles of 72 women. Using the Piper Fatigue Scale, CRF was measured at the start and midpoint of each chemotherapy cycle. The results indicated that women who were less active and had increased night awakenings reported higher CRF at all three cycle midpoints. During the third chemotherapy cycle, women who were less active during the day, took more naps, and spent more time resting during a 24-hour period experienced higher CRF. The implication is that interventions that promote daytime activity and nighttime rest should be key considerations in managing fatigue.

FATIGUE AND QUALITY OF LIFE

Regardless of the age of the patient, fatigue has a profound effect on an older adult's quality of life. Incapability in carrying out role performance tasks can result in decreased self-esteem, social isolation, depression, increased health care utilization and costs, and increased morbidity (Ferrell et al., 1996). Vogelzang et al. (1997) recruited 419 cancer patients from 100,000 randomly selected U.S. households and found that 71% of these patients reported that fatigue affected their activities of daily living and 61% reported that fatigue affected their daily lives more than pain (19%) did. The daily routines that were affected "very much" or "somewhat" by fatigue were ability to work (61%), physical well-being (61%), ability to enjoy life in the moment (57%), emotional well-being (51%), intimacy with partner (44%), ability to take care of the family (42%), relationships with family and friends (38%), and concerns about mortality and survival (33%). As a goal of care and an outcome variable in palliative care, quality of life is a priority of patients, families, and health profession-

als. Research indicates that, in order to promote quality of life, fatigue, as a symptom, must be appropriately assessed and effectively treated.

ASSESSMENT OF FATIGUE

As a subjective symptom, practitioners most often rely on the elder's self-report of fatigue to evaluate its severity. However, fatigue does include observable characteristics and has an impact on quality of life. A comprehensive assessment of a patient with fatigue, obtained through a health history, review of systems (including a specific fatigue assessment), physical examination, and laboratory data, can assist the practitioner in discriminating between physiologic and psychogenic fatigue, depression, and the presence of correctable causes of fatigue. Appendix A reviews the characteristics of the commonly used fatigue assessment tools.

Health History

The health history should include a medical, psychiatric, family, social, and medication history, which may reveal associated conditions such as diabetes, hypothyroidism, sleep apnea, anxiety or depressive disorders, inherited metabolic disorders, or a history of alcohol or illegal drug use, as well as the possibility of sexually transmitted infections, which are often associated with fatigue and occur even in older populations.

Review of Systems

A review of systems with regard to fatigue focuses on changes in other body systems that may indicate potential health problems associated with fatigue, such as respiratory disorders (e.g., dyspnea), cardiac problems, anemia, cancers, depression, or electrolyte disorders. In older adult populations, including those with chronic, incurable illness, fatigue may also be a side effect of medical treatments, including both prescription and over-the-counter medications. Furthermore, in speaking with the patient, it is important to determine his or her emotional status, particularly whether the person speaks of his or her own death or has suicidal ideations.

The Fatigue Assessment

The fatigue assessment includes questions related to the six dimensions of fatigue (Piper, 1997) (Fig. 20-1):

Instructions: Many individuals can experience a sense of unusual or excessive tiredness whenever they become ill, receive treatment, or recover from their illness/treatment. This unusual sense of tiredness is not usually relieved either by a good night's sleep or by rest. Some call this symptom "fatigue" to distinguish it from the usual sense of tiredness.

For each of the following questions, please fill in the space provided for that response that best describes the fatigue you are experiencing now or for today. Please make every effort to answer each question to the best of your ability. If you are not experiencing fatigue now or for today, fill in the circle indicating "0" for your response. Thank you very much!

1. How long have you been feeling fatigue? (Check one response only).
   ☐ 1. Not feeling fatigue
   ☐ 2. Minutes
   ☐ 3. Hours
   ☐ 4. Days
   ☐ 5. Weeks
   ☐ 6. Months
   ☐ 7. Other (Please describe)

2. To what degree is the fatigue you are feeling now causing you distress?

No Distress										A Great Deal
☐	☐	☐	☐	☐	☐	☐	☐	☐	☐	☐
0	1	2	3	4	5	6	7	8	9	10

3. To what degree is the fatigue you are feeling now interfering with your ability to complete your work or school activities?

None										A Great Deal
☐	☐	☐	☐	☐	☐	☐	☐	☐	☐	☐
0	1	2	3	4	5	6	7	8	9	10

4. To what degree is the fatigue you are feeling now interfering with your ability to socialize with your friends?

None										A Great Deal
☐	☐	☐	☐	☐	☐	☐	☐	☐	☐	☐
0	1	2	3	4	5	6	7	8	9	10

5. To what degree is the fatigue you are feeling now interfering with your ability to engage in sexual activity?

None										A Great Deal
☐	☐	☐	☐	☐	☐	☐	☐	☐	☐	☐
0	1	2	3	4	5	6	7	8	9	10

6. Overall, how much is the fatigue, which you are now experiencing, interfering with your ability to engage in the kind of activities you enjoy doing?

None										A Great Deal
☐	☐	☐	☐	☐	☐	☐	☐	☐	☐	☐
0	1	2	3	4	5	6	7	8	9	10

7. How would you describe the degree of intensity or severity of the fatigue that you are experiencing now?

Mild										Severe
☐	☐	☐	☐	☐	☐	☐	☐	☐	☐	☐
0	1	2	3	4	5	6	7	8	9	10

8. To what degree would you describe the fatigue that you are experiencing now as being?

Pleasant										Unpleasant
☐	☐	☐	☐	☐	☐	☐	☐	☐	☐	☐
0	1	2	3	4	5	6	7	8	9	10

9. To what degree would you describe the fatigue that you are experiencing now as being?

Agreeable										Disagreeable
☐	☐	☐	☐	☐	☐	☐	☐	☐	☐	☐
0	1	2	3	4	5	6	7	8	9	10

10. To what degree would you describe the fatigue that you are experiencing now as being?

Protective										Destructive
☐	☐	☐	☐	☐	☐	☐	☐	☐	☐	☐
0	1	2	3	4	5	6	7	8	9	10

11. To what degree would you describe the fatigue that you are experiencing now as being?

Positive										Negative
☐	☐	☐	☐	☐	☐	☐	☐	☐	☐	☐
0	1	2	3	4	5	6	7	8	9	10

12. To what degree would you describe the fatigue which you are experiencing now as being:

Normal										Abnormal
☐	☐	☐	☐	☐	☐	☐	☐	☐	☐	☐
0	1	2	3	4	5	6	7	8	9	10

13. To what degree are you now feeling:

Strong										Weak
☐	☐	☐	☐	☐	☐	☐	☐	☐	☐	☐
0	1	2	3	4	5	6	7	8	9	10

14. To what degree are you now feeling:

Awake										Sleepy
☐	☐	☐	☐	☐	☐	☐	☐	☐	☐	☐
0	1	2	3	4	5	6	7	8	9	10

15. To what degree are you now feeling:

Lively										Listless
☐	☐	☐	☐	☐	☐	☐	☐	☐	☐	☐
0	1	2	3	4	5	6	7	8	9	10

16. To what degree are you now feeling:

Refreshed										Tired
☐	☐	☐	☐	☐	☐	☐	☐	☐	☐	☐
0	1	2	3	4	5	6	7	8	9	10

Fig. 20-1 Piper Fatigue Scale (PFS). (From Piper, B. F., Dibble, S. L., Dodd, M. J., Weiss, M. C., Slaughter, R. E., & Paul, S. M. [1998]. The revised Piper Fatigue Scale: Psychometric evaluation in women with breast cancer. *Oncology Nursing Forum, 25,* 677-684.)

17. To what degree are you now feeling:

Energetic   Unenergetic

☐ ☐ ☐ ☐ ☐ ☐ ☐ ☐ ☐ ☐ ☐
0 1 2 3 4 5 6 7 8 9 10

18. To what degree are you now feeling:

Patient   Impatient

☐ ☐ ☐ ☐ ☐ ☐ ☐ ☐ ☐ ☐ ☐
0 1 2 3 4 5 6 7 8 9 10

19. To what degree are you now feeling:

Relaxed   A Great Deal

☐ ☐ ☐ ☐ ☐ ☐ ☐ ☐ ☐ ☐ ☐
0 1 2 3 4 5 6 7 8 9 10

20. To what degree are you now feeling:

Exhilarated   Depressed

☐ ☐ ☐ ☐ ☐ ☐ ☐ ☐ ☐ ☐ ☐
0 1 2 3 4 5 6 7 8 9 10

21. To what degree are you now feeling:

Able to Concentrate   Unable to Concentrate

☐ ☐ ☐ ☐ ☐ ☐ ☐ ☐ ☐ ☐ ☐
0 1 2 3 4 5 6 7 8 9 10

22. To what degree are you now feeling:

Able to Remember   Unable to Remember

☐ ☐ ☐ ☐ ☐ ☐ ☐ ☐ ☐ ☐ ☐
0 1 2 3 4 5 6 7 8 9 10

23. To what degree are you now feeling:

Able to Think Clearly   Unable to Think Clearly

☐ ☐ ☐ ☐ ☐ ☐ ☐ ☐ ☐ ☐ ☐
0 1 2 3 4 5 6 7 8 9 10

24. Overall, what do you believe is *most* directly contributing to or causing your fatigue?

25. Overall, the *best* thing you have found to relieve your fatigue is:

26. Is there anything else you would like to add that would describe your fatigue better to us?

27. Are you experiencing any other symptoms right now?

SCORING PIPER FATIGUE SCALE (PFS) SURVEY RESULTS:

PFS current format and scoring instructions:

1. The PFS in its current form is composed of 22 numerically scaled, "0" to "10" items that measure four dimensions of subjective fatigue: behavioral/severity (6 items; nos. 2-7); affective meaning (5 items: nos. 8-12); sensory (5 items: nos. 13-17); and cognitive/mood (6 items: nos. 18-23). These 22 items are used to calculate the four sub-scale/dimensional scores and the total fatigue scores.
2. Five additional items (no. 1 and nos. 24-27) are not used to calculate subscale or total fatigue scores but are recommended to be kept on the scale as these items furnish rich, qualitative data. Item no. 1, in particular gives a categorical way in which to assess the duration of the respondent's fatigue.
3. To score the PFS, add the items contained on each specific subscale together and divide by the number of items on that subscale. This will give you a subscale score that remains on the same "0" to "10" numeric scale. Should you have missing item data, and the respondent has answered at least 75%-80% of the remaining items on that particular subscale, calculate the subscale mean score based on the number of items answered, and substitute that mean value for the missing item score (mean-item substitution).
4. Recalculate the subscale score. To calculate the total fatigue score, add the 22 item scores together and divide by 22 in order to keep the score on the same numeric "0" to "10" scale.

Severity Codes:

| 0 | NONE | 4-6 | MODERATE |
| 1-3 | MILD | 7-10 | SEVERE |

Fig. 20-1, cont'd.

1. Temporal dimension, which includes the assessment of the timing of fatigue (when it occurs), onset (from seconds to years), duration (chronic, i.e., for more than 6 months), and pattern (waking up fatigued, evening fatigue, transient, etc.), and changes in this dimension over time.
2. Sensory dimension, which focuses on how the fatigue feels. For example, is the fatigue localized (e.g., tired eyes, arms, legs), or generalized (e.g., whole-body tiredness, weariness, weakness, lethargy)? What is the intensity or severity of fatigue (using a 0 to 10 scale)? Additional assessment questions cover what exacerbates the fatigue (e.g., pain, nausea, vomiting, environmental heat, noise) and what helps the patient feel better or alleviates the symptoms (e.g., rest, food, listening to music).
3. Mental/cognitive dimension, which examines the patient's ability to concentrate and focus,

his or her attention span and recall, and if he or she reports being "mentally tired."

4. Affective/emotional dimension, which assesses the patient's irritability, impatience, mood changes, and depression and the significance of the fatigue.

5. Behavioral dimension, which considers the effect that the fatigue has on the patient's ability to perform activities of daily living (e.g., bathing, dressing, cooking, socializing, sexual activity). Family and practitioner observations regarding the patient's posture, gait, appearance (e.g., drooping shoulders), and lack of energy should also be assessed. Acute behavioral manifestations can include a change in alertness; chronic manifestations may not be obvious to the practitioner because of the ability of many patients to adapt to their fatigue. If the patient also has a dementing illness, the behavioral dimensions may be the only clue that the practitioner has regarding the presence of fatigue and the

6. Physiologic dimension, which includes biologic mechanisms such as laboratory tests, a complete physical examination, and determining if comorbid conditions such as diabetes, cardiac illness, or other disease factors are present.

Table 20-1 provides additional questions related to the assessment of the pattern of sleep and rest, the elder's perceptions/expression of fatigue, and the impact on his or her quality of life (Cahill, 1999).

Physical Examination

Physical examination includes the following assessment parameters:

- Vital signs to determine if fever, low blood pressure, or weak pulse may be the cause of fatigue
- General appearance, including affect (anxious, depressed, agitated, tearful, angry, or flat), self-care behaviors, speech patterns, intonation, and general responsiveness
- Cardiac, respiratory, renal, musculoskeletal, and skin status to identify physiologic conditions, including signs of infection or dehydration/malnutrition that may be associated with fatigue
- Appropriate laboratory testing, such as complete blood count and other laboratory studies (e.g., electrolytes, blood gases, thyroid function tests), which may confirm diseases suspected

Assessment Instruments

Given its subjectivity and the general lack of consensus in the literature regarding a definition of fatigue, the measurement of fatigue remains a challenge. Early attempts at developing an instrument to measure fatigue focused on healthy populations. However, these instruments were less

Table 20-1 **Assessment of Patterns of Sleep/Rest, Perceptions/Expressions of Fatigue, and Impact on Quality of Life**		
Sleep/Rest Patterns	**Perceptions/Expressions of Fatigue**	**Impact on Quality of Life**
Do you nap?	What do you believe is the cause of your fatigue?	Do you feel the quality of your life has changed because of fatigue?
Do you feel rested after a nap?	Are you distressed by fatigue?	Can you work?
Do you have difficulty falling asleep at night or staying asleep?	What do you think is the meaning of this symptom?	Do you socialize?
Has the quality of your sleep at night changed?	Do you feel hopeful?	Has fatigue affected your relationship with others?
How do you feel when you awaken?	Has your appetite changed?	Are you able to enjoy life?
Has your sleeping environment changed?	Do you have other symptoms, such as pain?	Has fatigue affected your outlook?

than satisfactory in measuring fatigue in elder and chronically ill populations (Aaronson et al., 1999). More recently, self-assessments and self-reports have been developed to measure fatigue. However, construct validity is difficult to establish for an such an instrument because fatigue measures may examine various aspects of fatigue, such as its character, precursors, or causes, or the effects of fatigue, and each aspect can be addressed from a physiologic, psychosocial, or behavioral perspective. Aaronson and colleagues (1999) have identified significant characteristics to assess when measuring fatigue: (1) the subjective quantification of fatigue, (2) subjective distress because of fatigue, (3) subjective assessment of the impact of fatigue on activities of daily living, (4) correlates of fatigue, and (5) key biologic parameters. Researchers must consider the aspect of fatigue that they are interested in examining when selecting a specific measure. It is recommended, however, that researchers use the same multidimensional set of measures across clinical populations to limit possible discrepant findings among studies and to enhance the instrument's generalizability (Aaronson et al., 1999).

According to Aaronson et al. (1999), several instruments are available to assess the characteristics of fatigue. The Visual Analog Scale of Fatigue (VAS-F), developed by Lee, Hicks and Nino-Murcia (1991), has reported reliability and validity in subjectively quantifying fatigue. An 18-item scale, the VAS-F has a 5-item energy subscale and a 13-item fatigue subscale. The multiple items characterize fatigue as it is being presently experienced by the subject.

The first of Aaronson et al.'s characteristics of fatigue, subjective quantification, can be measured by the Multidimensional Assessment of Fatigue (MAF) measure (Tack, 1991), which examines the experience of fatigue in the past week and its severity, perceived distress, timing, and interference with activities of daily living. The MAF has been further refined into the Global Fatigue Index (Fig. 20-2) and developed to capture the subjective experience of fatigue for patients with rheumatoid arthritis (Belza, Henke, Yelin, Epstein, & Gilliss, 1993), and has been used with older adults (Belza, 1995). The Global Fatigue Index has also been shown to be a valid and reliable measure of fatigue in community-

living patients with HIV (Bormann, Shively, Smith, & Gifford, 2001).

The second characteristic of fatigue, subjective distress, can be measured by a single item on the MAF or by the Symptom Distress Scale (McCorkle & Young, 1978). This measure contains 13 items on symptoms causing distress that include an item on tiredness. A high correlation has been found between fatigue and other symptoms, and has identified the potentially confounding relationship between fatigue and other symptoms experienced by different clinical populations.

The effect of fatigue on activities of daily living (Aaronson et al.'s third characteristic of fatigue) can be measured by an 11-item subscale of the MAF. The report of activity interference may provide a more sensitive measure for assessing changes in fatigue or evaluating the success of an intervention.

The fourth characteristic of fatigue, correlates of fatigue, can be measured by instruments that assess sleep disturbance and depression. Synder-Halpern and Verran's (1987) Sleep Scale assesses the previous night's sleep, sleep disturbance, effectiveness, and supplementation. The Profile of Mood States (POMS) (McNair, Lorr, & Droppleman, 1992) is also a well-established measure of mood disturbance and includes subscales that measure fatigue and vigor.

The above fatigue rating scales are best used in research studies. A verbal rating scale (example in the fatigue journal) is often the most efficient assessment tool for clinical practice. Clinicians should consistently use the same scale and give the same instructions each time. The patient should be asked to rate his or her fatigue at the time of assessment and in the last 24 hours. The same scale, using a 0 (no symptom) to 10 (as bad as they can imagine it) rating, can be used for all symptom assessments, giving the patient and the clinician a common mode of communication.

Lastly, key biologic parameters of fatigue, Aaronson et al.'s fifth characteristic, can be assessed using standard blood tests to identify pathologic states commonly associated with fatigue, such as hypothyroidism, renal failure, and anemia. However, specific biologic measures should be selected based on the clinical population under study.

Instructions: These questions are about fatigue and the effect of fatigue on your activities.

For each of the following questions, circle the number that most closely indicates how you have been feeling during the past week.

For example, suppose you really like to sleep late in the mornings. You would probably circle the number closer to the "a great deal" end of the line. This is where I put it:

Example: To what degree do you usually like to sleep late in the mornings?

`1  2  3  4  5  6  7  (8)  9  10`

Not at all · · · · · · · · · · A great deal

Now please complete the following items based on *the past week*.

───────────────────────

1. To what degree have you experienced fatigue?

`1  2  3  4  5  6  7  8  9  10`

Not at all · · · · · · · · · · A great deal

If no fatigue, stop here.

2. How severe is the fatigue which you have been experiencing?

`1  2  3  4  5  6  7  8  9  10`

Mild · · · · · · · · · · · · · · Severe

3. To what degree has fatigue caused you distress?

`1  2  3  4  5  6  7  8  9  10`

No distress · · · · · · · · A great deal
of distress

Circle the number that most closely indicates to what degree fatigue has interfered with your ability to do the following activities *in the past week*. For activities you don't do, for reasons other than fatigue (e.g. you don't work because you are retired), check the box.

In the past week, to what degree has fatigue interfered with your ability to:

(NOTE: Check box to the left of each number if you don't do activity)

☐ 4. Do household chores

`1  2  3  4  5  6  7  8  9  10`

Not at all · · · · · · · · · · A great deal

☐ 5. Cook

`1  2  3  4  5  6  7  8  9  10`

Not at all · · · · · · · · · · A great deal

☐ 6. Bathe or wash

`1  2  3  4  5  6  7  8  9  10`

Not at all · · · · · · · · · · A great deal

☐ 7. Dress

`1  2  3  4  5  6  7  8  9  10`

Not at all · · · · · · · · · · A great deal

☐ 8. Work

`1  2  3  4  5  6  7  8  9  10`

Not at all · · · · · · · · · · A great deal

☐ 9. Visit or socialize with friends or family

`1  2  3  4  5  6  7  8  9  10`

Not at all · · · · · · · · · · A great deal

(NOTE: Check box to the left of each number if you don't do activity)

☐ 10. Engage in sexual activity

`1  2  3  4  5  6  7  8  9  10`

Not at all · · · · · · · · · · A great deal

☐ 11. Engage in leisure and recreational activities

`1  2  3  4  5  6  7  8  9  10`

Not at all · · · · · · · · · · A great deal

☐ 12. Shop and do errands

`1  2  3  4  5  6  7  8  9  10`

Not at all · · · · · · · · · · A great deal

☐ 13. Walk

`1  2  3  4  5  6  7  8  9  10`

Not at all · · · · · · · · · · A great deal

☐ 14. Exercise, other than walking

`1  2  3  4  5  6  7  8  9  10`

Not at all · · · · · · · · · · A great deal

15. Over the past week, how often have you been fatigued?

`4` Every day

`3` Most, but not all days

`2` Occasionally, but not most days

`1` Hardly any days

16. To what degree has your fatigue changed during the past week?

`4` Increased

`3` Fatigue has gone up and down

`2` Stayed the same

`1` Decreased

Fig. 20-2 Multidimensional assessment of fatigue (MAF) scale. (From Belza, B. L. (2000). *Multidimensional assessment of fatigue: User's guide.* Seattle: University of Washington. *http://www.son.washington.edu/research/maf.*)

MANAGEMENT OF FATIGUE

The goal of the management of fatigue for elder palliative care patients is to achieve the best quality of life that is possible given their specific circumstances. Having the energy to do what is important to the elder so that he or she may finalize specific tasks or interact in special relationships is a valuable outcome for treatment. Within the context of palliative care, the management of fatigue must be considered in relation to the age and developmental stage of the patients, in accordance with their wishes and preferences, and with regard to the extent of disease and coexisting symptoms (Dean & Anderson, 2001). Interventions for fatigue may focus on treating symptoms that exacerbate fatigue, preventing fatigue by balancing rest with activity, and identifying those activities that increase fatigue, as well as those restoring energy. Management of fatigue includes nonpharmacologic and pharmacologic interventions, and these are selected in accordance with the underlying cause of the fatigue.

Learning to cope with fatigue is important to promoting quality of life. In a study by Small and Lamb (1999), patients with COPD considered their fatigue as a natural consequence of their condition and identified a number of emotion-focused and problem-focused strategies to enhance their sense of coping. Emotion-focused strategies helpful in managing the emotional response to the problem included being positive with an upbeat outlook on life; accepting the physical limitations by living within the limits imposed; use of distraction by not dwelling on fatigue (e.g., taking things one day at a time, listening to music); and normalizing their condition by attempting to live life normally and fully while maintaining independence. Problem-focused coping strategies were used to manage and alter the fatigue, specifically energy conservation strategies, such as avoiding any unnecessary or excessive use of energy and pacing themselves; and energy restoration strategies, such as using their energy in such a way as to avoid further deconditioning and deterioration in physical functioning by keeping their muscles strong through exercising, continuing to be self-reliant (only asking for help when necessary), and rejuvenating their energy through relaxation strategies (e.g., "sitting down and resting," "putting your feet up with a cup of tea") and resting before activities by reading, watching television, or taking relaxing baths.

Nonpharmacologic Interventions

Nonpharmacologic interventions for fatigue include education/cognitive interventions, exercise, energy balance and conservation techniques, and nutritional considerations. Education/cognitive interventions include providing the elder with preparatory information and anticipatory guidance regarding the likelihood of fatigue as a side effect of many treatment options, the disease itself, or the emotional reaction to the disease. It should be a standard of care that older adults are educated about CRF in order to help them recognize and anticipate fatigue patterns (Escalante, 2002).

Older adults are often comforted to know that fatigue is often an expected outcome, and not a sign of disease progression. An analogy that can be helpful in conceptualizing fatigue is of fatigue as a depletion of a "bank account" of energy. Within the context of a person's lifestyle and expectations, strategies can be employed that attempt to "increase deposits" and "minimize withdrawals" (Abbey, 2000). Patients may be encouraged to keep a daily fatigue journal to identify the factors and activities associated with the depletion and restoration of energy. Such a journal will also help the older adult communicate with the health care provider regarding various concerns, which may be alleviated by effective symptom management. The journal provides the practitioner with objective evidence of how the patient is doing on a day-to-day basis and helps the older adult plan his or her schedule to optimize peak energy times.

Exercise is another effective intervention for older adults who are fatigued. Movement can prevent loss of muscle tone that is difficult to regain, and helps reduce the incidence of falls. Endorphins are released with even the slightest activity, resulting in increased mood and well-being. Exercise that utilizes the entire body will help maintain tone, strength, and flexibility. Exercise can take place in a structured rehabilitation/physical therapy department, particularly for patients with neuromusculoskeletal deficits or for those who are fatigued as a result of cardiac or respiratory problems and who would benefit from

EVIDENCE-BASED PRACTICE

Reference: Conn, V. S., Tripp-Reimer, T., & Maas, M. L. (2003). Older women and exercise: Theory of planned behavior beliefs. *Public Health Nursing, 20,* 153-163.

Research Problem: Despite well-documented benefits of exercise, elder women remain largely sedentary. Further understanding of beliefs associated with exercise could result in more effective public health interventions to increase exercise in this vulnerable population. This study examined the relationships between theory of planned behavior constructs and exercise behavior and exercise intention in older women.

Design: Face-to-face interviews.

Sample and Setting: 225 women ages 65 and older, living in one community.

Methods: Constructs from the theory of planned behavior (behavioral beliefs, perceived control beliefs, and normative beliefs) were examined.

Exercise was measured with the Baecke Physical Activity Scale. All women were interviewed, to prevent literacy and vision problems from hampering participation.

Results: Significant predictors of exercise behavior were perceived control beliefs and behavioral beliefs. Significant predictors of exercise intentions were perceived control beliefs, behavioral beliefs, and normative beliefs. Specific belief items predicting exercise behavior were that exercise is good for health and that exercise is difficult because of tiredness, as well as the lack of commitment and time.

Implications for Nursing Practice: These findings provide partial support for the application of the theory of planned behavior to exercise in older women.

Conclusion: The findings suggest that interventions should focus on increasing women's confidence that they can overcome barriers to exercise.

related rehabilitation therapy. For others, there may be simply a personal commitment to walk outdoors on a regular basis. Whichever is chosen, the exercise program should be individualized with consideration for the patient's physical condition and other medical problems. Patients should be instructed not to exercise to exhaustion, but reminded that the activity should be done on several days each week to be beneficial. Walking, swimming, gardening, or golf are all good considerations; the patient should be encouraged to exercise at least 6 hours before his or her typical bedtime so that he or she will not have difficulty falling asleep.

For patients with progressive illness, Potter (1998) suggested that, rather than admitting patients to rehabilitation centers (which have a daily exercise program of 4 hours a day) admission of these patients to a palliative care unit is more appropriate. On the palliative care unit, the majority of time can be devoted to promoting

quality of life and comfort, and the older adult does not have to watch others improve dramatically while he or she is just too tired to participate. This approach balances quality of life and a limited amount of therapy, which may be better tolerated.

Energy balance and conservation involves finding a balance between rest and exercise that will give patients the most energy to do the things that they would like to do. Suggesting that the older person sleep no longer than is necessary will help to establish a more solid, less fragmented sleep pattern. Waking up and going to sleep at the same time each day strengthens the circadian cycles and will assist in establishing and maintaining a regular sleep cycle, as does exposure to light daily (Dean & Anderson, 2001). The patient should be encouraged to establish a specific bedtime (with routines to prepare for sleep) and wake time. In addition to an established bedtime, a light bedtime snack and something

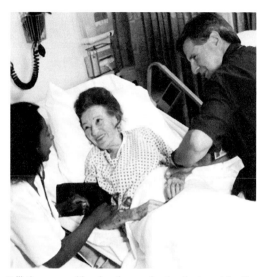

Palliative care: addressing the needs of patients and families. (Courtesy Mathy Mezey.)

warm to drink promotes sleep. Bedtime routines can help the reticular activating system in the brain shut down, readying the body for sleep. Strategies to promote a restful sleep also include the reduction of environmental stimuli (e.g., noise, light), diversional activities to encourage sleep (e.g., music, aromatherapy, massage), and the avoidance of alcohol and stimulants (e.g., caffeine, nicotine, steroids). Adjusting the room temperature and humidity, as well as pillow use, may also be helpful in providing support and comfort. If the patient is unable to fall asleep in 20 minutes, he or she should get out of bed and go into another room to read with a dim light, returning to bed when he or she gets sleepy.

Fatigue is not a sequestered symptom but one that will affect all aspects of the older adult's life. Therefore, the patient at the end of life will need to save energy and plan for activities that are very important to him or her. Patients should be asked what activities they enjoy most and be encouraged to schedule those activities for the time of the day when they have the most energy. Breaks should be scheduled during activities to help restore energy levels, as well as short naps (15 to 20 minutes), which tend to be more restoring than long ones. Energy conservation techniques

should be reinforced with the older adult; these include doing activities sitting down, using a power scooter for grocery shopping, storing frequently used items at chest level to avoid bending and stretching, putting on a terry robe after a shower instead of using energy to dry off with a towel, and wearing slip-on shoes. Providing devices such as a raised toilet seat, a reaching device, and walker can also help conserve energy for elders with progressive fatigue.

Older adults should also be encouraged to ask for help with specific chores. Some elders will see this type of interdependence as very threatening; they need to see their energy as something to be "budgeted" and used for something that they enjoy or that is very important for them to do. The elder should always feel that he or she has the option to "spend" energy on anything that he or she wishes, while being mindful of energy as a limited resource. Often reframing their fatigue in this way gives them the enfranchisement that they need to ask for help. Spending time with family and friends is also very important in promoting a sense of well-being, which may lessen the perception of fatigue. Prioritizing the individuals with whom they would like to visit can be helpful, as can planning such visits at a time of day when they have the most energy to avoid excessive fatigue. Health professionals may also assist in addressing the negative impact of psychological and social stressors and how to avoid or modify them (Winningham et al., 1994).

Nutritional status is also an important consideration; low-fat foods and small meals might be metabolized more easily, resulting in less energy used for digestion. Given that nutrition and hydration are important in preventing fatigue, increasing fluids may be of benefit, unless contraindicated by other medical problems. Protein intake and supplements can also be encouraged if the elder is having trouble with regular food. Recent data suggest that, for patients with advanced cancer, foods rich in omega-3 polyunsaturated fatty acids, such as flax seed oil and fish oil, may decrease cytokines such as tumor necrosis factor and interleukin-1 beta, which may increase weight and appetite and decrease fatigue (Kalman & Villani, 1997). Megestrol acetate may also stimulate appetite and provide energy, thereby lessening fatigue (Abbey, 2000).

Pharmacologic Interventions

Palliative care for fatigue in the elder is different from the management typically provided for other symptoms. In the pharmacologic management of other symptoms in palliative care, medications are often available to treat the actual cause of the symptom. Yet with fatigue, the cause may not be treatable, and in many cases medications may not be the primary intervention for this symptom (Matzo & Sherman, 2001). Furthermore, each medication that the patient receives should be reviewed for its potential for producing sedation and fatigue. Symptoms such as vomiting and pain should be optimally treated because their relief often decreases associated fatigue. Elders should be made aware that the fatigue experienced with opioid therapy will decease as tolerance to opioids develops. Optimizing the use of nonopioid analgesics and adjuvant therapies may also reduce fatigue associated with pain management.

In addition to treating symptoms that induce fatigue, such as pain, vomiting, or dyspnea, the use of other medications, such as corticosteroids, stimulants, and antidepressants, has been of benefit (see Table 20-2). Indeed, even modest improvements in fatigue can improve the older adult's ability to cope with suffering and thereby improve his or her quality of life (Abbey, 2000). There is empirical support for the use of low-dose corticosteroids for patients with multiple symptoms and advanced disease (Tannock et al., 1989); however, there are insufficient data on optimal type and dosage. Corticosteroids can improve appetite and elevate mood, resulting in an improved sense of well-being, although the duration of effect may be limited. Most commonly, dexamethasone, 1 to 2 mg twice daily, or prednisone, 5 to 10 mg twice daily, is prescribed. However, to date there have been no comparative studies (Portenoy, 2000).

Although the use of psychostimulants to treat CRF has not been empirically tested, anecdotal evidence indicates that the use of psychostimulants is worth considering with elders whose clinical profile would not contraindicate a trial (Breitbart et al., 1997). There is also clinical experience in using these drugs to treat depression in the older adult population (Breitbart & Mermelstein, 1992). Although there have been no controlled comparisons of dextroamphetamine and pemoline, pemoline is reported to have fewer sympathomimetic effects (Portenoy, 2000). Pemoline is available in a chewable formulation that will absorb through the buccal mucosa for those who are no longer able to swallow. However, given a risk of hepatotoxicity from pemoline that is not seen with other psychostimulants, methylphenidate is suggested for initial treatment (Breitbart et al., 1997). The initial dose of methylphenidate is usually 2.5 to 5 mg given at 8:00 AM and noon. The dose can be gradually increased until favorable effects occur or until toxicities, such as anorexia, insomnia, anxiety, confusion, tremor, or tachycardia, supervene. To limit toxicities in the medically ill population, dose escalation should be undertaken with caution, and over longer intervals (Portenoy, 2000).

When fatigue is associated with clinical depression, a trial of an antidepressant drug is appropriate. Antidepressants such as selective serotonin reuptake inhibitors are preferred because they are more likely to be activating (Portenoy, 2000). However, a sedating antidepressant can provide peaceful sleep as well as mitigating the depression; potential neurologic and cardiac disadvantages are of lesser concern for the dying elder (Beers & Berkow, 2000).

If the elder has had chemotherapy, the fatigue may be a result of anemia. Treatment with recombinant erythropoietin has been shown in randomized studies to increase the hemoglobin level, which improves the energy levels and quality of life of the patient with CRF (Glaspy et al., 1997). When the elder's hemoglobin level returns to 11 to 12 g/dL, many of the symptoms of anemia are assuaged. Anemia can also be treated with blood transfusions, but this intervention is not without risk to the patient's health and carries the potential of increasing health care costs. Risks associated with blood transfusions include systemic infections (e.g., HIV; hepatitis A, B, and C) from inadequate screening of the blood supply, acute hemolytic reactions, bacterial contamination, and allergic reactions (e.g., urticaria, anaphylaxis) (Labovich, 1997).

It is important to evaluate the efficacy of both pharmacologic and nonpharmacologic fatigue interventions on a regular basis. Systematic documentation regarding the assessment, management, and evaluation of the success of the

Table 20-2 Pharmacologic Therapies for the Treatment of Fatigue

Class of Drug	Examples	Mechanism of Action	Comments
Corticosteroids	Dexamethasone (1-2 mg bid) Prednisolone (5-10 mg bid) Methylprednisolone	Mechanism of action is unclear; can improve appetite and elevate mood. Duration and benefits limited to weeks.	May mask the signs of acute infections.
Psychostimulants	Methylphenidate (2.5-5 mg qd or bid) Dextroamphetamine (2.5-5 mg qd or bid) and pemoline (18.75 mg qd or bid) have been used anecdotally.	Stimulate CNS and respiratory centers, increase appetite and energy levels, improve mood, reduce sedation (Bruera, Chadwick, & Brennis, 1985).	Titrate to effect. Rapid onset of action, fewer side effects than many antidepressants. May cause agitation (Beers & Berkow, 2000). Risk of toxicity increases with dose. No controlled comparisons between efficacy of each of these drugs. Response to one does not predict response to others. Use of sequential trials to determine the most useful drug is suggested (Breitbart et al., 1997).
Antidepressants Selective serotonin reuptake inhibitors (SSRIs)	Trazodone (25-50 mg at bedtime, increase to 25-50 mg/day as tolerated to a maximum of 300 mg/day) (Beers & Berkow, 2000). Paroxetine (10 mg) Fluoxetine (10 mg) Sertraline (25 mg)	Inhibit serotonin reuptake. Reduce depressive symptoms associated with fatigue. Can improve sleep. Primary choice for treatment of depression in cancer patients.	Give once daily in the morning. Some SSRIs have long half-lives and should be used cautiously in the terminally ill older adult.
Tricyclic antidepressants	Amitriptyline (10-25 mg q hs) Nortriptyline (25 mg 3-4 times daily)	Block reuptake of various neurotransmitters at the neuronal membrane. Can improve sleep.	Amitriptyline contraindicated in patients on MAOIs or post-MI. Use with caution in elders with cardiovascular disease; adverse reactions include arrhythmias.
Erythropoietin	Epetin alfa, 150 U/kg sq 3 times a week	Increases hemoglobin with effects on energy, activity & overall quality of life while decreasing transfusion requirements (Krammer, Muir, Gooding-Gellar, et al., 1999).	Monitor hematocrit and reduce dose if it approaches 36% or increases by > 4 points in 2 wk.

CNS, central nervous system; *MAOIs*, monoamine oxidase inhibitors; *MI*, myocardial infarction.

interventions in relieving fatigue is essential to quality care.

FATIGUE IN FAMILY CAREGIVERS

Family caregivers are often profoundly fatigued by the stressors inherent in caregiving. Caregivers bear the physical and emotional burden of assisting elders with activities of daily living, as well as with treatments. They often must assume new roles and responsibilities and at times deal with additional financial distress (Abbey, 2000). As a result, family caregivers may also develop anxiety or depressive disorders associated with fatigue. Severe family fatigue is commonly experienced in four situations: (1) inadequate relief of the patient's pain and suffering, (2) inadequate resources to cope with home care, (3) unrealistic expectations of family caregivers by themselves or by the professional health care team, and (4) emotional distress that persists even when there is adequate relief of patient suffering (Cherny, 2000).

Palliative care recognizes the patient and family as the unit of care, and therefore assessment and interventions to relieve caregiver burden are essential. Validating the needs and concerns of family caregivers is important. Helping family caregivers to set priorities with regard to competing demands, optimizing stress and coping strategies, and encouraging relaxation and rest, while assisting caregivers with respite care, are important interventions in preventing or alleviating caregiver fatigue (Abbey, 2000).

Case Study Conclusion

Ms. L.'s fatigue was managed through several therapeutic approaches. Laboratory data revealed a persistent anemia, which was treated with iron supplements. Discussion also focused on eating a well-balanced diet and daily multivitamin supplementation. Ms. L. agreed to make a personal commitment to regular exercise by walking outdoors for 20 minutes each day to promote muscle tone, increase endorphin levels, and improve mood and sense of well-being. The palliative care nurse helped Ms. L. to learn to balance rest with activity, shortening her workday, prioritizing activities, and carrying out activities when she had the greatest energy. Ms. L. was comforted by an understanding that fatigue is a normal response to chemotherapy and radiation, rather than considering her fatigue as indicative of disease progression.

Psychological assessment also indicated that Ms. L. suffered from depression, which exacerbated her perception of fatigue. To treat her depression, Ms. L. met with a cancer center psychologist to discuss her feelings and fears, and was prescribed a selective serotonin reuptake inhibitor by the palliative care nurse practitioner. Ms. L. was encouraged to join a breast cancer support group and recognized the value of accepting help from willing friends. She was counseled regarding strategies to promote a restful night's sleep, including establishing regular bedtime routines and a quiet, relaxing environment. The plan of care involved continual evaluation of the efficacy of such interventions for fatigue. If necessary, a trial of dexamethasone would also be considered to decrease the sense of fatigue and promote maximal sense of well-being. On follow-up evaluation, Ms. L. expressed a lessening of fatigue, greater sense of control, and improved quality of life.

CONCLUSION

To the health care professional, fatigue represents a clue to illness, a treatment side effect, progressive illness, the residual physical change of illness and its treatment, or the emotional strain of illness or caregiving. To the older adult and his or her family, fatigue is a symptom that keeps them from moving forward fully with life (Greenberg, 1998). Health professionals can be supportive by acknowledging fatigue as real and taking fatigue and its frustrations seriously. Understanding the possible etiology of fatigue and the meaning of the symptom to the patient is important in determining its management. Assisting older adults to live fully as they move along the illness trajectory may require consideration of nonpharmacologic as well as pharmacologic therapies to comprehensively and effectively treat fatigue. Learning how to prevent fatigue and/or restore energy is important to improving the elder patient's function, his or her ability to socialize, and ultimately his or her adjustment to a "new normal" baseline as he or she lives with a life-limiting or chronic illness (Harpham, 1999).

REFERENCES

Aaronson, L. S., Teel, C. S., Cassmeyer, V., Neuberger, G. B., Pallikkathayil, L., Pierce, J., et al. (1999). Defining and measuring fatigue. *Image: Journal of Nursing Scholarship, 31*, 45-50.

Abbey, S. (2000). Psychiatric aspects of fatigue in the terminally ill. In H. M. Chochinov & W. Breitbart (Eds.), *Handbook of psychiatry in palliative medicine* (pp. 175-185). New York: Oxford University Press.

Adinolfi, A. (2001). Assessment and treatment of HIV-related fatigue. *Journal of the Association of Nurses in AIDS Care, 12*(Suppl.), 28-38.

Beers, M. H., & Berkow, R. (2000). Care of the dying patient. In *Merck manual of geriatrics* (3rd ed., pp. 115-127). Whitehouse Station, NJ: Merck.

Belza, B. L. (1995). Comparison of self-reported fatigue in rheumatoid arthritis and controls. *Journal of Rheumatology, 22*, 639-643.

Belza, B. L., Henke, C. J., Yelin, E. H., Epstain, W. V., & Gillis, C. L. (1993). Correlates of fatigue in older adults with rheumatoid arthritis. *Nursing Research, 42*, 93-99.

Berger, A. M., & Farr, L. (1999). The influence of daytime inactivity and nighttime restlessness on cancer-related fatigue. *Oncology Nursing Forum, 26*, 1663-1671.

Bormann, J., Shively, M., Smith, T. L., & Gifford, A. L. (2001). Measurement of fatigue in HIV-positive adults: Reliability and validity of the Global Fatigue Index. *Journal of the Association of Nurses in AIDS Care, 12*(3), 75-83.

Breitbart, W., Esch, J. F., & Portenoy, R. K. (1997). *Fatigue in cancer and AIDS: The Network Project.* New York: Memorial Sloan-Kettering Cancer Center.

Breitbart, W., McDonald, M., Rosenfeld, B., Monkman, N. D., & Passik, S. (1998). Fatigue in ambulatory AIDS patients. *Journal of Pain and Symptom Management, 15*, 159-167.

Breitbart, W., & Mermelstein, M. V. (1992). An alternative psychostimulant for the management of depressive disorders in cancer patients. *Psychosomatics, 33*, 352-356.

Breslin, E., van der Schans, S., Breukink, S., Meek, P., Mercer, K., Volz, W., et al. (1998). Perception of fatigue and quality of life in patients with COPD. *Chest, 114*, 958-964.

Bruera, E., Chadwick, S., & Brenneis, C. (1985). Methylphenidate associated with narcotic treatment of cancer pain. *Cancer Treatment Reports, 70*, 295-297.

Cahill, C. (1999). Differential diagnosis of fatigue in women. *Journal of Obstetric, Gynecologic, & Neonatal Nursing, 28*, 81-86.

Cauch-Dudek, K., Abbey, S., Stewart, D. E., Heathcote, E. J. (1998). Fatigue in primary biliary cirrhosis. *Gut, 43*, 705-710.

Cherny, N. I. (2000). The treatment of suffering in patients with advanced cancer. In H. M. Chochinov & W. Breitbart (Eds.), *Handbook of psychiatry in palliative medicine* (pp. 375-396). New York: Oxford University Press.

Chochinov, H., & Breitbart, W. (2000). *Handbook of psychiatry in palliative medicine.* New York: Oxford University Press.

Darko, D. R., McCutchan, J. A., Kripke, D. F., Gillin, J. C., & Golshan, S. (1992). Fatigue, sleep disturbance, disability and indices of progression of HIV infection. *American Journal of Psychiatry, 149*, 514-520.

Dean, G. E., & Anderson, P. R. (2001). Fatigue. In B. R. Ferrell & N. Coyle (Eds.), *Textbook of palliative nursing* (pp. 91-100). New York: Oxford University Press.

Escalante, C. P. (2002). Treatment of cancer-related fatigue: An update. *Supportive Care in Cancer, 11*, 79-83.

Ferrell, B. R., Grant, M., Dean, G. E., et al. (1996). Bone tired: The experience of fatigue and its impact on quality of life. *Oncology Nursing Forum, 23*, 1539-1547.

Fobair, P., Hoppe, R. T., Bloom, J., Cox, R., Varghese, A., & Spiegel, D. (1986). Psychosocial problems among survivors of Hodgkin's disease. *Journal of Clinical Oncology, 4*, 805-814.

Frazer, D. W., Leicht, M. L., & Baker, M. D. (1996). Psychological manifestations of physical disease in the elderly. In L. L. Carstensen, B. A. Edelstein, & L. Dornbrand (Eds.), *Practical handbook of clinical gerontology* (pp. 217-235). Thousand Oaks, CA: Sage.

Friedman, M., & King, K. (1995). Correlates of fatigue in older women with heart failure. *Heart & Lung: Journal of Critical Care, 24*, 512-518.

Glaspy, J., Bukowski, R., Steinberg, D., Taylor, C., Tchekmedyian, S., & Vadhan-Raj, S. (1997). Impact of therapy with epoetin alfa on clinical outcomes in patients with nonmyeloid malignancies during cancer chemotherapy in community oncology practice. *Journal of Clinical Oncology, 15*, 1218-1234.

Greenberg, D. (1998). Fatigue. In J. Holland (Ed.), *Psycho-oncology* (pp. 485-493). New York: Oxford University Press.

Groenwald, S. L., Frogge, M. H., Goodman, M., & Yarbo, C. H. (1993). *Cancer nursing: Principles and practice.* Sudbury, MA: Jones and Bartlett.

Harpham, W. (1999). Resolving the frustration of fatigue. *CA: A Cancer Journal for Clinicians, 49*, 178-189.

Ingles, J. L., Eskes, G. A., & Phillips, S. J. (1999). Fatigue after stroke. *Archives of Physical Medicine and Rehabilitation, 80*, 173-178.

Irvine, D. M., Vincent, L., Bubela, N., Thompson, L., & Graydon, J. (1991). A critical appraisal of the research literature investigating fatigue in the individual with cancer. *Cancer Nursing, 14*, 188-199.

Jenkins, C. A., Schulz, M., Hanson, J., & Bruera, E. (2000). Demographic, symptom, and medication profiles of cancer patients seen by a palliative care consult team in a tertiary referral hospital. *Journal of Pain and Symptom Management, 19*, 174-184.

Kalman, D., & Villani, L. J. (1997). Nutritional aspects of cancer-related fatigue. *Journal of the American Dietetic Association, 97*, 650-654.

Karlsen, K., Larsen, J. P., Tandberg, E., & Jorgensen, K. (1999). Fatigue in patients with Parkinson's disease. *Movement Disorders, 14,* 237-241.

Krammer, L., Muir, C., Gooding-Gellar, N., et al. (1999). Palliative care and oncology: Opportunities for nursing. *Oncology Nursing Update, 6,* 1-12.

Labovich, T. M. (1997). Transfusion therapy: Nursing implications. *Clinical Journal of Oncology Nursing, 1,* 61.

Lee, K. A., Hicks, G., & Nino-Murcia, G. (1991). Validity and reliability of a scale to assess fatigue. *Psychiatry Research, 36,* 291-298.

Liao, S., & Ferrell, B. A. (2000). Fatigue in an older population. *Journal of the American Geriatrics Society, 48,* 426-430.

Loge, J. H., Abrahamsen, A. F., Ekeberg, O., & Kaasa, S. (2000). Fatigue and psychiatric morbidity among Hodgkin's disease. *Journal of Pain and Symptom Management, 19,* 91-99.

Magnusson, K., Moller, A., Ekman, T., & Wallgren, A. (1999). A qualitative study to explore the experience of fatigue in cancer patients. *European Journal of Cancer Care, 8,* 224-232.

Mast, M. (1998). Correlates of fatigue in survivors of breast cancer. *Cancer Nursing, 21,* 136-142.

Matzo, M. L., & Sherman, D. W. (Eds.). (2001). *Palliative care nursing: Quality care to the end of life.* New York: Springer.

McCorkle, R., & Young, K. (1978). Development of a symptom distress scale. *Cancer Nursing, 3,* 248-256.

McNair, D. M., Lorr, M., & Droppleman, L. F. (1992). *EdITS manual for the Profile of Mood States.* San Diego: EdITS/Educational Testing Service.

Miaskowski, C., & Lee, K. A. (1999). Pain, fatigue, and sleep disturbances in oncology outpatients receiving radiation therapy for bone metastasis: A pilot study. *Journal of Pain and Symptom Management, 17,* 320-322.

Neuenschwander, H., & Bruera, E. (1998). Pathophysiology of cancer asthenia. In E. Bruera, & R. K. Portenoy (Eds.), *Topics in palliative care: Vol. 2* (pp. 171-181). New York: Oxford University Press.

Piper, B. F. (1989). Fatigue: Current bases for practice. In S. G. Funk, E. M. Funk, M. T. Champagne, et al. (Eds.), *Key aspects of comfort: Management of pain, fatigue, and nausea* (pp. 187-198). New York: Springer.

Piper, B. F.(1997). Measurements of fatigue. In M. Frank-Stromberg & K. Olsen (Eds.), *Instruments for clinical health-care research* (2nd ed.). Boston: Jones and Bartlett.

Portenoy, R. (2000). Physical symptom management in the terminally ill. In H. M. Chochinov & W. Breitbart (Eds.), *Handbook of psychiatry in palliative medicine* (pp. 116-119). New York: Oxford University Press.

Potter, P. (1998). The fatigue of cancer. *Canadian Medical Association Journal, 159,* 921.

Richardson, A., & Ream, E. (1996). Research and development: Fatigue in patients receiving chemotherapy for advanced cancer. *International Journal of Palliative Nursing, 2,* 199-204.

Sarna, L., & Brecht, M. (1997). Dimensions of symptom distress in women with advanced lung cancer: A factor analysis. *Heart & Lung, 26,* 23-30.

Schwartz, A. H. (2002). Validity of cancer-related fatigue instruments. *Pharmacatherapy, 22,* 1433-1441.

Schwartz, A. L. (1998). Patterns of exercise and fatigue in physically active cancer survivors. *Oncology Nursing Forum, 25,* 485-491.

Small, S., & Lamb, M. (1999). Fatigue in chronic illness: The experience of individuals with chronic obstructive pulmonary disease and with asthma. *Journal of Advanced Nursing, 30,* 469-478.

Snyder-Halpern, R., & Verran, J. A. (1987). Instrumentation to describe subjective sleep characteristics in healthy subjects. *Research in Nursing and Health, 10,* 155-163.

Swain, M. G. (2000). Fatigue in chronic illness. *Clinical Science, 99,* 1-8.

Tack, B. (1991). *Dimensions and correlates of fatigue in older adults with rheumatoid arthritis.* Unpublished doctoral dissertation, University of California, San Francisco.

Tannock, I., Gospodarowicz, M., Meakin, W., Panzarella, T., Stewart, L., & Rider, W. (1989). Treatment of metastatic prostatic cancer with low-dose prednisone: Evaluation of pain and quality of life as pragmatic indices of response. *Journal of Clinical Oncology, 7,* 590-597.

Tiesinga, L. J., Dassen, T. W. N., & Halfens, R. J. G. (1996). Fatigue: A summary of the definitions, dimensions and indicators. *Nursing Diagnosis, 7,* 51-62.

Vainio, A., & Auvinen, A. (1996). Prevalence of symptoms among patients with advanced cancer: An international study. *Journal of Pain and Symptom Management, 12,* 3-10.

Vogelzang, N. J., Breitbart, W., Cella, D., Curt, G. A., Groopman, J. E., Horning, S. J., et al. (1997). Patient, caregiver, and oncologist perceptions of cancer-related fatigue: Results of a tripart assessment survey. *Seminars in Hematology, 34,* 4-12.

Winningham, M. L., Nail, L. M., Burke, M. B., Brophy, L., Cimprich, B., Jones, L. S., et al. (1994). Fatigue and the cancer experience: The state of the knowledge. *Oncology Nursing Forum, 21,* 23-36.

Woo, B., Dibble, S. L., Piper, B. F., Keating, S. B., & Weiss, M. C. (1998). Differences in fatigue by treatment methods in women with breast cancer. *Oncology Nursing Forum, 25,* 915-920.

APPENDIX A: CANCER-RELATED FATIGUE INSTRUMENTS*

The following assessment instruments were used in validating the various CRF instruments listed in this appendix: Beck Depression Scale (BDS); Center for Epidemiological Studies–Depression Scale (CES-D); Eastern Collaborative Oncology Group Performance Status Rating (ECOG-PSR); Functional Assessment of Chronic Illness Therapy (FACIT); Marlowe-Crowne Social Desirability Scale (MC-20); Health Outcomes Study Short Form (SF-36); Satisfaction with Life Domains Scale–Cancer (SLDS-C); State–Trait Anxiety Inventory (STAI); and Visual Analog Scale of Fatigue (VAS-F).

Brief Fatigue Inventory (BFI)

Description
- 9-item questionnaire
- 11-point Likert scale
- Evaluation period: past week, current, and past 24 hours

Administration
- Self-report
- Second party (interview)
- Estimated time for completion: 5 minutes

Validity
- Validated in men and women
- Internal reliability verified
- Test–retest reliability: not evaluated
- Construct verified
- Convergent: Functional Assessment of Cancer Therapy Fatigue Subscale (FACT-F) and Anemia Subscale (FACT-An); Profile of Mood States Fatigue Subscale (POMS-F) and Vigor Subscale (POMS-V)
- Divergent: not evaluated
- Discriminators: albumin, hemoglobin, and ECOG-PSR

Comments
- Able to capture physical and psychological aspects
- Useful for screening and outcome assessments
- Able to distinguish severe fatigue, but less reliable when differentiating mild to moderate symptoms

*Adapted from Schwartz, A. H. (2002). Validity of cancer-related fatigue instruments. *Pharmacotherapy, 22,* 1433-1441, with permission.

Cancer Fatigue Scale (CFS)

Description
- 15-item questionnaire
- 5-point Likert scale
- Subscales: physical, affective cognitive
- Evaluation period: current

Administration
- Self-report
- Second party (interview)
- Estimated time for completion: 2 to 3 minutes

Validity
- Validated in men and women
- Internal reliability verified
- Test–retest reliability verified up to 8 days
- Construct: no healthy controls
- Convergent: VAS-F and Hospital Anxiety and Depression Scale
- Divergent: Mini-Mental State Examination
- Discriminators: ECOG-PSR (physical and affective subscales)

Comments
- Able to capture physical and psychological aspects
- Validation performed in Japanese population, which may affect generalization
- Telephone test–retest: lower mean values but retained validity

Fatigue Symptom Inventory (FSI)

Description
- 14-item questionnaire
- 11-point Likert scale (12 questions)
- Remaining questions pertain to number of days per week (0 to 7) fatigue is experienced and the pattern of daily fatigue (4-point Likert scale)
- Evaluation period: past week, current

Administration
- Self-report
- Second party (interview)
- Estimated time for completion: 5 minutes

Validity
- Validated in men and women
- Internal reliability: interference subscale
- Test–retest reliability: low-to-moderate correlations
- Construct verified
- Convergent: POMS-F, SF-36, SLDS-C, and CES-D
- Divergent: MC-20
- Discriminators: not evaluated

Comments

- Questions similar to those on BFI
- Able to capture physical and psychological aspects
- Useful for screening and outcome assessments (single assessments only, not repeated measures)
- Identified a second version of this tool that used a 5-point Likert scale for the final question pertaining to daily pattern of fatigue

Functional Assessment of Cancer Therapy General Subscale (FACT-G)

Description

- 27-item questionnaire
- 5-point Likert scale
- General cancer assessment tool derived from FACIT database
- Evaluates physical, functional, emotional, and social well-being (quality of life); two questions regarding patient–physician relationships
- Evaluation period: past week

Administration

- Self-report
- Second party (interview)
- Estimated time for completion: 5 minutes

Validity

- Validated in men and women
- Internal reliability verified
- Test–retest reliability verified
- Construct: no healthy controls
- Convergent: POMS, SF-36, SLDS-C, and CES-D
- Divergent: MC-20
- Discriminators: ECOG-PSR

Comments

- General focus
- Useful for screening and outcome assessments

Functional Assessment of Cancer Therapy Fatigue Subscale (FACT-F)

Description

- 13-item questionnaire administered with FACT-G
- 5-point Likert scale
- Evaluation period: past week

Administration

- Self-report
- Second party (interview)
- Estimated time for completion: 5 to 10 minutes

Validity

- Validated in men and women
- Internal reliability verified
- Test–retest reliability: 3 to 7 days

- Construct: no healthy controls
- Convergent: Piper Fatigue Scale (PFS), POMS-F, and POMS-V
- Divergent: MC-20
- Discriminators: hemoglobin and ECOG-PSR

Comments

- Able to capture physical and psychological aspects
- Useful for screening and outcome assessments

Functional Assessment of Cancer Anemia Subscale (FACT-An)

Description

- 20-item questionnaire (13 of which are identical to FACT-F) administered with FACT-G
- 5-point Likert scale
- Assesses symptoms associated with anemia
- Evaluation period: past week

Administration

- Self-report
- Second party (interview)
- Estimated time for completion: 5 to 10 minutes

Validity

- Validated in men and women
- Internal reliability verified
- Test–retest reliability: 3 to 7 days
- Construct: no healthy controls
- Convergent: PFS, POMS-F, and POMS-V
- Divergent: MC-20
- Discriminators: hemoglobin and ECOG-PSR

Comments

- Able to capture physical and psychological aspects
- Useful for screening and outcome assessments

Lee Fatigue Scale (LFS or VAS-F)

Description

- 18-item visual analogue scale
- Fatigue subscale: 13 items
- Energy subscale: 5 items
- Evaluation period: current

Administration

- Self-report
- Second party (interview)
- Estimated time for completion: less than 5 minutes

Validity

- Validated in men and women
- Internal reliability verified
- Test–retest reliability: limited data
- Construct verified
- Convergent: POMS-F, POMS-V; and Stanford Sleepiness Scale

- Divergent: not evaluated
- Discriminators: not evaluated

Comments
- Able to capture physical and psychological aspects
- Useful for screening and outcome assessments
- Although used to assess CRF, original validation performed in patients with sleep disorders

Multidimensional Fatigue Inventory (MFI-20)
Description
- 20-item questionnaire
- 5-point Likert scale
- Scales: general, physical, mental, reduced motivation, reduced activity
- Evaluation period: past 24 hours

Administration
- Self-report
- Second party (interview)
- Estimated time for completion: 5 to 10 minutes

Validity
- Validated in men and women
- Internal reliability verified
- Test–retest reliability: not evaluated
- Construct verified
- Convergent: VAS (single item), BDS, and Rhoten Fatigue Scale
- Divergent: not evaluated
- Discriminators: not evaluated

Comments
- Able to capture physical and psychological aspects
- Useful for screening and outcome assessments

Multidimensional Fatigue Symptom Inventory (MFSI)
Description
- Developed by same group as FSI
- 83-item questionnaire
- 5-point Likert scale
- Rational subscale: global, somatic, affective, cognitive, and behavioral aspects
- Empirical subscale: general, physical, emotional, mental, aspects; also evaluates vigor
- Short form (MFSI-SF): developed to evaluate only empirical information
- Evaluation period: past week

Administration
- Self-report
- Second party (interview)
- Estimated time for completion: 10 minutes

Validity
- Validated in women
- Internal reliability: both subscales
- Test–retest reliability: significant and equivalent correlations noted for both subscales
- Construct verified
- Convergent: POMS-F, SF-36 (vitality), STAI, and CES-D
- Divergent: MC-20
- Discriminators: ECOG-PSR

Comments
- Able to capture physical and psychological aspects
- Validation performed in women only, which may affect generalization
- Useful for screening; however, may be too long or cumbersome for outcome assessments

Piper Fatigue Scale (PFS)
Description
- 27-item questionnaire
- 22 items: 11-point Likert scale used to estimate fatigue scores
- 5 items: open-ended
- Subscales: behavioral/severity, affective/meaning, sensory, and cognitive/mood
- Evaluation period: current

Administration
- Self-report
- Second party (interview)
- Estimated time for completion: 5 minutes

Validity
- Validated in women
- Internal reliability verified
- Test–retest reliability: not evaluated
- Construct: no healthy controls
- Convergent: demographic profile (investigator developed), POMS, and Fatigue Symptom Checklist
- Divergent: POMS-V
- Discriminators: not evaluated

Comments
- Able to capture physical and psychological aspects
- Useful for screening and outcome assessments
- Used clinically to assess CRF in men; however, formal validation efforts not yet published

Profile of Mood States (POMS)
Description
- 65-item questionnaire
- 5-point Likert scale
- Subscales: tension-anxiety, anger-hostility, vigor-activity, fatigue-inertia, and confusion-bewilderment

- Short form: 30 items (derived from the six subscales); developed for the elderly and individuals with medical disorders or disabilities
- Evaluation period: past week

Administration
- Self-report
- Second party (interview)
- Estimated time for completion: 5 to 7 minutes (some individuals may require more time)

Validity
- Validated in men and women
- Internal reliability: all subscales
- Test–retest reliability: all subscales
- Construct verified
- Convergent: Hopkins Symptom Distress Scale, Manifest Anxiety Scale, BDS, and Interpersonal Behavior Inventory
- Divergent: MC-20
- Discriminators: not evaluated

Comments
- Only able to capture psychological aspects
- Useful for screening; however, may be too long or cumbersome for outcome assessments
- Flexible scoring: entire document or individual subscales

Schwartz Cancer Fatigue Scale (SCFS) [original version]
Description
- 28-item questionnaire
- 5-point Likert scale
- Subscales (factors): physical, emotional, cognitive, and temporal
- Evaluation period: past 2 to 3 days

Administration
- Self-report
- Second party (interview)
- Estimated time for completion: 5 minutes

Validity
- Validated in men and women
- Internal reliability verified
- Test–retest reliability not evaluated
- Construct: limited evaluation
- Convergent: VAS-F
- Divergent: not evaluated
- Discriminators: not evaluated

Comments
- Able to capture physical and psychological aspects
- Described validation under experimental conditions, but validation was not maintained when used in a clinical setting

Schwartz Cancer Fatigue Scale (SCFS-6) [revised version]
Description
- 6-item questionnaire
- 5-point Likert scale
- Subscales (factors): physical and perceptual
- Developed because further testing was unable to confirm validation of original version
- Evaluation period: past 2 to 3 days

Administration
- Self-report
- Second party (interview)
- Estimated time for completion: 1 to 2 minutes

Validity
- Validated in men and women
- Internal reliability verified
- Test–retest reliability: not evaluated
- Construct verified
- Convergent: not evaluated
- Divergent: not evaluated
- Discriminators: limited evaluation

Comments
- Able to capture physical and psychological aspects
- Requires further validation (in the clinical setting)
- Items are identical to those in POMS
- Computerized version has been developed

PAIN ASSESSMENT AND MANAGEMENT

Elizabeth Ford Pitorak and Bridget Montana

Case Study

Mrs. H., a 78-year-old cognitively intact, African American female, was admitted to a hospice program after experiencing a 40-pound weight loss secondary to the primary diagnosis of esophageal cancer. She has chosen not to be treated because of personal experiences of watching family and friends undergo radiation therapy and chemotherapy. Comorbid conditions included rheumatoid arthritis (RA) with severe multiple deformities, congestive heart failure and coronary artery disease treated with coronary artery bypass surgery and a pacemaker, and chronic obstructive pulmonary disease (COPD).

Mrs. H.'s daughter died 2 years ago in the emergency room following an acute asthmatic attack. Six months later, the daughter's husband died of a massive myocardial infarction, leaving three children who are Mrs. H.'s only grandchildren, one of whom is estranged as a result of chemical dependency. The patient has a history of both smoking and drinking alcohol to excess. She is very connected to her church community; three times a week she goes to an adult day care center.

Mrs. H.'s presenting pain problems were joint pain in the feet and hips caused by RA, which she rated as 8 to 10 at its worst on a scale of 0 to 10. This pain had been controlled with prednisone, 10 mg every other day, until recently. Initially the prednisone was increased to every day and oxycodone, 10 mg at bedtime, was added. After a steady state was reached, the oxycodone was converted to OxyContin, 30 mg twice a day, plus OxyFast, 5 mg every 2 hours as needed (PRN) for breakthrough pain. A bowel regimen of senna and docusate sodium (Senokot-S) 2

tablets every day, was initiated at the same time oxycodone was started. Nonpharmacologic interventions included repositioning, heat, relaxation techniques, distraction, and counseling. Six months into care, Mrs. H. complained of "heartburn" assumed to be due to the esophageal malignancy; therefore, the doses of both OxyContin and prednisone were increased and nitroglycerin, two 4-mg tablets every day, was added to relieve esophageal spasm.

Issues to be addressed include the following:
Initially, how was her RA pain going to be controlled?
Why was the patient's pain not controlled? Why did she not consistently take opioids?
How were her spiritual needs going to be addressed when she no longer could leave the house?
The patient became confused. Why?
Who was going to be her caregiver?
The patient was unable to swallow; how would she take her steroid?

INTRODUCTION

Pain, an unpleasant sensory and emotional experience (Merskey, 1996), is common in older adults (Fujimoto, 2001). Frequently, pain is associated with a pathologic process that causes discomfort, or an uncomfortable experience because it may be associated with injury. There is no objective biologic marker of pain; the older adult's description and self-report of pain usually provides accurate, reliable, and sufficient evidence for the presence and intensity of pain (American Geriatric Society [AGS] Panel on Persistent Pain in Older Persons, 2002). McCaffery and Pasero (1999) defined pain as whatever the experiencing person says it is, and existing whenever he or she says it does. Inadequate pain assessment and treatment is a significant health care problem for older adult patients. Assessment and management of pain is important in the care of all patients and especially in palliative care programs that care for dying elder patients. The management of pain in the older adult can be challenging because of the complexity of multiple disease processes, social issues related to being independent, and potential financial constraints.

This chapter discusses "total pain" as conceptualized by Dame Cicely Saunders (Clark, 1999), who founded the modern hospice and palliative care movement in England in 1967. The concept of treating the patient and the family (or caregiver) as a unit of care is the foundation on which holistic pain management was built. Saunders stressed the importance of understanding and recognizing all domains of total pain, incorporating the physical, psychological, social, emotional, and spiritual elements. From that perspective, it is clear that no one discipline or professional domain is adequate on its own to ensure comfort from pain, freedom from distressing symptoms, and relief from suffering. To fully understand and deal with total pain, the team approach provides the expertise and range of skills necessary to deal with the multiple facets of pain that older patients experience.

Clinical manifestations of persistent (chronic) pain are commonly multifactorial because of the complex interplay among these factors across several domains (physiologic, psychosocial, and spiritual). Determining which factors are most important for the purpose of treatment can be very challenging. Further complicating this task is the fact that underreporting, fears of addiction, polypharmacy, cognitive impairment, and legal concerns regarding prescribing have an impact on the ability to relieve pain for older adults (AGS Panel on Persistent Pain in Older Persons, 2002).

Assessment of pain in the older adult includes parameters similar to those in younger individuals, such as the description of pain, clinical observation, identification of alleviating factors, and social history. In addition, the functional status must be assessed because pain in older adults may severely restrict mobility, impact their ability to perform activities of daily living (ADLs), and cause increased dependence.

The pain experience of older adults continues to be debated by health care practitioners, and myths of aging also contribute to the inadequacy of pain management in the older population. Aging is a normal physiologic process of life, not a disease. Older individuals often have comorbid medical conditions that contribute to the challenge of symptom management in palliative care and necessitate special approaches for nursing care (Williams, 1994). The major cause of pain in the elder appears to be musculoskeletal, with osteoarthritis (OA) as the predominant complaint of pain in the older adult. Arthritis may affect as many as 80% of people over the age of 65, and most report significant pain (Davis, 1988). Cancer is another frequent cause of pain; Foley (1994) reported that as many as 80% of all cancer patients over age 65 have substantial pain.

Currently pain in elder persons is receiving increasing attention by researchers. Desbiens, Mueller-Rizner, Connors, Hamel, and Wenger (1997) found that the "oldest old" (over 85 years of age) hospitalized patients had verbalized frequency of pain similar to that of younger hospitalized patients. The study concluded that pain is extremely common among older adult patients. Harkins (1996) reviewed several studies that involved inducing pain in experimental subjects. From these studies, it was concluded that changes in pain perception with age probably do not occur. In a final analysis, the consequences of stereotyping elder individuals as experiencing less pain may be an inaccurate assessment that results in needless suffering (Ferrell, 1991).

The implications of pain vary with each elder. The consequences of unrelated, undertreated pain may be depression, decreased socialization, sleep disturbance, impaired ambulation, and the inability to complete ADLs. Although less explored, an increase in gait impairment, falls, polypharmacy, cognitive dysfunction, and malnutrition are among the geriatric conditions that may worsen with poorly managed pain (Ferrell, 1991).

BARRIERS TO EFFECTIVE PAIN MANAGEMENT

The Agency for Health Care Policy and Research (AHCPR) clinical practice guidelines have done much to educate consumers as to their basic

---

Box 21-1 Patient/Caregiver Barriers to Effective Pain Management

- Belief that pain is a normal consequence of aging and must be accepted
- Reluctance to report pain
- Reluctance by patient or caregivers to follow treatment recommendation
- Fear of tolerance or addiction
- Concern about treatment-related side effects
- Fears regarding disease progression
- Patient's inability to report pain related to cognitive impairment
- Frail caregiver who is willing to care for loved one, but is managing his or her own comorbidities
- Limited financial resources, which result in the inability to purchase medication
- Polypharmacy
- Addiction to alcohol or other substances

Box 21-2 Clinician-Related Barriers to Effective Pain Management

- Age-related perception of pain resulting in unusual presentation of illness (e.g., painless abdominal diseases and the painless myocardial infarction leading to controversy as to whether these clinical observations are age related [Ferrell, 1991])
- Clinician's inability to assess the aging process versus chronologic age
- Clinician's inaccurate assessment of the older patient, and the impact on pain as it affects the "young-old" (65-74 years), the "middle-old" (75-84 years), and the "frail-old" (over 85 years)
- Inaccurate health history to identify presence of comorbidities and disabilities that render individuals more susceptible to complications of new treatments for pain management
- Inability to assess delirium versus dementia
- Inaccurate assessment of pain in cognitively impaired persons
- Lack of assessment of pain and its impact on functional status
- Lack of knowledge of theory and practice in managing pain in the older adult
- Lack of understanding of sociocultural domain of pain

---

right to receive aggressive pain management. Unfortunately, many older adults are not aware of this right, and even those who have this awareness are often reluctant to exercise it for fear of bothering or angering their caregivers. Instead, they have a greater desire to be seen as the "good patient," resulting in underreporting of pain and unnecessary stoic suffering of pain.

Barriers to effective pain management can be categorized into three major areas: patient/caregiver related, clinician related, and health care system related. Patients and/or caregivers may complicate the process of pain assessment because of misconceptions (Box 21-1). Clinician-related barriers are similar to patient-related barriers (Box 21-2). For example, in clinical practice, there is a tendency to group patients into one category referred to as "elder," which spans over two decades of one's life. However, there is no direct correlation between chronologic age and level of frailty and decline. Clinicians should assess individuals more specifically over each decade of their lives. Other clinician-related barriers to adequate pain management in elder patients with advanced cancer include inadequate knowledge of pain management, concerns about patient addiction,

and tolerance (AHCPR, 1994). Traditionally health care professionals have had little or no training in pain management, and knowledge deficits in pain assessment and management have been well documented (Foley, 1998). The potential side effects of analgesics and misconceptions regarding their use in the older adult population are significant factors that prevent health professionals from prescribing analgesics in appropriate doses (AHCPR, 1994; McCaffery & Pasero, 1999).

The third major category that presents barriers to pain management is the health care system (Box 21-3). Undertreated pain may promote a decline in the individual's ability to be independent, resulting in the need for placement in alternative care settings such as nursing homes, which can create substantial challenges to medical care and pain management. Limited

Box 21-3 **Health Care System Barriers to Effective Pain Management**

- Rising cost of medications and limited income creating barriers to the ability to purchase medications
- Frequent "physician hopping" fragmenting care and creating polypharmacy side effects
- Clinicians who are not trained in assessment of pain management of older adults
- Decreased access to health care, which includes hospice, related to isolation or social economics
- Increased placement of older adults in nursing facilities, leading to logistical barriers such as lack of availability of physician, laboratory, and radiographic evaluations
- Nursing shortage resulting in increased caseloads
- Lack of common language to describe pain
- Lack of commitment to pain management
- Failure to use validated tools for pain management in practice
- Lack of team approach to address multidimensional approach to pain management
- Legal factors and restrictions to drug prescribing and availability further impeding the process of pain management

medical resources, polypharmacy, limited access to physicians, and frequent turnover of nursing staff all contribute to fragmented oversight of the plan of care that is focused on pain management. These patients are often sent to outside clinics and emergency rooms, where they are evaluated and cared for by personnel who are not familiar with the elder's medical history, baseline status, and goals of care. Often the health care worker lacks interest and training in the care of frail adults (Ferrell & Ferrell, 1995).

Recently, the Joint Commission on Accreditation of Healthcare Organizations (JCAHO) issued pain management standards in an effort to hold institutions accountable (JCAHO, 2000). In addition, to raise awareness about the importance of pain management, the American Pain Society (1992) has recommended that pain be incorporated into the assessment data as the fifth vital sign.

GENERAL CONSIDERATIONS
Roles of Family

Caring for older persons requires holistic assessment of the individual, his or her environment, and the support system. One of the first factors to determine is whether the older person is independent and, if so, to what extent. If he or she is not independent, who is the identified caregiver for the patient? If the caregiver is a professional nurse or nursing assistant, it is important to determine his or her level of competency with regard to pain management. Also, the patient–caregiver relationship needs to be evaluated. Goals of care should be identified so all individuals involved in the patient's care are aware of the patient's wishes and the plan of care.

In the role of caregiver, the family member may take on responsibilities requiring education. The caregiver may have a knowledge deficit regarding the patient's disease process, disease progression, and symptoms of pain. Observation of pain and rating of the pain level need to be taught. If the patient is cognitively impaired, assessment of pain will be more difficult. The caregiver needs basic education regarding medication and dosing used to treat each symptom. He or she also needs to be encouraged to verbalize any fears and concerns regarding addiction and tolerance. Another important task of caregiving is to keep a record of medication administration, which provides documentation to share with the primary care team.

Sensory Changes That May Affect Pain Assessment and Management

As a normal part of aging, individuals will experience changes in auditory and visual senses, including changes in depth perception, color perception, and visual acuity. With increasing age, the ability to discriminate sounds diminishes. Background noises impede the ability to filter sound. In addition, older individuals often complain of a "ringing" sensation (tinnitus), and they may have difficulty hearing high-pitched sounds. These problems can complicate pain assessment and treatment efforts. Communication between the health care team and the patient can be challenging. Patients may have difficulty reading handouts, prescriptions, and other pain management material because of changes in vision.

Oftentimes, individuals are embarrassed and fail to report the changes or difficulties they experience with vision and hearing.

Substance Abuse and Dependence

The use of alcohol to such an extent that it causes physical or psychological harm needs to be assessed. Physiologic dependence implies tolerance (increasing amounts are needed to get the same effect), and signs of withdrawal symptoms may occur when consumption ceases. If the patient is chemically dependent, including on alcohol, levels of opioids and analgesics might need to be titrated higher because of tolerance. Thus use of alcohol is an important part of the total pain assessment.

The Subcommittee on Health and Long-Term Care of the Select Committee on Aging reported that alcohol is the leading drug of choice for the elder. Widowers over the age of 75 have the highest rate of alcoholism in the country (Glass, Prigerson, Kasl, & Mendes de Leon, 1995). Elder drinkers are less likely to consume large quantities because fewer drinks are needed to raise blood alcohol levels. The best way to assess alcohol consumption in the older adult is to interview the patient. The patient may be reluctant to report alcohol misuse or may be unaware that a problem exists. Using a direct, nonjudgmental, and nonthreatening approach may elicit accurate information.

As part of a total pain assessment, practitioners are encouraged to look for subtle, unexplained conditions such as incontinence, malnutrition, malaise, insomnia, cognitive impairment, and social isolation. These may be evidenced by unexplained injuries from falls, cigarette burns, and short-term memory loss, and may provide an indication of alcohol misuse (Geroldi, Rozzini, Frisoni, & Trabucchi, 1994).

Drugs commonly used by the older adult can interact adversely with alcohol. The clinician should not assume that somnolence, imbalance, and delirium are side effects from medications because these symptoms may be caused by increased alcohol use. Nonsteroidal anti-inflammatory drugs (NSAIDs) frequently are a major part of the pain regimen for older adults. If these drugs are consumed with alcohol, prolonged bleeding time and increased gastric inflammation may occur. Also, acetaminophen, which is commonly used in pain management, may lead to liver failure when used in combination with alcohol.

Use of illegal drugs is uncommon among the current generation of older adults. This may change as the "baby boomers" age. There are few studies of opiate abuse and dependence among the older adult; substance abuse involving over-the-counter and other prescription drugs tends to occur frequently.

Holistic Pain Management Using an Interdisciplinary Team

The clinical presentation of pain, especially persistent pain, commonly involves the physical, social, psychological, and spiritual domains. Thus the complex interplay of these multiple factors creates a challenge when attempting to accomplish good pain management. Nurses and physicians are naive if they believe that they are capable of accomplishing pain management without involving the various members/disciplines of the team, including the patient and family.

Both the patient and family, as members of the team, should be encouraged to express their concerns regarding a pain regimen and methods that can be used to control side effects, should they occur. For example, if the patient or family member has experienced side effects from the use of opioids that were not controlled well in the past, there will be reluctance to accept their use to control pain now. Drowsiness, nausea, and constipation are very predictable potential side effects that commonly occur with the initiation of opioids but can be controlled. Patients deserve to know that side effects can be controlled and, if not, that other medications will be prescribed. Not only should the health care professional be monitoring the patient for the effectiveness of the intervention and immediately addressing any side effects, but the patient also needs to be educated in regard to possible side effects and the need to report them immediately. Although pharmacists give patients written information regarding side effects, from conversations with patients, it appears that many do not read it. Regardless, giving written material without follow-up discussion is not an effective teaching methodology with any patient.

Ferrell (1996) developed a conceptual model that depicts the impact of pain on the various

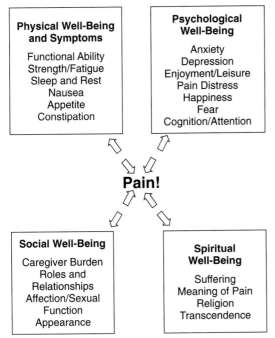

Physical Well-Being and Symptoms	Psychological Well-Being
Functional Ability Strength/Fatigue Sleep and Rest Nausea Appetite Constipation	Anxiety Depression Enjoyment/Leisure Pain Distress Happiness Fear Cognition/Attention

Pain!

Social Well-Being	Spiritual Well-Being
Caregiver Burden Roles and Relationships Affection/Sexual Function Appearance	Suffering Meaning of Pain Religion Transcendence

Fig. 21-1 The impact of pain on the dimensions of quality of life. (Developed by B. R. Ferrell, 1996.)

dimensions of quality of life. According to this model, pain involves the dimensions of physiologic well-being, including symptoms and function; psychological well-being, such as anxiety and depression; social well-being, including roles and relationships; and spiritual well-being, including aspects such as suffering and the meaning of pain (Fig. 21-1). This conceptual model serves as an excellent basis on which to approach pain management in the older adult and is complemented by the interdisciplinary team approach.

Spiritual Care Counselor's Role in Pain Management

Determining the meaning of pain for the individual patient and incorporating an intervention into the plan of care is the role of a spiritual care counselor. Patients frequently assume that pain denotes progression of disease when, in fact, it is often a sign that the medications need to be titrated higher. If the spiritual care counselor is an active participant on the interdisciplinary team, that information can be relayed to the

appropriate member of the team, the pain can be decreased with appropriate adjustment of medications, and, most importantly, the patient's fears can be allayed.

The element of suffering is more difficult to correct. Statements such as "It is God's will" or "God will not give me more pain than I can handle" indicate the need for the intervention of spiritual care. There are some patients who truly believe they must suffer before they die and persist in this belief despite multiple approaches. This is an example of a situation in which an interdisciplinary team can become extremely frustrated. If the team is certain that all approaches have been tried, individual team members must ask themselves the fundamental question regarding their desire to alleviate the patient's pain: "Whose need is it? Is it the patient's need or my need?" To force a patient to accept an intervention would be disrespectful and would violate the basic ethical principle of autonomy. In addition, to remove a patient's pain against his or her will could potentially create more suffering for the patient.

Social Worker's Role in Pain Management

One potential area of concern for the older adult is finances, especially in relation to the cost of medications. The social worker is only one member of the team and can only advocate for the patient if the other members of the team share information regarding needs. To illustrate, frequently the opioid prescribed for pain will be the one that is best marketed by the drug company representative. Physicians do not always know the cost of an individual drug; it may be more likely that the nurse is aware of medication costs. If limited income is a problem, the first option would be to advocate for a less expensive drug. If there is none, the social worker may know of a drug assistance program. Table 21-1, which presents the equianalgesic doses for various opioids for 24 hours with the associated costs, illustrates the wide variation in the cost of opioids.

PAIN ASSESSMENT

Many definitions of pain exist. Pain is an unpleasant sensory and emotional experience associated with actual or potential tissue damage or described in terms of such damage (International

Table 21-1 Daily Equianalgesic Costs of Opioids

Drug	Dose	Cost*
Methadone	10 mg q12h	$0.30
Morphine IR	30 mg q4h	$1.86-$6.21
Morphine SR	90 mg q12h	$11.16
Oxycodone IR	30 mg q4h	$8.64-$10.33
Duragesic Patch	100 µg/hr	$16.09
Oxycodone SR	80	$17.16

IR, immediate release; *SR*, sustained release.
*Based on product formulation.
Cost based on average wholesale price obtained from RED BOOK (2003): Thomson PDR, Montvale, NJ.

Association for the Study of Pain Task Force on Taxonomy, 1994). However, in the nursing world, probably the most common mantra is, "Pain is whatever the experiencing person says it is and exists whenever he/she says it does" (McCaffery & Beebe, 1989, p. 8). From this definition, one would assume that determining whether a patient has pain would be straightforward, given a cognitively intact population. Research findings demonstrate just the opposite. Katsma and Souza (2000) conducted a study with 89 long-term care nurses to determine their knowledge base regarding pain assessment and management for the older adult. They were given two patient scenarios, one in which the patient was smiling and showing no objective signs of pain, and the other in which the patient was grimacing. The nurses were asked to indicate their pain assessment on a 0-to-10 scale and to choose the correct pain medication and dose. The findings indicated that nurses were more likely to interpret grimacing as a manifestation of pain than smiling. Older nurses with more experience were less likely to believe or document their patient's self-reports of pain than nurses with few years of experience. Less than half of the nurses would increase the analgesic dose for either patient scenario. This same study has been replicated with nurses in other settings with similar results.

Determining if a patient is experiencing pain is the most crucial step in the assessment process. Regardless of age, many patients will deny they are experiencing pain if asked directly, "Are you in pain?" or "Do you have pain?" The average person, regardless of age, does not realize that such descriptors as "burning," "tingling," and "electric" are signs of pain. The first part of a total pain assessment is to determine the older patient's preferred pain terminology. It is not uncommon for elders to deny pain when asked if they have it, but to respond in the affirmative to other terms such as "hurt," "ache," "discomfort," or "sore" (AGS Panel on Chronic Pain in Older Persons, 1998; Feldt, Ryden, & Miles, 1998; Sengstaken & King, 1993). "Hurt" is one of the most commonly used terms by older adults to describe pain. Of the 78 pain descriptors in the McGill Pain Questionnaire, the most frequently selected were "hurting," "tiring," "exhausting," "nagging," and "annoying" (Ferrell, Ferrell, & Rivera, 1995). Thus, after the denial of pain, suggested rewording of questions would include "Do you hurt anywhere?" or "Are you uncomfortable?" to verify the absence of discomfort. As with any aspect of assessment, the information should be documented so all members of the health care team are cognizant of the patient's preferred terminology.

Pain History: Previous Pain Experience

A careful history regarding previous pain experiences is essential to determine approaches that have been used in the past, both pharmacologic (including over-the-counter drugs, herbs, and home remedies) and nonpharmacologic interventions. Another part of a pain history is taking a drug profile. It is necessary to determine exactly what the drugs, doses, and outcomes have been in the past because memories of previous undesirable side effects (nausea, sedation, or constipation) can be difficult to erase. Although the patient might report having been prescribed multiple medications, he or she may not report nonadherence to a prescribed regimen. It is not uncommon for older adults to decrease the dose or discontinue the drug because of undesirable side effects.

Another factor contributing to degree of nonadherence is the cost of medications. Older adults may not be able to afford to have the prescription filled, or they may take the drug less frequently than prescribed to make the prescription last longer. Another factor can be going to multiple physicians for treatment of each disease; the primary physician may be unaware of the complete drug profile. Therefore, when a physician prescribes a full dose of a known (or unknown) drug, an adverse event may result.

A second part of the history is determining alcohol consumption; if the use of alcohol is not specifically addressed when a drug profile is taken, patients may not include it (see "Substance Abuse and Dependence" above). Alcohol use that is not reported or is underreported by older adults can complicate a hospitalization as a result of changes in liver metabolism and/or development of withdrawal symptoms. Although this issue is not unique to the older adult, it can be overlooked and result in life-threatening effects.

Assessing the Disease Process and Possible Causes of Pain

In the older adult population, the incidence of cancer increases with increased age; many of the malignancies (breast, lung, and prostate) occurring in the older adult metastasize to bones, particularly the femur and ribs. Metastatic lesions in the bone can be very painful, and can be the cause of pathologic fractures precipitated by an activity as simple as a sneeze. Pain in patients with colon cancer is much less likely to be due to metastatic bone disease; rather, it is more commonly associated with a bowel obstruction causing a distended abdomen. Herpes is another common occurrence in this population, with resulting pain even after the skin eruptions have healed. Ultimately, some patients are left with postherpetic neuralgia.

Assessing Components of Pain

Location

Older adult patients are likely to have more than one type of pain, especially if it is cancer related. A simple and important technique to use when assessing the site(s) of pain is to ask the patient to point to each pain location as it is discussed, because each one could have an entirely different pathophysiology and require a different intervention. An example is a patient with lung cancer with metastases to the brachial plexus, resulting in neuropathic pain, as well as a metastatic lesion to the femur, resulting in somatic pain. Using the above method enhances the ability to assess and reassess pain accurately (Twycross & Lack, 1983).

Intensity

Patients should be asked to rate their pain "right now," "at best," "at worst," and "on average." Without the final step of asking what the pain is "on average," the rating of the pain intensity could be a totally inaccurate picture of the overall pain intensity. The Wisconsin Brief Pain Questionnaire accurately assesses the global picture of pain (Daut, Cleeland, & Flanery, 1983). An example of this pain tool can be found in the text *Management of Cancer Pain: Adults* (AHCPR, 1994).

Quality

It is important to ask the older adult for specific descriptors of the quality of the pain. Each pain mechanism has specific word descriptors. For example, somatic pain is described as "aching," "gnawing," or "throbbing," and the cognitively intact patient will be able to point to the site of the pain. Visceral pain is poorly localized and described as "squeezing," "deep," and "boring." Neuropathic pain is "burning" or "numb," and sometimes described as "shooting" or "electric." As discussed later in the chapter, each type of pain requires a different pharmacotherapy for management.

Onset/Duration

Another important component of the pain assessment process is determining if the pain is constant, intermittent, or both. Interventions will be different depending on the type of pain. If the patient has intermittent pain related to an activity, such as physical therapy, the patient will need to be medicated prior to therapy and may not require any medication the remainder of the day. In contrast, a patient with persistent pain, such as with RA, will require ongoing intervention for pain. There are specific questions to ask: "When did the pain begin?" "How long does it last?" "Are you ever free of pain?" and "What is the frequency of the pain episodes?"

Factors that Exacerbate and Alleviate Pain

A thorough pain assessment includes not only noting when the pain started, but also what activities exacerbate the pain and if there any other symptoms, such as nausea and vomiting, associated with the pain. Including the family in the history taking can be helpful to the older adult regarding the facts of his or her current situation. Pain usually does not occur at just one moment in time; therefore, when conducting a pain assessment on any new pain, it is imperative to get a more global picture of the pain experience. Pain needs to be assessed not only at rest, but also with movement. How does the pain affect ADLs? Does the pain prevent doing activities the patient enjoys? The nurse should assess the present pain regimen and how well it is working.

Pain Scales

The measurement of pain over time requires some method of benchmarking. The most frequent objective method to determine pain intensity as an indicator of the effectiveness of pain intervention is to use a pain scale.

A variety of tools are available to quantify pain intensity. Psychometric evaluation of pain intensity scales suggests that variations of the verbal descriptor scale (VDS), the visual analogue scale, the numeric rating scale (NRS), and the Faces Pain Scale, can be used with older adults. Herr and Mobily (1993) compared five pain intensity scales in a sample of 49 elders (age > 65 years) who reported pain. The largest percentage perceived the VDS to be the easiest to complete and the measure that best described their pain. The VDS consists of a series of phrases describing different levels of pain intensity (e.g., "no pain," "mild pain," "moderate pain," "severe pain," "extreme pain," and "the most intense pain imaginable"). It has shown good reliability and validity when used with older adults.

The NRS involves asking people to rate their pain from 0 to 10, with 0 representing no pain and 10 the worst pain imaginable. The NRS can be presented either vertically or horizontally; however, studies indicate that the older adult population prefers the vertical presentation. An analogy to a thermometer can be made for the elder patient. Conceptually, it is understood that, as temperature rises, the number becomes larger, with the same being true of pain. As the pain becomes worse, the number becomes larger.

The Wong Faces Pain Scale is occasionally used with adults, including the older adult population. This scale was originally developed and tested in the pediatric population, so there is concern regarding its validity with adults. Some

of the questions that need to be answered are "How well does a person who is very stoic respond to this tool?" and "Does it measure pain or feelings in the adult?"

Physical Examination

When completing a physical examination on an older adult, special attention should be given to the neuromuscular and musculoskeletal systems. Neurologic impairment, weakness, allodynia, numbness, and paresthesia should be assessed in the neuromuscular system. In the musculoskeletal system, one should palpate for tenderness, inflammation, deformity, and trigger points (AGS Panel on Chronic Pain in Older Persons, 1998). The interdisciplinary team can be an asset in the ongoing assessment of pain; frequently, it is the nursing assistant who will be able to report if the patient complains of pain when joints are moved while providing personal care.

INFERRED PATHOPHYSIOLOGY OF PAIN

Pain is classified under two major types, nociceptive and neuropathic; each of these is further divided into two subtypes. Nociceptive pain is subdivided into either somatic or visceral pain. Somatic pain occurs as a result of activation of pain-sensitive structures, or nociceptors, in either cutaneous or musculoskeletal tissues. It is described as gnawing, aching, or throbbing, and patients can frequently point to the exact location of the pain. Examples of somatic pain seen in the older population would be arthritis (both RA and OA), myalgias, decubitus ulcers, ischemic disorders, incisional pain, and metastatic bone pain. Conversely, visceral pain is caused by processes such as infiltration of tumor, gastric paralysis secondary to diabetes, and stretching of the viscera of organs. Typically, visceral pain is related to stimulus of thoracic, abdominal, or pelvic organs. For example, the liver could be enlarged as a result of metastatic cancer, and this may result in stretching of the hepatic capsule, which contains visceral pain fibers. Visceral pain is poorly localized and described as deep, boring, squeezing, or cramping. Frequently this pain is felt in areas remote from the original site, and is therefore called referred pain. The patient may experience pain on touching the original site, as well as tenderness at the referred site. Both somatic and visceral pain responds to NSAIDs and opioids. Occasionally, steroids are added to the regimen for visceral pain.

Neuropathic pain is much more complex and difficult to manage than nociceptive pain, and is subdivided into pain generated either peripherally or centrally. Neuropathic pain resulting from a pathophysiologic process that involves the peripheral nervous system is described as burning, tingling, and shocklike or electric. Examples are postherpetic neuralgia, diabetic neuropathy, and trigeminal neuralgia. In the older cancer patient, neuropathic pain commonly occurs with tumor infiltration or compression of nerves, surgical trauma, or chemotherapy- or radiation-induced injury. Examples would be brachial or lumbosacral plexopathy, spinal cord compression, and post-thoracic or mastectomy incisional pain. Centrally generated pain occurs at the spinal cord level and results from hyperexcitability. Because of the hyperexcitability, otherwise nonpainful stimuli are perceived as painful (allodynia). An example would be poststroke pain.

A third classification, which merits consideration in the geriatric population, is mixed or undetermined pathophysiology. Under this category are chronic recurrent headaches (e.g., tension headaches, migraine headaches, mixed headaches) and vasculopathic pain syndromes (e.g., painful vasculitis) (AGS Panel on Chronic Pain in Older Persons, 1998).

ACUTE PAIN

A holistic approach should be utilized to adequately assess pain in any population; this is especially true for older adult patients. Pain is a multidimensional experience with sensory, affective, and cognitive evaluative components that interact and contribute to the final pain response (Ferrell, 1996). The nurse must never underestimate the important role psychological distress plays in the total pain experience for the older patient. Some patients carry the burden of a lifetime of previous pain experiences. As the underlying disease progresses (especially cancer), all the unfinished business of one's life work can become integrated into the pain experience (Stein, 1996).

Perioperative Setting

Pain management during the perioperative period is challenging because most older adult patients have at least one chronic condition and take multiple medications in addition to those associated with the surgery. Compounding the problem, the prevalence of cognitive impairment in the older adult increases the likelihood of poor pain management at the time of surgery. Phillips (2000) reported that appropriate pain management results in quicker clinical recovery, shorter hospital stays, fewer readmissions, and improved quality of life. Yet older patients hospitalized for surgery tend to receive less aggressive treatment. The problem of poor pain management in the United States is beginning to be addressed by the JCAHO and their pain management guidelines; these algorithms emphasize the need for both pharmacologic and nonpharmacologic interventions, especially in the elder population (JCAHO, 2000).

Assessment is a vital component of giving good care at the time of surgery. Distinguishing between pain from a chronic condition versus pain from an acute process, which may be limited to the surgical wound, is the important first step. Questions remain regarding the perception of pain by the older adult and thereby the reporting of pain. Because of some age-related changes in the integrity of the skin, sensation of the skin may change with time; however, it is not clear if nociception also changes. Certain types of visceral pain may be perceived less intensely by the older adult; for example, the "surgical abdomen" may present without leukocytosis or marked pain. "Silent" myocardial infarctions may be more common in older adults. Not only is the incidence of headache lower in older adults, but it is also much more serious when it does occur; serious conditions such as temporal arteritis, congestive heart failure, subdural hematoma, and electrolyte disturbances are more likely the etiologies (Gordon, 1979).

Preoperative Management

Informing patients about the surgical procedure and the planned postoperative activities is fairly routine; however, the initiation of prophylactic pain measures is not. Older adult patients should be informed regarding exactly what to expect with regard to pain postoperatively. Included in the instructions should be the type of pain, what it will feel like, how to report the pain, what pain scale will be used, to whom the pain should be reported, what method of administering the medication will be used (patient-controlled analgesia pump, injections, or oral), and when to expect relief after being medicated. Part of the preoperative preparation should also involve suggesting to older adult patients that they appoint a family member or friend who can advocate for aggressive pain management if they are unable to speak for themselves after surgery.

Another important consideration is clarifying PRN dosing. Frequently, older adult patients do not understand that, when medication is prescribed PRN, they are responsible for requesting to be medicated when pain occurs. They may assume, unless instructed differently, that medication is automatically administered and, conversely, that, if medication is not being given, this means that they must not need it. The earlier section "Pain Scales" provides information on what pain scales have been tested and are valid for use in the older adult population.

Postoperative Management

Regardless of the etiology of the pain, both pharmacologic and nonpharmacologic interventions should be considered. In the elder population, in whom the risk of adverse events is higher with pharmacologic interventions, the nonpharmacologic options may be first-line choices because they have fewer side effects and are usually less costly. Several factors can influence how well the older adult patient will do postoperatively. A thorough drug history should be taken upon admission to prevent untoward experiences following surgery, because polypharmacy is a known occurrence and a concern when working with the older adult population.

Symptoms commonly associated with analgesics may develop with a completely different etiology in the postoperative state. For example, sleep is to be expected, especially when pain is controlled. However, careful assessment needs to be performed to differentiate between normal sleep and oversedation from opioids; this is discussed further in the section "Opioids" below. Postoperative delirium may manifest itself for a host of reasons in the older adult patient that are not typical in younger patients. Urinary tract infections, pneumonia (commonly overlooked in the older adult), drugs, and urinary retention (which may or may not be related to some analgesics) are some causes of delirium in this population (Blackburt & Dunn, 1990).

PERSISTENT (CHRONIC) PAIN

Guidelines for treating pain in older adult patients were released by the AGS in May of 2002 (AGS Panel on Persistent Pain in Older Persons, 2002). A significant change in these guidelines is the use of the term *persistent pain* rather than chronic pain (which connoted negative images). It is believed that the term *persistent pain* will promote a more positive attitude for both patients and professionals.

Persistent pain is common among older adults because they have many comorbid disorders that contribute to their pain (Ferrell, 1991; Gallagher, Verma, & Mossey, 2000); these disorders often include OA, cancer, diabetic neuropathy, herpes zoster, and osteoporosis. Although persons ages 65 and older are more likely to experience persistent pain, they are less likely to obtain pain relief than younger people. Achieving good pain relief is complicated by three main factors: comorbid diseases; increased risk of adverse drug reactions; and physician factors, including lack of knowledge in pain management and fear of prescribing opioids for the elder patient (Gloth, 2000).

By definition, persistent pain has a duration of greater than 3 months. By the time pain becomes persistent, adaptation of the autonomic nervous system occurs and the objective signs of an elevated blood pressure and rapid pulse, which occur with acute pain episodes, are absent. People with chronic pain usually do not "look like" they are in pain, as compared to people with acute pain, who might grimace or demonstrate other behaviors more likely to be associated with pain. To further complicate the picture, family caregivers may not believe the person is experiencing pain because they "don't look like they are in pain," and may be unlikely to advocate for their family member. Over the past 16 years, B. R. Ferrell and colleagues have done research related to pain management in the home and to the role of family caregivers. One consistent finding is that the fears, inappropriate knowledge, and beliefs of family caregivers frequently are more disruptive to care than those of patients (Ferrell, 2001). For the geriatric patient experiencing chronic pain, the greatest fear is the potential

EVIDENCE-BASED PRACTICE

Reference: Given, C. S., Gwen, B., Azzoriz, F., Kozachik, S., & Stommel, N. (2001). Predictors of pain and fatigue in the year following diagnosis among elderly cancer patients. *Journal of Pain and Symptom Management, 21*, 456-466.

Research Problem: Pain and fatigue are prevalent symptoms that occur throughout the course of cancer. The majority of research has focused on the consequences of pain and fatigue related to a single site of cancer. Clarification is needed regarding the roles that pain and fatigue play with respect to the co-occurrence with other symptoms commonly associated with cancer.

Design: Descriptive longitudinal investigation.

Sample and Setting: Inception cohort of 841 patients 65 years of age or older and newly diagnosed with breast, colon, lung, or prostate cancer, recruited from the Lower Peninsula of Michigan, including the Detroit metropolitan area, and from one community in Indiana.

Methods: The co-occurrence and patterns of change among combinations of pain and fatigue, and the number of other symptoms reported by patients with four different types of cancer, were examined. Data were collected at four observation periods between 6 and 52 weeks.

Results: During the year, patients improved with respect to their reports of pain and/or fatigue. Stage, more comorbidity, and lung cancer were related to both pain and fatigue. Chemotherapy was related to reports of fatigue, but did not have an extended effect on fatigue.

Implications for Nursing Practice: Pain and fatigue did have a substantial independent effect on the presence of other symptoms. This alone speaks very strongly to the importance of managing these two symptoms and to their centrality to patients' comfort and quality of life.

Conclusion: Among patients 65 years of age or older with these four diagnoses of cancer, the model indicates a greater risk of reporting pain and/or fatigue if the patient has three or more comorbid conditions, lung cancer compared with breast cancer, late-stage disease, and any treatment within 40 days.

loss of independence and dignity (McElhaney, 2001).

Osteoarthritis: A Common Persistent Pain

OA is a common chronic problem experienced by the geriatric population. OA involves weight-bearing joints and, until recently, was not considered to have an inflammatory component; however, low-grade inflammation without systemic symptoms has been found (Brandt, 1995). As previously discussed, the older adult patient tends to underreport pain. As a result of underreporting, pain is undertreated, resulting in increased catabolic demands and muscle breakdown, impaired healing, weakness, and undue suffering (McCarberg & Herr, 2001). To combat these issues, caregivers of older adult patients must perform consistent and complete pain assessments in patients with arthritis.

Pharmacologic interventions, such as analgesics and anti-inflammatory medications, help control pain and disability when used in conjunction with a holistic approach that addresses the physical, psychological, and spiritual needs of the patient. Acetaminophen is considered first-line therapy for OA. Although it is not thought to have useful anti-inflammatory activity, its analgesic effect is comparable to that of ibuprofen and naproxen, and it has a lower side effect profile (Williams, Ward, & Egger, 1993). NSAIDs are effective in treating rest pain, nighttime pain, and pain associated with significant inflammation. As discussed later in this chapter, NSAIDs should be prescribed with caution for the older adult patient because the potential adverse effects in this population are extremely high. Opioids are part of the pain regimen in the treatment of chronic nonmalignant pain, including OA, when other agents have failed to relieve symptoms. Despite clear evidence of a positive value of opioids in selected patients with moderate to severe OA pain, debate continues over their efficacy and safety (Portenoy, 1996).

Breakthrough Pain

Breakthrough pain is an intermittent episode of moderate to severe pain that occurs between scheduled doses of opioids. Anytime that opioids are scheduled around the clock, breakthrough doses of a short-acting opioid should be prescribed. The breakthrough dose is calculated as 10% to 15% of the 24-hour dose and can be given as frequently as every 1 to 2 hours because the oral peak effect is 1 hour (McCaffery & Pasero, 1999). Until a dose that controls the pain is reached, breakthrough pain can occur anytime between dosing intervals. Patients should never be forced to "wait until the next dose" because it is "not time." Another common scenario is when breakthrough pain occurs close to the next sustained-release dose. Usually that indicates one of two problems: either the dose is too low or the interval between doses is too long. Ideally, pain should be controlled for a 24-hour period without breakthrough doses unless there is incidental pain associated with a specific activity or procedure. Until such control is achieved, patients should be encouraged to keep a pain diary in relation to the time of breakthrough dosing and the related activity. Normally adding all the breakthrough doses for the past 24 hours to the present 24-hour dose creates a new 24-hour dose. However, if the breakthrough represents incidental pain, that should not be included in creating a new 24-hour dose. For example, if the patient requires a daily dressing change that is painful, but pain is well-controlled the rest of the day, that breakthrough dose should not be included in the 24-hour total; instead, the patient should be premedicated before the daily dressing change.

PHARMACOLOGIC INTERVENTIONS

Lack of knowledge with regard to pain management is a commonly cited reason for undertreatment of pain. Ferrell, Virani, and Grant (1999) analyzed 50 nursing textbooks for nine areas of end-of-life content. Only 2% of the overall content was on end-of-life care, and much of it was inaccurate. Pain was often discussed in the textbooks, but usually in the context of acute

rather than persistent pain. Content on pain management during the end of life was virtually absent. A similar lack of information was found when medical textbooks were analyzed. In addition to lack of knowledge as a reason for poor pain management, confusion still exists for some professionals and patients regarding the terms *addiction, tolerance,* and *physical dependence*.

Terminology
Addiction

Addiction is defined as a pattern of compulsive drug use characterized by continued craving for an opioid, loss of control, and continued use despite harm (Coyle & Layman-Goldstein, 2001). A classic study done by Porter and Jick (1980) demonstrated that addiction is rare in patients without a history of drug abuse who are using opioids for cancer pain. Tolerance and physical dependence, both of which are expected with long-term treatment with opioids, should not be confused with addiction. Because of lack of knowledge, some health care professionals and lay people assume the presence of tolerance and physical dependence equates to addiction, which it does not.

Tolerance

Tolerance is defined as the need to increase the dosage of an opioid over time to maintain pain relief (American Pain Society, 1999). As part of the assessment process, patients should be asked directly if they have ever been chemically dependent on any drugs, including alcohol. The nurse should explain why the question is being asked: "The reason I am asking if you have ever been chemically dependent is so we can do good pain control. If you are or have been chemically dependent, you may require a higher dose of drug to receive good pain relief." The first sign of tolerance would be a need to increase the opioid dosage. However, increasing dose requirements are most consistently correlated with progressive disease, which produces increased pain intensity, rather than to tolerance to the analgesic effect of opioids. Patients who have stable disease usually do not require increasing doses (Foley, 1993; Levy, 1989).

Physical Dependence

Physical dependence is the physical reliance on an opioid, evidenced by withdrawal symptoms if the opioid is stopped abruptly or an antagonist is administered (McCaffery & Pasero, 1999). It can occur even if a patient is prescribed an opioid for only a few weeks. However, there will be no signs of physical dependence unless the drug is abruptly stopped. Typically the signs of withdrawal resemble "flulike" symptoms, including chills, hot flushes, joint pain, lacrimation, rhinorrhea, diaphoresis, nausea, vomiting, abdominal cramps, "goose bumps," agitation (inability to sleep), and diarrhea. Opioids should never be abruptly stopped; instead, the dosage of the opioid should be reduced by 50% every 2 to 3 days as part of the gradual weaning process (Emanuel, von Gunten, & Ferris, 1999).

One of the most frequent times when health care professionals unintentionally put patients into withdrawal is during the dying process. Even if the patient is nonresponsive, he or she requires some level of opioid if he or she is opioid dependent. Otherwise, the patient could be put into withdrawal. Therefore, at the end of life, a portion of the daily dose of opioid is given to alleviate pain and dyspnea and prevent withdrawal.

Pharmacologic Intervention for Acute Pain

Meperidine is used to treat acute pain, but is not recommended in treating persistent pain because of its short half-life and its neurotoxic metabolite, normeperidine. Meperidine is commonly used in the immediate postoperative period and deserves special caution because a host of adverse events in the older adult patient have been associated with its use (Stein, 1996). Meperidine is one of the few opioids that has a ceiling dose. The accumulation of normeperidine beyond the analgesic duration of the parent compound causes central nervous system (CNS) stimulation that may lead to seizures.

If meperidine must be used, the older adult patient should be assessed every 8 to 12 hours for signs of neurotoxicity, specifically tremors and myoclonus. With the patient holding out his or her hands straight in front of the body, if a tremor is evident that was not present prior to the administration of meperidine, this is highly suspicious for normeperidine accumulation. The patient should be switched immediately to another mu receptor agonist such as morphine or hydromorphone because further accumulation of

normeperidine can cause seizures (Pasero & McCaffery, 1996).

Meperidine has poor oral absorption and therefore requires high oral doses compared to parenteral dosing. For example, if a patient receives 50 mg of meperidine parenterally, 150 mg would be required for an equivalent oral dose because there is a 1:3 ratio when converting from parenteral to oral dosing.

Chronic Pain: The World Health Organization's Analgesic Ladder

The World Health Organization's (WHO's) three-step ladder approach, as presented in the AHCPR guidelines for the management of cancer pain, is applicable to the older adult patient with pain (AHCPR, 1994) (Fig. 21-2). It involves a framework for pain management that uses a stepped approach to move from mild to severe pain. For mild pain, step I analgesics such as aspirin, acetaminophen, or a NSAID are prescribed.

If the pain progresses to a moderate level despite dose increase, a change to step II analgesics is indicated. Among these drugs are low-dose oxycodone or weaker opioids (codeine or

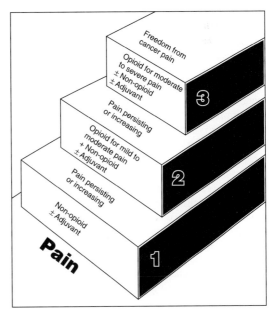

Fig. 21-2 WHO three-step analgesic ladder. (From World Health Organization. [1996]. *Cancer pain relief* [2nd ed.]. Geneva: WHO.)

hydrocodone), used either alone or in combination with step I drugs. For severe pain, step III opioids such as morphine, oxycodone, hydromorphone, methadone, and fentanyl are prescribed. It is now understood that the step of the WHO ladder must be matched to the severity of pain. If a patient is experiencing severe pain, opioids on step III of the ladder should be administered with or without nonopioids and adjuvants. It is now recognized that opioids previously described as "weak," such as oxycodone, can also be administered for severe pain at higher doses.

Analgesics should be given by mouth, by the clock, by the ladder, and for the individual when treating persistent pain (WHO, 1986). This summarizes the need to administer medications orally if the gut works; to schedule medications around the clock, not PRN; to use the WHO analgesic ladder; and to titrate the dose until the pain is relieved. Opioids alone will rarely control pain, so at each step of the pain ladder, adjuvant drugs may be added depending on the pathophysiology. Three categories of analgesics are included in the three-step ladder model: nonopioids, opioids, and adjuvant analgesics. Figure 21-3 is an example of a pain management care path that includes the WHO analgesic ladder.

Nonopioids: Nonsteroidal Anti-inflammatory Drugs

For mild pain and step I of the analgesic ladder, the nonopioid drug of choice is a NSAID; however, special consideration must be used when prescribing for the older adult patient because of the potential side effects. Acetaminophen is often classified in this group, although it seems to lack significant anti-inflammatory properties and has a different side effect profile.

Before discussing the mechanism of action of NSAIDs, an explanation of what happens to tissue at the time of injury should be considered. When tissue damage occurs, inflammatory mediators, such as bradykinin and prostaglandins, are released at the site of injury; these in turn activate nociceptors that transmit pain. An enzyme called cyclooxygenase (COX), which has two forms (COX-1 and COX-2), breaks down arachidonic acid to produce prostaglandins (Pasero & McCaffery, 2001). COX-1 is involved in the production of prostaglandins that preserve platelet

function and protect gastric mucosa, while COX-2 produces prostaglandins that cause pain.

Conventional NSAIDs are extremely effective in treating somatic pain, such as bone pain, because the periosteum of the bone is rich in prostaglandins, which modulate pain. NSAIDs are not selective in blocking prostaglandins just at the site of injury; they also deplete the protective layer of prostaglandins in the gastrointestinal tract. When the protective layer of gastric prostaglandin is depleted, gastrointestinal side effects such as indigestion, nausea, heartburn, ulceration, perforation, and hemorrhage can occur. Studies have identified a correlation between advanced age and risk of ulceration (Popp & Portenoy, 1996).

Conventional NSAIDs, such as ibuprofen, nonspecifically block both COX-1 and COX-2, thus providing pain relief but increasing the potential for bleeding. For long-term use of NSAIDs, prophylactic treatment with misoprostol is recommended to reduce the incidence of NSAID-induced ulcers by replacing gastric prostaglandin (Raskin et al., 1995). COX-2 inhibitors, such as celecoxib and rofecoxib, selectively block or inhibit only COX-2 and theoretically have a more favorable side effect profile than conventional NSAIDs. The decision to use the more expensive COX-2 inhibitors should be based on the individual patient's risk of gastrointestinal tract hemorrhage (Noble, King, & Olutade, 2000).

NSAIDs that are highly protein bound cause significant toxicity in older adults and severely ill patients, who may have low levels of serum albumin. Older adults taking NSAIDs may develop dizziness, confusion, and excessive salt and water retention (Abraham, 2000). NSAID-related side effects that occur with increased frequency in the elder population include renal impairment, cardiovascular events (e.g., exacerbation of congestive heart failure), and hematologic effects (e.g., decreased platelet function resulting in bleeding). The renal clearance of drugs, including analgesics, declines with increasing age; therefore, the use of NSAIDs generally should be avoided in patients with an elevated serum creatinine level or decreased creatinine clearance.

Although thought to be lacking in anti-inflammatory effect, acetaminophen frequently is

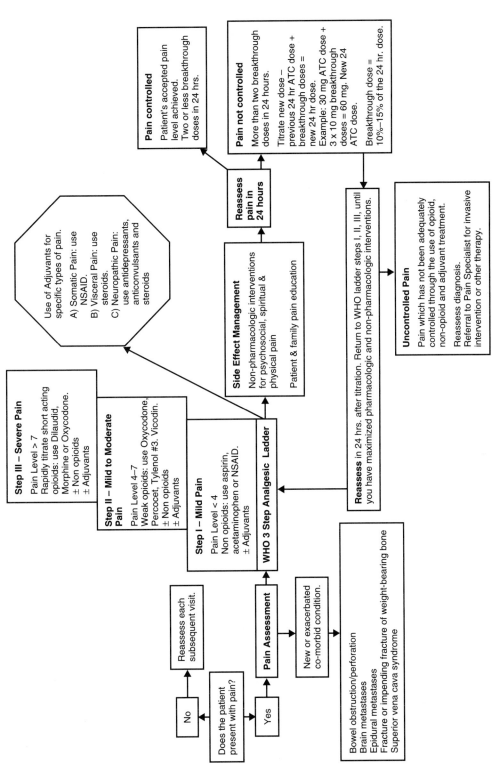

Fig. 21-3 Pain management care path. *ATC*, around the clock; *NSAID*, nonsteroidal anti-inflammatory drugs; *WHO*, World Health Organization. (Created by the Safe Conduct Team of the Safe Conduct Project–Ireland Cancer Center and The Hospice of the Western Reserve, Cleveland, OH. Copyright © 2000 Robert Wood Johnson Foundation Demonstration Project.)

classified with the NSAIDs and is part of the pain regimen. The major side effect of acetaminophen is hepatic toxicity. Patients with chronic alcoholism and liver disease can develop severe hepatotoxicity even when the drug is prescribed within the usual therapeutic doses (Whitcomb & Block, 1994). Caution must be used when prescribing acetaminophen because there is a ceiling dose of 4000 mg/24 hours.

In step II of the analgesic ladder, there are many combinations of acetaminophen with another analgesic. Among these are Percocet (oxycodone), Darvon and Darvocet N (propoxyphene), and Vicodin (hydrocodone), which all contain acetaminophen. For example, if a patient is prescribed two Percocet, equaling 10 mg oxycodone with 650 mg acetaminophen, every 4 hours around the clock, the acetaminophen ceiling dose of 4 g in 24 hours will be reached. All additional dosing of acetaminophen, whether it is given for an elevated temperature or additional breakthrough pain, must be added to this 24-hour dose. With Vicodin, there is even a greater danger of overdose because each tablet contains 500 mg of acetaminophen. Careful evaluation of the amount of acetaminophen contained in all medications—both prescribed and over the counter—must take place because some over-the-counter medications also contain large amounts of acetaminophen. For example, Nyquil contains 1000 mg acetaminophen/30 mL. However, to avoid acetaminophen overdosage, nonopioids can be administered as single agents with opioids to create an additive effect, often decreasing the amount of opioids needed for pain relief.

Opioids

Opioids are prescribed when pain progresses from a mild to a moderate level (step II) or to a severe level (step III). The mechanism of action for opioids is their ability to bind to mu receptors in the brain and spinal cord, thereby preventing the release of the neurotransmitters, such as substance P, required for the transmission of pain (Paice, 1999). Appropriate nonopioids and/or adjuvant medications are continued depending on the classification of pain. Polypharmacy is becoming commonplace in geriatric pain management because of the ability to capitalize on the synergistic effects of drugs, often used at lower doses with fewer side effects, to obtain a therapeutic effect.

Health care professionals have fears and misinformation regarding the use of opioids. Experience has shown that nurses sometimes confuse Cheyne-Stokes breathing patterns, which are not unusual in elders during sleep, with signs that the patient is in the dying process or experiencing a side effect of opioids. Opioid analgesics do not need to be discontinued unless unacceptable degrees of arterial oxygen desaturation (to <85%) occur (AHCPR, 1992). Opioids have no ceiling effect or dosage with the exception of propoxyphene and meperidine. Propoxyphene is a controversial opioid that tends to be overprescribed for the older adult; its efficacy is no greater than that of aspirin or acetaminophen, and it has significant potential for addiction as well as renal damage. Propoxyphene has a metabolite, norpropoxyphene, that can produce severe CNS toxicity (Herr, 2002). This is similar to the situation with meperidine, which was discussed previously. Thus propoxyphene and meperidine, two opioids that have ceiling doses, are not recommended for treating pain in the older adult (Forman, 1996).

Certain physiologic changes can occur with the aging process. Among these changes are decreases in hepatic clearance, glomerular filtration rate, renal tubular function, plasma protein binding, and body water, while body fat stores may be relatively increased (Popp & Portenoy, 1996). As a result, the older adult may be more sensitive to the analgesic effects of opioids, with a higher peak effect and longer duration of action secondary to decreased elimination. Because of these physiologic changes, there are major implications for prescribing opioids for the older adult. For example, an older adult who receives oral morphine may experience unexpected drug effects because of an increase in oral bioavailability. Normally, with the oral administration of morphine, a significant amount of the drug's effect is lost because of the "first-pass effect" as it is cleared through the liver. With aging, a diminished first-pass effect, secondary to decreased hepatic function, leaves more circulating drug. Similarly, when drugs that are cleared primarily by the kidneys are administered to an older adult, the resultant effect could be slower elimination and higher circulating drug concentration. The nursing implication for these physiologic changes is in relationship to dosing intervals. Morphine, 10 mg, would normally be prescribed every 4 hours. The older adult patient may be able to tolerate the same dose of 10 mg, but would need it prescribed every 6 hours because of decreased kidney function with a slower elimination time. In the very old adult patient (85+ years), morphine should be titrated even more slowly, on an every-8-hours basis, because of the accumulation of morphine 6-glucuronide, which is more potent than morphine (Twycross, 1999).

A second point related to the distribution of drugs in the older adult needs to be made. As the lean body mass decreases, the volume of distribution for hydrophilic drugs decreases and the volume of distribution for lipophilic drugs increases (Popp & Portenoy, 1996). Because of these changes, there is a clinical implication in relationship to a single dose. For example, if morphine, which is relatively hydrophilic, is administered as a loading dose, a higher peak concentration–time curve and slower fall in concentration will result, perhaps one reason some drugs appear to have a greater effect on older adult patients than on younger patients (Popp & Portenoy, 1996).

Morphine, hydromorphone, codeine, oxycodone, hydrocodone, methadone, and fentanyl are classified as full agonists because there is no "ceiling" dose to their effectiveness. A full agonist will not reverse or antagonize the effect of another full agonist if given simultaneously, whereas an agonist-antagonist, such as pentazocine, will reverse the effect of a full agonist. If a full agonist and an agonist-antagonist are given simultaneously, withdrawal will be precipitated and the patient will experience a sudden increase in pain.

Morphine. Morphine is the prototype opioid mu receptor agonist; examples of other commonly used mu agonists are oxycodone and hydromorphone. The advantage to using morphine is its availability in tablet, elixir, suppository, and parenteral form. Thus, if the patient is unable to take oral medications at some point in time, many other forms of the same drug are available. Patients can be initially titrated with immediate-release morphine and, when a steady state is obtained, converted to a long-acting controlled-release preparation of morphine. For example, morphine has a half-life of 4 hours, and it takes five to six half-lives of a drug to reach a steady state. Thus, if morphine is administered every 4 hours around the clock, a steady state will

take place in 24 hours. Once a steady state is reached with less than three breakthrough doses, the morphine can be converted to a sustained-release form. An equianalgesic chart should be used to convert routes within the same drug or to convert from one analgesic to another (see Table 21-2 and Box 21-4).

Other Opioids. Hydromorphone and oxycodone are both strong analgesics, with each having limitations as compared to morphine. Hydromorphone is available in various forms, but to date a sustained-release form is not available. Oxycodone comes in both immediate- and sustained-release forms, but it is one of the most costly opioids available. Health care providers have a responsibility to be concerned about the resources of patients, especially older adults, who may have a limited income. The following case illustrates this point well:

An older adult patient was seen in an outpatient clinic with the chief complaint of pain. A review of the prescribed medications included what was a very appropriate dose of OxyContin for pain; however, she experienced persistent pain. Upon further questioning by the social worker, the patient admitted that she had never had the prescription filled because she needed to make a choice between paying her rent and paying for the prescription. To address the concern over cost, methadone, which is extremely inexpensive, was instead ordered for pain, and she was able to accomplish both goals of paying her rent and obtaining good pain relief.

TRANSDERMAL FENTANYL. Transdermal fentanyl is particularly useful when patients cannot swallow, do not remember to take medications, or experience adverse effects with other opioids. However, fentanyl has a long half-life, which makes it more difficult to use in the geriatric population. Fever, diaphoresis, and cachexia, all of which are often present in the older adult, may significantly impact the absorption, predictability of blood levels, and clinical effects of transdermal fentanyl; this form of administration may not be appropriate in these conditions (Newshan, 1998).

Transdermal fentanyl is frequently used in the long-term care population. This practice needs to be evaluated very carefully because elder patients, who are frequently opioid-naive, cannot tolerate fentanyl. It is not uncommon to see confusion and sedation as side effects. Also, at the end of life, when the patient's condition can decline rapidly, it is almost impossible to decrease a long-

Table 21-2 Opioid Reference Table

Drug Name (Available Dosage)	Appropriate Opioid Equianalgesic Dose		Oral to Parenteral Dose Ratio	Oral Dosing Interval (hours)	Strengths of Products/ Comments
	PO/SL (mg)	SO/IV (mg)			
Morphine	30	10	3:1	CR 12	Oramorph 15, 30, 60, 100 mg tablets MS Conth 15, 30, 60, 100, 200 mg tablets
				CR 24	Kadian 20, 30, 60, 80, 100 mg sprinkle caps (LU)
	30	10	3:1	IR 4	MSIR 10, 15, 30 mg tablets Roxanol 20 mg/ml, solution 10 mg/sec (peds)
Hydromorphone	7.5	1.5	5:1	IR 4	Dilaudid 1, 2, 3, 4, 8 mg tablets
Oxycodone	20	N/A	N/A	CR 12	OxyContin 10, 29, 40, 80 mg tablets (LU)
	20	N/A	N/A	IR 4	OxyIR 6 mg caps Roxicodone 5, 15, 30 mg tablets Oxyfast, Roxicodone 29 mg/ml Percocet 5/325 = 5 mg oxycodone + 325 mg acetaminophen
Hydrocodone	30	N/A	N/A	4-6	Vicodin 5/550 = 5 mg hydrocodone + 500 mg acetaminophen
Codeine	200	130	1.5:1	6-8	15, 30, 60 mg tablets High constipation potential
Meperidine	300	180	3:1	N/A	Demeral 50, 100 mg tablets Contraindicated in cancer pain management
Levorphanol	4	2	2:1	6-8	Levo-Dromoran 2 mg tablets Long half-life: must be used with caution to avoid delayed accumulation.
Methadone	Variable	Variable	2:1	9-24	5, 10, 40 mg tablets Long half-life: must be used with caution to avoid delayed accumulation. Highly variable dosing. Morphine:Methadone ratio dependent on total 24 hr dose of MS: <100 mg = 4:1; 100-300 mg = 8:1; 300 mg = 12:1
Fentanyl (25 mcg/hr)	25 mcg/hr = 45 mg PO MS	Refer to conversion	N/A	72 hr	Duragesic 25, 50, 75, 100 mcg/hr patch (LU)

Copyright © 2001, Hospice of the Western Reserve, Cleveland, OH.
CR, continuous release; *IR,* immediate release; *LU,* Limited use.

Box 21-4 **Equianalgesic Conversion**

- Reading down the column in the Opioid Reference Table* titled "Appropriate Opioid Equianalgesic Dose" gives you the accepted equianalgesic dose between the different opioids for the applicable route.

Ex: 30 mg PO MS Contin = 7.5 mg PO hydromorphone

- Reading across a row gives you the accepted equivalence between routes of the same drug.

Ex: 30 mg PO MS Contin = 10 mg parenteral (SQ/IV) MS Contin

Conversion Equation:

$$\frac{x \text{ Desired Drug Dose/24 hours}}{\text{Current Drug Dose/24 hours}} = \frac{\text{Desired Drug Equianalgesic Dose from Table}}{\text{Current Drug Equilanalgesic Dose from Table}}$$

Ex: Patient on MS Contin 30 mg PO bid needs to convert to hydromorphone PO.

$$\frac{x \text{ hydromorphone/24 hours}}{60 \text{ mg PO MS/24 hours}} = \frac{7.5 \text{ mg PO hydromorphone}}{30 \text{ mg PO MS}}$$

$$30x = 450$$

$$x = 15 \text{ mg PO hydromorphone/24 hours}$$

- Finalize dosing schedule by utilizing appropriate oral dosing interval.
- Recommended breakthrough dose = 10-15% of the 24-hour total.
- When switching between opioids, consider decreasing the calculated total of the new opioid by 1/3 to account for incomplete cross-tolerance between agents.

Copyright © 2001, Hospice of the Western Reserve, Cleveland, OH.
*See Table 21-2.

acting opioid that is already in an older adult's system.

Fentanyl patches should not be prescribed until the appropriate dose of an immediate-release opioid to achieve pain relief is determined. When switching from an immediate-release dosage to a fentanyl patch, the immediate-release opioid needs to be continued for 12 to 18 hours until the peak plasma level of fentanyl is achieved. Patches are never cut and are normally changed every 48 to 72 hours.

TRANSMUCOSAL FENTANYL. Oral transmucosal fentanyl citrate (OTFC) is lipid soluble and therefore absorbed through the mucosa of the mouth when given buccally. It is given for breakthrough pain because it has a rapid onset. Other opioids, such as morphine, oxycodone, and hydromorphone, are hydrophilic, and therefore not appropriate for administering through the buccal or sublingual route. However, in the home environment, morphine is sometimes administered sublingually. Because the pharmacokinetics of morphine does not support this practice, it is assumed that absorption takes place in the lower gastrointestinal tract with varying resulting absorption rates.

Many factors need to be evaluated before OTFC is prescribed for the older adult because fentanyl is a strong opioid and therefore the same principles apply for OTFC as for any strong opioid. It should never be prescribed for a patient who is opioid naive because severe side effects could result. Also, the oral mucosa and the mouth need to be carefully assessed prior to the administration of oral fentanyl. Is the mucosa too dry for the patient to suck on the lozenge? Is the older adult capable of sucking? Is the patient alert or confused?

Route of Administration
Oral

Confusion exists among the lay population as well as some professionals regarding the route of administration of medications and their analgesic effect. This confusion especially exists concerning opioids. A common misconception is that drugs given parenterally result in better pain management. However, the route of administration does not determine the effectiveness of the drug; instead, health care providers need to remember the principle that the correct dose must be used for the route of administration. To illustrate, it takes three times the amount of morphine orally as compared to parenterally to result in an equianalgesic dose, hence the saying, "if the gut works, use it." The oral route is preferred provided there is no pathology of the gastrointestinal tract because it is convenient and noninvasive, and usually oral opioids are less expensive.

Rectal and Transdermal

If the patient is unable to take oral medications, other less invasive routes (e.g., rectal or transdermal) should be considered before advancing to parenteral methods, which are more demanding for professional caregivers and usually more expensive. A word of caution is given regarding both the rectal and transdermal routes. Before suggesting the rectal route, a careful evaluation of the patient should be done. For many patients, not just the older adult patient, the rectal route is not always culturally acceptable and may not be practical (e.g., in an obese patient or if the caregiver is a family member, such as a son or daughter). Although transdermal (fentanyl) patches tend to be a popular route of administration of opioids in long-term care facilities, for the older adult patient the potential for adverse side effects is great (see "Opioids" above for further details).

Parenteral: Intravenous and Subcutaneous

The parenteral route of administration of drugs may be the route of choice if a rapid onset of action is required. In the older adult patient, the intravenous rather than the intramuscular route is preferred. Because of changes in the body that can occur with aging, older adults frequently have more muscle wasting and increased fatty tissue than younger patients. In the very old adult population, another shift takes place in the ratio of fatty tissue to muscle mass if there is a reduction in the proportion of body fat (Popp & Portenoy, 1996).

If a parenteral route is required for a patient who resides at home or in a hospice facility, the subcutaneous route is more convenient than the intravenous route. A 25- or 27-gauge "butterfly"

needle can be inserted subcutaneously and left in place for up to 7 days before rotating sites. In addition, multiple sites—anterior thigh, abdomen, upper arms, and upper back—are available. As part of discharge planning from an acute care hospital to home or a long-term care facility, the route of medication administration should be converted to subcutaneous prior to the patient leaving the hospital to provide for a smooth transition.

Invasive Analgesic Techniques

Prescribing systemic medications in any age group requires a conscious decision based on whether the benefit of the drug outweighs the risk of the potential side effects for a given patient. When the older adult patient is given systemic medications, the side effects can result in major changes in cognitive level and functional status. With visceral pain, the nociceptive pathways from the abdomen and thoracic viscera accompany the efferent sympathetic nerves. Once these nerves are stimulated, skeletal muscle spasm or sympathetic hyperactivity results. Systemic narcotic agonists, such as morphine, have limited usefulness in treating the resulting pain. If other therapies have failed to provide relief of visceral pain, sympathetic blockade may produce a satisfactory response. The three most common sympathetic blockades performed are those involving the stellate ganglion (cervicothoracic), the lumbar sympathetic area, and the celiac plexus (Prager, 1996).

Side Effects of Opioids

Occasionally, patients will say they are allergic to morphine when they have experienced a common side effect of nausea and vomiting, drowsiness, or constipation. If a patient had a true allergic reaction, the symptoms would more likely be a rash, wheezing, or difficulty breathing. The side effects associated with initial dosing can be treated effectively and usually resolve within a few days as tolerance to them develops. However, tolerance does not develop to constipation; therefore, prophylaxis is required when an opioid regimen is instituted.

Constipation

Any time opioids are prescribed, the potential for opioid-induced constipation must be anticipated and prevented. In fact, constipation is the only side effect to which patients do not become tolerant. Opioids bind to the opioid mu receptor in the gut, slowing peristalsis and increasing the transit time of the feces. Because of this, the length of time for water and sodium to be reabsorbed across the intestinal mucosa is prolonged, resulting in dry, hard stool. Secondly, opioids increase the tone and decrease the sensitivity of the anorectal sphincter. As a result, the anorectal sphincter does not relax appropriately. For the elder population, this effect of opioids further predisposes them to opioid-induced constipation because they may already have decreased sphincter sensitivity (Abraham, 2000). To further compound the incidence of constipation, drug regimens for pain management frequently include such adjuvant drugs as tricyclic antidepressants used for neuropathic pain and/or antiemetics for opioid-induced nausea and vomiting, both of which have anticholinergic side effects, one of which is constipation.

Usual interventions include increasing fluid intake, activity level, or dietary fiber intake. Even if the patient can increase water intake and exercise, the slowed transit time makes fiber therapy much less effective, and patients frequently complain of feeling "full" and "bloated." In addition, bulk laxatives that contain psyllium or increased fiber are not recommended, especially if the fluid intake is less than 2 L/day, because they can exacerbate opioid-induced constipation (Plaisance & Ellis, 2002).

At the initiation of opioids, a daily bowel regimen of a stool softener and large bowel stimulant may need to be prescribed. The challenge is getting patients to follow a daily regimen consistently. Even without opioids, the elder population (especially those who are confused) is particularly susceptible to impaction because of decreased rectal sensitivity, which permits large rectal masses to form. From the pressure of the fecal mass, the two most common resulting symptoms are urinary incontinence and diarrhea, which is a sign of fecal impaction.

Respiratory Depression

The fear of respiratory depression is the overwhelming concern of both physicians and nurses who are inexperienced in using morphine, especially at high doses. In most patients, tolerance

to respiratory depression develops in 5 to 7 days. There are three situations when respirations are more likely to become depressed with the use of morphine: first dose in a narcotic-naive patient, the elder patient over the age of 70, and patients with COPD.

Many health care professionals fear giving the last dose of morphine before the patient dies; the fact is, there will always be a "last dose." To allay that fear, a discussion of the principle of double effect is warranted. This principle distinguishes between the primary intent to relieve pain and suffering, and the unavoidable untoward consequence of the potential to hasten death (Latimer, 1991). Thus this principle is predicated on the axiom that *intent* (to relieve pain and suffering) is the critical ethical concern. In short, giving a patient who is dying and in pain sufficient opioid to control the pain is good palliative care, not euthanasia (Schwarz, 2001). This double effect with morphine could be compared to that with the use of NSAIDs for pain, which may result in the patient coming into the emergency room with a frank gastrointestinal bleed for which there was no warning. The intent was to relieve pain and the gastrointestinal bleed was the unintended, but predictable effect.

Sedation

Part of a good pain assessment includes assessing for the level of sedation; sedation will always occur prior to depressed respirations. The nurse will never see patients with depressed respirations up and walking because they would become too sedated to do so. Also, it would be rare for respirations to be depressed in the presence of severe pain because pain antagonizes CNS depression. Opioid-induced respiratory depression can occur if the pain is abruptly eliminated, as in the case of radiation therapy to relieve the pain of bone metastases, and the level of opioid is not decreased. In such a situation, when the pain stimulus is no longer present, respiratory depression can occur.

When patients are initially prescribed opioids, some level of sedation is not uncommon. Why this occurs is unclear, but one probable reason is that patients who have previously been unable to achieve restful sleep because of pain are finally able to catch up on their rest. Regardless of the cause of sedation, patients usually develop tolerance to the sedation in a few days. Good clinical assessment must occur to differentiate between the expected acceptable level of sedation and an unacceptable level indicative of too much opioid in the elder's system. For the elder patient, hourly assessments may be necessary initially. There are four levels of sedation (Box 21-5). If a patient reaches level 3, the opioid should be decreased. Figure 21-4 is an example of a pain management flow sheet that includes assessing for level of sedation every time the patient is assessed for pain.

The use of naloxone, an opioid antagonist, in a physically dependent patient will result in a pain crisis unless the drug is carefully titrated. Therefore, only in the most severe case of respiratory depression should it be considered. The American Pain Society (1999) recommends using a dilute solution of naloxone (0.4 mg in 10 mL of normal saline solution), which may be administered every 1 to 3 minutes until the symptom of respiratory depression subsides. In most situations, decreasing the dosage and/or the

---

Box 21-5 Levels of Sedation

1 = Awake and alert
2 = Slightly drowsy, easily aroused
3 = Frequently drowsy, arousable, drifts off to sleep (consider decreasing opioid)
4 = Somnolent, minimal or no response to physical stimulation, sleeps during conversation

---

Location of Pain	Type of Pain	Sedation Scale
A. _____ B. _____ C. _____ D. _____ Acceptable pain level _____	B = Bone (dull, aching, localized tenderness) NC = Neuro-anticonvulsants (shooting, lancinating) ND = Neuro-antidepressants burning, tingling) V = Visceral (deep, boring, poorly localized)	4 = Somnolent, minimal or no response to physical stimulation, sleep during conversation 3 = Frequently drowsy, arousable, drifts off to sleep (consider decreasing opioid) 2 = Slightly drowsy, easily aroused 1 = Awake and alert S = Sleep, easy to arouse

Side Effects		Non-Pharmacologic Interventions	
A = Anxiety Cf = Confusion C = Constipation E = Epigastric distress H = Hallucinations	M = Motor weakness N = Nausea P = Pruritus U = Urinary retention V = Vomiting	C = Cold D = Distraction E = Exercise EB = Energy-based therapy ET = Expressive therapy	GI = Guided imagery/meditation H = Heat M = Massage PR = Progressive relaxation S = Spiritual care

Date/ Time/ Initial	Location of pain	Type of pain	Pain rating: 0–10	Opioids	Antidepressant Anticonvulsant NSAIDs Steroids	Level of sedation	Side effects	Nondrug intervention	Last BM (bowel protocol)	Comments

Pain will be reassessed every 24 hours any time a change in medication dose or type occurs as noted by an asterisk.

Fig. 21-4 Pain management flow sheet.

frequency of the opioid administration is the only intervention required. However, if the undesired sedation persists, a different opioid or route of administration can be initiated. Also, if the analgesic is effective, consider adding a psychostimulant (e.g., methylphenidate, 5 mg every morning and noon, titrated to effect) (Emanuel et al., 1999).

Nausea and Vomiting

Nausea and vomiting are other troublesome side effects that can occur in opioid-naive individuals when opioids are initially prescribed. These symptoms are common with opioids because of their activation of the chemoreceptor trigger zone in the medulla and increased vestibular sensitivity. In addition, there is a direct effect on the gastrointestinal tract, including increased gastric antral tone, decreased motility, and delayed gastric emptying (Portenoy et al., 1994). An antiemetic that has worked for the patient in the past can be prescribed around the clock (not PRN) for 2 to 3 days, followed by gradual tapering of the dose and weaning. Constipation should always be considered as a contributing factor until ruled out or treated. The pain and nausea and/or vomiting associated with constipation can be more distressing than the underlying pathology. Pharmacologic intervention should be individualized to the most likely mechanism in each patient with nausea and/or vomiting. Low-dose metoclopramide is effective for patients with apparent gastric stasis problems who are tolerant of taking medications by mouth. Phenothiazines such as prochlorperazine (Compazine) or chlorpromazine (Thorazine) are useful for opioid-induced symptoms but must be dosed very carefully because older adults tend to have more extrapyramidal side effects. Antihistamines such as meclizine can be added if movement exacerbates the symptoms; low-dose haloperidol is a good general intervention if the cause is unclear. Box 21-6 presents a listing of antiemetics with dosages. Nausea and vomiting usually subside within a few days if related to the initiation of opioids.

ADJUVANT INTERVENTIONS

Adjuvant interventions are medications originally formulated and approved for other disease processes, but that are used as part of a pain regimen. Included in this category are antidepressants and anticonvulsants, which are essential drugs in the treatment of neuropathic pain. As part of the WHO's three-step analgesic ladder, adjuvants are used as coanalgesics or single agents at any step of the ladder. Table 21-3 lists details on adjuvant medications with dosage.

Antidepressants

Tricyclic antidepressants (TCAs) are prescribed to treat the burning and tingling component of neuropathic pain in such conditions as infiltrating tumors, diabetic neuropathy, and postherpetic neuralgia. Other chronic painful conditions for which TCAs have been proven to be effective are fibromyalgia and headaches (Magni, 1991).

The analgesic effect of TCAs is independent of their antidepressant effect. Normally endogenous neurotransmitters, including norepinephrine and serotonin, transmit pain. TCAs inhibit the reuptake of norepinephrine and serotonin, and decrease pain transmission through afferent nerve fibers (Lipman, 1996). The use of TCAs in older adults is limited because of anticholinergic side effects: dry mouth, constipation, blurred vision, tachycardia, urinary retention, and delirium. Nortriptyline, a secondary amine, is preferred over amitriptyline, a tertiary amine, because it induces less orthostatic hypotension with its resultant danger of falls. TCAs are relatively contraindicated in patients with coronary artery disease because they can worsen ventricular arrhythmias (Portenoy, 1998). As in all situations, the risk:benefit ratio must be considered. For those elders with coronary artery disease, a TCA with less cardiotoxicity, such as desipramine, would be an alternative. Selective serotonin reuptake inhibitors have thus far been found to be less effective as adjuvants for neuropathic pain than the TCAs (Emanuel et al., 1999). It appears that the inhibition of both norepinephrine and serotonin is needed for an analgesic effect (Lipman, 1996).

Dosing with TCAs should be "low and slow" to allow elder patients to become tolerant to the prominent side effects. The typical starting dose for the elder should be no more than 10 mg/day given at bedtime; increases in 10-mg increments can be ordered as tolerance to side effects develops (Lipman, 1996).

Box 21-6 Pharmacologic Interventions for Nausea and Vomiting (N/V)

I: CHEMORECEPTOR TRIGGER ZONE (CTZ)

N/V caused by chemical imbalances (opioids, chemotherapy)

PHENOTHIAZINES

- Prochlorperazine (Compazine), 5-10 mg PO/25 mg PR q8h pm
- Chlorpromazine (Thorazine), 10-100 mg PO/PR/SL q6h pm

BUTYROPHENONES

Haloperidol (Haldol) 0.5-5 mg PO/SL/PR q4-12h pm

II. VESTIBULAR AGENTS

N/V caused by movement

ANTIHISTAMINES

- Meclizine (Antivert), 12.5-50 mg PO bid–tid pm
- Dimenhydrinate (Dramamine), 50-100 mg PO q4-6h pm

ANTICHOLINERGICS

- Hyoscyamine (Levsin), 0.125-0.25 PO/SL q4-6h pm
- Glycopyrrolate (Robinul), 1-2 mg PO q4-12h pm

III. GASTRIC STASIS TRIGGER ZONE

PROKINETIC AGENT

- Metoclopramide (Reglan), 5-20 mg PO qid

Don't use if suspected complete obstruction

IV: CEREBRAL CORTEX AGENTS

Anxiety-induced nausea

BENZODIAZEPINES

Quick onset of action

- Lorazepam (Ativan), 0.5-2 mg PO/SL/PR q4-6h pm
- Alprazolam (Xanax) 0.25-1 mg PO/SL/PR q4-6h pm
- Diazepam (Valium) 2-10 mg PO/SL/PR q6-8h pm

BUTYROPHENONES

- Haloperidol (Haldol), 0.5-5 mg PO/SL/PR q4-12h pm

FOR HYPERCALCEMIA

Consider pamidronate (Aredia), 60-90 mg IV over 4h

FOR INTRACRANIAL PRESSURE

Consider dexamethasone (Decadron)

Anticonvulsants

Anticonvulsant drugs are used to control the sharp, shooting, electric qualities of neuropathic pain. Their analgesic effect is believed to be related to the slowing of peripheral nerve conduction in primary afferent fibers, thereby decreasing the painful sensory information transmitted to the CNS (Leo & Singh, 2002). Several different anticonvulsants have been used for neuropathic pain management, including carbamazepine, gabapentin, phenytoin, and valproic acid. Until recently, the greatest success was reported to be with carbamazepine; however, one of the side effects of this drug is blood dyscrasias (Lipman, 1996). Gabapentin has received approval from the U.S. Food and Drug Administration for use in the treatment of neuropathic pain. This drug offers numerous advantages over other anticonvulsants because it is unlikely to produce the serious side effects associated with other anticonvulsants. The most commonly reported side effects of gabapentin are somnolence, dizziness, ataxia, tremor, and fatigue (Leo & Singh, 2002). In addition, gabapentin is a gamma-aminobutyric acid (GABA) receptor agonist (see below), which may enhance pain management.

Gamma-aminobutyric Acid Agonists

Some of the more recent research in pain management has led to new approaches. Among these is the use of GABA agonists. GABA is a modulating substance secreted via the descending neuronal pathways; it is believed that, when the inhibitory action of GABA is lost, certain neuropathic pain symptoms such as allodynia

Table 21-3 **Adjuvant Analgesics**				
Pain Classification	Pain Descriptor	Drug Classification	Selected Drugs	Additional Information
Bone	Aching, dull. localized tendemess	NSAIDs	Ibuprofen (Motrin, Advil), 400-800 mg PO/PR q6-8hrs Naproxen (Naprosyn), 250-500 mg PO q12h	• May cause GI upset • Maximum dose 3200 mg/day • Less frequent dosing
		Salicylate	Choline Mg^{2+} trisalicylate (Tritisate), 500-1500 mg PO q8-12h	• Less GI upset • No effect on platelets
Visceral	Deep, boring, referred, poorly localized	Steroids	Dexamethasone (Decadron), 2-24 mg PO/PR per day (Prednisone), 10-80 mg PO/PR, per day	• May increase blood glucose levels • May cause GI upset • Can cause euphoria and/or dysphoria • Higher doses for cerebral edema and spinal cord compression • Doses greater than 80 mg qd are rare
Neuropathic	Burning, tingling, allodynia	Antidepressants	Amitriptyline (Elavil), 10-150 mg PO hs Desipramine (Norpramin), 10-150 mg PO hs	• Monitor sedation and anticholinergic effects • Caution with methadone • Orthostatic hypotension with geriatric patients • Start with a low dose • Fewer side effects than amitriptyline • Relative contraindication with methadone
	Shooting, lancinating, chronic neuralgias	Anticonvulsants	Carbamazepine (Tegretol), 100-400 mg PO/PR bid-old Divalproex sodium (Depakote), 250-500 mg PO bid-qid	• Sedating • Frequent drug interactions • Start with low dose & titrate • Do not crush, split or chew • Can dose every hs

Table 21-3 **Adjuvant Analgesics—cont'd**				
Pain Classification	Pain Descriptor	Drug Classification	Selected Drugs	Additional Information
			Gabapentin (Neurontin), 100 mg tid, then titrate to 300-900 mg PO/PR tid	• Sedating
	Inclusive	Steroids	Dexamethasone (Decadron), 2-24 mg PO/PR per day (used for nerve compression)	• May increase blood glucose levels • May cause GI upset • Doses greater than 20 mg od are rare
General	Generalized headache, musculoskeletal	Nonopioid	Acetaminophen (Tylenol) 650-1000 mg PO/PR q6-8 h (routine) or q4 h PRN	• Celling dose 4000 mg qd • Caution in hepatic disease (cirrhosis, alcohol abuse) • Used for osteoarthritis and degenerative joint disease

Copyright © 2001, Hospice of the Western Reserve, Cleveland, OH.

GI, gastrointestinal; NSAIDs, nonsteroidal anti-inflammatory drugs.

occur. To treat this symptom, a GABA agonist such as gabapentin is given to increase the activity at the GABA receptor site and thereby decrease pain. The principle of "go low and go slow" applies to initiating gabapentin. Initially the dose is 100 mg three times a day, with the dose escalating every 1 to 2 days by 100 mg until effective (Emanuel et al., 1999). In the younger population, 300 mg orally can be given at bedtime, but in the older adult, 100 mg three times a day is recommended because of the side effect of drowsiness in larger single doses and the concern that older adults may get up during the night to use the bathroom.

N-Methyl-D-Aspartate Receptor Antagonists

One of several receptors involved in neurotransmission at the spinal cord level is the N-methyl-D-aspartate (NMDA) receptor, which is proposed to be involved in neuropathic pain. Medications that inhibit this receptor interfere with the transmission of pain across the synaptic area.

Methadone

Methadone is believed to have NMDA receptor antagonistic effects plus opioid effects. For several years methadone was not used because it was difficult to titrate as a result of its long half-life. In the last few years, with a better understanding of its benefit for use with neuropathic pain and increased knowledge of drug titration, methadone has come back into favor; however, caution should always be used if it is prescribed for the older adult because of the long half-life and unpredictable individual kinetics of absorption and elimination. Also, methadone does not have a 1:1 equianalgesic conversion to morphine; the conversion varies according to the level of dosage of morphine (see Table 21-2 and Box 21-4).

Ketamine

Ketamine is another NMDA antagonist that may have a role in refractory pain management (Portenoy & Prager, 1999). In the medically frail patient at the end of life, it is used to control refractory neuropathic pain (Coyle & Layman-Goldstein, 2001). However, it must be used with great caution because undesirable psychomimetic side effects of delirium, nightmares, hallucinations, and dysphoria can occur. Ketamine normally is used as an anesthetic agent, but for the purpose of analgesia, it is prescribed in subanesthetic doses.

Dextromethorphan

Another NMDA antagonist, dextromethorphan, had mixed results when clinical trials were performed. It is hypothesized that dextromethorphan is particularly beneficial in patients with ongoing peripheral neuron damage, as seen in diabetic neuropathy, but not in patients with fixed lesions, which are common in postherpetic neuralgia (Nelson, Park, Robinovitz, Tsigos, & Mas, 1997).

Corticosteroids

Corticosteroids inhibit prostaglandin synthesis and decrease edema surrounding neural tissues (Watanabe & Bruera, 1994). This category of drug is particularly useful for neuropathic pain resulting from plexopathies and visceral pain such as that associated with stretching of the liver capsule from metastases. Dexamethasone rather than prednisone is used because it produces the least amount of mineralocorticoid effect, resulting in less potential for Cushing's syndrome. It is the drug of choice for pain secondary to CNS inflammation or swelling. Corticosteroids also provide adjuvant relief for nausea and vomiting associated with opioid use, as well as with increased intracranial pressure. Corticosteroids and NSAIDs should not be used in combination because they both use the same pathways, which increases bleeding tendencies.

With any drug therapy, a careful history is required before prescribing a new drug. This is true regarding the use of corticosteroids in any population, but especially with older adults. It is not uncommon for older adults to have diabetes as a comorbid condition, and the control of their diabetes can be greatly impacted with concomitant use of corticosteroids. Although there can be dramatic improvement in symptoms when corticosteroids are prescribed, the risk of adverse effects increases with the duration of use. As a result, they tend to be prescribed more often for patients with a limited life expectancy, and, when the pain is controlled, the dose is tapered as much as possible. Starting dosages range from 1 to 2 mg dexamethasone or 5 to 10 mg prednisone once or twice a day (Portenoy & Prager, 1999) to 10 mg dexamethasone twice a day, with tapering to the minimal effective dose (Watanabe & Bruera, 1994).

COMPLEMENTARY AND ALTERNATIVE THERAPIES FOR PAIN MANAGEMENT

Managing pain requires a holistic approach. Interventions for pain management include noninvasive or nonpharmacologic pain relief measures, which can provide cost-effective pain relief without the side effects of medications. These interventions may be beneficial and may decrease the need for analgesics. Nonpharmacologic interventions are best used as adjuvants to medications (Jacox et al., 1994). In a study conducted by Ferrell (1994) on a sample of 66 older cancer patients living at home, patients preferred heat, massage, and distraction as therapies, and were less familiar with therapies such as healing touch or guided imagery.

Over the past few decades there has been an increased interest by Americans in integrating complementary therapy into their plans of care. The use of complementary alternative medicine (CAM) has grown from 33.8% in 1990 to 42.1% in 1998. Congress established the National Center for Complementary and Alternative Medicine to support research and disseminate information on CAM to professional health care workers and the general public (Eisenberg et al., 1998).

Complementary therapies are used for symptom management and to enhance well-being. The philosophy is based on a wellness model that focuses on the inner resources of each individual rather than disease treatment. "Health" is obtained from achieving a balance between the patient's internal resources and the influences of the external physical and social environment. It is a holistic approach to care that emphasizes the whole person rather than body systems. CAM has become a part of the palliative care model because it is consistent with the focus on healing. It is rooted in reaching a balance by utilizing complementary therapies as adjuncts to mainstream care. The therapies are integrated within a patient's plan of care to be comfort oriented so as to enhance a patient's quality of life (Cassileth, 2002).

Complementary therapies are safe, nontoxic, easy to use, and inexpensive. Many of these therapies can be self-managed, meaning that licensed practitioners are unnecessary. This promotes the opportunity for patients to maintain a measure of control over their well-being. Older adults may need to be encouraged to use complementary therapies in their daily routine to promote comfort.

Guided Imagery/Relaxation

There are several interventions that are well known and accepted in palliative care; guided imagery techniques have been used for years. Often guided imagery is used in conjunction with relaxation techniques. With imagery, the mind focuses on the balance within the body and the effects of the mind on the body, a relationship proposed over a century ago (Micozzi, 1996). Messages such as feelings, beliefs, and attitudes are suggested to the right hemisphere of the brain before they can be interpreted by the autonomic nervous system (Dossey, 1995).

The primary purposes of guided imagery include (1) inducing physiologic changes, (2) raising psychological insight, and (3) increasing emotional awareness. Imagery also serves as a distraction for use in pain management. Relaxation from imagery may reduce muscular tension, promote rest, and enhance sleep. In guided imagery or visualization, the patient creates pleasant mental images that involve the five senses, for example, being at a beach, hearing the waves crash against the rocks, feeling the cool water on their feet, and smelling and tasting the salty ocean water. These images are used to substitute a nonpainful sensation for pain.

The older patient may need assistance and encouragement to use these techniques. Although guided imagery has been shown to be an effective modality, Juarez and Ferrell's (1996) research suggested that elders are not very likely to use nondrug methods, especially guided imagery. They attributed this reluctance to unfamiliarity with nontraditional interventions.

Energy-Based Healing

Healing touch is a technique that uses the caregiver's hands for the purpose of providing comfort. When using healing touch, caregivers balance a patient's energy field, resulting in the promotion of comfort and healing. The philosophy supporting this technique is based on the theory of universal energy, in which human beings are recognized as being energy fields that are integrated with other energy fields in their environment, including the fields of other human beings (Rogers, 1992). Many cultures support this theory, and healing touch is gaining acceptance within many medical settings. In addition to healing touch, therapeutic touch and Reiki are examples of energy-based interventions. Healing touch is a combination of techniques for therapeutic intervention appropriate for use in care of the older adult experiencing pain; it is gentle and noninvasive.

Healing touch is learned by attending an educational program that incorporates teachings of many modalities, one of which is therapeutic touch. The program consists of several levels of training leading to the option of national certification. Healing touch is endorsed by the American Holistic Nurses' Association. Despite the name, healing touch does not require physical touch; the techniques can be used within inches of the body. The tools are the caregiver's hands, and the techniques can be applied through meditation and prayer.

Massage Therapy

Massage can be done by use of hands or with electric massagers. When used in conjunction with soft lighting, comforting music, and aromatherapy, it can be very relaxing physically and psychologically. Benefits include relaxation, reduced swelling, decreased stress, relief of fatigue, improved sleep, and decreased pain (Ferrell, Wisdom, & Wengl, 1989).

Using massage therapy with older patients experiencing pain has numerous benefits for the receiver and the giver. Many of the physical benefits for massage include softening and releasing tight muscles, improving circulation, reducing generalized aches and pains, nurturing, and calming. Massage therapy is convenient and requires little instruction to caregivers, and is an intervention that is widely accepted by the older population; caregivers or health professionals can do it. In offering therapeutic massage to older persons, a conscious, caring pressure combined with a gentle touch is as important as any specific massage technique. Unconditional human contact in the form of touch acknowledges the reality of the situation, reminding the patient that he or she is still an individual, regardless of his or her frail body or health condition. Touch may help reduce a person's feelings of isolation and loneliness; this physical contact reassures individuals that they are not alone (Zuberbueler, 1996).

In a study of the effects of therapeutic massage on perception of pain intensity, anxiety, and relaxation, Ferrell-Torry and Glick (1993) found that the use of massage in patients with cancer reduced their perception of pain and anxiety and enhanced relaxation. A decrease in sympathetic nervous system activity, such as heart rate, blood pressure, and respiratory rate, was also noted.

Physical Therapy

When caring for older patients with pain, physical therapy is a natural adjunct. Physical therapists are trained to work with individuals with acute and persistent pain with the goal of relieving pain and maximizing mobility and function. Physical therapy involves the use of exercise, functional training, and assistive devices. Caregivers are part of the plan of care; with appropriate instruction, caregivers play a key role in assisting older patients with their home therapy, which may include passive range-of-motion, assistive, active, and resistive exercise.

Music Therapy

According to the American Music Therapy Association's 1999 Member Sourcebook, "music therapy" is the use of music in the accomplishment of therapeutic goals: the restoration, maintenance, and improvement of mental and physical health. Munro (1984) defined music therapy as "the controlled use of music, its elements and their influences on human beings to aid in the physiologic, psychological, and emotional integration of the individual during treatment of illness or disability." Kenny (1989, p. 54) defined music therapy as "the process and form which combines the healing aspects of music with the issues of human needs for the benefit of the individual and hence, society."

Older patients experiencing pain may benefit from music therapy that focuses on the emo-

tional, spiritual, and physical well-being of the individual. An older person's well-being may depend on such quality-of-life issues as the ability to interact or participate in personal relationships, to communicate information or emotions to enjoy maximum levels of personal growth, to reduce pain, and to promote comfort (Haghighi & Pansch, 2001).

Music therapists assess the patient's and caregiver's needs. Various instruments are used along with verbal discussion to examine feelings and emotions in relation to the healing process. Music therapy is an excellent intervention for older adults; as with any intervention, the music needs to be geared to the individual.

Art Therapy

Art therapy is an effective intervention for patients experiencing pain; this form of therapy focuses on the creative process as a healing process, and on resulting artwork as a form of communication. Art therapy promotes comfort and healing. The art therapist offers art to the older adult to engage him or her in a process that taps into the person's inner world through the making of art. Using art can be a catalyst for verbal communication and can be especially effective with individuals who have difficulty expressing themselves verbally. When pain may be related to anxiety or fear, art therapy is one effective way to identify and explore the fears and anxieties with a positive impact on pain management (Trauger-Querry, 2001).

Aromatherapy

Aromatherapy is a CAM intervention in which aromatic plant extracts are inhaled or applied to the skin as a means of treating illness or promoting beneficial changes in mood and outlook. The benefit of these aids comes from their effects on the limbic system, which coordinates mind and body activity (Allison, 1999). The limbic system is very sensitive to odors and encodes them into memories. When awakened, these associations can trigger a response in basic physical functions such as heart rate, blood pressure, breathing, and hormone level.

Hundreds of plants are used in aromatherapy. The ones most commonly used when caring for the seriously ill are lavender and capsicum for pain relief, enhanced mood, increased vitality, and promotion of relaxation (Robins, 1999). Although these plants and oils can be found in natural or health food stores, elder patients and their families need information and education in order to safely and effectively use aromatherapy.

Meditation/Prayer

Another useful technique in managing pain in older adults is the process of quietly turning inward, commonly referred to as meditation or prayer. This practice is the focusing of an individual's attention internally to achieve clearer consciousness and inner stillness. There are numerous ways to practice meditation; however, all methods focus on emptying the mind and letting go of the mind's clutter.

Meditation originates in Eastern traditions and has been in existence for centuries. Many elder patients may be familiar with the concept but may not know how to practice it. Using meditation and prayer together may help in understanding the process; in recent years, many religions have incorporated meditation as common practice. The method involves the focusing of attention on something such as breathing, an image, or a word or action, such as Tai Chi or Qigong. It is important to support the older adult through the process; meditation is often difficult for the cognitively impaired elder. If the patient is able, participation in Tai Chi can assist to relieve discomfort by means of gentle movement.

There are many reasons to use meditation and prayer as an intervention for pain management. Research studies have demonstrated that relaxed forms of meditation decrease heart rate and blood pressure and increase breathing volume (Gatchel & Maddrey, 1998). It is believed that meditation and prayer activate the right cerebral hemisphere and the parasympathetic nervous system, quieting the nerves and allowing intuitive, wordless thinking to occur (Payne, 1998). The older patient who participates in meditation may be left with a sense of relaxation and inner peace.

Physical Approaches to Pain Relief in Older Adults

Superficial Heat and Cold

The use of dry and moist superficial heat and cold are effective in providing pain relief from muscle spasms, stiffness, and inflammation of joints. The older adult population will typically feel comfortable utilizing this therapeutic approach. It is considered the most used nondrug therapy and is perceived by elders to be most effective (Ferrell, 1996).

Both cold and heat have direct effects on local muscle spasm and can provide analgesia. Superficial heat can increase local blood flow and metabolic rate. Therapy using cold compresses enhances relief of pain by numbing nerve endings and decreasing inflammation. Older patients prefer heat therapy to cold, but cold is thought to be most effective and to relieve pain faster than heat (Pitorak, 1999). According to McCaffery (1990), however, alternating heat and cold is most effective. Physical therapy using heat and cold may be beneficial in older patients with pain of muscular origin (Patt, 1993).

Transcutaneous Electrical Nerve Stimulation

Transcutaneous electrical nerve stimulation (TENS) is a frequently discussed adjunct for pain relief in older adults. This technique is used for selected pain syndromes such as persistent back pain. TENS involves stimulating nerves below the surface of the skin by placing electrodes on the skin surface. The impulse causes both an excitation and an inhibition of sensory nerve impulses in the CNS (Ferrell, 1996).

Patients have experienced relief of discomfort from neuropathic origins, such as pain from bursitis and fractured ribs, using TENS. There have been mixed responses in elders who use TENS for persistent back pain. Patients who are cognitively impaired may require frequent assessment to determine if the electrode is in place and not causing skin irritation. Although TENS may be effective in managing pain, it is not commonly used in older patients because of the lack of accessibility and affordability as compared to other methods.

Biofeedback

Biofeedback requires the utilization of equipment that can detect, record, and amplify the body's internal electronic impulses and provide a corresponding signal that can be interpreted by the patient (Ferrell, 1996). The advantage of this equipment is that it monitors information that the patient is ordinarily unaware of, such as heart rate, blood pressure, and temperature. Older patients can experience the physiologic benefits of biofeedback when it is used in conjunction with pain management interventions such as relaxation techniques. Patients are able to see the information (feedback) displayed on a unit so that they can learn to control their physiologic responses and achieve greater relaxation and comfort. A major limitation in utilizing this therapy with older patients is the availability of the equipment, cost, and accessibility to trained personnel.

Acupuncture

Acupuncture is a Chinese medical procedure involving the insertion of fine needles through the skin, adjacent to or distant from the painful area. It is believed that acupuncture creates analgesia by activating "endogenomas," or pain-modulating pathways, through direct stimulation of peripheral nerves (Melzach & Wall, 1984). The use of acupuncture for managing pain in elders has been limited primarily by their limited willingness to accept the intervention.

Conclusion

Comprehensive, holistic care of the older adult patient can incorporate CAM as part of the nondrug options for care. It does require patient and caregiver education regarding the various therapies and their benefits in pain relief. There are many misconceptions that may be a barrier to utilization of CAM in the current generation of elders. As the baby boomers reach their elder years, it is predicted that CAM will be integrated into traditional practice as part of routine health care. In the meantime, we need to resource these options of care to promote comfort and enhance quality of life in the older adult.

OTHER CONSIDERATIONS
Anticipatory Grief

As with pain, grief affects multiple domains—physical, social, cognitive, and emotional. Assessing grief is never easy, especially because many of the symptoms could be discounted as side effects of medications or a change in disease state. To illustrate, patient X has lung cancer that has metastasized to the brachial plexus. Part of his pain regimen is amitriptyline for neuropathic

pain, which has anticholinergic side effects. One of his chief discomforts is a dry mouth. His condition is gradually deteriorating, and he is experiencing a loss of appetite and not sleeping well. He is demonstrating three physical symptoms—dry mouth, loss of appetite, and inability to sleep—that could be side effects of amitriptyline and/or signs of deterioration, but could also be signs of a normal grief response. The lesson is twofold: always include the signs of anticipatory grief as part of a total pain assessment, and do not assume that all symptoms are either side effects of medications or disease process related when doing a complete pain assessment.

Depression as a Potential Consequence of Persistent Pain

Depression commonly occurs secondary to chronic/persistent pain. Older adults with chronic pain have an increased likelihood of becoming depressed, leading physicians to suspect an emotional cause of their pain. However, pain and depression share the same neural circuitry and hormones, as demonstrated through functional imaging scans, which show similar disturbances in brain chemistry in both conditions. According to Breitbart (2002), "Chronic pain uses up serotonin like a car running out of gas. If the pain persists long enough, everybody runs out of gas" (p. 1).

Depression, an often-overlooked entity in the older adult patient, should always be considered when managing a patient with chronic pain. Cohen-Mansfield and Marx (1993) found (using multiple regression analysis) that increasing level of pain, number of medical conditions, and lack of social support are predictors of depression, with pain being the strongest predictor. In another study, older adult patients with depression and anxiety reported pain more frequently, and reported more pain complaints, than nondepressed older adults (Parmelee, Katz, & Lawton, 1991). Investigation of the association between depression and pain complaints in older adult patients has revealed that the initial control of depression greatly facilitates pain management. Needless to say, nurses should not assume that pain is the sole cause of depression, such that, if the pain is controlled, the depression will be eliminated. Pain is holistic and influenced by many factors, one of which could be depression.

If the depression is not addressed aggressively, the interventions to manage pain are unlikely to work. TCAs are adjuvant medications commonly used as part of the pain regimen for neuropathic pain. For example, if a patient is depressed and is experiencing neuropathic pain, nortriptyline or desipramine may be used as part of the pain regimen; at the same time, they may be effective in treating depression, provided the dosage is at a therapeutic level to treat depression (AGS Panel on Chronic Pain in Older Persons, 1998).

Assessing Delirium in Pain Management

Delirium can be a prevalent symptom for older adults; it is frequently overlooked, and reversible. This condition not only is a source of distress to patients and families, but also presents significant medical challenges in pain management. The hallmarks of delirium are acute onset, alterations in level of consciousness, and deficits in attention. Although many different causes can trigger delirium, they can be broadly divided into localized CNS conditions and non-CNS systemic conditions. CNS conditions include tumors, either primary or metastatic, and drugs, including anesthetics, neuroleptics, antidepressants, sedative-hypnotics, anticonvulsants, opioids, and alcohol. Additional medications that can contribute to delirium include anti-inflammatory agents (both steroids and nonsteroidal) and antihistamines, particularly histamine$_2$ blockers. The non-CNS systemic conditions include infections (e.g., sepsis, pneumonia, urinary tract infection, osteomyelitis), decompensation related to heart and lung disease, and endocrine and electrolyte imbalances. Another assessment factor to be considered is the possibility of sensory deprivation resulting from impaired hearing or vision or environmental disruptions such as hospitalization.

Pain assessment of elders should include an assessment for delirium because it often goes undetected. There is a tendency to attribute the elder patient's symptoms to dementia and to assume that this is a normal consequence of aging. One way to avoid this pitfall is to use a standardized evaluation instrument with any elder patient who exhibits symptoms of an alteration in cognition.

Once delirium has been diagnosed, the cause should be identified and treated. Managing pain for elder patients requires special attention to the medication treatment plan. Older individuals metabolize and excrete medication at a slower rate than their younger counterparts, which can lead to a buildup of medication at sometimes toxic levels. It is typically good practice to introduce one new medication at a time to differentiate between side effects of a single drug or the combination of drugs. All nonessential drugs should be discontinued when opioid-induced delirium appears to be the likely diagnosis. It may be useful to institute a switch from one opioid to another. Although no opioid has been shown to have a more favorable CNS side effect profile than any other, this practice may identify a drug with a more favorable balance between analgesia and the side effects in an individual patient. Bruera, Franco, Maltoni, Watanabe, and Suarez-Almazor (1995) suggested that, in elder terminal cancer patients, careful monitoring of cognitive function, attention to dehydration, and opioid rotation can reduce the incidence of agitated delirium and the need for neuroleptic medication for older adult patients. Documentation of behaviors and symptoms should be noted.

Cognitive Impairment

Dementia frequently coexists with painful medical conditions such as degenerative joint disease, arthritis, cancer, back pain, and headaches, all of which tend to occur more with increasing age. As is well known, there is no objective method to measure a person's pain, and the best pain assessment takes place when the patient can subjectively self-report his or her pain. Unfortunately, elders who have a dementing illness are typically unable to report pain accurately because of memory loss, concentration difficulties, or confusion. These cognitive problems affect the whole pain experience; not only are these patients unable to identify and anticipate painful sensations, but they are typically unable either to recall a painful experience or to evaluate the effectiveness of the treatment (Buff, Miaskowski, Sands, & Brod, 2001).

Nonverbal, cognitively impaired older adults are at high risk for undertreatment of pain. Short-term memory loss may result in elder patients with dementia forgetting that they have had pain once they are immobile and comfortable at rest. The nursing staff can become frustrated because the patient will respond "no" to questions about pain even though he or she may have experienced pain

EVIDENCE-BASED PRACTICE

Reference: Allen, R. S., Haley, W. E., Small, B. J., & McMillan, S. C. (2002). Pain reports by older hospice patients and family caregivers: The role of cognitive functioning. *The Gerontologist, 42,* 507-514.

Research Problem: Research in nursing homes shows that cognitive impairment may reduce self-reported pain, but this relationship has not been systematically explored among hospice patients. In the hospice population, little is known about how cognitive functioning may impact the self-report of pain or the report of care recipient pain by family caregivers.

Design: Cross-sectional, correlational.

Sample and Setting: 176 dyads of caregivers and cancer care recipients, drawn from a hospice located in Florida that has an average daily census of 1000 patients.

Methods: The associations between pain, cognitive functioning, and gender among cancer patients and their family caregivers during in-home hospice were studied. Initial assessment interviews with the care recipient–caregiver dyad were conducted within 48 hours after admission to hospice. The following areas were screened and measured: gross cognitive function, independence in self-care, functional status, and pain.

Results: More intense self-reports of pain among care recipients were associated with more intense reports of care recipient pain by the family caregivers. Care recipient self-reported pain was also significantly associated with lower Short Portable Mental Status Questionnaire score (more cognitively impaired) and lower education. Better cognitive functioning was associated with self-reports of less intense pain.

Implications for Nursing Practice: Proxy pain report by caregivers in conjunction with hospice care recipients' self-report of pain should be considered. Research is needed to examine the impact of care recipient cognitive impairment on self-reported pain and caregiver-reported care recipient pain over time. Such evidence-based research will provide data to use in the development of educational interventions in pain management for use by hospice staff with family caregivers.

Conclusion: Care recipients with cognitive impairment reported more intense pain than their cognitively intact counterparts. Consistent with other studies, family caregivers reported higher levels of pain relative to the cognitively impaired care recipients' own self-report of pain.

---

with movement just a few minutes prior to the assessment (Feldt et al., 1998).

Sengstaken and King (1993) did retrospective chart reviews and interviews to detect pain among geriatric nursing home residents. Sixty-six percent of the communicative residents were identified as having chronic pain, but the treating physicians did not detect pain in 34% of these residents. Physicians detected pain in only 17% of noncommunicative residents. Of these nonverbal patients, only 4% were receiving regularly scheduled analgesics, in contrast to 21% of the communicative patients.

A classic study done by Ferrell and Rivera (1995) examined the pain experiences of 325 residents of skilled nursing homes, where typically there is a high prevalence of cognitive impairment. They documented that cognitively impaired patients were able to describe the pain they were presently experiencing and that 83% of the subjects who had pain could complete at least one of the assessment scales.

Cognitively impaired elders typically have limited attention spans and are easily distracted. In addition, they also require more time to assimilate questions and make a response. Data from a study of 758 residents of a single long-term care facility suggested that, although cognitively impaired elder patients may slightly underreport their pain experiences, their self-reports are usually just as valid as reports from patients who are cognitively intact (Parmelee, Smith, & Katz, 1993). Two principal nursing implications can be derived from the work of Ferrell and Rivera and Parmelee et al.: first, this group of patients requires frequent and constant assessment of pain; and second, it is important to determine what pain scale each person is capable of completing as part of the routine pain assessment. Verbal reports of pain should always be believed; however, the absence of a verbal report does not equal an absence of pain.

Elders who are cognitively impaired may retain some ability to comprehend and verbally communicate. Nonverbal or severely confused elder patients are unable to verbally communicate their pain experience; for these individuals, observing a change in nonverbal behavior is the primary method used to assess pain. An observation of a patient in pain, noting facial grimaces and agitation, is an important qualitative assessment technique (Ferrell & Ferrell, 1990). Other nonverbal behaviors that may be indicative of pain are increased confusion, decreased decision-making skills, decreased communication, combative behavior, and impaired mobility. Marzinski (1991) concluded that experienced nursing staff members working with patients diagnosed with Alzheimer's disease could detect subtle behavioral cues that implied pain using what was normal behavior for each individual patient as a baseline. To illustrate, one nonverbal patient displayed rapid blinking with slight grimacing during pain episodes. Another patient whose normal behavior was moaning and rocking would become quiet and withdrawn when in pain.

In response to the difficulties in identifying a reliable and valid instrument for measuring pain in cognitively impaired elders, the Checklist of Nonverbal Pain Indicators (CNPI) was developed (Fig. 21-5). This instrument was piloted in a study that examined the treatment of pain in cognitively impaired compared with cognitively intact older adults after surgery for hip fracture

Date _____ Patient Name _____		
(Write a 0 if the behavior was not observed, and a 1 if the behavior occurred even briefly during activity or rest.)	**With Movement**	**Rest**
1. Vocal complaints: Nonverbal (Expression of pain, not in words, moans, groans, grunts, cries, gasps, sighs)	_____	_____
2. Facial grimaces/winces (Furrowed brow, narrowed eyes, tightened lips, dropped jaw, clenched teeth, distorted expressions)	_____	_____
3. Bracing (Clutching or holding onto siderails, bed, tray table, or affected area during movement)	_____	_____
4. Restlessness (Constant or intermittent shifting of position, rocking, intermittent or constant hand motions, inability to keep still)	_____	_____
5. Rubbing (Massaging affected area) (In addition, record verbal complaints)	_____	_____
6. Vocal complaints: Verbal (Words expressing discomfort or pain ["ouch," "that hurts"], cursing during movement, or exclamations of protest, ["stop," "that's enough"])	_____	_____
Subtotal Scores	_____	_____
Total Score	_____	

Fig. 21-5 Checklist of nonverbal pain indicators. (Data from Feldt, K. S. [1996]. Treatment of pain in cognitively impaired versus cognitively intact post hip fractured elders. [Doctoral dissertation, University of Minnesota, 1996]. *Dissertation Abstracts International, 57-09B,* 5574; and Feldt, K. S. [2000]. Checklist of nonverbal pain indicators. *Pain Management Nursing, 1*[1], 13-21.)

(Feldt, 1996; Feldt et al., 1998). The CNPI has good face validity based on literature regarding pain behaviors in elders with dementia (Marzinski, 1991; Raway, 1994; Sengstaken & King, 1993). Feldt (2000) also reported other validity testing outcomes when the CNPI was compared with pain intensity (VDS) scores. The CNPI proved to be an initially reliable and simple tool to measure pain behaviors in postoperative elders, but, because of low frequencies of observed behaviors at rest, the tool is less useful during rest and may be more useful for observing activities such as transfers, standing, or ambulation during physical therapy (Feldt, 2000). The findings also indicated that, while at rest, both cognitively impaired and intact patients appear fairly comfortable, and, unless asked if they are in pain or having discomfort, they appear not to need to be medicated for pain. The nursing implication is that impaired patients may forget their pain while at rest and therefore be less likely to request medication. However, movement seems to be an instant, and perhaps surprising, reminder that they are experiencing pain.

Total Sedation

Total sedation, also referred to as end-of-life sedation, is a topic that can arouse emotion among health care professionals. To totally sedate a patient at the end of life should not be the first option considered, but the last. This topic may be raised when a patient is dying and within hours or days of the end of life. Anecdotally, some expert clinicians who are frequently at the bedside with the dying patient question how frequently this is required. Some of the questions to be asked and answered are "Whose need is it, the patient's or the caregiver's (professional and family) need?" "Has the patient's end-of-life work been accomplished?" "Have all the benefits and burdens of sedation been addressed?" "Is there an underlying spiritual need creating the suffering?" At the end of life, it is not uncommon for older adult patients to have unfinished business, and only in the very last hours of life are they able to close their life book. Certainly there are medications that can be prescribed if the elder is extremely restless, but that is different from totally sedating a patient. In rare situations, when the older adult is experiencing intractable pain at the end of life that is not responding to

therapy, the kind and appropriate intervention might be to sedate him or her.

If the decision is to totally sedate a patient regardless of the cause of suffering, there are resources available that explain how this is done. The reader is referred to an excellent resource guide on total sedation published by the National Hospice and Palliative Care Organization (2001). Included in the guide is an outline for in-service programs, case studies, and an annotated bibliography plus handouts and overheads.

Case Study Conclusion

Mrs. H. had RA from the time she was a young adult and was severely deformed from it. When she first entered the hospice program, she was still going to an adult day services facility three times a week, which was no easy feat on her part. A nursing assistant went into the home early in the morning, bathed Mrs. H., applied heat to her joints, and made sure she took her medications. Mrs. H. would then go back to bed for 1 hour before going to the day services facility. The nonpharmacologic intervention of heat was an extremely important part of the plan of care.

Multiple issues regarding the management of pain occurred throughout the time Mrs. H. was in the hospice program. She demonstrated some of the barriers that patients have regarding pain. Because her grandson was chemically dependent, she had a fear of taking opioids for pain; thus the interdisciplinary team had to constantly reassure her and reinforce that it was okay to take them. Also, because of her own history of alcoholism, she was fearful of taking "drugs," as she called them. As her physical condition deteriorated, she became confused and was not capable of remembering to take her medications as prescribed. This resulted in the need for placement in a nursing facility, which was not what she wanted, but there was no 24-hour caregiver.

In the last few days of her life, she was unable to swallow, which presented multiple problems regarding the administration of medications. How was her prednisone going to be administered for her long-standing joint pain? How was she going to take her OxyContin and OxyFast? The prednisone could not be given rectally; however, it could be replaced with dexamethasone, which can be given rectally. OxyContin cannot be administered rectally. Normally, OxyFast could be increased and given orally, but Mrs. H. developed nausea and vomiting from the size of the tumor, so that was not an option. OxyContin was converted to MS Contin and administered rectally. Although absorption rate cannot be guaranteed when MS Contin is administered rectally, it is acceptable in the home environment when a patient is actively dying. Lastly, Compazine per rectum controlled the nausea and vomiting.

Over the months, Mrs. H.'s condition had declined, resulting in the loss of independence and inability to go to church. She became depressed and was treated with nortriptyline. The social worker and spiritual care counselor counseled her regarding the depression and spirituality. Also contributing to the depression was the severity of the pain; persistent pain and depression are interrelated because they both use the same neurocircuitry. Although Mrs. H. was not able to die in her own home, which was her goal, she died comfortably surrounded by her grandchildren.

CONCLUSION

The management of all types of pain was presented with special emphasis on the unique aspects of pain management for an older adult population. A holistic approach was used as the conceptual model for assessing, planning, and intervening in pain management.

REFERENCES

Abraham, J. (2000). *A physician's guide to pain and symptom management in cancer patients.* Baltimore: The Johns Hopkins University Press.

Agency for Health Care Policy and Research. (1992). *Acute pain management: Operative or medical procedures and trauma* (AHCPR Publication No. 92-0032). Rockville, MD: U.S. Department of Health and Human Services.

Agency for Health Care Policy and Research. (1994). *Management of cancer pain: Adults* (AHCPR Publication No. 94-0593). Rockville, MD: U.S. Department of Health and Human Services.

Allison, N. (1999). Guided imagery. In N. Allison (Ed.), *The illustrated encyclopedia of body mind disciplines* (pp. 71-73). New York: The Rosen Publishing Group, Inc.

American Geriatrics Society Panel on Chronic Pain in Older Persons. (1998). Clinical practice: The management of chronic pain in older persons. *Journal of the American Geriatrics Society, 46,* 635-651.

American Geriatrics Society Panel on Persistent Pain in Older Persons. (2002). The management of persistent pain in older persons. *Journal of the American Geriatrics Society, 50,* 1-20.

American Music Therapy Association. (1999). *AMTA member sourcebook.* Silver Spring, MD: Author.

American Pain Society. (1992). *Principles of analgesic use in the treatment of acute and chronic cancer pain* (3rd ed.). Glenview, IL: Author.

American Pain Society. (1999). *Principles of analgesic use in the treatment of acute pain and cancer pain* (4th ed.). Glenview, IL: Author.

Blackburt, T., & Dunn, M. (1990). Cystocerebral syndrome: Urinary retention as confusion. *Archives of Internal Medicine, 150,* 2577.

Brandt, K. D. (1995). Toward pharmacologic modification of joint damage in osteoarthritis [editorial]. *Annals of Internal Medicine, 122,* 874-875.

Breitbart, W. (2002). Chronic pain defined as a disease. *OHPCO News, 6*(1), 1.

Bruera, E., Franco, J. J., Maltoni, M., Watanabe, S., & Suarez-Almazor, M. (1995). Changing pattern of agitated impaired mental status in patients with advanced cancer: Association with cognitive monitoring, dehydration and opioid rotation. *Journal of Pain and Symptom Management, 10,* 287-291.

Buff, M. D., Miaskowski, C., Sands, L., & Brod, M. (2001). A pilot study of the relationship between discomfort and agitation in patients with dementia. *Geriatric Nursing, 22,* 80-85.

Cassileth, B. R. (2002). Complementary and alternative approaches. In A. Berger, R. K. Portenoy, & D. E. Weissman (Eds.), *Palliative care and supportive oncology* (2nd ed, pp. 1007-1015). Philadelphia: Lippincott Williams & Wilkins.

Clark, C. (1999). *Encyclopedia of complementary health practice.* New York: Springer.

Cohen-Mansfield, J., & Marx, M. S. (1993). Pain and depression in the nursing home: Corroborating results. *Journal of Gerontology, 48,* 96-97.

Coyle, N., & Layman-Goldstein, M. (2001). Pain assessment and management in palliative care. In M. Matzo & D. Sherman (Eds.), *Palliative care nursing: Quality care to the end of life* (p. 422). New York: Springer.

Daut, R. L., Cleeland, C. S., & Flanery, R. C. (1983). Development of the Wisconsin Brief Pain Questionnaire to assess pain in cancer and other diseases. *Pain, 17,* 197-210.

Davis, M. A. (1988). Epidemiology of osteoarthritis. *Clinics in Geriatric Medicine, 4,* 241-255.

Desbiens, N. A., Mueller-Rizner, N., Connors, A. F., Jr., Hamel, M. B., & Wenger, N. S. (1997). Pain in the oldest-old during hospitalization and up to one year later. *Journal of the American Geriatrics Society, 45,* 1167-1172.

Dossey, B. (1995). Imagery: awakening the inner healer. In *Holistic nursing: A handbook for practice* (pp. 609-666). Gaithersburg, MD: Aspen.

Eisenberg, D. M., Davis, R. B., Ettner, S. L., Appel, S., Wilkey, S., Van Rompay, M., et al. (1998). Trends in alternative medicine use in the United States 1990-1997: Results of a follow-up national survey. *Journal of the American Medical Association, 280,* 1569-1575.

Emanuel, L. L., von Gunten, C. F., & Ferris, F. D. (Eds.). (1999). *The education for physicians on end-of-life care (EPEC) curriculum.* Princeton, NJ: The Robert Wood Johnson Foundation.

Feldt, K. S. (1996). Treatment of pain in cognitively impaired versus cognitively intact post hip fractured elders (Doctoral dissertation, University of Minnesota, 1996). *Dissertation Abstracts International, 57-09B,* 5574.

Feldt, K. S. (2000). The checklist of nonverbal pain indicators (CNPI). *Pain Management Nursing, 1*(1), 13-21.

Feldt, K. S., Ryden, M. B., & Miles, S. (1998). Treatment of pain in cognitively impaired compared with cognitively intact older patients with hip fracture. *Journal of the American Geriatrics Society, 46,* 1079-1085.

Ferrell, B. A. (1991). Pain management in elder people. *Journal of the American Geriatrics Society, 39,* 64-73.

Ferrell, B. A., & Ferrell, B. R. (1990, July/August). Easing the pain. *Geriatric Nursing, 11*(4), 175-178.

Ferrell, B. A., Ferrell, B. R., & Rivera, L. (1995). Pain in cognitively impaired nursing home patients. *Journal of Pain and Symptom Management, 10,* 591-598.

Ferrell, B. R. (1996). Patient education and nondrug interventions. In B. R. Ferrell & B. A. Ferrell (Eds.), *Pain in the elder* (pp. 35-44). Seattle: IASP Press.

Ferrell, B. R. (2001). Pain observed: The experience of pain from the family caregiver's perspective. *Clinics in Geriatric Medicine, 17,* 595-609, viii-ix.

Ferrell, B. R., & Ferrell, B. A. (1995). Pain in elderly persons. In D. B. McGuire, C. Henke Yarbro, & B. R. Ferrell (Eds.), *Cancer pain management* (2nd ed., pp. 273-287). Boston: Jones and Bartlett.

Ferrell, B. R., Virani, R., & Grant, M. (1999). Analysis of end of life content in nursing textbooks. *Oncology Nursing Forum, 26,* 869-876.

Ferrell, B. R., Wisdom, D., & Wengl, C. (1989). Quality of life as an outcome variable in the management of cancer pain. *Cancer, 63,* 2321-2327.

Ferrell-Torry, A. T., & Glick, O. J. (1993). The use of therapeutic massage as a nursing intervention to modify anxiety and the perception of cancer pain. *Cancer Nursing, 16,* 93-101.

Foley, K. M. (1993). Changing concepts of tolerance to opioids: What the cancer patient has taught us. In C. R. Chapman & K. M. Foley (Eds.), *Current and emerging issues in cancer pain: Research and practice* (pp. 331-350). New York: Raven Press.

Foley, K. M. (1994). Pain in the elderly. In W. R. Hazzard, E. L. Bierman, J. P. Blass, W. H. Ettinger, Jr., & J. B. Halter (Eds.), *Principles of geriatric medicine and gerontology* (pp. 347-351). New York: McGraw-Hill.

Foley, K. M. (1998). Pain assessment and cancer syndromes. In D. Doyle, G. W. D. Hanks, & N. MacDonald (Eds.), *Oxford textbook of palliative medicine* (2nd ed., pp. 310-331). Oxford, UK: Oxford University Press.

Forman, W. B. (1996). Opioid analgesic drugs in the elder. *Clinics in Geriatric Medicine, 12,* 489-499.

Fujimoto, D. (2001). Regulatory issues in pain management. *Clinics in Geriatric Medicine, 17,* 537-551, vii.

Gallagher, R. M., Verma, S., & Mossey, J. (2000). Chronic pain: Sources of late life pain and risk factors of disability. *Geriatrics, 55,* 40-47.

Gatchel, R., & Maddrey, A. (1998). Clinical outcome research in complementary and alternative medicine: An overview of experimental design and analgesics. *Alternative Therapies, 4*(5), 36-43.

Geroldi, C., Rozzini, R., Frisoni, G., & Trabucchi, M. (1994). Assessment of alcohol consumption and alcoholism in the elderly. *Alcohol, 11,* 513-516.

Glass, T. A., Prigerson, H., Kasl, S. V., & Mendes de Leon, C. F. (1995). The effects of negative life events on alcohol consumption among elderly men and women. *Journals of Gerontology. Series B, Psychological Sciences and Social Sciences, 50,* 5205-5216.

Gloth, F. M., III. (2000). Geriatric pain: Factors that limit pain relief and increase complications. *Geriatrics, 55*(10), 46-48, 51-54.

Gordon, R. S. (1979). Pain in the elder. *Journal of the American Medical Association, 241,* 2491.

Haghighi, K., & Pansch, B. (2001). Music therapy. In *Complementary therapies in end-of-life care* (pp. 53-60). Alexandria, VA: National Hospice and Palliative Care Organization.

Harkins, S. A. (1996). Geriatric pain: Pain perceptions in the old. *Clinics in Geriatric Medicine, 12,* 435-459.

Herr, K. (2002). Chronic pain in the older patient: Management strategies. *Journal of Gerontological Nursing, 28*(2), 28-34.

Herr, K. A. & Mobily, P. R. (1993). Comparison of selected pain assessment tools for use with the elderly. *Applied Nursing Research, 6*(1), 39-46.

Inouye, S. K., van Dyck, C. H., Alessi, C. A., Balkin, S., Siegal, A. P., & Horwitz, R. I. (1990). Clarifying confusion: the confusion assessment method. A new method for detection of delirium. *Annals of Internal Medicine, 113,* 941-948.

International Association for the Study of Pain Task Force on Taxonomy. (1994). *Classification of chronic pain* (2nd ed.). Seattle: IASP Press.

Jacox, A., Carr, D. B., Payne, R., et al. (1994). *Management of cancer pain* (Clinical Practice Guideline No. 9). Rockville, MD: Agency for Health Care Policy and Research.

Joint Commission on Accreditation of Healthcare Organizations. (2000). *Pain assessment and management: An organizational approach.* Washington, DC: Joint Commission Resources, Inc.

Juarez, G., & Ferrell, B. R. (1996). Family and caregiver involvement in pain management. *Clinics in Geriatric Medicine, 12,* 531-547.

Katsma, D. L., & Souza, C. H. (2000). Elder pain assessment and pain management knowledge of long-term care nurses. *Pain Management Nursing, 1*(3), 88-95.

Kenny, C. (1982). *The mystic artery.* Atascadero, CA: Ridgeview Publishing Company.

Latimer, E. J. (1991). Ethical decision-making in the care of the dying and its application to clinical practice. *Journal of Pain and Symptom Management, 6,* 329-336.

Leo, R. J., & Singh, A. (2002). Pain management in the elder: Use of psychopharmacologic agents. *Annals of Long-Term Care, 10*(2), 37-45.

Levy, M. H. (1989). Integration of pain management into comprehensive cancer care. *Cancer, 63,* 2328-2335.

Lipman, A. G. (1996). Analgesic drugs for neuropathic and sympathetically maintained pain. *Clinics in Geriatric Medicine, 12,* 501-515.

Magni, G. (1991). The use of antidepressants in the treatment of chronic pain: A review of the current evidence. *Drugs, 42,* 730-748.

Marzinski, L. R. (1991). The tragedy of dementia: Clinically assessing pain in the confused, nonverbal elder. *Journal of Gerontological Nursing, 17*(6), 25-28.

McCaffery, M. (1990). Nursing approaches to nonpharmacological pain control. *International Journal of Nursing Studies, 27,* 1-5.

McCaffery, M., & Beebe, A. (1989). *Pain: Clinical manual for nursing.* St. Louis: Mosby.

McCaffery, M., & Pasero, C. (1999). *Pain: Clinical manual for nursing* (2nd ed., pp. 15-54). St. Louis: Mosby.

McCarberg, B. H., & Herr, K. A. (2001). How to manage pain and improve patient function. *Geriatrics, 56*(10), 14-24.

McElhaney, J. (2001, March). Chronic pain in older adults: Strategies for control. *Consultant,* pp. 337-338.

Melzack, R., & Wall, P. D. (1984). *The challenge of pain.* New York: Basic Books.

Merskey, H. (1996). Classification of chronic pain: Description of chronic pain syndrome and definition of pain terms. *Pain. Supplement, 3,* S217.

Micozzi, M. S. (1996). Characteristics of complementary and alternative medicine. In M. S. Micozzi (Ed.), *Fundamentals of complementary and alternative medicine* (pp. 3-8). New York: Churchill Livingstone.

Munro, S. (1984). *Music therapy in palliative/hospice care.* St. Louis: Magnamusic, Baton.

National Hospice and Palliative Care Organization. (2001). *Total sedation: A hospice and palliative care resource guide.* Alexandria, VA: Author.

Nelson, K. A., Park, K., Robinovitz, E., Tsigos, C., & Mas, M. B. (1997). High-dose oral dextromethorphan versus placebo in painful diabetic neuropathy and postherpetic neuralgia. *Neurology, 48,* 1212-1218.

Newshan, G. (1998). Heat-related toxicity with the fentanyl transdermal patch. *Journal of Pain and Symptom Management, 16,* 277-278.

Noble, S. L., King, D. S., & Olutade, J. I. (2000). Cyclooxygenase-2 enzyme inhibitors: Place in therapy. *American Family Physician, 61,* 3669-3676.

Paice, J. A. (1999). Symptom management. In C. Miaskowski & P. Buchsel (Eds.), *Oncology nursing: Assessment and clinical care.* St. Louis: Mosby.

Parmelee, P. A., Katz, I. R., & Lawton, M. P. (1991). The relation of pain to depression among institutionalized aged. *Journal of Gerontology, 46,* 15-21.

Parmelee, P. A., Smith, B. D., & Katz, I. R. (1993). Pain complaints and cognitive status among elder institution residents. *Journal of the American Geriatrics Society, 41,* 517-522.

Pasero, C., & McCaffery, M. (1996). Postoperative pain management in the elder. In B. R. Ferrell & B. A. Ferrell (Eds.), *Pain in the elder* (pp. 45-68). Seattle: IASP Press.

Pasero, C., & McCaffery, M. (2001). Selective COX-2 inhibitors. *American Journal of Nursing, 101*(4), 55-56.

Patt, R. B. (1993). Classification of cancer pain and cancer pain syndromes. In R. B. Patt (Ed.), *Cancer pain.* Philadelphia: Lippincott.

Payne, R. (1998). *Relaxation techniques: A practical handbook for the healthcare professional.* New York: Churchill Livingstone.

Phillips, D. M. (2000). JCAHO pain management standards are unveiled. *Journal of the American Medical Association, 284,* 428-429.

Pitorak, E. (1999). The challenge of pain management in the elderly patient in hospice care. *Journal of Hospice and Palliative Nursing, 1*(1), 9-20.

Plaisance, L., & Ellis, J. (2002). Opioid induced constipation. *American Journal of Nursing, 102*(3), 73.

Popp, B., & Portenoy, R. K. (1996). Management of chronic pain in the elder: Pharmacology of opioids and other analgesic drugs. In B. R. Ferrell & B. A. Ferrell (Eds.), *Pain in the elder* (pp. 21-34). Seattle: IASP Press.

Portenoy, R. K. (1996). Opioid therapy for nonmalignant pain: A review of the critical issues. *Journal of Pain and Symptom Management, 11,* 203-217.

Portenoy, R. K. (1998). Adjuvant analgesics in pain management. In D. Doyle, G. W. C. Hanks, & N. MacDonald (Eds.), *Oxford textbook of palliative medicine* (2nd ed., pp. 361-390). Oxford, UK: Oxford University Press.

Portenoy, R. K., & Prager, G. (1999). Pain management: Pharmacological approaches. In C. F. von Gunten (Ed.),

Palliative care and rehabilitation of cancer patients (pp. 1-29). Boston: Kluwer Academic Publishers.

Portenoy, R. K., Thaler, H. T., Kornblith, A. B., Lepore, J. M., Friedlander, I. H., & Coyle, N. (1994). Symptom prevalence, characteristics and distress in a cancer population. *Quality of Life Research, 3,* 183-189.

Porter, J., & Jick, H. (1980). Addiction rare in patients treated with narcotics. *New England Journal of Medicine, 302,* 123.

Prager, J. P. (1996). Invasive modalities for the diagnosis and treatment of pain in the elder. *Clinics in Geriatric Medicine, 12,* 549-561.

Raskin, J. B., White, R. H., Jackson, J. E., Weaver, A. L., Tindell, E. A., Lies, R. B., et al. (1995). Misoprostol dosage in the prevention of non-steroidal anti-inflammatory drug induced gastric and duodenal ulcers: A comparison of three regimens. *Annals of Internal Medicine, 123,* 344-350.

Raway, B. (1994). Pain behaviors and confusion in elder patients with hip fracture (Doctoral dissertation, Catholic University of America, 1994). *Dissertation Abstracts International, 55-02B* (University Microfilms No. AA194-18593).

Robins, J. (1999). The science and art of aromatherapy. *Journal of Holistic Nursing, 12*(1), 5-17.

Rogers, M. (1992). Therapeutic touch. Part 1. *Theory and research: healing through human energy fields.* New York: National League for Nursing.

Rummans, T. A., Evans, J. M., Krahn, L. E., & Fleming, K. C. (1995). Delirium in elderly patients: Evaluations and management. *Mayo Clinic Proceedings, 70,* 989-998.

Schwarz, J. (2001). Ethical aspects of palliative care. In M. Matzo & D. Sherman (Eds.), *Palliative care nursing: Quality care to the end of life* (pp. 140-179). New York: Springer.

Sengstaken, E. A., & King, S. A. (1993). The problem of pain and its detection among geriatric nursing home residents. *Journal of the American Geriatrics Society, 41,* 541-544.

Stein, W. (1996). Cancer pain in the elder. In B. R. Ferrell & B. A. Ferrell (Eds.), *Pain in the elder* (pp. 69-80). Seattle: IASP Press.

Trauger-Querry, B. (2001). Art therapy. In *Complementary therapies in end-of-life care* (pp. 87-108). Alexandria, VA: National Hospice and Palliative Care Organization.

Twycross, R. (1999). *Introducing palliative care* (3rd ed.). Abingdon, Oxon, UK: Radcliff Medical Press.

Twycross, R., & Lack, S. A. (1983). *Symptom control in the far advanced cancer patient.* London: Pitman Books.

Watanabe, S., & Bruera, E. (1994). Corticosteroids as adjuvant analgesics. *Journal of Pain and Symptom Management, 9,* 442-445.

Whitcomb, D. C., & Block, G. D. (1994). Association of acetaminophen toxicity with fasting ethanol use. *Journal of the American Medical Association, 272,* 1845-1850.

Williams, H. F., Ward, J. R., & Egger, M. J. (1993). Comparison of naproxen and acetaminophen in a two-year study of treatment of osteoarthritis of the knee. *Annals of the Rheumatic Diseases, 36,* 1196-2206.

Williams, M. E. (1994). Clinical management of the elderly patient. In W. R. Hazzard, E. L. Bierman, J. P. Blass, W. H. Ettinger, Jr., & J. B. Halter (Eds.), *Principals of geriatric medicine and gerontology* (pp. 195-201). New York: McGraw-Hill.

World Health Organization. (1986). *Cancer pain relief.* Geneva: Author.

Zuberbueler, E. (1996). Complementary therapies in terminal care. Massage therapy: an added dimension in terminal care. *American Journal of Hospice and Palliative Care, 13*(2), 50.

22 SKIN CARE NEEDS OF PALLIATIVE CARE PATIENTS

Elizabeth A. Ayello

Case Study

Mrs. A. is a 72-year-old female with metastatic colon cancer. She has a descending colostomy for which she has been doing her own self-care. Following her radiation treatments, she has had difficulty with liquid stools, and a tumor is now beginning to appear on her abdomen. The wound is oozing exudates and stool. With progression of her disease, she now spends most of her time in bed; she states that her body has a terrible odor, and that she has pain on her sacrum from lying in one position. She is no longer letting her friends visit because of her weakened state and her feelings of shame regarding the smell. She hardly talks to her husband, who is doing his best to care for her despite his own cardiac problems. A son lives 2 hours away and visits on alternate weekends.

Issues to be addressed include the following:
What changes in her ostomy care are needed?
How can the odor and drainage from the tumor wound on her abdomen be handled?
What is the best treatment plan for the pressure ulcer on her sacrum?
How can communication and quality of life be improved for Mrs. A. and her family?

INTRODUCTION

The visible changes in the skin are typically very apparent to an elder palliative care patient and his or her family because it is the largest externally organ. The physical appearance of skin wounds and/or damage to the skin from drainage, as well as the odor, can be physically and emotionally upsetting. Skin injuries not only cause pain, but also may require changes in other aspects of the elder's overall management as part of the treatment plan.

Skin assessment is an important part of care of the older adult who is at the end of his or her life. Prevention of skin injury may need to be balanced against the overall goals of care. Actual observation of the skin and of the total patient is needed to identify patients at risk for skin injury and to begin prevention protocols. However, there is no consensus in the literature as to what constitutes a minimum skin assessment. Baranoski and Ayello (2004) have suggested five elements to include in a basic skin assessment. They are skin temperature, color, moisture, and turgor, and whether the skin is intact or has areas of injury, such as open areas.

Educating elders about skin care is an important part of nursing interventions. Ideally, this type of teaching will occur prior to any skin injury. For example, Haisfield-Wolfe and Rund (2002) created a booklet for cancer patients with guidelines for skin care. The 30 female oncology patients in their study who were receiving chemotherapy found the booklet helpful in doing their own self-assessment for perineal skin changes.

Once areas of skin injury are identified, it is imperative to determine the correct etiology of the type of skin wound. In palliative care, the goal may not be wound healing, but rather wound maintenance; control of wound odor, exudates, infection, and bleeding; and alleviation of wound pain. This knowledge will guide the clinician in developing the proper treatment plan. In this chapter, several common skin problems (skin tears, pressure ulcers, tumor- and treatment-related skin injuries, ostomy skin, and fistulas) are discussed.

Table 22-1 **Incidence of Pressure Ulcers by Location**		
Location	% of Cases	% of Ulcers
Hospital	44.3%	44.6%
Nursing home	37.8%	40.2%
Family home	14.2%	12%

Date from Eckman, K. (1989). The prevalence of pressure ulcers among persons in the U.S. who have died. *Decubitus*, 2(2), 36-41.

PRESSURE ULCERS

Pressure ulcers are common occurrences during the dying process. Eckman (1989) reported the results of a randomized study of 130 funeral homes across the United States. Among 1378 deceased persons, 1 of 4 (23.6%) had a pressure ulcer. The number of ulcers ranged from 1 to 14; 31% had one ulcer while 68.6% had more than one ulcer. Table 22-1 shows the number of cases by location when location, of death was known.

Kennedy (1989) reported that 56% of patients who died in an intermediate care facility developed a pressure ulcer within the 6 weeks prior to their death. Furthermore, Kennedy has described the following characteristics of the Kennedy terminal ulcer, which appears when death is imminent: pear shaped; located on the coccyx or sacrum; red, yellow, or black; and of sudden onset. The idea that the pressure ulcer "complicates care, increases costs, and threatens quality of life" for hospice patients was proposed by Colburn (1987). The incidence of pressure ulcers may be higher in hospice patients (Hanson et al., 1991). "Time in bed increases as their condition deteriorates, which occurs concomitantly as multisystem failure and growing weakness predispose them to risk factors including decreased activity and mobility, depleted nutrition and hydration, incontinence, and changes in sensory perception and consciousness" (Langemo, Bates-Jensen, & Hanson, 2001, p. 143). It is unclear exactly what protocols are best to use when the goals of care are comfort rather than cure or healing, preventing extension of the wound, and limiting impact of the wound on the elder's quality of life. "Strategies used to prevent pressure ulcers in

Box 22-1 **NPUAP Research Implications and Recommendations**
RECOMMENDATIONS
• Significant gaps in knowledge
• Large multisite studies of hospice patients needed
• Extent and nature of ulcers need clarification
• Pressure ulcer prevention at end of life
QUESTIONS
• To what extend can pressure ulcer be attributed to the "dying condition"?
• What are "best practices" for pressure ulcer prevention at the end of life?
• What is palliative pressure ulcer care?
• When does palliative care replace the goal of healing the wound?

Data from Cuddigan, J., Ayello, E. A., & Sussman, C. (Eds.), *Pressure ulcers in America: Prevalence, incidence, and implications for the future*. Reston, VA: National Pressure Ulcer Advisory Panel.

other populations may seem to be in direct conflict with palliative care strategies" (Langemo et al., p. 143).

The National Pressure Ulcer Advisory Panel (NPUAP) (Cuddigan, Ayello, & Sussman, 2001) reviewed studies done over a 10-year period to determine the prevalence and incidence of pressure ulcers in the palliative care/hospice patient population. This report reviewed the existing evidence base of seven studies on hospice or palliative care; Box 22-1 presents a summary of the report's implications and recommendations. Incidence rates ranged from a low of 8% (Olson, Tkachuk, & Hanson, 1998) to 85% (Waltman, Bergstrom, Armstrong, Norvell, & Braden, 1991). The majority of the patients in these studies had cancer. Hanson and colleagues (1991) reported an incidence of 13% for stages I and II pressure ulcers. Locations of these pressure ulcers were the sacrum (38.4%), elbows (30.7%), and heels (15.4%). Pressure ulcers occurred within 2 weeks of death. Waltman and colleagues (1991) found a higher incidence of pressure ulcers in elder patients with cancer (85%) compared to a matched group without cancer (70%).

In this prospective study, average time to death after developing a pressure ulcer was 3 weeks.

Pressure Ulcer Locations

The sacrum is the number one location for pressure ulcer occurrence; the heels are second (Baldwin, 2001; Cuddigan, Hollinger, Brown, & Horslen, 2001). In specific palliative care patients, other sites may be at risk for pressure ulcer breakdown. For example, in elders with chronic obstructive pulmonary disease who are on long-term oxygen therapy, the part of the ears underneath the oxygen tubing must be checked for pressure ulcers.

Pressure Ulcer Staging

Pressure ulcers are staged based on the visible assessment of the depth of tissue that has been damaged in the wound bed. If eschar is present, the pressure ulcer cannot be staged. Bennett (1995) has urged clinicians to use appropriate lighting sources such as natural or halogen lighting as well as evaluating skin temperature and consistency to detect stage I pressure ulcers in clients with darkly pigmented skin. The NPUAP staging definitions, available from its website, are as follows:

Stage I: Observable pressure-related alteration of intact skin, whose indicators as compared to an adjacent or opposite area on the body may include changes in one or more of the following:
- skin temperature (warmth or coolness)
- tissue consistency (firm or boggy feel) and/or
- sensation (pain, itching)

The ulcer appears as a defined area of persistent redness in lightly pigmented skin, whereas, in darker skin tones, the ulcer may appear with persistent red, blue, or purple hues.

Stage II: Partial-thickness skin loss involving epidermis and/or dermis. The ulcer is superficial and presents clinically as an abrasion, blister, or shallow crater.

Stage III: Full-thickness skin loss involving damage to or necrosis of subcutaneous tissue that may extend down to, but not through, underlying fascia. The ulcer presents clinically as a deep crater with or without undermining of adjacent tissue.

Stage IV: Full-thickness skin loss with extensive destruction, tissue necrosis, or damage to muscle, bone, or supporting structures (e.g., tendon, joint capsules).

Preventing Pressure Ulcers

Risk Assessment

The use of risk assessment scales to identify patients at risk for pressure ulcers is recommended by the Agency for Health Care Policy and Research (AHCPR) Clinical Practice Guidelines (Panel for the Prediction and Prevention of Pressure Ulcers in Adults, 1992). Most studies that have used risk assessment scales have been conducted in long-term care, hospital, or home care settings. Unfortunately, these studies do not always report whether the older adults in these settings are palliative care patients. A widely used scale in the United States is the Braden Scale. This scale has six factor subscales—sensory perception, moisture, activity, mobility, nutrition, and friction/shear—which are ranked to provide a total risk score. The Braden Scale is considered to have good reliability and specificity (Panel, 1992). One study by Hanson, Langemo, Olson, Hunter, and Byrd (1994) reported on the use of data from the Braden Scale to identify pressure ulcer risk in hospitalized cancer patients. Incidence was 8%, sensitivity 82%, and specificity 84% (Hanson et al., 1994). Based on patients on a palliative care unit in England, Chaplin (2000) is developing a pressure ulcer risk assessment tool.

The AHCPR pressure ulcer guidelines (Panel, 1992) recommend that patients be evaluated on admission to a care setting and at periodic intervals. Guidelines for reassessment for pressure ulcer risk by specific settings have been suggested (Ayello & Braden, 2001). Box 22-2 lists these recommendations; however, just how applicable these are to palliative care patients is not known.

Prevention Interventions

The purpose of doing a risk assessment is to identify which older adults need prevention interventions. The goal of reducing risk factors is the prevention of pressure ulcers; the utilization of prevention strategies for at-risk older adults is to spare them painful and sometimes tiresome treatments. Older adults are considered to be "at risk" when their Braden Scale score reaches 18,

Box 22-2 **Intervals for Pressure Ulcer Risk Assessment**

ACUTE CARE
- Initial assessment on admission
- Reassessment every 48 hours or whenever the patient's condition changes

LONG-TERM CARE
- Initial assessment on admission
- Reassessment weekly for first 4 weeks, then monthly to quarterly or whenever the patient's condition changes

HOME HEALTH CARE
- Initial assessment on admission
- Reassessment with every RN visit

Box 22-3 **AHCPR Pressure Ulcer Prevention Protocol**

INSPECTION AND CARE OF SKIN
- Frequency of inspection—daily & document
- Bathing—avoid hot water, soaps
- Use moisturizers to treat dry skin
- Avoid low-humidity environment
- Do not massage reddened bony prominences
- Manage incontinence (see AHCPR incontinence guidelines)

MECHANICAL LOADING AND SUPPORT SURFACES
1. Turning and positioning schedules—reposition q2h—use a written schedule
2. Full position changes, use positioning devices
3. 30° lateral position
4. "Pillow bridging"
5. Small shift changes
6. No donuts
7. Use lifting devices
8. Use protective devices and support surfaces
9. Do range-of-motion exercises
10. Keep head of bed <30°
11. Use of support surfaces

From Panel for the Prediction and Prevention of Pressure Ulcers in Adults. (1992, May). *Pressure ulcers in adults: Prediction and prevention.* (Clinical Practice Guideline No. 3, AHCPR Publication No. 92-0047). Rockville, MD: Agency for Health Care Policy and Research.

and intervention protocols have been linked to levels of risk (Ayello & Braden, 2001). Attention to an elder's scores on subscales can also help to target prevention interventions to the specific factor that is most placing the patient at risk. Based on the AHCPR guidelines, Box 22-3 gives pressure ulcer prevention guidelines.

The AHCPR guidelines may need to be modified based on the overall goals of the older adult's care. For palliative care patients, following the recommended every-2-hour repositioning schedule may cause the patient undue pain, and nursing staff may decide not to follow this usual standard of practice. The patient and the family need to clearly understand the implications for skin injury. These changes in a standard treatment plan also need to be documented in the patient's record.

Teaching the patient and his or her family about pressure ulcer prevention is very important (Ayello, Mezey, & Amella, 1997). Patient teaching booklets developed by the AHCPR may not be appropriate for all patients because the reading level is higher than the usual recommended grade 5 to 6 reading level (Ayello, 1993). An "easy reading" patient booklet written by the NPUAP is available from their website.

Pressure Ulcer Treatment
The AHCPR pressure ulcer treatment guidelines (Bergstrom et al., 1994) recommend using

normal saline and some commercially available wound cleaners to cleanse the ulcer. Unlike cytotoxic agents such as Dakin's solution (sodium hypochlorite solution) and acetic acid, these solutions do not kill cells. Cytotoxic agents are typically not recommended for cleaning of pressure ulcers. For palliative care patients, use of these solutions may be warranted because the goal is no longer healing. The benefits of odor control from these solutions may make them an appropriate choice for older adults who are at the end of their lives. Gentle irrigation (4 to 15 psi) to irrigate pressure ulcers can be achieved by using a 19-gauge needle with a 35-mL syringe. The psi from a bulb syringe is below 4, so it may not provide adequate pressure to clean the pressure ulcers.

Box 22-4 Selected Wound Dressings

LOW EXUDATE ABSORPTION
FILM DRESSINGS
- Easily applied
- Can see the wound site
- Waterproof, good for incontinent patients
- Adhesive may cause skin injury during removal
- Generally not recommended for use with infected wounds

HYDROGEL DRESSINGS
- Available as sheets or gels
- Effective for painful wounds
- High water content, so effective to use for wounds that are dry
- Require a secondary dressing to keep in place

HYDROCOLLOID DRESSINGS
- Available in many shapes and sizes
- Very moldable
- Some are adhesive, some are not
- Can remain in place for many days

MODERATE TO HIGH EXUDATE ABSORPTION
CALCIUM ALGINATE DRESSINGS
- Made from seaweed
- Available in sheet and rope forms
- Effective for packing wounds

- Be aware that the wound may have the odor of "low tide"
- Switch to another dressing if exudates diminish, because dressing can dry out a wound with low exudates
- Requires a secondary dressing to hold in place

FOAM DRESSINGS
- Very useful for wet, weepy wounds
- Effective for packing deep wounds
- Requires a secondary dressing
- Can be used underneath compression stockings and multiple-layer bandaging systems

NEGATIVE PRESSURE DRESSINGS (VACUUM-ASSISTED CLOSURE [VAC]
- Great for wounds with large amounts of exudate
- Requires learning the technique for placing the specialized foam into the wound, positioning the tubing, applying the specialized drape, and attaching to the vacuum source

ANTIMICROBIAL DRESSINGS
- Effective for infected wounds
- Requires a secondary dressing
- Cannot perform magnetic resonance imaging if silver dressings used

Pressure ulcers may need ongoing débridement of necrotic tissue. Autolytic débridement can be achieved by using film, hydrocolloid, hydrogel, or other dressings (Ayello, Cuddigan, & Kerstein, 2002). Débridement using enzymes is another method that is effective in the palliative care setting because there is little pain associated with this intervention. Surgical débridement may be best for infected wounds with advancing cellulitis. Mechanical débridement accomplished by wet-to-dry dressings is painful and can cause additional damage as well as bleeding of the tissue, so it is not generally recommended for use with palliative care patients, when comfort is the goal.

Beginning with the discovery of moist wound healing by Winter (1962), many types of dressings have been developed over the years. With the hundreds of different types of dressings now available, selecting the right dressing can be confusing for the clinician. A good way to approach this decision is by assessing the pressure ulcer wound characteristics and then matching the dressing to those needs. For many clinicians, the key determining factor is the amount of exudate in the pressure ulcer wound. For example, wounds with low amounts of exudates can be managed by a dressing with low absorbent capabilities. If the wound bed were dry, then using dressings that add moisture to the wound would be indicated. Box 22-4 presents a brief summary of selected dressings.

Quality-of-Life Issues, Including Pressure Ulcer Pain

Although they are few in number, some studies have provided clinicians with insights into quality-of-life issues for patients with pressure ulcers (Langemo, Melland, Hanson, Olson, & Hunter, 2000) and their caregivers (Baharestani, 1994). Themes common to both of these studies were pain, lack of knowledge, the meaning of the pressure ulcer, and lifestyle changes imposed by the pressure ulcer. Pain is common for older adults with pressure ulcers, yet pain management is often inadequate (Dallam et al., 1995). Total management for the older adult with a pressure ulcer will also require attention to nutritional needs. Adequate nutrition may be difficult for elders experiencing anorexia from cancer or other chronic diseases. It also may be inconsistent with the elder's wishes and/or advance directives, and the goals of management.

Pressure ulcers are a result of unrelieved pressure. Providing an adequate pressure-relieving support cushion, mattress, or bed may greatly decrease the older adult's pain, prevent skin breakdown, or prevent further tissue destruction in an existing pressure ulcer. Use of static support surfaces should be initiated if the patient can turn (Panel, 1992). Always check to see if the support surface is "bottoming out" by placing a hand under the support surface. If the patient's bottom can be felt, then the support surface is not adequate. If this is the case, dynamic support surfaces should be obtained.

SKIN TEARS
Scope of Problem
Unlike chronic wounds such as pressure ulcers, skin tears are acute wounds. Malone, Rozario, Gavinski, and Goodwin (1991) have defined a skin tear as a "traumatic wound resulting from separation of the epidermis from the dermis." Although the exact number of skin tears is unknown, Thomas, Goode, LaMaster, Tennyson, and Parnell (1999) have reported that 1.5 million skin tears occur each year in institutionalized adults.

Effect of Aging on Skin
Aging predisposes a patient to skin tears as a result of many changes that are normal aspects of the aging process. As skin ages, there is a decrease in the dermal thickness leading to a thinning of the skin, especially over the legs and forearms. With the decrease in fatty layers and subcutaneous tissues, the bony prominences are less protected. The skin's elastin fibers lose their ability to recoil. Sensation, metabolism, and sweat gland production are also diminished, resulting in dry skin that lacks some of the normal protection mechanisms. An important change that translates into skin tear injury risk is the decrease in the size of the rete ridges in the basement membrane of the skin. As these ridges become flatter with aging, it becomes easier to accidentally separate the epidermis from the dermis (Kaminer & Gilchrest, 1994; Mason, 1997).

Location and Cause
Most skin tears (80%) occur on the arms and hands over areas of senile purpura (Malone et al., 1991; McGough-Csarny & Kopac, 1998; Payne & Martin, 1990). Skin tears on the back and buttocks can be mistaken for stage II pressure ulcers. For about half of skin tears, there is no apparent cause. When the cause is known, 25% are from wheelchair injuries, 25% are caused by accidentally bumping into objects, 18% result from transfers, and 12.4% result from falls (Malone et al., 1991). Long-term steroid use and decreased hormone levels in older females may also be risk factors for skin tears (O'Regan, 2002).

A retrospective study by White, Karam, and Cowell (1994) identified dependent patients who required total care for all activities of daily living as being most at risk for skin tears. The skin tears occurred during routine activities of dressing, bathing, positioning, and transferring. Next at risk were independent ambulatory residents, whose skin tears were mostly found on the lower extremities. Least at risk were slightly impaired residents, whose skin tear injuries resulted from hitting furniture or equipment such as wheelchairs (White et al., 1994).

The method of skin cleansing in routine bathing practices may affect the occurrence of skin tears. Soap increases skin pH to an alkaline level rather than preserving the normal "acid mantle" of the skin (Mason, 1997). Mason (1997) found a lower rate of skin tears in long-term residents (34%) who were bathed every other day with emollient soap. Use of the newer no-rinse bathing products may also be advantageous. Birch and Coggins (2003) have reported a decline of skin tears from 23% to 3% in a long-term care facility when a no-rinse, one-step bed bath protocol, rather than the traditional soap and water bath, was used.

Risk Factors

White and colleagues (1994) developed a skin integrity risk assessment tool to identify persons at risk for skin tears. The tool utilizes three groups (I, II, and III) for evaluating the risk of skin tear occurrence. Implementation of a skin tear risk prevention plan of care depends on the number of criteria that a patient meets in a specific group or a combination of criteria in groups II or III. Additional research with this assessment tool would be valuable in establishing its reliability and validity.

In their 6-month study of residents in a Veterans Administration (VA) nursing home care unit and nine community nursing homes, McGough-Csarny and Kopac (1998) identified 10 risk factors for skin tears; 6 of these accounted for skin tears in 65% of their sample. They were advanced age, sensory loss, compromised nutrition, history of previous skin tear, cognitive impairment, and dependency. Fifty percent of the sample had bruising and poor locomotion as contributing factors. Two other factors present in 40% of the sample were polypharmacy and assistive device use. Using these 10 identified risk factors, the authors reported a plan to develop an instrument to assess skin tear risk.

Classifying Skin Tears

The Payne-Martin classification system for assessing skin tears (Payne & Martin, 1990, 1993) is used to identify the type of skin tear. It has three categories. Category I tears are skin tears without any tissue loss. Category II skin tears have a partial tissue loss of the epidermal flap. Skin tears with complete tissue loss, where the epidermal flap is absent, are designated as category III (Payne & Martin, 1993).

The Payne-Martin classification system has been used in subsequent studies. McGough-Csarny and Kopac (1998) used this system in their study of residents in a VA nursing home care unit and nine community nursing homes. These authors reported that category I and category III were the easiest tears for staff to identify. Thomas and colleagues (1999) utilized this system in their study comparing the healing of skin tears with foam versus transparent film

dressings. Although the Payne-Martin classification system has been used in these studies, further research to determine the tool's efficacy in documentation of skin tears is warranted.

Plan of Care to Prevent or Treat Skin Tears

Once a patient has been identified as being at risk for developing skin tears, a protocol to prevent skin injury should be implemented. There is no universal agreement as to the best practice to prevent or treat skin tears in the literature; one example of suggested best practice can be found in Figure 22-1. The prevention and treatment protocols suggested in Box 22-5 and Box 22-6, respectively, are based on information in the literature (Baranoski, 2000, 2001a, 2001b; Camp-Sorrell, 1991; Krasner, 1991; Malone et al., 1991;

Box 22-5 Skin Tears Prevention Protocol

- Use proper position, turning, lifting, and transferring techniques.
- Use a lift sheet to move and turn patients.
- Have the patient wear long sleeves and pants to add a layer of protection.
- Pad bed rails, wheelchair arm, leg supports, and any other equipment that the patient may use.
- Use nonadherent dressings on frail skin. Be gentle when removing these products to prevent skin injury.
- Use stockinettes, gauge wrap, or some of the commercially available drain holders to secure dressings and drains. If you use tape, use only paper tape.
- Support dangling arms and legs with pillows or blankets.
- Consider use of waterless, no-rinse cleansers. Use emollient soaps. Avoid using alcohol on the skin because it is drying.
- Pat dry skin instead of rubbing while bathing patients.
- Use moisturizing agents on dry skin.
- Keep the environment well lit to prevent falls.
- Educate staff and caregivers to practice gentle care. This includes being careful that their nails do not scratch an elder's vulnerable skin and not sliding watches or jewelry over the arm of an at-risk person.

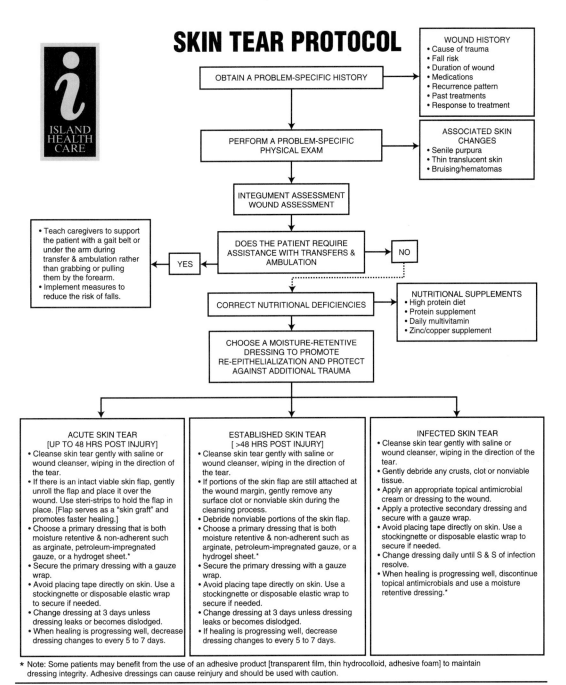

Fig. 22-1 Skin tear protocol. (From Cuzzell, J. [2002].Wound assessment and evaluation: Skin tear protocol. *Dermatology Nursing, 14*[6], 405.)

Box 22-6 Skin Tears Treatment Protocol

- Continue using the skin tear prevention protocol.
- Gently clean the skin tear with normal saline.
- Let the area air dry or pat dry carefully.
- Approximate the skin tear flap.
- Apply petroleum-based ointment, Steri-Strips, or a moist nonadherent wound dressing.
- Use caution if using film dressings because skin damage can occur when removing this dressing.
- Consider putting an arrow on the dressing to indicate the direction of the skin tear to minimize any further skin injury during dressing removal.
- Always assess the size of the skin tear, and consider doing a wound tracing.
- Document assessment and treatment findings.

Mason, 1997; McGough-Csarny & Kopac, 1998; O'Regan, 2002; Payne & Martin, 1990; Thomas et al., 1999; White et al., 1994) and expert clinical opinion.

PERISTOMAL (OSTOMY) SKIN

Secondary to the original course of treatment or because of complications such as obstruction from recurrent tumor, some older adults may require urinary or fecal diversions. Once a patient develops an incontinent ostomy, protecting the skin around the stoma—the peristomal skin—and preventing its breakdown become important nursing goals. A certified wound, ostomy, and continence nurse (CWOCN, formerly an enterostomal therapist [ET]) is an excellent resource in planning and implementing care for these elders. The website of the Wound, Ostomy, and Continence Nurses Society maintains a directory of these nurses by geographic area who are available for clinical consults.

Assessing Peristomal Skin

Peristomal skin must be assessed with each pouching system change. Normal peristomal skin should be intact without discoloration and with no difference between the peristomal skin and adjacent skin surfaces. Peristomal skin damage may be evidenced by erythema, maceration, denudation, skin rash, ulceration, or blister formation. In darkly pigmented patients, the damaged skin may appear lighter or darker than the surrounding skin (Erwin-Toth 2001).

Protecting the peristomal skin from the damaging effects of urinary or fecal effluent is paramount. The proteolytic enzymes found in the effluent from small bowel stomas can rapidly erode the skin. If the urine from a urinary diversion becomes alkaline, it is more damaging to the skin than normally acidic urine. Large amounts of liquid effluent can result in maceration, if allowed to pool on the skin.

Maintaining Peristomal Skin Integrity

Maintaining the integrity of peristomal skin can be accomplished, in part, by observing correct pouching principles. Similarly, peristomal skin must be protected from mechanical trauma, which can occur from inappropriate cleaning. To avoid skin stripping, adhesive removers should be used to remove skin barriers and pouching systems. The adhesive barriers are gently peeled off the skin by stretching the skin taut with one hand, and using adhesive remover along the edge of the barrier where it is attached to the skin. Application of skin sealants prior to application of skin barriers of the pouching system can provide protection for the peristomal skin. Too-frequent or unnecessary changing of the pouch/skin barrier should be avoided.

The nurse should be sure to use the correct products on peristomal skin. Alcohol-based products should never be used, especially if the peristomal skin is denuded. If solvents are used, the skin should be cleaned and the solvent removed before applying the ostomy pouch. The older adult should be assessed for sensitivity to any ostomy product *prior* to using the product; this includes assessing for latex sensitivity.

Skin sealants come in a variety of forms— wipes, gels, and sprays. These products, when dried, provide a thin film over the skin surface, and thus decrease the chance of skin stripping. Some skin sealants contain alcohol, so care should be taken not to use them on denuded skin because they can cause the elder additional pain or burning on application.

A variety of skin barriers can be used to protect the peristomal skin from effluent. These are available as rings, wafers, pastes, and powders.

EVIDENCE-BASED PRACTICE

Reference: Lyon, C. C., Smith, A. J., Griffiths, C. E. M., & Beck, M. H. (2000). The spectrum of skin disorders in abdominal stoma patients. *British Journal of Dermatology, 143,* 1248-1260.

Research Problem: Skin integrity is essential for the normal usage of a stoma appliance. However, there is little published information on the prevalence, nature, or management of stoma-related skin disorders. This study was conducted to document stoma-related skin disorders in a large cohort of patients.

Design: Questionnaire, assessment

Sample and Setting: 525 surviving patients who had had abdominal stoma surgery at Hope Hospital, Salford, United Kingdom, in the 10 years from January 1, 1989.

Methods: A mail questionnaire was sent to all surviving patients, and those reporting skin disease were invited to attend a clinic run by a dermatologist and a stoma-care specialist nurse. All lesions were categorized and swabs taken for microbiologic examination.

Results: Of 525 surviving patients, 325 (62%) replied to the questionnaire. Of these, 73% reported a skin problem that had affected normal stoma bag use. Dermatoses included irritant reactions, particularly from leakage of urine or feces (42%); preexisting skin diseases, principally psoriasis, seborrhoeic dermatitis, and eczema (20%); infections (6%); allergic contact dermatitis (0.7%); and pyoderma gangrenosum (0.6% annual incidence). A further 15% of patients with skin problems had persistent or recurrent dermatitis not explained by allergy, frank infection, or fecal irritation. This dermatitis responded to short-term treatment with topical corticosteroids. Further investigation is under way into its pathogenesis.

Implications for Nursing Practice: Patients receiving new stomas should be educated about potential skin disorders, signs/symptoms, and when a health care provider should be consulted.

Conclusion: Skin disorders are common in stoma patients, and various patterns can be recognized and effectively treated.

In addition to protecting the skin, they also create a level pouching surface, which can prevent leakage of effluent underneath the pouch seal in "difficult-to-fit" stomas. A properly sized and applied skin barrier can protect the skin from the damaging effects of ostomy effluent. Skin barriers vary in their resistance to breakdown by urine or feces. Karaya dissolves with urine, so it should not be used with urinary diversions.

Skin barriers that are powders can be "dusted" onto the denuded skin. Using a skin sealant product over this powder can help provide an absorptive protective layer for the peristomal skin. Some skin barriers can cause pain when used on denuded skin. The nurse should check that the skin sealant product does not have alcohol in it, because this can be painful when applied to denuded and irritated skin. Some companies make "no sting" skin barriers that do not

cause pain or "burning" when applied to irritated, denuded skin.

Selecting the right ostomy pouching system for the patient may require the assistance of a CWOCN (ET) nurse. Pouching systems are provided as one or two pieces. A one-piece system has the skin barrier permanently attached to the ostomy pouch. A two-piece ostomy pouching system has the advantage of the skin barrier remaining on the skin for several days with the ease of snapping the pouch off the skin barrier for emptying of contents. Pouches can be drainable or closed ended.

Pouches should be selected that are correct for the type of drainage coming from the ostomy. For example, fecal pouches will not work for urinary diversions. Urinary ostomy pouches have a spout on the bottom for proper emptying of the urine. For fecal pouches, the opening is wide and is closed, in most cases, with a special ostomy clamp. Most modern-day ostomy pouching systems are odor proof when correctly closed and the seal is intact. If the elder has an unusually large amount of drainage, one of the high-output pouches should be used. Treatments such as chemotherapy or radiation may affect the patient's stool consistency and amount of output. Adjustments in the size of the pouch, more frequent emptying of the pouch, and changes in ostomy irrigations may need to be implemented. It is imperative, when selecting the appropriate pouch, that it is the correct size for the ostomy stoma. A pouch opening size that is too large or too small can cause leakage and/or trauma to the stoma (Bryant & Fleischer, 2000).

Total Ostomy Care Management

Care of the older adult patient with an ostomy involves more than just assessing the peristomal skin and pouching system. The elder's emotional and psychosocial acceptance of the stoma is important; for some people, the creation of a diverting ostomy may bring relief from the symptoms of obstruction, but may also serve as a permanent reminder of the progression of their disease. Supporting the patient to adjust to this change in body image, overcome concerns about odor, learn new psychomotor self-care skills, and make necessary dietary adjustments are just some of the comprehensive care elements that may require the consultation of a CWOCN (ET) nurse to meet the patient's needs.

FISTULAS

Fistulas are abnormal passages between two organs or between an organ and the skin. An internal fistula is contained inside the body while an external fistula tracts outside the body to the skin surface, most commonly through the gastrointestinal tract or bladder but sometimes through the vagina or rectum. Fistulas can occur with certain diseases (e.g., malignancies including obstructions, Crohn's disease, diverticulitis) or from treatment modalities such as radiation therapy or surgery, including postoperative adhesions. A high-output fistula can release more than 200 mL of effluent in 24 hours (Rolstead & Bryant, 2000). Assessment of the perifistula skin is critical because continual irri-

gation by the effluent can be caustic to the skin and result in irritation and erosion. The perifistula skin should be assessed for signs of fungal infections as well as for redness, papular rash, and satellite lesions.

Identification of the fistula to determine its origin is important for developing the plan for closure, which can be spontaneous (about 50%) or surgical. Goals of management for an older adult with a fistula should include maintaining fluid and electrolyte balance (the patient should be assessed for dehydration and metabolic acidosis), protection of the perifistula skin, odor control, effluent containment and measurement, nutritional management, and patient comfort. Holistic care of an elder with a fistula might include total parenteral nutrition to meet the patient's nutritional needs, therapeutic communication to respond to the patient's emotional needs from having a foul-smelling fistula, protecting the skin from injury from the effluent, and eliminating odor.

Older adult females who have pelvic radiation can subsequently develop vaginal fistulas, which are often distressing to the patient and challenging to the nurse. Containment of the feces and odor are difficult and require frequent dressing changes. For nonambulatory patients, urinary incontinence pouches, commercially available vaginal drain devices, or a breast shield or vaginal diaphragm attached to a Malecot catheter may be used (Rolstead & Bryant, 2000).

Management Options
Pouching

A pouching system may be the primary choice for management for older adults with odorous fistulas. Using a clear pouch will enable the caregiver or nurse to easily see the type and amount of effluent. Pouching is superior to dressings because it provides better protection for the skin. A pouch with a spout on the bottom works well for fistulas with thin effluent drainage; for thicker drainage, a fecal pouch that can be closed with a clamp is a better choice. Wound management pouches come in a variety of sizes and are useful for treating abdominal fistulas (Schaffner, Hocevar, & Erwin-Toth, 1994). For patients with odorless fistulas and moderate output (100 ml/24 hr), dressings may be used. A dressing that is absorbent, such as foams, calcium alginates, or hydrocolloids (see Box 22-4 for an overview of dressings), should be used. In these cases, a petroleum- or zinc-based ointment will protect the perifistula skin from maceration or breakdown. Some patients have such large wounds with enterocutaneous fistulas that the usual commercially available pouches are too small and will not fit. O'Brien, Landis-Erdman, and Erwin-Toth (1998) have described the management of one such fistula and large wound using a surgical isolation bag with a skin barrier while packing the wound with moistened gauze.

The higher the enzyme content and liquidity of the fistula output, the greater the need to place additional skin barrier seals around the fistula opening prior to placing a high-output pouch. For older adults who have abdominal fistulas with irregular skin surfaces, skin barrier pastes or strips may need to be placed around the fistula opening in order to "build it up" so the abdominal plane can be "filled in" and then a pouch placed over it. Sometimes, a patient has two fistula openings; if they are close together, one pouch may fit over both fistula orifices. If not, "saddle bagging" two pouches may be the best option.

Tubes and Suction

Another way to manage fistulas is to use drainage tubes, with or without suction. Beitz and Caldwell (1998) have described the management of a high-output enterocutaneous fistula using a drain tube (Jackson-Pratt), connected to low wall suction (60 mm Hg pressure), that was covered with saline-soaked gauze and a large surgical plastic drape. When using this technique, care must be taken in placing the catheter tube so it does not inadvertently cause injury to the tissue. Harris and Komray (1993) have used a similar system to manage a pharyngocutaneous fistula. This system should not be confused with the vacuum-assisted closure (VAC) negative-pressure system previously discussed in the section on pressure ulcers. According to the manufacturer, the VAC should not be used for fistulas.

Trough

Another method of managing enterocutaneous fistulas is by using the trough procedure. This technique is used for fistulas that are deep

within wounds (Wiltshire, 1996). It is made up of several layers of transparent dressing with an ostomy pouch placed at the bottom of the wound (Rolstead & Bryant, 2000).

Patient Comfort

Promoting patient comfort is a major priority in caring for a patient with a fistula. The amount of pain or discomfort that a particular management option may cause a patient should influence the decision regarding which management option to select. The goal is to choose the method that will cause the least discomfort and disruption to the patient and caregiver. Medicating the patient prior to removal or application of fistula containment measures is essential.

TUMOR NECROSIS AND SKIN CARE

In some older adults with advanced cancer, the tumor can invade the skin, which results in ulcerated fungating wounds. For example, in patients with breast cancer, the tumor can grow outward onto the skin in a blackened, cauliflower-like appearance. This results in maceration of the surrounding skin as well as extensive odor from bacterial infection caused by organisms such as *Pseudomonas aeruginosa*, *Staphylococcus*, *Proteus*, and *Klebsiella* (Haisfield-Wolfe & Baxendale-Cox, 1999; Haisfield-Wolfe & Rund, 1997). Nodules may enlarge and erupt spontaneously through the abdominal skin in patients with carcinomatosis. Although the majority of metastatic skin lesions are found on the anterior trunk, they may also be found on the pelvis, flank, head and neck, and posterior trunk (Bauer, Gerlach, & Doughty, 2000). Haisfield-Wolfe and Baxendale-Cox (1999) have suggested the use of a staging classification for assessment of malignant cutaneous wounds. Parameters to include are wound depth, color of the wound, drainage, pain, odor, and presence of tunneling or undermining.

Management Strategies

In an effort to palliate symptoms, radiation therapy or chemotherapy may be used to shrink tumors that have grown onto the skin. Goals of care for these patients include controlling the infection, odor, bleeding, and pain.

Although the evidence base for management of such extensive wounds is limited, options for addressing patient care needs are anecdotally reported. Frequent irrigation of the wound with large amounts of fluid is important to reduce the bacterial burden on the wound surface (Bauer et al., 2000). For patients who can get into the shower, cleansing these fungating wounds may provide physical as well as psychological benefits. The nurse should instruct the patient not to aim the shower water directly at the wound, but rather to aim it above the ulcerated area so the water can trickle down over the wound without undue force. Use of a handheld shower device might be preferred by some patients (Bauer et al., 2000). For patients who cannot tolerate being showered or in cases where the tissue is very friable, gentle cleaning with saline may be substituted.

Management of these wounds can be challenging. They generally have large amounts of exudate because of the tumor's hyperpermeability to fibrinogen and colloids, but primarily as a result of the secretion of vascular permeability factor by the tumor (Bauer et al., 2000). There may also be drainage of fecal material in the case of patients with abdominal carcinomatosis. Dressings should be used that are absorbent (foam, calcium alginate, or cotton absorbent dressing pads). Often there is much necrotic tissue in these wounds, and débridement is required. Autolytic débridement techniques such as the use of calcium alginate dressings, hydrogel dressings, or other nonadherent modern dressings are advocated. Others (Bauer et al., 2000) recommend using a petroleum-impregnated gauze dressing. The skin area around the fungating wound can be "picture framed" with protective skin barriers such as hydrocolloid dressing strips. Use of Montgomery straps to hold the secondary dressing in place will also reduce damage to skin that can be caused by the frequent removal of tape. Cutting the crotch off mesh underpanties and placing the panties around the chest wall like a tube top will also hold the bulky dressings in place (Bauer et al., 2000). Mechanical débridement, such as wet-to-dry dressings, should be avoided because of the obvious risk of causing more bleeding and increasing the older adult's pain.

Bleeding commonly occurs in these types of wounds because tumor cells take over the function of platelets, and the growth and clotting factors that they secrete damage normal tissue

(Bauer et al., 2000). Preventing the dressings from drying out can minimize tissue trauma from the removal of soiled dressings. Calcium alginate dressings (Haisfield-Wolf & Rund, 1997) have a hemostatic effect and are a good choice for bleeding wounds. Silver nitrate sticks can be used to control small amounts of blood.

Pain also results from the tumor growing on the skin and from treatment procedures. Seaman (1995) suggested using ice packs or a topical anesthetic aerosol spray (Hurricane) to alleviate wound pain. Some clinicians have reported using the VAC dressing system solely for pain management and comfort for elders with these types of extensive wounds. Topical opioids have also been used to relieve wound pain.

Odor may be one of the most distressing problems for the patient and his or her caregivers. Seaman (1995) suggested first using one of the commercially available wound gel deodorizers; some patients may experience burning with application of these products. The use of MetroGel (0.8% topical antibiotic wound deodorizing gel) (Newman, Allwood, & Oakes, 1989; Rice, 1990; Seaman, 1995) to control even the most horrific odors has been reported. Metronidazole tablets can be dissolved into normal saline and used to irrigate the wound (McMullen, 1995). Metronidazole tablets (250 or 500 mg) can be crushed and sprinkled directly onto the wound bed (Bauer et al., 2000). Taking metronidazole systemically is also recommended. Topical application of yogurt or buttermilk has been used to combat the extensive odors from tumor necrosis (Schulte, 1993; Welch, 1981). The newer antimicrobial cadexomer iodine or silver dressings are also excellent at reducing odor, with the added benefit of controlling the bacterial burden in the wound. Another advantage is that some of these dressings can stay in place for up to 7 days, which reduces the pain from dressing changes. Odor control within the patient's environment may be achieved by utilizing aromatherapy products, such as peppermint oils/sprays, or placing activated charcoal under the bed (Cormier, McCann, & McKeithan, 1995).

Quality-of-Life Issues

The clinician should be aware of his or her nonverbal and verbal communications to the older

Reference: Wallace, M., & Fulmer, T. (2002). Fulmer SPICES: An overall assessment tool of older adults. *Dermatology Nursing, 14*(2), 142.

Research Problem: Normal aging brings about inevitable and irreversible changes. These normal aging changes are partially responsible for the increased risk of developing health-related problems within the elderly population. Prevalent problems experienced by older adults include sleep disorders, problems with eating or feeding, incontinence, confusion, evidence of falls, and skin breakdown. The most appropriate instrument for obtaining the information necessary to prevent health alterations in SPICES, an acronym for the common syndromes of the elderly requiring nursing intervention:

S is for Sleep disorders
P is for Problems with eating or feeding
I is for Incontinence
C is for Confusion
E is for Evidence of falls
S is for Skin breakdown

Target Population: The problems assessed through SPICES occur commonly among the entire elderly population. Therefore, the instrument may be used for both healthy and frail older adults.

Validity/Reliability: The instrument has been used extensively to assess the elderly population. Notably, members of the Geriatric Nurse Resource Project at Yale University Medical Center use the tool to assess and prevent the most frequent health problems of older adults. It is also being used at New York University Medical Center. Psychometric testing has not been done.

Implications for Nursing Practice: Familiarity with these commonly occurring disorders helps the nurse prevent unnecessary iatrogenesis and promote optimal function of the aging patient. Flagging conditions for further assessment will allow the nurse to implement preventive and therapeutic interventions.

Conclusion: The SPICES acronym is easily remembered and may be used to recall the common problems of the elderly population in all clinical settings. It provides a simple system for flagging areas in need of further assessment and provides a basis for standardizing quality of care around certain parameters. SPICES is an alert system and refers to only the most frequently occurring health problems of older adults. Through this initial screen, assessments that are more complete are triggered. It should not be used as a replacement for a complete nursing assessment.

adult during dressing changes. Patients and/or family members may have difficultly coping with wound odor or appearance, and will look to the clinician to see his or her reaction. Seeing the extensive death of their own bodies, coupled with overpowering smells and weeping feces, may be extremely overwhelming to patients. The clinician's resolve to problem-solve and provide the patient the physical comfort by means of appropriate wound management is vital in helping these patients overcome their (sometimes self-imposed) isolation and social avoidance.

SKIN CARE NEEDS FROM FECAL INCONTINENCE

Changes in bowel habits may occur in older adults undergoing cancer treatments such as radiation therapy or chemotherapy. Bliss, Larson, Burr, and Savik (2001) tested the reliability of a four-picture, word definition stool consistency classification system, and found it to be a valid tool for use by nurses and lay caregivers. Precision in describing the characteristics of the stool is important for clinicians. By understanding if a patient truly is having diarrhea or loose stools, the clinician can then develop an appropriate plan to protect the skin. For example, Grogan and Kramer (2002) have described the use of the "rectal trumpet" (nasopharyngeal airway) to contain fecal incontinence in critically ill and geriatric patients. This technique proved to be less traumatic than other methods of fecal containment (diapers, perineal incontinence pouches, and balloon catheters).

Case Study Conclusion

There are many interventions that can help Mrs. A. to be more comfortable as she comes to the end of her life. Given the increased liquid consistency of her colostomy, the nurse might suggest that she stop doing the colostomy irrigations, switch her to a high-output pouch, and alert her to empty the pouch more frequently. Checking the peristomal skin for any signs of skin breakdown and reassessing that she is wearing the correct size of skin barrier and pouch are important nursing considerations.

Odor control is important for this patient. Making sure Mrs. A. is wearing a correctly applied ostomy pouch should eliminate the odor from the colostomy except when emptying the pouch, and she can use aromatherapy. The fecal and exudate drainage from the tumor on her abdominal skin can be contained by using a wound pouch and applying crushed metronidazole tablets directly to the tumor wound to reduce the odor; alternatively, the wound could be irrigated with a solution of dissolved metronidazole tablets. The nurse should ensure that pain medications are provided prior to dressing changes.

Mrs. A. and her family should be taught about pressure ulcer prevention using the NPUAP easy reading booklet, which can be downloaded from the NPUAP website. Mr. and Mrs. A. and their son should understand the importance of turning so that her pressure ulcers do not get worse. Arranging for a nursing attendant to come to the house will enable Mr. A. to have some respite for activities that he might enjoy, or just to rest. Mr. and Mrs. A. also might wish to talk to a social worker or might like their pastor to call to provide additional spiritual support.

CONCLUSION

The nurse can be faced with multiple skin problems when caring for older adults receiving palliative care. By focusing on the wound etiology, and providing appropriate local wound care based on the particular wound etiology, wound characteristics, and individual needs of the patient, the physical needs of the elder's wound can be met. Comprehensive care, however, requires attention to the total needs of the older adult, including quality of life, psychosocial impact of the wound, and the meaning and significance of the wound to the older adult patient.

RESOURCES

- European Pressure Ulcer Advisory Panel (EPUAP) (*www.epuap.org*): This panel was created to lead and support all European countries in the efforts to prevent and treat pressure ulcers.
- National Pressure Ulcer Advisory Panel (NPUAP) (*www.npuap.org*): The NPUAP provides multidisciplinary leadership for improved patient outcomes in pressure ulcer prevention and management through education, public policy, and research.
- Wound, Ostomy, and Continence Nurses Society (WOCN) (*www.wocn.org*): WOCN is an international society of more than 3700 nursing professionals who are experts in the care of patients with wound, ostomy, and continence problems.

REFERENCES

Ayello, E. A. (1993). A critique of the AHCPR's "Preventing pressure ulcers—a patient's guide" as a written instructional tool. *Decubitus, 6*(3), 44-50.

Ayello, E. A., & Braden, B. (2001). Why is pressure ulcer risk assessment so important? *Nursing 2001, 31*(11), 75-79.

Ayello, E. A., Cuddigan, J., & Kerstein, M. (2002). Skip the knife: Debriding wounds without surgery. *Nursing 2002, 32*(9), 58-63.

Ayello, E. A., Mezey, M., & Amella, E. J. (1997). Educational assessment and teaching of older clients with pressure ulcers. *Clinics in Geriatric Medicine, 13*, 483-496.

Baharestani, M. M. (1994). The lived experience of wives caring for their frail, home bound, elderly husbands with pressure ulcers. *Advances in Wound Care, 7*(3), 40-52.

Baldwin, K. (2001). Incidence and prevalence of pressure ulcers in children. *Advances in Skin & Wound Care, 15*(3), 121-124.

Baranoski, S. (2000). Skin tears: The enemy of frail skin. *Advances in Skin & Wound Care, 13*(3), 123-126.

Baranoski, S. (2001a). Skin tears: Guard against this enemy of frail skin. *Nursing Management, 32*(8), 25-31.

Baranoski, S. (2001b, September). *Skin: The forgotten organ.* Presented at the 16th Annual Clinical Symposium of Advances in Skin & Wound Care, Lake Buena Vista, FL.

Baranoski, S., & Ayello, E. A. (2004). *Wound care essentials: Practice principles.* Philadelphia: Lippincott.

Bauer, C., Gerlach, M. A., & Doughty, D. (2000). Care of metastatic skin lesions. *Journal of Wound, Ostomy Continence Nursing, 27*, 247-251.

Beitz, J. M., & Caldwell, D. (1998). Abdominal wound with enterocutaneous fistula: A case study. *Journal of Wound, Ostomy Continence Nursing, 25,* 102-106.

Bennett, M. A. (1995). Characteristics of intact dark skin. *Advances in Wound Care, 8*(6), 34-35.

Bergstrom, N., Bennett, M. A., Carlson, C. E., et al. (1994, December). *Treatment of pressure ulcers* (Clinical Practice Guideline No. 15, AHCPR Publication No. 95-0652). Rockville, MD: Agency for Health Care Policy and Research.

Birch, S., & Coggins, T. (2003). No-rinse, one-step bed bath: the effects on the occurrence of skin tears in a long term care facility. *Ostomy/Wound Management 49*(1), 64-67.

Bliss, D. Z., Larson, S. J., Burr, J. K., & Savik, K. (2001). Reliability of a stool consistency classification system. *Journal of Wound, Ostomy Continence Nursing, 28,* 305-313.

Bryant, D., & Fleischer, I. (2000). Changing an ostomy appliance. *Nursing 2000, 30*(11), 51-53.

Camp-Sorrell, D. (1991). Skin tears: What can you do? *Oncology Nursing Forum, 18,* 135.

Chaplin, J. (2000). Pressure sore risk assessment in palliative care. *Journal of Tissue Viability, 10*(1), 27-31.

Colburn, L. (1987). Pressure ulcer prevention for the hospice patient: Strategies for care to increase comfort. *American Journal of Hospice Care, 4*(2), 22-6.

Cormier, A. C., McCann, E., & McKeithan, L. (1995). Reducing odor caused by metastatic breast cancer skin lesions. *Oncology Nursing Forum, 22,* 988-999.

Cuddigan, J., Ayello, E. A., & Sussman, C. (Eds.). (2001). *Pressure ulcers in America: Prevalence, incidence, and implications for the future.* Reston, VA: National Pressure Ulcer Advisory Panel.

Cuddigan, J., Hollinger, K., Brown, C., & Horslen, S. P. (2001). Pressure ulcers in infants and children. In J. Cuddigan, E. A. Ayello, & C. Sussman (Eds.), *Pressure ulcers in America: Prevalence, incidence, and implications for the future* (pp. 163-166). Reston, VA: National Pressure Ulcer Advisory Panel.

Dallam, L., Smyth, C., Jackson, B. S., Krinsky, R., O'Dell, C., Rooney, J., et al. (1995). Pressure ulcer pain: Assessment and quantification. *Journal of Wound, Ostomy Continence Nursing, 22,* 211-218.

Eckman, K. (1989). The prevalence of pressure ulcers among persons in the U.S. who have died. *Decubitus, 2*(2), 36-41.

Erwin-Toth, P. (2001). Caring for a stoma is more than skin deep. *Nursing 2001, 31*(5), 36-40.

Grogan, T. A., & Kramer, D. J. (2002). The rectal trumpet: Use of a nasopharyngeal airway to contain fecal incontinence in critically ill patients. *Journal of Wound, Ostomy Continence Nursing, 29,* 193-201.

Haisfield-Wolfe, M. E., & Baxendale-Cox, L. M. (1999). Staging of malignant cutaneous wounds: A pilot study. *Oncology Nursing Forum, 26,* 1055-1064.

Haisfield-Wolfe, M. E., & Rund, C. (1997). Malignant cutaneous wounds: A management protocol. *Ostomy/Wound Management, 42*(1), 56-66.

Haisfield-Wolfe, M. E., & Rund, C. (2002). The development and pilot testing of a teaching booklet for oncology patients' self assessment and perineal skin care. *Journal of Wound, Ostomy Continence Nursing, 29,* 88-92.

Hanson, D., Langemo, D. K., Olson, B., Hunter, S., & Burd, C. (1994). Evaluation of pressure ulcer prevalence rates for hospice patients post-implementation of pressure ulcer protocols. *American Journal of Hospice & Palliative Care, 11*(6), 14-19.

Hanson, D., Langemo, D. K., Olson, B., Hunter, S., Sauvage, T. R., Burd, C., et al. (1991). The prevalence and incidence of pressure ulcers in the hospice setting: Analysis of two methodologies. *American Journal of Hospice & Palliative Care, 8*(5), 18-22.

Harris, A., & Komray, R. R. (1993). Cost-effective management of pharyngocutaneous fistulas following laryngectomy. *Ostomy/Wound Management, 39*(8), 36-44.

Kaminer, M., & Gilchrest, B. (1994). Aging of the skin. In W. Hazzard (Ed.), *Principles of geriatric medicine and gerontology* (pp. 411-415). New York: McGraw-Hill.

Kennedy, K. L. (1989). The prevalence of pressure ulcers in an intermediate care facility. *Decubitus, 2*(2), 44-45.

Krasner, D. (1991). An approach to treating skin tears. *Ostomy/Wound Management, 32,* 56-58.

Langemo, D., Bates-Jensen, B., & Hanson, D. (2001). Pressure ulcers in individuals at the end of life: Palliative care and hospice. In J. Cuddigan, E. A. Ayello, & C. Sussman (Eds.), *Pressure ulcers in America: Prevalence, incidence, and implications for the future* (pp. 143-151). Reston, VA: National Pressure Ulcer Advisory Panel.

Langemo, D., Melland, H., Hanson, D., Olson, B., & Hunter, S. (2000). The lived experience of having a pressure ulcer: A qualitative analysis. *Advances in Skin & Wound Care, 13*(5), 225-235.

Malone, M. L., Rozario, N., Gavinski, M., & Goodwin, J. (1991). The epidemiology of skin tears in the institutionalized elderly. *Journal of the American Geriatrics Society, 39,* 591-595.

Mason, S. (1997). Types of soap and the incidence of skin tears among residents of a long-term care facility. *Ostomy/Wound Management, 43*(8), 26-41.

McGough-Csarny, J., & Kopac, C. A. (1998). Skin tears in institutionalized elderly: An epidemiological study. *Ostomy/Wound Management, 44*(3A), 14S-24S.

McMullen, D. (1992). Topical metronidazole, part II. *Ostomy/Wound Management, 38*(3), 42-47.

Newman, V., Allwood, M., & Oakes, R. A. (1989). The use of metronidazole gel to control the smell of malodorous lesions. *Palliative Medicine, 3,* 303-305.

O'Brien, B., Landis-Erdman, J., & Erwin-Toth, P. (1998). Nursing management of multiple enterocutaneous fistulae located in the center of a large open abdominal wound: A case study. *Ostomy/Wound Management, 44*(1), 20-24.

Olson, B., Tkachuk, L., & Hanson, J. (1998). Preventing pressure sores in oncology patients. *Clinical Nursing Research, 7*(2), 207-224.

O'Regan, A. (2002). Skin tears: A review of the literature. *WCET Journal, 22*(2), 26-31.

Panel for the Prediction and Prevention of Pressure Ulcers in Adults. (1992, May). *Pressure ulcers in adults: Prediction and prevention* (Clinical Practice Guideline No. 3, AHCPR Publication No. 92-0047). Rockville, MD: Agency for Health Care Policy and Research.

Payne, R. L., & Martin, M. L. (1990). The epidemiology and management of skin tears in older adults. *Ostomy/Wound Management, 26*(1), 26-37.

Payne, R. L., & Martin, M. L. (1993). Defining and classifying skin tears: Need for a common language. *Ostomy/Wound Management, 39*(5), 16-24.

Rice, T. (1990). Metronidazole use in malodorous skin lesions. *Rehabilitation Nursing, 17,* 244-245.

Rolstead, B. S., & Bryant, R. (2000). Management of drain sites and fistulas. In R. Bryant (Ed.), *Acute and chronic wounds: Nursing management* (2nd ed., pp. 317-341). St. Louis: Mosby.

Schaffner, A., Hocevar, B. J., & Erwin-Toth, P. (1994). Small bowel fistulas complicating midline surgical wounds. *Journal of Wound, Ostomy Continence Nursing, 21,* 161-165.

Schulte, M. J. (1993). Yogurt helps to control wound odor. *Oncology Nursing Forum, 20,* 1262.

Seaman, S. (1995). Home care for pain, odor, and drainage in tumor-associated wounds. *Oncology Nursing Forum, 22,* 987.

Thomas, D., Goode, P., LaMaster, K., Tennyson, T., & Parnell, L. K. S. (1999). A comparison of an opaque foam dressing versus a transparent film dressing in the management of skin tears in institutionalized subjects. *Ostomy/Wound Management, 45*(6), 22-28.

Waltman, N. L., Bergstrom, N., Armstrong, N., Norvell, K., & Braden, B. (1991). Nutritional status, pressure sores, and mortality in elderly patients with cancer. *Oncology Nursing Forum, 18,* 867-873.

Welch, L. B. (1981). Simple new remedy for the odor of open lesions. *RN, 44*(2), 42-43.

White, M., Karam, S., & Cowell, B., (1994). Skin tears in frail elders: A practical approach to prevention. *Geriatric Nursing, 15*(2), 95-99.

Wiltshire, B. L. (1996). Challenging enterocutaneous fistula: A case presentation. *Journal of Wound, Ostomy Continence Nursing, 23,* 297-301.

Winter, G. D. (1962). Formation of scab and the rate of epithelialization of superficial wounds in the skin of domestic pig. *Nature, 193,* 293-294.

23

NUTRITION AND HYDRATION

Patricia Hess

Mr. R., 80, was admitted to the acute care medical unit for the third time in 2 months with congestive heart failure and venous stasis ulcers. It is apparent that, with each admission, his condition has rapidly deteriorated despite his adherence to the prescribed medical regimen. On this admission, he was too breathless to talk, and was fatigued and lethargic. Pulmonary crackles were heard, and there was marked edema to the knees and a slight increase in abdominal girth. His laboratory values revealed a moderate hypernatremia and a serum albumin of 3.2 g/dL.

Mr. R. was placed in a recliner chair and was started on a slow isotonic intravenous (IV) drip with orders for the addition of a diuretic twice a day. His heart function was no more than 25% and his heart failure was listed as New York Heart Association functional class IV. Mr. R.'s wife of 60 years was a nervous woman who was fearful of being left alone. She had tried making foods that would tempt Mr. R. to eat, but to no avail. She has watched him become frailer by the week and is concerned that her husband will starve to death.

INTRODUCTION

Nutrition and hydration become a passionate and thorny end-of-life issue, particularly as the final weeks and days near (Hoefler, 2000; Welk, 1999). During the living–dying trajectory, a series of changes occur in which an individual's health progresses along a downward slope (Corbin & Strauss, 1988; Glasser & Strauss, 1968; Project on Death in America, 2002). Despite significant life changes, the goal of palliative care is to help the older adult to live life to the fullest, from his or

her own perspective. Twycross and Licher (1993) believe that life should be maintained as normally as possible by and for the dying person.

Throughout the stages of a serious illness such as heart disease, stroke, pulmonary disease (emphysema), kidney disease, or cancer, food and fluids are considered medical treatment modalities. During this time, nutrition and hydration may be a matter of following a prescribed dietary regimen. The elder can usually maintain his or her normal intake of food and fluid, or a decision may be made to discontinue dietary restrictions if they interfere with the quality of life that remains. As the person's health changes with increasing physical and/or mental symptoms or disabilities, adaptive responses must be made, particularly in the last months and days of life. Table 23-1 lists some of the triggers that indicate the end stage of an illness; however, palliative care should begin at the time of diagnosis with a life-threatening, progressive illness.

"Thirty years ago, chronically ill patients who became dehydrated simply died. Twenty-five years ago, tube feeding became routinely available and nearly universally applied" (Hoefler, 2000, p. 249). Since the early 1990s, decision making regarding the benefits and burden of maintaining artificial nutrition and hydration for individuals with end-stage illnesses, including the older adult with end-stage chronic diseases and/or dementia, has been discussed and clarified by the courts (Dubler, 2000; Luce & Alpers, 2001).

Anxiety is generated for the family, professionals, and ancillary caregivers when the foregoing of food and fluid is considered in end-of-life care. The natural desire to offer food and fluids represents not only a basic need, frequently

Table 23-1 **End Stages of Chronic Conditions**

Condition and Data	Triggers
GENERAL	Progressive weight loss Nonremedial functional decline Recurrent hospitalization
CONGESTIVE HEART FAILURE Most common in those 65 yr and older Increased prevalence with age One-third readmissions in 60 days One-half readmissions in 90 days	Hospitalization >7 days Low ejection fraction without correction Recurrent hospitalization
CHRONIC OBSTRUCTIVE PULMONARY DISEASE Fifth leading cause of death Initiation of use of O_2: mean survival 3 yr Use of mechanical ventilation: mean survival 5 mo	Hospitalization >7 days Initiation of O_2 therapy Any decompensation resulting in ventilator use
RENAL FAILURE (END-STAGE RENAL DISEASE) Increase in elder population: 5%-8%/yr Mortality increase: 6% New patients die within 90 days of treatment First year mortality: 20%	Symptoms of renal insufficiency Any discussion of dialysis
LIVER FAILURE (END-STAGE LIVER DISEASE)	80%-90% of liver must be damaged Active hepatitis a contributing factor
NEURODEGENERATIVE DISEASE (PARKINSON'S, DEMENTIA, ALS, MS) Cause of mortality: nutritional and pulmonary complications	Difficulty swallowing Continued weight loss Respiratory illnesses (pneumonia)

ALS, amyotrophic lateral sclerosis; MS, multiple sclerosis. Adapted from McGrew, D. M. (2001). Chronic illness and end-of-life. *Primary Care, 28,* 339-347.

referred to as a life-support intervention, but a demonstration of love, compassion, and caring (Lawton & Cyster, 2000; Welk, 1999). For the professional, providing or ordering the administration of food and fluids signifies to the patient, family, and the professional him- or herself that they are caring, compassionate, and hopeful (realistic or not). Strong symbolic, cultural, and religious meanings and beliefs influence decisions regarding when and what foods should be eaten (Callahan 1987; Justice, 1995).

Those who are very experienced in end-of-life care are more comfortable with decisions regard-

ing withholding or withdrawal of food and fluids or providing artificial nutrition and hydration (ANH) as appropriate to the situation (Hoefler, 2000; Welk, 1999). Consensus groups of 10 organizations have published statements about withholding and withdrawing food and fluids from the dying patient at the end of life (Hoefler, 2000). These organizations concur that nutrition and hydration are medical interventions that can be foregone like any other treatments, in accordance with the patient's preference, expressed either directly or through a surrogate (American College of Physicians, 1993; American Medical

EVIDENCE-BASED PRACTICE

Reference: Callahan, C., Haag, K. M., Weinberger, M., Tierney, W. M., Buchanan, N. N., Stump, T. E., et al. (2000). Outcomes of percutaneous endoscopic gastrostomy among older adults in a community setting. *Journal of the American Geriatrics Society, 48,* 1048-1054.

Research Problem: Percutaneous endoscopic gastrostomy (PEG) has become the preferred method to provide enteral tube feeding to older adults who have difficulty eating, but the impact of PEG on patient outcomes is poorly understood. The objective of this study was to describe changes in nutrition, functional status, and health-related quality of life among older adults receiving PEG.

Design: Prospective cohort study.

Sample and Setting: 150 patients ages 60 years and older receiving PEG from one of the four gastroenterologists practicing in a small community of approximately 60,000 residents served by two hospital systems.

Methods: Patients were assessed at baseline and every 2 months for 1 year to obtain information on clinical characteristics, process of care data, physical and cognitive function, subjective health status, nutritional status, complications, and mortality.

Results: Over a 14-month period, 150 patients received PEG tubes in the targeted community; the mean patient age was 78.9. The most frequent indications for PEG were stroke (40.7%), neurodegenerative disorders (34.7%), and cancer (13.3%). All measures of functional status, cognitive status, severity of illness, comorbidity, and quality of life demonstrated profound and life-threatening impairment; 30-day mortality was 22% and 1-year mortality was 50%. Among patients surviving 60 days or more, at least 70% had no significant improvement in functional, nutritional, or subjective health status. Serious complications were rare, but most patients experienced symptomatic problems that they attributed to the enteral tube feeding.

Implications for Nursing Practice: The issues raised in this descriptive study provide stimulus for a randomized trial of PEG tube feeding compared with alternative methods of patient care for older adults who have difficulty eating.

Conclusion: PEG tube feeding in severely and chronically ill older adults coould be accomplished safely. However, there were important patient burdens associated with PEG, and there was limited evidence that the procedure improved functional, nutritional, or subjective health status in this cohort of older adults.

Association, 1994; American Thoracic Society, 1991; Catholic Health Association of the United States, 1993; Hafemeister and Hannaford, 1996; Hastings Center, 1987; Meissel, Snyder, & Quill, 2000; National Center for State Courts, 1991). The American Nurses Association (1998), in *Ethics in Nursing: Position Statement and Guidelines,* stated that "A nurse is morally obliged to withhold food and fluids when it is more harmful to administer them than to withhold them" (p. 2). "It is morally as well as legally permissible for nurses to honor the refusal of food and fluids by competent patients in their care" (p. 3).

It is difficult to separate nutrition and hydration when discussing end-of-life patient care. Usually these two needs are considered together, but, for the sake of a better understanding of the dynamics of each, they are discussed separately in the first part of this chapter, and are then presented collectively in the discussion of assessment and interventions.

HYDRATION
Definition

Hydration is merely adequate water in the body or added to the body to maintain a balance that is measured by comparing intake and output. *Dehydration* is the deprivation or loss of water from the body or tissues. In the clinical sense, it is a consequence of negative fluid balance with output greater than intake. Dehydration may be isotonic, hypertonic, or hypotonic (Felver, 2000; Guyton & Hall 1996; Kee & Paulanka, 2000; Kuebler & McKinnon, 2002).

Symptoms

Isotonic dehydration is the depletion of both water and sodium. Electrolytes remain unchanged, but there is a decrease in skin turgor, dry mucous membranes, a decline in urine output, weight loss, and often a low-grade fever. Thirst complaints may be an issue. Serum concentrations may reflect an elevated hematocrit and hemoglobin, as well as an elevated blood urea nitrogen. Studies have shown that nearly half the patients at the end stage of life are either in isotonic or hypernatremic dehydration (Ellershaw, Sutcliffe, & Saunders, 1995; Waller, Hershkowitz, & Adunsky, 1994).

Hypertonic dehydration is reflected in the loss of fluid and an elevation in sodium concentration above 150 mEq/L. Total water deficit (intracellular) is always hypernatremic (Sarhill, Walsh, Nelson, & Davis, 2001). Hospitalized and frail elders are at high risk for developing hypernatremia as a result of lack of thirst response and dependence on others to offer and provide fluids (Adeleye, Faulkner, Adeola, & ShuTangyie, 2002).

Water excess, which dilutes the sodium concentration of plasma below 130 mEq/L, creates a hypotonic state (Guyton & Hall, 1996; Kee & Paulanka, 2000; Palm, Reimann, & Gross, 2000). In hypotonic dehydration, tachycardia and delayed capillary refill are early signs. Dry mucous membranes, decline in urine output, a noticeable loss of weight, and thirst occur as dehydration progresses. Thirst, as stated above, may not be prominent in older adults. Similarly, decreased skin turgor is not a reliable sign in elders because their skin hydration is normally slightly decreased. In addition, a flushed appearance, low-grade fever, hypotension, delirium or confusion, restlessness, myoclonus, and seizures are possible (Kee & Paulanka, 2000).

Incidence and Prevalence of Dehydration

It has been noted that older adults are in a state of slight dehydration because of a lack of thirst drive or as a consequence of chronic conditions or the associated therapies instituted to treat those conditions (Ritz, 2001). Normal dehydration in older adults is considered a matter of shifting of cellular fluids between compartments or alterations in membrane permeability, concentration of fluids transported, or the energy required for transport (Flear & Singh, 1973; Ritz, 2001; Timaris, 1994).

In 1996, an average hospital stay was 6.5 days, at an average cost of $1006 a day, for people 65 years of age and older who were diagnosed with dehydration from causes other than end-stage illness. Mortality for patients who were dehydrated was seven times greater than for those who were not dehydrated (Bloom, 2000).

Etiology

General physiology tells us that the older adult has approximately 23% less body fluid by weight than a newborn and 6% less than an adult under the age of 55 (Felver, 2000; Guyton & Hall, 1996; Kee & Paulanka, 2000). Therefore, hydration is an important component of maintaining wellness and is particularly important under conditions of illness. Hydration can be maintained through administering fluids orally or through parenteral routes.

The total body fluid intake and output must be in balance for homeostasis to exist. This means that daily intake of water either from ingestion of liquids or foods is necessary. Water can be obtained from ingested foods through oxidation of carbohydrates. It is important to keep in mind that the intake of fluid is highly individual among people, and is affected by climate, habits, and levels of physical activity. Often forgotten is insensible loss of fluid, which occurs through skin diffusion from large lesion or wound areas and through respiratory evaporation, which is different from sweating. Additional fluid loss occurs through the kidneys via urine.

In seriously ill elders, it is difficult to maintain adequate fluid hydration in both intra- and extracellular compartments. Osmotic pressure is responsible for the change in cell volume that result in an isotonic, hypotonic, or hypertonic state. A variety of physiologic changes can create fluid imbalance, as depicted in Box 23-1. Intracellular edema may result when the metabolism of the tissues is diminished or from lack of nutrition. Generally this occurs when oxygen delivery to the tissues is reduced and blood flow becomes too low for normal metabolism of the tissues to be maintained. Sodium leaks into cells and there is not enough force to pump it out of the cell.

Extracellular edema is the reverse; it occurs when extracellular spaces receive fluid leaking from the plasma to interstitial spaces and the lymphatics fail to return fluid back to the blood. Lymphatic blockage also causes edema and can become a problem because there is no way to return the fluid back to the blood. This occurs with certain cancers when lymph vessels have been surgically removed or by lymph vessel obstruction (Felver, 2000; Guyton & Hall, 1996; Kee & Paulanka, 2000; Timaris, 1994).

NUTRITION
Definition
Nutrition encompasses all the processes of taking in and utilizing food by the body through ingestion, digestion, absorption, and cellular metabolism ("Taber's," 1997). When one is not able to eat, nutritional adequacy can be attained through artificial means such as enteral feeding (nasogastric or gastrostomy tube) or total parenteral nutrition. These options provide caloric and vitamin intake in an attempt to maintain or enhance sources for the body's need for energy when in a compromised state.

The general perception of an individual who does not or will not eat (anorexia) is that they will waste away (cachexia) by starving. This is true for healthy well individuals, but, when an individual is in the end stage of his or her disease, death is due to dehydration (which is relatively quick and painless) rather than starvation. Cranford (1991); Shils, Olson, and Shike (1994); and Meares (1994) indicated that all "natural deaths"—those not associated with trauma or infection—occur because of dehydration and not starvation. The difference between starvation in healthy well individuals and lack of food and fluids in the dying is quite significant.

Death by starvation in the healthy person is a long, arduous process that involves drastic weight loss and body wasting. One associates this type of starvation with gruesome images of emaciated children and adults in Third World countries and of individuals who deliberately go on "hunger strikes." As this type of starvation progresses, immunity is compromised, organs shrink, and bodily function deteriorates, producing uncomfortable and painful symptoms and death from cardiac arrest. This process can continue for weeks.

Conversely, the dying individual who refuses food and fluids, or from whom food and fluids are withheld or withdrawn when deemed appropriate, dies not in this way but by dehydration, which can lead to the production of natural analgesics. Specifically, the body's breakdown of fat results in ketosis and other chemical changes that lead to the release of endorphins, which are naturally produced pain killers (Zerwekh, 1997).

Prevalence
Food intake naturally declines as one ages as a result of alterations in body composition and changes in energy and protein metabolism, which are directly associated with aging and the effects of age-related diseases (Morley, 2001). Morley suggested the term *physiologic anorexia of aging* because it is seen in adults 70 years of age and older who lose body mass. Three processes of nutritional concern are responsible: loss of adipose tissue and muscle mass (sarcopenia), loss of appetite (anorexia), and loss of fat and body mass with little or no weight loss (cachexia) (Roubenoff, 1999). In addition, depression, fatigue, and isolation may affect a person's desire to take in nutrients.

Etiology

Satiety involves a peripheral and a central feeding system. These systems are mediated by a hormonal feedback mechanism that transmits information on an organ's nutrient status. The stomach plays a key role in deciding meal size; food enters the fundus, where it is stored. The decrease in fundus adaptability with age results in a more rapid filling of the antrum, and antral stretching sends back a strong signal of fullness. In addition, signals relating a decline in available endogenous kappa-opioid feeding peptides (e.g., dynorphin), a decline in the function of orexigenic peptides (e.g., neuropeptide Y), and an increase in anoretic peptides are fed back to the hypothalamus, with the resultant loss of appetite.

Many elders have recurrent disease processes that result in the release of powerful anoretic cytokines such as interleukin-1, interleukin-6, ciliary neurotropic factor, and tumor necrosis factor-alpha, all of which lead to loss of appetite (Thomas & Morley, 2001). In addition, catabolic effects on muscle and decreased circulating albumin levels cause loss of albumin from intravascular spaces (Konsman & Dantzer, 2001; Kotler, 2000; Meguid, Yang, & Gleason, 1996; Plata-Salaman, 2000; Roubenoff et al., 1994; Thomas & Morley, 2001; Yeh & Schuster 1999). Table 23-2 notes the systems that control neurotransmitter and hormonal control of food intake. Figure 23-1 diagrams how these factors lead to anorexia.

End-stage illness represents a broad spectrum of incurable diseases (Huang & Ahronheim, 2000; McGrew, 2001), with each disease presenting its own triggers for initiating palliative care decisions. Current literature suggests that instinctively giving food and fluids to dying patients should not be a routine practice, nor should they be automatically withheld. What is essential is to establish the goals of care and the assessment of patient comfort. Quill and Byock (2000) identified criteria necessary for making decisions not only for food and fluids but for other aspects of the patient's condition (Box 23-2).

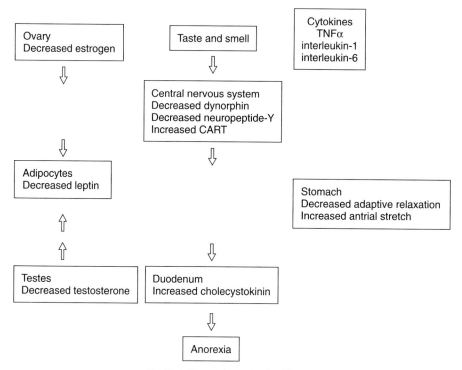

Fig. 23-1 Factors decreasing food intake.

Table 23-2 Neurotransmitters and Hormonal Control of Food Intake

Food Intake Control Systems	Stimulate	Inhibit	Action of Neurotransmitters/Hormones
Peripheral	Motilin (↓ gherlin)		Peptide growth hormone in stomach. Decreases feeding drive but increases metabolic efficiency. Levels increase during fasting. Stimulates food intake, reduces fat utilization.
		Cholecystokinin (major component of high-density food)	Released into duodenum in fat-rich meals; limits ability to ingest fats; potent satiating agent.
		Leptin (men only)	Peptide hormone released from adipose cells; decreases food intake, increases resting metabolic rate. Leptin decreases with age; associated with weight loss in elder men as a result of andropause; proportional to body adipose tissue; increase from subcutaneous tissue rather than visceral fat.
		Cytokines: Interleukin-1 Interleukin-6 Ciliary neurotropic factor Tumor necrosis factor-alpha	Catabolic effect on muscle; decreased circulating albumin from intravascular space.
Hormones	Thyroid (↓ testosterone)		Catabolic effect on muscles; decreases circulating albumin from intravascular space.
	Cortisol Progestins	Estrogen (female only)	Anoretic in older women
Central	Kappazopioid peptides (↓ dynorphin)		Decreases feeding drive to activate receptors.
	(↓ neuropeptide Y) Orexin A Melanin-concentrating hormone Dopamine Norepinephrine Histamine (↓ Nitric oxide)	CART	Decreases the level and function of neuropeptide Y Anoretic peptide in hypothalamus

Box 23-2 **Criteria for Decision Making for Patient Care**
<ul><li>Palliative care must be available to relieve suffering.</li><li>Usual patient characteristics: persistent, unrelenting, otherwise unrelieveable symptoms that are unacceptable to the patient, such as fatigue, weakness, and disability.</li><li>Terminal prognosis of weeks to months.</li><li>Patient should be fully informed, competent, and give consent.</li><li>Participation of the family in decisions for those who are incompetent.</li><li>Food and drink orally must not be withheld from incompetent persons who are willing to and able to eat.</li><li>Second opinion should be obtained from an expert in palliative care, a mental health expert, and a specialist in the patient's underlying disease.</li><li>Participation of medical staff (with their consent) in decision making if they are immediately involved in the care of the patient.</li></ul>

From Quill, T. E., & Byock, I. R. (2000). Responding to intractable terminal suffering: The role of terminal sedation and voluntary refusal of food and fluids. ACP-ASIM End of Life Care Consensus Panel. American College of Physicians-American Society of Internal Medicine. *Annals of Internal Medicines, 132,* 408-414.

ASSESSMENT

Assessment will guide interventions, which can benefit or hinder patient care. It establishes whether the lack of eating is due to obstacles to eating, anorexia associated with the dying process, or the deliberate decision not to eat. One of the first things that should be done is to ascertain that the elder person has an advance directive that indicates a stated wish that food and fluids be withheld or withdrawn under certain conditions. It is also important to identify barriers to eating. One question the clinician should ask is "Why is there anorexia?" It might be due to chemotherapy, loss of taste and smell, a deliberate choice, oral health, or the dying process per se. Improperly fitting dentures may be caused by weight loss, which shrinks the gums and allows denture slippage and nonadherence to the gums. This may cause irritation and ulceration of the

Box 23-3 **Providing Hydration and Nutrition**
<ul><li>Will artificial food and fluids enhance the elder's well-being?</li><li>Are there symptoms that can be relieved by providing or withholding food and/or fluid?</li><li>Are there symptoms that will be aggravated by either giving or withholding food and/or fluids?</li><li>Could hydration or dehydration enhance mental status or level of consciousness?</li><li>Will food and fluid temporarily prolong the patient's life or the dying process?</li><li>Is food and fluid desired by the patient and family based on cultural, spiritual, or personal perspective?</li></ul>

From Zerwekh, J. V. (1997). Do dying patients really need IV fluids? *American Journal of Nursing, 97*(3), 26-30.

gums from rubbing and result in difficulty chewing food. Assessing the elder's ability to hold utensils, raise food to the mouth, chew food, and swallow, as well as assessing the pace of eating, are essential.

Exploring the meaning of food with the older adult, and determining what the individual eats during the day, the timing and sequence of meals, and with whom they usually eat, may identify barriers to adequate nutrition and hydration. Knowledge of the person's religious beliefs, cultural and ethnic food preferences (e.g., hot/cold), and medically indicated dietary restrictions is also an important aspect of the nutritional assessment.

The older adult must also be assessed as to whether he or she is competent or incompetent to make decisions regarding nutrition and hydration if an advance directive has not been completed. If the patient is incompetent, as in the case of dementia or a decreased level of consciousness, the family will play an important role in the decision making as to food and fluid intake (Burke & Laramie, 2000; Lueckenotte, 1996; Munro, Suter, & Russell, 1987).

Some dying older adults may benefit from hydration; others may not. Answering the questions in Box 23-3 is the key to providing hydration and nutrition and can serve as clarification for the professional and family. The overall medical picture should be considered when considering diet therapy (Dorner, Gallagher-Allred,

EVIDENCE-BASED PRACTICE

Reference: Meier, D. E., Ahronheim, J. C., Morris, J., Baskin-Lyons, S., & Morrison, S. R. (2001). High short-term mortality in hospitalized patients with advanced dementia: Lack of benefit of tube feeding. *Archives of Internal Medicine, 161,* 594-599.

Research Problem: Does tube-feeding hospitalized patients with advanced dementia improve survival? This study evaluated long-term survival of patients related to tube feeding placement during hospitalization.

Design: Descriptive

Sample and Setting: 99 hospitalized patients with advanced dementia and an available surrogate decision maker.

Methods: Patients were followed during and after hospitalization for mortality and placement of a feeding tube. Other variables measured were advance directive status, presence of a long-term primary care physician, level of involvement of the surrogate decision maker, diagnosis on admission, prior hospitalizations, comorbidities, and diagnosis-related group category.

Results: A new feeding tube was placed in 50% (51/99) of the study patients during the hospitalization, 31% (31/99) left the hospital without a feeding tube, and 17% (17/99) were admitted with a feeding tube already in place. By stepwise logistic regression analysis, predictors of new feeding tube placement included African American ethnicity (odds ratio, 9.43; 95% confidence interval, 2.1 to 43.2) and residence in a nursing home (odds ratio, 4.9; 95% confidence interval, 1.02 to 2.5). Median survival of the 99 patients was 175 days. Eighty-five (85%) survived the index hospitalization, and 28 (28%) were still alive at last follow-up, a range of 1.3 to 4.2 years after enrollment in the study. Tube feeding was not associated with survival ($p = .90$). An admitting diagnosis of infection was associated with higher mortality (odds ratio, 1.9; 95% confidence interval, 1.01 to 3.6).

Implications for Nursing Practice: Consider efficacy of tube placement, advocate comfort measures, allow patient to consume or refuse foods and/or liquids, and educate care givers about pros and cons of feeding tube placement.

Conclusion: In this study of hospitalized patients with advanced dementia, risk of receiving a new feeding tube was high, and was associated with African American ethnicity and prior residence in a nursing home. Feeding tube placement had no measurable influence on survival. With or without a feeding tube, these patients had a 50% 6-month median mortality.

Deering, & Posthauer, 1997), because therapy can complicate the quality of the elder's remaining days.

INTERVENTIONS

Data gathered during assessment guides the approach to nutrition and hydration in end-of-life care. Nutrients may be provided; however, anorexia and cachexia can occur in many end-stage illnesses, such as chronic obstructive pulmonary disease, congestive heart failure, Parkinson's disease, rheumatoid arthritis, and cancer, and increased nutrition does not improve nutritional status (Roubenoff et al., 1994). Feeding or hydrating the older adult who is near the end of life will depend on where he or she is

in the dying process: years, months, weeks, or days from death. Regardless, it is the nurse's role to promote patient autonomy and establish goals of care based on assessment data regarding nutrition and hydration (Chippendale, 2001).

The complications from over- and underfeeding (see Box 23-4) and the benefits and burdens of nutrition and hydration (see Box 23-5) must be taken into account to ensure the quality of the patient's remaining days of life (Burke & Laramie, 2000; Daly, 2000). Various factors must also be weighed when discussing the appropriate and inappropriate use of either enteral or parenteral avenues of ANH. Both of these available technologies are considered medically and ethi-

---

Box 23-4 Complications from Over- and Underfeeding

OVERFEEDING
- Hyperglycemia
- Increased CO_2 production
- Increased respiratory rate
- Electrolyte imbalance
- Uremia
- Fatty liver
- Abdominal distention
- Vomiting

UNDERFEEDING
- Muscle wasting
- Loss of diaphragmatic mass
- Decreased capacity and minute ventilation
- Delayed wound healing
- Long hospital stays
- Skin breakdown

Box 23-5 Benefits and Burden of Artificial Hydration and Nutrition

BENEFIT
- May increase life span
- Increase ability to regain strength and return to useful function
- Improve quality of life
- Improve psychologic and physiologic states
- Increase resistance to infection
- Improve healing of skin and wounds

BURDEN
- Physical pain
- Spiritual and emotional pain and suffering
- Denial of a peaceful death
- Invasive procedures
- Indignity
- Emotional and financial burden on family
- Prolong dying

---

cally indefensible when nutrition and hydration is refused. ANH may increase suffering without the sought-for improvement in the quality of life (Winter, 2000). Hypodermoclysis (the injection of fluid into subcutaneous tissue such as the thighs, under the breasts, or the buttocks) and proctoclysis (a continuous infusion of fluid into the rectum and colon), which are sometimes used in palliation of thirst, may also increase patient discomfort. Oral nutrition should be the only form of sustenance intervention considered in late terminal care. If the person can swallow safely, he or she should be allowed desired substances or sips of clear liquids. At this point, the goal of eating is for pleasure, but the nurse should be aware of the risks of aspiration. The use of percutaneous endoscopic gastrostomy tubes was not found to improve the status of terminally ill patients for any significant length of time (Daly, 2000; Mitchell, Kiely, & Lipsitz, 1998; Rabeneck, Wary, & Peterson, 1996). The pros and cons of artificial nutrition and hydration are listed in Box 23-6.

Nonpharmacologic Interventions

At the time an older adult is diagnosed with advanced illness, the goal of care may be the maintenance of weight and caloric intake so that the patient can continue an acceptable quality of life. Whether to feed and hydrate a person who has an end-stage illness will depend on where he or she is in the dying process and the related goals of care agreed upon by the patient/family and members of the interdisciplinary team. If the individual wants to eat and can eat, strategies to improve or maintain nutritional status include the removal of the assessed barriers, enlisting the family's assistance, offering snacks and supplemental booster foods, and providing supplemental vitamins and minerals. Meals should be small and served on small tableware so that portions are not overwhelming. Frequent meals may also be helpful, as are flexible eating times. The use of a favorite alcoholic cocktail 30 minutes before eating the dinner meal often stimulates appetite. The provision of comfort foods, also called "soul foods," may entice an individual to eat. Continually coaxing the elder to eat may create frustration for both the patient and family member who is assisting with the feeding, and may unintentionally cause digestive discomfort if the patient eats more than is naturally desired.

Pharmacologic Interventions

The use of specific medications is an option to improve appetite. Low-dose corticosteroids such

Box 23-6 Pros and Cons of Artificial Hydration

PROS
- Corrects fluid and electrolytes
- Decreases symptoms of dehydration
- When patisir not quite end stage: Reverses hyper-calcemia, diarrhea, diuretic treatment
- May prolong life
- May reduce disorientation
- May reduce restlessness

CONS
- Exacerbates fluid accumulation
- Increases gastrointestinal motility, possibly leading to vomiting:
  - hard to control
  - may need negative suction tube placement
- Increases respiratory secretions:
  - produce cough
  - hard to catch breath
  - suctioning may be hard to avoid
- Parenteral fluid administration:
  - can cause or aggravate ascites with congestive heart failure, liver disease, kidneys (third spacing)
  - worsens edema
  - increases wound or fistula drainage
  - expands tissue edema around tumor, causing more pain
  - distracts from spiritual needs of patient because of focus on technology
  - may interfere with natural analgesia

Adapted from Zerwekh, J. V. (1997). Do dying patients really need IV fluids? *American Journal of Nursing*, 97(3), 26-30.

as megestrol acetate (e.g., Megace) may be used as appetite stimulants, and medications such as metoclopramide (Reglan) and methylphenidate (Ritalin) may be prescribed (Lynn, 2000; Thomas & Morley, 2001). Each drug has a different means of action for stimulating the appetite, but each comes with adverse effects (see Table 23-3).

It is important to understand that older adults at the end of their illness respond differently to food and fluids than do healthy persons (Institute of Palliative Care, 2001). National data indicate that, in the last 6 months of life, the very old may be repeatedly in and out of the hospital (Goodlin, Fisher, Patterson, & Wasson, 1998). During the weeks or days before death, the natural loss of desire for food and fluids may become more intense and perhaps more disturbing to families (Ashby & Stoffell, 1995).

For elders who are imminently dying, food and fluids may be withheld or withdrawn for the comfort of the patient. At this stage, extra attention to good oral hygiene is needed. Brushing of teeth, removal of mouth debris, frequent moistening of the mucous membranes, application of balm to the lips to prevent cracking, and the offering of ice chips to keep the buccal cavity moist are essential. These interventions are actions interpreted by the family as caring and provide both physical and psychological comfort to the patient and family (Institute of Palliative Care, 2001; Lynn, 2000). The older adult may indicate thirst, which can be relieved by sips of fluid and oral care. Administering parenteral fluids may be ineffective and may increase physical discomfort given that body processes are shutting down. As stated earlier, suffering rather than comfort may be the outcome of hydration. Box 23-7 states the benefits of dehydration.

PSYCHOSOCIAL AND EMOTIONAL ASPECTS

Dying is a process that involves the interplay of emotions that affect the elder, his or her family, and significant others, as well as the nurse. Not everyone is at the same emotional place at the same time when dealing with the dying process. When an elder patient is not eating and drinking, caregivers often feel helpless.

Family

When caring for the family, great sensitivity is needed by the nurse throughout the dying process. Providing the family members and significant others with clear and simple explanations of what is happening and what to expect allows them to process the information individually and with each other. By keeping the family and significant others informed of the patient's level of comfort and involving them in planning and implementing care, anxiety and fear are allayed. Showing family members the most

Table 23-3 **Pharmacotherapy for Anorexia**

Medication	Action	Adverse Action
Megestrol (Megace)* 160-800 mg/day	Improvement of appetite and sense of smell	Fluid retention, nausea, vomiting Thrombus/pulmonary embolism
Metoclopramide (Reglan) 10 mg PO ac meals	Enhances stomach emptying (gastric status) by reducing esophageal sphincter tone and increasing gastric peristalsis, relieving fullness, bloating, and nausea. Increases small intestine transit time. Benefit may take 1-2 wk before effective.	Extrapyramidal symptoms, tardive dyskinesia (especially females) if used in early anorexia
Methylphenidate (Ritalin)* 2.5-5 mg every morning before 9:00 AM; increase every 2-3 days as tolerated to maximum of 20 mg/day May divide dose to be given e.g., 7:00 AM and noon	Increases attention, interest, and motivation to improve appetite	Dysphoric agitation, confusion

*Unlabeled use, meaning does not appear in pharmacology references as an indication for anorexia in end stages of life.

Box 23-7 **Benefits of Dehydration**

Decrease in urine output
- Less use of bedpan, commode, urinal
- Less need for a urinary catheter
- Fewer incontinent episodes

Decreased gastrointestinal fluids
- Eliminates negative suction tube for decompression
- Less vomiting

Decreased respiratory secretions
- Less or no coughing

- Decreased lung and bronchial congestion

Decreased pharyngeal secretions
- Less swallowing of secretions
- Decrease in or elimination of choking and drowning in own secretions
- Decrease in or elimination of pharyngeal, tracheal suctioning

Natural analgesia
- Blood chemistry changes
- Increase opioid effect

Adapted from Printz L. A. (1992), Terminal in hydration: A compassionate treatment. *Archives of Internal Medicine, 152,* 597-700.

effective way to administer small sips of fluid and bites of food, if the elder is conscious and able to chew and swallow, can decrease their sense of helplessness.

If the patient cannot chew or swallow or is in an altered state of consciousness, showing the family or significant other how to moisten the mouth with swabs or gauze pads or administer artificial saliva allows them a caregiving role. It is important for the family to comprehend that the cessation of food and fluid intake is a natural process and that the use of nutrition and

EVIDENCE-BASED PRACTICE

Reference: McAulay, D. (2001). Dehydration in the terminally ill patient. *Nursing Standards, 16* (4), 33-37.

Research Problem: The study sought to learn about staff nurses' attitudes toward, interpretation of, understanding of, and discomfort with dehydration in unconscious patients in their last few days of life.

Design: Survey research.

Sample and Setting: Convenience sample of all those currently working or who had worked with dying patients on the researcher's ward in the past 12 months.

Methods: The researcher created a hypothetical situation based on an older adult who had a massive stroke and was unconscious and nonresponsive for 4 days. Nineteen nurses and eight physicians agreed to participate in the study and were given the situation and questionnaire to complete and return with anonymity. Ten (53%) of the nurses and all of the physicians returned the completed questionnaire.

Results: The nurses indicated that they would ask the physician to prescribe subcutaneous fluids for the patient, indicating it was ultimately the physician's decision. Both nurses and physicians agreed that stopping all treatment would aid comfort and that possible hydration of semicomatose or comatose terminally ill patient should be individually assessed. Seven nurses indicated that they had insufficient knowledge to answer relatives' questions. Physicians would not prescribe subcutaneous fluids; six would comply with relatives' wishes, two would discuss the pros and cons of dehydration and would not treat fever but would maintain comfort measures.

Implications for Nursing Practice: Nurses need knowledge about dehydration in end-of-life care and must educate themselves in order to support families regarding hydration decisions and prevent misconceptions about terminal dehydration.

Conclusion: The researcher concluded that colleagues had little understanding of the effects of dehydration and that caregivers lacked knowledge regarding dehydration.

hydration may be more of a burden to the elder's comfort than a benefit as multi-organ system failure occurs (Kazanowski, 1995). It is also important to point out that giving IV fluids may help for a short time, but IV fluids are not food and do not help to prolong life in advanced illness (Institute of Palliative Care, 2001), and may actually create discomfort or pain (see Box 23-6 for the burdens of artificial hydration).

Perhaps one of the strongest psychosocial aspects of dying for which the nurse can be instrumental is to listen to the family and significant others as they express their concerns, fears, sorrow, anger, and sense of loss. The nurse can help them to explore these feelings, and support their anticipatory grief work (Ebersole & Hess, 1998).

Nurses' Perceptions of Withdrawing and Withholding Nutrition and Hydration

Nurses have their own perceptions of withholding and withdrawing food and fluids from dying patients. Unless the nurse has worked with many dying patients and has seen the beneficial effects of withholding food and fluids, he or she may have difficulty justifying this action. There may be fear of its legality, ethics, and morality. It is important for the nurse to know that the American Nurses Association's (1994, 1998) position statements affirm these actions, as previously mentioned. The dying process itself also affects the nurse. It is difficult for the nurse to watch a person dying before his or her eyes, but there are many other supportive nursing measures that can be used to relieve suffering and promote comfort.

The nurse brings to the dying experience his or her values regarding life and death, past experiences with dying, and perpetuated myths, as well as cultural, religious, and societal beliefs. The nurse may maintain an acute care philosophy, with a focus on aggressive interventions that are not appropriate when caring for the dying elder. All of these factors influence the nurse's approach and response to the patient and the family. The nurse must be cognizant of his or her feelings and, if unable to provide the care needed, seek out someone who can meet the needs of the patient and family.

The Older Adult Patient

The older adult may or may not have difficulty facing his or her death. Those who welcome death have often resolved outstanding issues in their life and have placed their lives in order as best as they could. Those who have difficulty may have unfinished business from the past and/or present or may be dissatisfied with the life they have lived. Fear, anxiety, and uncertainty may manifest in a variety of behaviors such as withdrawal, agitation, depression, verbal outbursts, crying, or selective listening; some elders refuse to eat or drink.

The nurse may assist the patient by affirming that the elder's needs will be met, explaining what is happening and what to expect, encouraging the patient to do what he or she feels capable of doing as appropriate, and telling the patient that uncomfortable symptoms will be relieved. This lessens the sense of helplessness and hopelessness that the elder may feel.

Listening to the patient's concerns and exploring their significance is useful. Listening to and, in whatever manner is appropriate, acknowledging the legitimacy of the individual's psychological as well as physical distress indicates to the person that the nurse really cares about him or her. Reminiscing with the older adult often reveals pleasures long cherished or long forgotten. This can at times be a diversion from the sensation of thirst and other symptoms that the patient may find to be annoying. Giving the patient permission to "let go" when there is no family, or supporting the family in suggesting to the patient to "let go," is a precious gift that the nurse can give the dying elder patient.

Case Study Conclusion

Mr. R. is in the end stage of his disease. Not only is he third spacing fluid as a result of his heart disease but he is also retaining fluid because of his low serum albumin. It is questionable whether an IV should be continued because this may increase his symptoms and discomfort. There is a question regarding his kidney function and the need to increase his use of the diuretic.

The nursing and medical staff talked with Mr. and Mrs. R. regarding withdrawal of food and fluids because these could intensify his symptoms. They clarified that Mr. R. would not be "starving to death," but rather that the changing chemistry of his body was providing natural pain relief and that he had little desire for food. The staff offered comfort measures to lessen his distress of breathing and for reducing or eliminating the "hurting" of his legs. They also discussed the reality of his death and assured the family that Mr. R would die with dignity and peacefully.

The nurses gave Mrs. R. the opportunity, if she wished, to add to his comfort by keeping his mouth and lips moistened with cool wet gauze. When he was awake enough to swallow, they showed her how to give him ice chips or sips of fluid. The nurses reassured Mrs. R. that they would be in every 40 minutes to check on both of them so she would not feel alone.

Mr. R. died peacefully 36 hours after admission, with his wife at his side. Though she was deeply saddened by her husband's death, she was grateful she had been given the chance to contribute to his care and for the support given by the nursing staff to both of them.

CONCLUSION

Understanding the dynamics of providing versus withholding or withdrawing nutrition and hydration, as well as the benefits and burden to the older adult patient, particularly at the end of life, helps the nurse make appropriate decisions concerning end-of-life care. Knowledge that withholding or withdrawing food and fluids is not the same as starvation is important to decision making for patients, their families, and health care professionals. Withdrawing or withholding hydration and nutrition in many instances can lessen or alleviate distressing physical symptoms associated with the dying process. The nurse should ascertain whether an advance directive has been prepared because this will help in determining the goals of care as they relate to hydration and nutrition. At the end of life, oral food and fluids should be considered, given that parenteral fluids are short lived and generally ineffective, many times only adding to symptom burden. In all circumstances, attention to excellent mouth care is imperative. Continuous evaluation of comfort is important, with adjustments of interventions made during the dying process.

The end of life is a difficult time not only for the family and significant others but also for the professional caregiver. Personal experiences, biases, and lack of knowledge about the ethical, moral, and legal implications can influence the nurse's approach to care. Knowledge and sensitivity are essential when explaining to family and significant others what to expect and the need or value of withholding or withdrawing nutrition and hydration. It is also necessary to be available to the family and significant others to help them cope with this major life event. Keeping the elder and family informed, facilitating identification of the goals of care, and supporting their decision making often reduces the anxiety, fear, and helplessness that can occur at the end of life.

REFERENCES

Adeleye, O., Faulkner, M., Adeola, T., & ShuTangyie, G. (2002). Hypernatremia in the elderly. *Journal of the National Medical Association, 94,* 701-705.

American College of Physicians, Ad Hoc Committee on Medical Ethics. (1993). *Ethics manual* (3rd ed.). Philadelphia: Author.

American Medical Association, Council on Ethical and Judicial Affairs. (1994). *Code of medical ethics: Current opinions with annotations, 1994 edition.* Chicago: Author.

American Nurses Association. (1994). *Position statement on nurse's role in end of life decisions, active euthanasia, assisted suicide.* Washington, DC: Author.

American Nurses Association. (1998). *Ethics in nursing: Position statements and guidelines.* Washington, DC: Author.

American Thoracic Society. (1991). *Bioethics task force report.* New York: Author.

Ashby, M., & Stoffell, B. (1995). Artificial hydration and alimentation at the end of life: A reply to Craig. *Journal of Medical Ethics, 21,* 135-140.

Bloom, S. (2000). Dehydration: Simple measures can lower risk in nursing facilities. *Caring for the Ages, 1,* (2), 1, 25-26.

Burke, M. M., & Laramie, J. A. (2000). *Primary care of the older adult: A multidisciplinary approach* (pp. 74-76). St. Louis: Mosby.

Catholic Health Association of the United States. (1993). *Caring for persons at the end of life: A facilitator's guide to educational modules for healthcare leaders.* St. Louis: Author.

Callahan, D. (1987). *Setting limits: Medical goals in an aging society.* New York: Simon & Schuster.

Chippendale, S. (2001). Ethical issues in palliative care. In S. Kinghorn & R. Gamlin (Eds.), *Palliative nursing* (pp. 213-229). London: Bailliere Tindall in association with Royal College of Nursing.

Corbin, J. M., & Strauss, A. (1988). *Unending work and care* (pp. 33-48, 253-288). San Francisco: Jossey-Bass.

Cranford, R. E. (1991). Neurological syndromes and prolonged survival: When can artificial nutrition and hydration be foregone? *Law, Medicine, and Health Care, 19,* 13-22.

Daly, B. J. (2000). Special challenges of withholding artificial nutrition and hydration. *Journal of Gerontological Nursing, 26* (9), 25-31.

Dorner, B., Gallagher-Allred, C., Deering, C. P., & Posthauer, M. E. (1997). The "to feed or not to feed" dilemma. *Journal of the American Dietetic Association, 97* (10 Suppl. 2), S172-S176.

Dubler, N. N. (2000). Legal and ethical issues. In M. H. Beers & R. Berkow (Eds.), *The Merck manual of geriatrics* (pp. 127-139). Whitehouse Station, NJ: Merck Research Laboratories.

Ebersole, P., & Hess, P. (1998). Death, dying, and grief. In *Toward healthy aging: Human needs and nursing response* (5th ed., pp. 939-970). St. Louis: Mosby.

Ellershaw, J. I., Sutcliffe, J. M., & Saunders, C. M. (1995). Dehydration and the dying patient. *Journal of Pain and Symptom Management, 10,* 192-197.

Felver, L. (2000). Fluid and electrolyte homeostasis and imbalances. In L. E. C. Copstead & J. L. Banasik (Eds.), *Pathophysiology: Biologic and behavioral perspectives* (2nd ed., pp. 524-537). Philadelphia: Saunders.

Flear, C. T. G., & Singh, C. M. (1993). Hyponatremia and sick cells. *British Journal of Anaesthesia, 45,* 976-994.

Glasser, B. B., & Strauss, A. (1968). *A time for dying.* Chicago: Aldine.

Goodlin, S. J., Fisher, E., Patterson, J. A., & Wasson, J. H. (1998). End of life care for persons age 80 years or older. *Journal of Ambulatory Care Management, 21* (3), 34-39.

Guyton, A. C., & Hall, J. E. (1996). The body fluid compartments: Extracellular and intracellular fluids; interstitial fluid and edema. In *Textbook of medical physiology* (9th ed., pp. 349-366). Philadelphia: Saunders.

Hafemeister, T. L., & Hannaford, P. L. (1996). *Resolving disputes over life-sustaining treatment: A health care provider's guide.* Williamsburg, VA: National Center for State Courts.

Hastings Center. (1987). *Guidelines on the termination of life-sustaining treatment and care of the dying: A report.* Briarcliff Manor, NY: Author.

Hoefler, J. M. (2000). Making decisions about tube feeding for severely demented patients at the end of life: Clinical, legal, and ethical considerations. *Death Studies, 24,* 233-254.

Huang, Z. B., & Ahronheim, J. C. (2000). Nutrition and hydration in terminally ill patients: An update. *Clinics in Geriatric Medicine, 16,* 313-325.

Institute of Palliative Care. (2001). *Palliative care—nutrition.* Retrieved November 24, 2001, from http://www.pallcare.org/nutritio.htm

Justice, C. (1995). The "natural" death while not eating: A type of palliative care in Banaras, India. *Journal of Palliative Care, 11* (1), 38-42.

Kazanowski, M. (1995). End-of-life care. In D. D. Ignatavicius & M. L. Workman (Eds.), *Medical-surgical nursing: Critical thinking for collaborative care* (2nd ed., pp. 106-114). Philadelphia: Saunders.

Kee, J. L., & Paulanka, B. J. (2000). *Handbook of fluid, electrolyte and acid-base balances* (pp. 1-41). New York: Delmar.

Kuebler, K. K., & Berry, P. H. (2002). End of life care. In K. K. Kuebler, P. H. Berry, & D. E. Heidrich (Eds.), *End of life care* (pp. 23-37). Philadelphia: Saunders.

Konsman, J. P., & Dantzer, R. (2001). How the immune and nervous system interact during disease-associated anorexia. *Nutrition, 17,* 664-668.

Kotler, D. P. (2000). Cachexia. *Annals of Internal Medicine, 17,* 622-634.

Lawton, S., & Cyster, D. (2002). Ethical issues. In J. Lugton & M. Kindlen (Eds.), *Palliative care: The nursing role* (pp. 262-265). Edinburgh: Churchill-Livingstone.

Luce, J. M., & Alpers, A. (2001). End of life care: What do the American courts say? *Critical Care Medicine, 29* (2 Suppl.), N40-N45.

Lueckenotte, A. G. (1996). *Gerontological nursing* (pp. 397-405). St. Louis: Mosby.

Lynn, J. (2000). Care of the dying. In M. H. Beers & H. Berkow (Eds.), *The Merck manual of geriatrics* (2nd ed., pp. 115-127). Whitehouse Station, NJ: Merck Research Laboratories.

McGrew, D. M. (2001). Chronic illness and end of life, *Primary Care, 28,* 339-347.

Meares, C. J. (1994). Terminal dehydration: A review. *American Journal of Hospice & Palliative Care, 11,* 10-14.

Meguid, M. M., Yang, Z. I., & Gleason, J. R. (1996). The gut-brain axis in anorexia: Toward an understanding of food intake regulation. *Nutrition, 12* (1 Suppl.), 557-562.

Meissel, A., Snyder, L., & Quill, T. (2000). Seven legal barriers to end-of-life care: Myths, realities, and grains of truth. *Journal of the American Medical Association, 284,* 2495-2501.

Mitchell, S. L., Kiely, D. K., & Lipsitz, L. A. (1998). Does artificial enteral nutrition prolong survival of institutionalized elders with chewing and swallowing problems? *Journals of Gerontology. Series A, Biological Sciences and Medical Sciences, 53,* M207-M213.

Morley, J. E. (2001). Anorexia, body composition, and ageing. *Current Opinion in Clinical Nutrition and Metabolic Care, 4* (1), 9-13.

Munro, H. N., Suter, P. M., & Russell, R. M. (1987). Nutritional requirements of the elderly. *Annual Review of Nutrition, 7,* 23-49.

National Center for State Courts. (1991). *Guidelines for state court decision making.* Williamsburg, VA: Author.

National Conference of Commissioners on Uniform State Laws. (1993). *Health—care decisions act.* Chicago: Author.

New York State Task Force on Life and the Law. (1992). *When others must choose.* New York: Author.

Palm, C., Reimann, D., & Gross, P. (2000). Hyponatremia—with comments on hypernatremia, *Therapeutische Umschau, 57,* 400-407.

Plata-Salaman, C. R. (2000). Central nervous system mechanisms contributing to the cachexia-anorexia syndrome. *Nutrition, 16,* 1009-1012.

Project on Death in America. (2002). *Research brief: Medical specialty societies adopt core principles for end-of-life care.* Retrieved from http://www.soros.org/death/Milbank_Memorial_Fund.htm

Quill, T. E., & Byock, I. R. (2000). Responding to intractable terminal suffering: The role of terminal sedation and voluntary refusal of food and fluids. ACP-ASIM End of Life Care Consensus Panel. American College of Physicians—American Society of Internal Medicine. *Annals of Internal Medicine, 132,* 408-414.

Rabeneck, L., Wary, N. P., & Peterson, N. J. (1996). Long-term outcomes of patients receiving percutaneous endoscopic gastrostomy tubes. *Journal of General Internal Medicine, 11,* 287-293.

Ritz, P. (2001). Chronic cellular dehydration in the aged patient. *Journals of Gerontology. Series A, Biological Sciences and Medical Sciences, 56,* M349-M352.

Roubenoff, J. R., Roubenoff, R. A., Cannon, J. G., Kehayias, J. J., Zhuang, H., Dawson-Hughes, B., et al. (1994). Rheumatoid cachexia: Cytokine-driven hypermetabolism accompanying reduced body cell mass in chronic inflammation. *Journal of Clinical Investigation, 93,* 2379-2386.

Roubenoff, R. A. (1999). The pathology of wasting in the elderly. *Journal of Nutrition, 129* (1 Suppl.), 256S-259S.

Sarhill, N., Walsh, D., Nelson, K., & Davis, M. (2001). Evaluation and treatment of cancer-related fluid deficits: Volume depletion and dehydration. *Supportive Care in Cancer, 9,* 408-419.

Shils, M. E., Olson, J. A., & Shike, M. (1994). *Modern nutrition in health and disease* (8th ed.). Philadelphia: Lea & Febiger.

Taber's Cyclopedic Medical Dictionary (19th ed.). (1997). Philadelphia: Davis.

Timaris, P. S. (1994). Degenerative changes in cells and cell death. In P. S. Timaris (Ed.), *Physiological basis of aging and geriatrics* (2nd ed, pp. 47-59). Boca Raton, FL: CRC Press.

Thomas, D. R., & Morley, J. E. (2001). Anorexia and weight loss in elderly outpatients: Part I. In *Nutrition literature resource compendium: Supplement to Annals of Long-Term Care* (pp. 21-30). Newtown Square, PA: Programs in Medicine, division of Multimedia Health Care/Freedom, LLC..

Twycross, R., & Licher, I. (1998). The terminal phase. In D. Doyle, G. W. C. Hanks, & N. MacDonald (Eds.), *Oxford textbook of palliative medicine* (pp. 979-981). New York: Oxford University Press.

Waller, A., Hershkowitz, M., & Adunsky, A. (1994). The effect of intravenous fluid infusion on blood and urine parameters of hydration and on state of consciousness in terminal cancer patients. *American Journal of Hospice & Palliative Care, 11* (6), 22-27.

Welk, T. A. (1999). Clinical and ethical considerations of fluid and electrolyte management in terminal clients. *Journal of Intravenous Nursing, 22* (1), 43-47.

Winter, S. M. (2000). Terminal nutrition: Framing the debate for the withdrawal of nutrition support in terminally ill patients. *American Journal of Medicine, 109,* 723-726.

Yeh, S. S., & Schuster, M. W. (1999). Geriatric cachexia: The role of cytokines. *American Journal of Clinical Nutrition, 70,* 183-197.

Zerwekh, J. V. (1997). Do dying patients really need IV fluids? *American Journal of Nursing, 97* (3), 26-30.

24

POLYPHARMACY

Sue E. Meiner

At age 86, Mrs. A. lives with her 60-year-old widowed daughter in a private home. Although Mrs. A. was fairly healthy until her mid-70s, she has declined in health steadily over the past 5 years. Her current list of diagnoses includes type 2 diabetes mellitus, hypertension, congestive heart failure, irregular heart rate and rhythm, gastroesophageal reflux (GERD), osteoarthritis, depression, chronic dehydration, and constipation. Last year she was diagnosed with stage II chondrosarcoma of the pelvis. After much discussion with her family and a second surgical and oncology opinion, Mrs. A. decided not to have surgical intervention. Radiation therapy and chemotherapy were not options because of an adverse risk:benefit ratio and the ineffective results of these therapies as reported in the current medical literature (Otto, 1995).

Her mobility has declined rapidly over the past 3 months. Using a walker, she slowly gets to the kitchen table, where she eats three small meals a day with very little liquid intake. She takes her pills with the food on her plate because of difficulty in swallowing medicines with water. She does not have an appetite and reports that the food is tasteless. She needs to rest for a few minutes after each meal before she has the energy to walk to her bedroom. Other than walking to the table, she is rarely out of her bedroom except to walk to the attached bathroom.

Symptoms that have become noticeable to her daughter include fatigue and weakness, pain after short walks in the house, increase in depression with episodes of anxiety, shortness of breath, increased swelling of both lower extremities, more frequent episodes of GERD, and two

episodes of fecal impaction over the last month. The daughter has asked for a home care nurse to help her with symptom control and care suggestions.

On the initial visit, all medicines, food supplements, herbs, and over-the-counter drugs were examined. Box 24-1 lists the items found by the home care nurse. The nurse estimated that Anne took between 22 and 35 doses of drugs daily.

The home care nurse prepares a written flow sheet of all of the items listed in Box 24-1 for the primary care provider. After the home visit, the nurse documents the health, psychosocial, and nutritional history; physical assessment; list of medications; current plan of care; and suggestions for new interventions. A call is made to the primary care provider to establish communication and discuss the patient's current condition. Box 24-2 presents the planned interventions aimed at improving issues related to polypharmacy.

INTRODUCTION

The relief of somatic distress during the months and weeks before death is a major part of pharmacotherapeutic support. The most common focus of treatment involves pain, dyspnea, fatigue, anxiety, agitation, nausea and/or vomiting, and constipation (Lubkin & Larsen, 2002). In addition to these symptoms that need management, other comorbid conditions may exist that require maintenance drug therapy. The interaction of all of the various medications can lead to unfavorable responses or even toxicity that can hasten the end of life. In general, older adults take an overwhelming number of prescribed drugs. At the same time, some reports indicate a trend toward underprescribing some drug therapies, such as beta-blockers following an acute myocardial

---

Box 24-1 Medications, Supplements, and Herbals Found in Mrs. A.'s House

All medicines identified as being part of Anne's regular regimen are taken orally. The drugs noted as taken on a prn basis were not able to be identified as to the amount and/or frequency of dosing. Unless marked as over-the-counter (OTC), all listed medications were prescribed by a primary care provider.

1. Hydrochlorothiazide, 25 mg daily; metoprolol, 100 mg twice a day; felodipine, 5 mg daily
2. Isosorbide dinitrate, 40 mg three times daily; digoxin, 0.25 mg daily; aspirin 81 mg daily
3. Glyburide, 20 mg daily
4. Ranitidine, 150 mg daily; cimetidine, 200 mg twice daily; omeprazole, 40 mg twice daily
5. MS Contin, 30 mg prn; Lortab, 5/500 prn

6. Sertraline, 50 mg daily; trazadone, 25 mg at bedtime
7. Clonazepam, 1 mg twice daily
8. Calcium, 800 mg with 400 IU vitamin D daily
9. K-Dur, 10 mg daily
10. Maalox (prn), 24-oz bottle; Gelusil (prn), 12-oz bottle; Tums antacid tablets (prn), 100/bottle (OTC)
11. Ex-lax suppositories prn; Correctol tablets prn; milk of magnesia (prn), 24-oz bottle (OTC)
12. St. John's wort, three tablets daily (OTC)
13. Glucosamine/chondroitin, 3 tablets daily (OTC)
14. Motrin IB, 200 mg prn; acetaminophen, 500 mg prn (OTC)

---

infarction (Schafer, 2001). This chapter addresses issues related to multiple medication use, also called polypharmacy, among elders at the end of life and strategies for adjusting medications where appropriate.

The term *polypharmacy* has several different definitions. Although some basic differences exist among the definitions, the underlying premise of overuse, misuse, mismatching, or obtaining prescription drugs improperly remains. Box 24-3 provides four basic definitions of polypharmacy. When medication misuse or abuse is suspected, characteristics that can identify this include medications that have no apparent indication, duplicated medicines, contraindicated medicines, inappropriate dosages, and concurrent use of interacting medications. Drugs prescribed for too long a time or drugs in exceedingly high doses for an older adult contribute to polypharmacy. Often additional prescriptions are added to the treatment plan to cover symptoms that are created by previously prescribed drugs (known as the "chasing phenomenon").

The number of persons 65 years of age or over is projected to reach 39.3 million by the year 2010 (AARP, 2001). The current population of older adults purchases approximately 35% of all prescription drugs. The amount of nonprescription medications taken by older adults is estimated to be 40%, which is greater than all other age groups. Nonprescription medicines are

commonly referred to as over-the-counter drugs. Nearly three fourths of ambulatory older adults take at least one prescription medication daily along with an unknown number of over-the-counter medicines (Corcoran, 1997). The older adult is particularly sensitive to the effects of drugs, yet numerous drugs are often necessary to manage the multiple medical problems that occur among this population. As new medicines are developed to treat or to prevent illnesses such as cancer, polypharmacy will continue to proliferate. The actual cost of prescription and over-the-counter drugs to the older adult is overwhelming for many elders with limited incomes. Even when the income is adequate, the cost of the drug therapy can consume all of the disposable monthly income and reduce the person's ability to engage in social activities that are an important component for a satisfactory quality of life.

POLYPHARMACY IN COMORBIDITY TREATMENT: BENEFITS AND RISKS

For some older adults with multiple comorbidities, polypharmacy (in the context of multiple medications being taken daily) may not be avoidable. In the case study, for example, medications for cardiovascular, endocrine, digestive, and elimination systems must be addressed, while offering palliative care for other symptoms of terminal illnesses. The overlapping of many of the symptoms

Box 24-2 **Changes to Pharmacotherapeutic Interventions Planned for Mrs. A.**

The following changes to Anne's pharmacotherapeutic regimen were recommended. These changes may not represent the ideal pattern of medications for other patients, but were the beginning of a plan to decrease the number and dosage of several medications prescribed for her multiple health deficits. Some were eliminated altogether for a variety of reasons, including (but not limited to) duplicate drugs, inappropriate for the reason used, and/or synergetic response when used with other medications on her list.

1. Hydrochlorothiazide, 25 mg daily—*reduce to 12.5 mg daily in AM; monitor blood pressure
2. K-Dur, 10 mg daily—continue as long as #1 is continued on regimen
3. Metoprolol, 100 mg bid—reduce the dosage over a 2-week period, then discontinue
4. Felodipine, 5 mg daily—discontinue completely (conflicts with #2, 5, 8, 9)
5. Isosorbide dinitrate, 40 mg tid—*discontinue completely (conflicts with #1)
6. Digoxin 0.25 mg daily—*reduce dosage to 0.125 mg daily after pulse is taken and > 60
7. Aspirin, 81 mg daily—no change
8. Glyburide, 20 mg daily—change to 10 mg bid and monitor blood glucose every 3 months
9. Ranitidine, 150 mg daily—continue, but to be taken as bedtime instead of in the morning
10. Cimetidine, 200 mg bid—discontinue completely (conflicts with #8)
11. Omeprazole, 40 mg bid—discontinue completely (use is for acute *Helicobacter pylori* infection times 4 weeks)

12. Sertraline, 50 mg daily—increase dose to 100 mg in the morning
13. Trazadone, 25 mg at bedtime—no change
14. St. John's wort—discontinue completely (conflicts with #11 & 12)
15. MS Contin, 30 mg prn—change to an every 3–4 hour schedule and evaluate for effective pain relief
16. Lortab, 5/500 prn—continue for severe breakthrough pain
17. Motrin IB, 200 mg prn—for minor aches and pain or pain of arthritis
18. Acetaminophen, 500 mg prn—discontinue in favor of #16
19. Calcium, 800 mg with 400 IU Vitamin D daily
20. Glucosamine/chondroitin, 3 tablets daily—continue if cost is not a concern
21. Clonazepam, 1 mg BID—*reduce by ½ the dose every 4 days until 0 dose, then discontinue
22. Maalox, Gelusil, & Tums antacid tablets—discontinue (conflict with #8); symptoms of upset stomach, belching, or sour taste should be reported to the primary care provider
23. Ex-lax suppositories prn, Correctol tablets prn, milk of magnesia—discontinue both of these OTC medicines; report constipation concerns to the primary care provider
24. Encourage eight 8-ounce glasses of water daily (not carbonated); suggest taking 4 ounces hourly while awake and keeping a chart to mark off daily

*Recommended changes in administration.
Sources: Deglin, J. H., & Vallerand, A. H. (2001). *Davis's drug guide for nurses* (7th ed.). Philadelphia: F. A. Davis; Semia, T. P., Beizer, J. L., & Gigbee, M. D. (2002). *Geriatric dosage handbook* (6th ed.). Cleveland: Lexi-Comp, Inc.; Wynne, A. L., Woo, T. M., & Millard, M. (2002). *Pharmacotherapeutics: For nurse practitioner prescribers*. Philadelphia: F. A. Davis.

can cause treatment confusion when no aggressive course of cancer treatment is desired. However, palliative care should include symptom relief from known pathophysiologic causes (Corcoran, 1997).

When an elder cancer patient with heart disease is receiving chemotherapy, the function of the heart may be affected. If the patient is taking cardiovascular medications to control the comorbid heart condition, the additional volume of fluid or toxicity of the drug may create an imbalance. Although these adverse events are taken into consideration prior to chemotherapy, complications can arise following treatment (American Society of Hospital Pharmacists, 1997).

Inaccurate diagnoses can hamper effective drug therapy. Many older adults underreport symptoms while presenting multiple vague complaints. The overlapping of symptoms of physical diseases and symptoms of psychological illness are common. Adding another factor to these potential problems are the atypical symptoms that are presented by older people. These elements can make the identification of the correct diagnoses, with appropriate prescribing, a most difficult task in the geriatric population (Kane, Ouslander, & Abrass, 1999).

The use of laxatives among older adults is quite common. Laxatives coupled with some chemotherapeutic agents with laxative effects can cause diarrhea, resulting in dehydration with fluid and electrolyte disturbances that may need emergency attention. Patient education in the form of verbal, written, and follow-up discussions (by phone) may prevent the use of laxatives when other drugs quite possibly will lead to loose stools.

Combining vitamin and mineral supplements, or herbal or natural products sold as alternatives to prescription drugs, with a therapeutic drug regimen may prove harmful. One example is taking an iron supplement when fatigue is thought to be from anemia. Iron products can inhibit the absorption of tetracyclines, quinolones, and some antihypertensive medications. When iron is taken with thyroxine, the serum concentration of thyrotropin (thyroid-stimulating hormone) decreases, and thus the signs and symptoms of hypothyroidism are increased. Another example is the use of calcium, which should be used with caution in older adults taking cardiac glycosides because of drug-drug interactions that might lead to arrhythmias (Schafer, 2001).

Vitamins are frequently taken by older adults because of their antioxidant effects, which are associated with cancer prevention. However, side effects may result from indiscriminate use by cancer patients. Mega-doses of vitamin C are known to cause the formation of kidney stones and can acidify the urine. Drugs such as methotrexate need an alkaline urine pH to be adequately excreted. In the presence of acidic urine, methotrexate may cause excess toxicity and damage the renal tubules (Corcoran, 1997).

When drug dose reduction is a goal of treatment, tapering or withdrawing only one medication at a time is preferred to acting more quickly and reducing or discontinuing more than one drug at once. Dose reduction of some drugs is recommended prior to discontinuation of the drug entirely. Adverse drug withdrawal reactions from beta-blockers and benzodiazepines can usually be avoided by gradually tapering the doses over a 4-week period. Both classes of drugs can be reduced by one fourth the daily dose at a 1- to 2-week interval. Finally, giving the lowest dose possible every other day for a final week prior to completely stopping the medication is suggested (Corcoran, 1997; Gerety, Cornell, Plichta, & Eimer, 1993; Stewart & Cooper, 1994). Throughout this reduction period, side effects of the reduced dose need to be reported to the primary care providers for evaluation.

When polypharmacy is necessary in order to treat comorbidities, the benefits of therapy outweigh the risks of untoward responses. However, all medications taken need to be listed in the medical chart with known side effects, previously reported adverse reactions, toxicity levels (if appropriate), and information on drug-drug and drug-food interactions. When this list is available to the primary care provider, in the event of a change in medications, there is less potential for adding a new agent that might cause drug potentiation, synergism, or an antagonistic effect. Box 24-4 provides a list of nine prescribing tips. The older patient should be provided with a medication list that is to be carried with him or her at all times. This list should contain information that will be helpful to other health care professionals in the event of an adverse drug reaction, side effect, or toxicity. Special instructions can be written on this list to serve as a reminder to adhere to prescribing directions. Figure 24-1 presents a sample form for providing suggested information.

Primary Care Provider "Shopping" and Polypharmacy

The importance of remaining functional with the highest possible quality of life is an important issue among older adults with chronic conditions. This can lead to seeking help from several sources. Different physicians may be consulted without knowing that another primary care provider has prescribed the same or similar drugs for treatment. Multiple pharmacies may be used

to fill prescriptions from different providers of care. While most chain drug stores now have computer records on customers, private pharmacies may not be able to interchange information with these chain pharmacies. Overprescribing of

Box 24-4 **List of Prescribing Tips**
1. Evaluate the patient's list of medications at each visit.
2. Have the patient carry a current list of medications with him or her at all times.
3. Maintain information on the name, purpose, and prominent side effects of each drug on both lists.
4. Obtain information about the use of over-the-counter medications, herbals, and food supplements each visit.
5. Review the major health goals with the patient and with the family when appropriate.
6. Schedule office visits or arrange for phone contacts to monitor medication adherence.
7. Discuss the method for contacting the palliative care practitioner when side effects or adverse effects are seen.
8. Begin all new prescriptions at the lowest possible dose and titrate upward slowly, if needed, from that point.
9. Decrease drug dosage slowly prior to discontinuing completely when possible.

Name: _____   Home phone: (_____) _____ - _____

Address: _____   Nearest relative: _____

Health care provider: _____   and phone: (_____) _____ - _____

Medicine name	Why is it used	Description	When is it taken a.m. noon p.m. hs				Notes
Digoxin 0.125 mg	Slows heart rate	Small white pill	X				Take pulse first Omit if under 60 bpm

Instructions: _____

Fig. 24-1 Sample medication data sheet.

medications needs to be avoided while balancing the benefits of each prescription in the treatment regimen. Monitoring the adherence to the pharmacotherapeutic treatment plan is essential for early identification of adverse effects (American Society of Hospital Pharmacists, 1997).

Psychopharmacology

Psychological symptoms such as depression, anxiety, agitation, insomnia, paranoia, and disruptive behaviors are often caused or exacerbated by comorbidities in older patients. A complete medical evaluation is needed prior to attributing the cause to a psychiatric condition alone and adding a psychotropic medication to prescriptive drug regimens. Some incidents have been reported that are directly related to the caregiver's interpretation of agitation and disruptive behaviors. Compliance with demands of caregivers may not be reasonable at times, and the behavior noted may be a natural response to being told to do something that the individual

---

EVIDENCE-BASE PRACTICE

Reference: Pharmacist review changed more repeat prescriptions for elderly patients than did usual general practice review. (2002, September-October). *ACP Journal Club, 137*(2), 73,.

Research Problem: In elderly patients who receive repeat prescriptions, is a clinical review of medications by a pharmacist more effective than usual general practice review for increasing medication changes and reducing costs?

Design: 12-month randomized (allocation concealed), unblinded, controlled trial.

Sample and Setting: 1188 patients who were 65 years of age or older (mean age 74 years, 56% women); were receiving one or more drug on repeat prescription as of 1 June 1999; and were from one of four general practices in Leeds, England, in which prescribing costs were average and that had four or more partners, computerized repeat prescribing, and no previous or current clinical pharmacist involvement. Patients were excluded if they lived in nursing or residential homes, had a terminal illness, or were enrolled in clinical trials. Follow-up was 95%.

Methods: A study group of 608 patients was allocated to pharmacist review, which had three components. In stage 1, the pharmacist evaluated the patients, their illnesses, and their medications, including adherence. In stage 2, the pharmacist evaluated the patients' medication regimen in terms of need for ongoing drugs, side effects, inadequate treatment, and cost. In stage 3, if necessary, the pharmacist

implemented changes. Any substantial changes were made with the cooperation of a general practitioner (GP). A control group of 580 patients was allocated to usual care from their GP, including a review of medications according to the practice's normal custom. The main outcome measure was the number of changes to repeat prescriptions. Secondary outcomes included changes in number of medications and cost.

Results: Analysis was by intention to treat. The pharmacist-reviewed group had a higher mean number of changes to repeat prescriptions per patient and a lower mean change from baseline in the number of repeat medications prescribed than did the usual-care group. The increase in mean medication cost per patient over 28 days was less in the pharmacist-reviewed group than in the usual-care group (change from baseline 1.80 vs. 6.52, 95% confidence interval for the 4.72 difference, 2.41 to 7.04).

Implications for Nursing Practice: All medications should be reviewed with every patient on every visit. The staff nurse review should look at all of the medicines being taken and keep an updated list for the physician review. The Advanced Practice Nurse review should look at a need to continue or to adjust any prescribed medications.

Conclusion: In elderly patients who receive repeat prescriptions, a pharmacist review of medications resulted in more prescription changes but fewer medications prescribed and lower medication costs than did usual general practice review.

does want to do. Therefore, asking questions of a caregiver to determine if the description of the action fits the definition of a true psychiatric concern that needs pharmacotherapeutic intervention is essential. Behavioral modification, environmental manipulation, supportive actions on the part of the caregivers, and other activities can be used instead of drug therapy, which may benefit the older patient (Kane et al., 1999).

Screening for depression, including in patients with dementia, is important at all stages of life, including the end of life. Chronic comorbidities are more likely to be complicated by a state of depression in older adults. Depression often accompanies debilitating chronic conditions of the heart, lungs, central nervous system, or musculoskeletal system. Among the more common illnesses associated with the treatment of depression are Parkinson's disease, Alzheimer's disease, thyroid disease, arthritis, and diabetes mellitus. A diagnosis of cancer or other terminal conditions can be highly associated with depression in many older adults. The signs and symptoms of dementia are frequently related to undiagnosed depression. When polypharmacy already exists, the primary care provider may be reluctant to add another medication to the list. Therefore, the patient may not be treated or may be inadequately treated for depression.

COORDINATION OF CARE WITH A FOCUS ON PHARMACOTHERAPEUTICS

End-of-life care often involves several primary care providers. Each provider usually focuses on an area of expertise that might require pharmacotherapy. When these providers do not have a rapid system of relaying changes in the treatment plans to the other providers, confusion and adverse polypharmacy can result. Transcription of office notes can further delay the transmittal of information in a timely manner. The current use of facsimile transmission is effective in the transfer of information from one primary care provider to another. A safety issue that should be in place when facsimile transmission is used is the return of a signed or initialed document to notify the sender of the receipt of the message by the other providers. Most major pharmacies now use computer database systems that record the names of

the health care providers and the medication details in a file with the patient's name. Some systems have an alert mechanism that will signal when a possible conflict exists with new prescriptions. The patient's database generally includes information on allergies and prior drug reactions as well as a way to contact the patient for additional information.

Appropriate Prescribing Criteria

A nationally recognized expert panel in geriatric care and geriatric pharmacology met to define criteria to determine inappropriate prescribing patterns for older adults (Beers, 1997). These prescribing patterns were for medications that resulted in adverse reactions caused by the processes of aging. Medications that should be avoided or used with caution in older adults are listed in Box 24-5. When these drugs are used, appropriate monitoring is essential. The monitoring is required because of an increase in sensitivity to side effects and toxicity; often much safer alternatives are available.

Adverse Drug Reactions

Adverse drug reactions are identified as undesired, dose-dependent reactions to medicines. They may be the result of changes in drug pharmacodynamics and pharmacokinetics in older adults. For example, the pharmacokinetics of cimetidine leads to a reduced hepatic metabolism of drugs such as warfarin, phenytoin, theophylline, propranolol, some benzodiazepines, and some tricyclic antidepressants. The reduction of hepatic metabolism increases the blood concentrations of these drugs while reducing drug elimination. Side effects are more frequently seen when cimetidine is taken concomitantly with phenytoin and theophylline. However, discontinuation of cimetidine can result in subtherapeutic levels of the same drugs (Graves et al., 1997). Adverse drug reactions also can be associated with changes in daily activities such as sleep patterns, food and fluid intake, and exercise (Wynne, Woo, & Millard, 2002).

The risk of an adverse drug reaction or a serious side effect can be directly tied to the aging process. Although aging produces a wide variation in physiologic changes and responses, some changes are predictable. The pharmacokinetics of absorption, distribution, biotransformation

Box 24-5 Medications to Avoid or Use with Caution in Older Adults

INCREASED SENSITIVITY TO SIDE EFFECTS
- Amitriptyline and combinations
- Antihistamines with potent anticholinergic effects
- Diphenhydramine
- Gastrointestinal antispasmodics
- Indomethacin
- Iron over 325 mg/day
- Long-acting benzodiazepines
- Pentazocine
- Phenylbutazone

INCREASED TOXICITY (SAFER ALTERNATIVES ARE AVAILABLE)
- Barbiturates, excluding phenobarbital
- Chlordiazepoxide
- Diazepam
- Digoxin
- Dipyridamole
- Disopyramide
- Doxepin
- Fluazepam
- Meperidine
- Meprobamate
- Methyldopa and combinations
- Propoxyphene and combinations
- Reserpine
- Ticlopidine

*Adapted from Beers, M. (1997). Explicit criteria for determining potentially inappropriate medication use by the elderly. *Archives of Internal Medicine, 157,* 1531.

(metabolism), and excretion as well as tissue sensitivity are important to the understanding of the risks associated with unavoidable polypharmacy. In the older adult, absorption is affected by a decrease in absorption surface, decreased splanchnic blood flow, altered gastrointestinal motility, and an increased gastric pH. Distribution is affected by a decrease in total body water, lean body mass, and adequate serum albumin. Metabolism is affected by a decrease in liver blood flow and enzyme fluctuation. Excretion is affected by a decrease in renal blood flow, glomerular filtration rate, and tubular secre-

tory function. Tissue sensitivity is altered in regard to the number and affinity of receptors, the second-messenger function, and cellular functions (Kane et al., 1999).

The "catch-up" pattern is responsible for some adverse drug reactions when a missed dose or doses are followed by overdosing to catch up. Symptoms of nausea and vomiting are often related to the catch-up pattern. When vomiting leads to dehydration, emergency visits or hospitalization may result (Chrischilles, Segar, & Wallace, 1992).

Adverse drug reactions are frequently seen in long-term care settings. A recent study of adverse drug reactions in nursing homes found that 50% of adverse drug reactions were preventable. The occurrence of an adverse drug reaction was defined as an event that had an observable impact on the resident's health status or function. These events had substantial impact on the residents, with symptoms that included delirium, lethargy, falls, gastrointestinal manifestation, and hemorrhage. Residents at the highest risk for adverse drug reactions were those with liver and/or kidney disease and residents with dementia. Delirium was the most frequently identified initial sign of an adverse drug reaction to medications in older residents (Field et al., 2001).

Renal function and measurement of creatinine clearance is often overlooked when prescribing renally excreted drugs to older long-term care residents. Potential adverse drug reactions may be due to drugs remaining in the blood at high levels for longer time periods, thus prolonging the half-life of each dose of a drug. The creatinine clearance is an excellent diagnostic indictor of renal function; the rate of clearance is expressed in terms of the volume of blood (in milliliters) that can be cleared of creatinine in 1 minute. Values for older persons normally decrease by 6 mL/min for each decade. Normal creatinine clearance for men ranges from 85 to 125 mL/min, while women have a normal range of 75 to 115 mL/min. These levels become abnormal when more than 50% of the total nephron units have been damaged (Springhouse Corporation, 1994). When the creatinine clearance is below 35 mL/min, drugs that are eliminated through the kidney need to be reevaluated for safety.

EVIDENCE-BASED PRACTICE

Reference: Triazolam caused sedation and impairment of psychomotor performance in elderly persons. (1991, November-December). *ACP Journal Club, 115,* 94.

Research Problem: To evaluate the pharmacologic properties of triazolam and determine if the clinical response to this drug is enhanced in elderly persons.

Design: Randomized, double-blind, crossover study.

Sample and Setting: 21 elderly persons (ages 62 to 83 years) and 26 younger persons (ages 21 to 41 years); all were healthy and not taking any medications. Participant recruitment methods were not described; the sample came from the New England Medical Center Hospital.

Methods: Participants were given single doses of placebo or triazolam (0.125 or 0.25 mg), in a double-blind fashion in random order, with 1 week or more between doses. The study drug was given at 9:00 AM after overnight fasting and a liquid breakfast. Plasma triazolam concentrations, percent change from baseline for degree of sedation as rated by subjects and by a blinded observer using a visual analogue scale, percent change from baseline on digit-symbol substitution scores, and percent change relative to scores after placebo on word-list free recall were assessed. Assessments were made before drug administration, every half hour for 3 hours following drug administration, and then at 4, 6, 8, and 24 hours thereafter.

Results: Peak plasma triazolam concentrations were higher (1.67 vs. 1.08 ng/mL after 0.125 mg; 3.06 vs. 2.02 ng/mL after 0.25 mg; $p < .002$ for both doses) and clearance was reduced (6.8 vs. 11.4 mL/min/kg for 0.125 mg [$p < .07$]; 5.8 vs. 10.5 mL/min/kg for 0.25 mg [$p < .001$]) in the older relative to the younger participants, respectively. Observer-rated degree of sedation for young and elderly participants paralleled plasma concentrations and was proportional to dose. Observer-rated degree of sedation was greater in the older than in the younger group at corresponding times with both triazolam doses; the interaction between age and study medication approached significance ($p < .07$). Although younger participants reported that the degree of sedation increased in proportion to dose, the older participants did not. Impairment on the digit-symbol substitution test was proportional to the dose for both groups, with an interaction between age and dose ($p < .05$). The subjects' ability to recall words presented 1.5 hours after drug administration 24 hours later was impaired by both doses; the percent decrease was similar in young and old participants.

Implications for Nursing Practice: Medication dosages need to be reviewed using evidence-based pharmacology reports when prescribing medications to older adults, especially sedating drugs due to the prolonged effect in aging persons as compared to younger persons.

Conclusion: Peak triazolam plasma concentrations were higher, and clearance was reduced in elderly compared with younger persons. Percent changes in the degree of sedation and psychomotor impairment were correspondingly greater.

When an older adult is treated for several comorbidities, larger numbers of medications are usually taken daily, which is associated with higher numbers of adverse drug reactions. About one half of all deaths related to adverse drug reactions occurred among elders (Schafer, 2001). An evaluation of the interactions and responses of the residents of long-term care facilities who are taking psychoactive drugs, antibiotics, opioids, or antiseizure drugs was highly recommended by Papaioannou, Clarke, Campbell, and Bedard (2000). The older population should have routine evaluations to identify changes in symptoms that may indicate a drug-related event (Field et al., 2001). Table 24-1 presents a comparison of common disease-drug interactions among older adults.

Table 24-1 **Common Disease–Drug Interactions among Older Adults**	
Disease or Condition	**Medications to Avoid**
Heart failure	Disopyramide and drugs with high sodium content
Diabetes mellitus	Beta-blockers in the care of patients receiving oral hypoglycemic drugs or insulin
Hypertension	Diet pills, amphetamines
Chronic obstructive pulmonary disease	Beta-blockers, sedative–hypnotic agents
Asthma	Beta-blockers
Ulcers	NSAIDs, potassium supplements, aspirin >325 mg/day
Seizures, epilepsy	Clozapine, chlorpromazine, thioridazine, chlorprothizene, metoclopramide
Peripheral vascular disease	Beta-blockers
Blood clotting disorders & anticoagulants	Aspirin, NSAIDs
Benign prostatic hypertrophy	Dipyridamole, ticlopidine
Incontinence	Anticholinergic antihistamines, gastrointestinal antispasmodics, muscle relaxants, opioids, alpha-blockers
Constipation	Anticholinergic drugs, narcotic drugs, tricyclic antidepressants
Syncope or falls	Beta-blockers, long-acting benzodiazepines
Arrhythmia	Tricyclic antidepressants
Insomnia	Decongestants, theophylline, desipramine, selective serotonin reuptake inhibitors, methylphenidate, monamine oxidase inhibitors, beta-agonists

NSAIDs, nonsteroidal anti-inflammatory drugs.
Adapted from Beers, M. (1997). Explicit criteria for determining potentially inappropriate medication use by the elderly. *Archives of Internal Medicine, 157,* 1531.

Side Effects

Side effects are frequently uncomfortable but usually do not require that the medication be discontinued. It is the treatment of the side effects that increases the risk of polypharmacy. Often a new primary care provider has difficulty identifying the rationale behind several drugs listed by an older patient during the health history and medication review. Trying to identify the specific medicine that is causing a particular side effect can be frustrating for the patient and the primary care provider. Many medications have similar indications and side effects. An example is combining the use of a tricyclic antidepressant and an opioid for pain relief; both may result in constipation. Adding a daily stool softener after a single use of a laxative might be confusing to an older adult who had recently experienced diarrhea with chemotherapy (Kazanowski, 2001).

The most common opioid-related side effects are constipation, sedation, nausea, vomiting, and cognitive disturbance. Less frequent side effects include urinary retention, perceptual distortion, respiratory depression, and myoclonus. Recognition of the symptoms of opioid-related side effects as opposed to those from causes such as a disease process, treatment approaches, or polypharmacy issues is vitally important. Differentiating the side effects of opioids from side effects with other causes can spare the patient the uncertainty of changing pain medications when the opioid may not be the cause of the problem (O'Mahony, Coyle, & Payne, 2001).

Nonadherence Issues

Adherence to a care plan for a positive outcome is the expected behavior when the primary care provider and the patient set mutual goals. Nonadherence to medication and/or treatment plans can compromise the efficacy and outcome of that plan, which more often than not can lead to a poor outcome. If the primary care provider is not aware of the nonadherence, alterations may be made in the treatment plan that could place the patient at risk for adverse drug reactions. Open communication in the patient-provider relationship is important in preventing complications of nonadherence.

Nonadherence is often associated with the number of medicines to be taken, and the frequency and timing of the medication schedule. When a medication schedule is complex, including drugs that must be taken before and/or after meals, between meals, without food, at bedtime, and every other day, then errors can be made. Hearing and visual impairments often lead to inadvertent nonadherence. Memory and cognitive factors along with knowledge base can affect adherence. Even swallowing difficulties can prevent adherence to medication regimens. When large tablets cannot be crushed or broken, they might be put aside and not taken. The older adult's quality of life can be affected when therapeutic effects of the medication require the person to be homebound for several hours each day. The most common drugs associated with such quality-of-life issues are diuretics, which often lead to increased frequency and volume of urination.

Another factor is related to the cost of prescriptions. With the ever-increasing cost of prescription medications, the older adult on a fixed income without a prescription assistance health plan may need to make financial decisions that limit the amount of medications purchased. The limitation can be in several forms. One form may be a decision not to refill one or more of multiple prescriptions during a time when heating or cooling bills are high. Another form may be to split pills in half in order to make them last longer before a refill is needed. The hard choice between food and medicine has been described in news accounts. None of these actions is beneficial to the patient, but in reality each is possible given certain circumstances. Therefore, the primary care provider needs to maintain current information related to the patient's ability to pay for prescriptions and other aspects of the treatment plan. Some pharmaceutical companies have programs for individuals unable to pay for essential prescriptions for products from their company. The primary care provider is the gatekeeper for these programs. Drug company representatives can provide the information related to their respective companies' services.

Taking prescription medicines less often than directed may be related to an unpleasant physiologic response or distress. Some drugs are frequently associated with adherence issues related to unpleasant symptoms such as dry mouth, blurred vision, constipation, and even mental impairment. These anticholinergic side effects can be anticipated and dealt with so that nonadherence does not occur (Kennedy-Malone, Fletcher, & Plank, 2000).

The prevention of mistakes leading to overdosing, underdosing, or missing doses followed by taking too large a dose to catch up with the daily amount of prescribed medicines can be a problem for many older adults. Caregivers and/or home health aides need to become involved in understanding and using adherence aids. Some simple adherence aids include a large daily or weekly calendar or medicine chart. Other adherence aids that have had success are the daily pill boxes/dispensers that can be prepared ahead of time for periods ranging from 1 week up to 1 month. Some of these containers have compartments for multiple daily doses. Advances in technology have produced the programmable alarm device with or without an attached medicine dispenser (Adelman & Daly, 2001).

PREVENTION OF POLYPHARMACY

Preventing polypharmacy can only be accomplished with the recognition of the problem. Simplifying the medication regimen by using once-a-day dosing schedules, where possible, is one method of reducing polypharmacy. Prescribing medicines that have more than one therapeutic indication to cover several conditions with one drug can be helpful (Cohen, 2000). Consulting with a clinical pharmacist may improve prescribing patterns for older adults. Maintaining a current information sheet on the primary care provider's most commonly prescribed drugs with classifications, dosage for geriatric patients, cost, adverse drug reactions, side effects, drug-drug interactions, and contraindications could assist with adherence issues (Lipton, Bero, Bird, & McPhee, 1992). Figure 24-1 shows a sample medication data sheet that can be given to the patient. Instructions need to include keeping a copy of the list at home and with the person (in a wallet or pocket for men, in a purse or pocket for women).

In some instances, polypharmacy cannot be avoided, but strides toward reducing the possibilities of adverse drug reactions and side effects should be considered. Baseline data for each patient must include a medication history and current usage of prescription, nonprescription (over-the-counter), and herbal medications, as well as food supplements and vitamins and minerals. An open-ended questionnaire completed by and reviewed with the patient on a periodic schedule might provide insight into the previous pharmacotherapeutic adherence patterns. Recording adverse drug reactions, side effects, and allergies to medications in the patient's chart is essential for future reference during visits, requests for refills, and empirical treatment. Placing this information in the front of the patient's chart and instructing anyone responsible for prescribing, administering, or dispensing medicines to review this information might reduce the incidence of polypharmacy and its negative outcomes.

Technology is currently available to support the recognition of potential adverse drug reactions. Computer software programs are being used in major pharmacies to alert the pharmacist of harmful drug-drug, drug-food, and drug-herb interactions. With or without computer capability, attention is needed to identify any potential for a newly prescribed drug to adversely interact with another currently used medication (Kane et al., 1999).

When a personalized medication schedule can be established for a patient, adherence is improved. The use of anticipatory guidance with educational needs and follow-up care that supports the provider and patient relationship is beneficial to medication schedule adherence. This pattern of care requires an understanding of the physical, psychological, and developmental stages and prior education of each patient (Ladebauche, 1997). When appropriate written treatment plans are combined with a follow-up review of adherence, misinformation can be corrected prior to an adverse drug reaction. Improved communication between patient, provider, and family members is ultimately the most significant factor to prevent negative outcomes from polypharmacy (Wynne et al., 2002).

EDUCATION AND FAMILY SUPPORT

Understanding the concept of palliative care can be confusing to family members whether they are direct caregivers or not. Addressing the symptomatic care instead of therapeutic care is the focus that should be taught to the family. Discussing issues that are geared toward keeping the patient's quality of life as high as possible through maintaining comfort while ensuring personal dignity must be a part of family education. Comfort measures often revolve around pain control. The perception of giving scheduled pain medication as being synonymous with drug addiction should be addressed early in the relationship with the family. Once an understanding of the benefits of maintaining a pain-free state are accepted by family members, regimens for giving narcotics or other pain-relieving medications are followed (Czenis, 1999; Springhouse Corporation, 2002).

The teaching methods used need to include an assessment of the family's health beliefs. This information can assist in the planning of the teaching sessions. During the initial sessions, pertinent information on palliative care can be added while physical care is discussed. Each discussion should be followed with handouts prepared specifically for each patient. Patient/family education needs to be in an understandable written format with a verbal review and follow-up visits or phone calls to determine adherence to the daily schedule of physical care and pharmacotherapeutics.

Case Study Conclusion

Mrs. A. did much better after her medications were reduced and she was able to talk about important family and personal issues. Although her physical condition declined toward the time when Mrs. A. became bedfast, she was alert until the final hours of life. The reduction of her pharmacotherapy allowed her to be comfortable while minimizing her difficulty in swallowing multiple medications daily. When she slipped into a coma, her family and minister were at her bedside. Mrs. A. died quietly and peacefully that day.

CONCLUSION

With the large number of medications being taken by older adults, often prescribed by several physicians, the misuse and/or abuse of drugs is common. Each year, drug misuse among older adults accounts for more than 9 million adverse drug reactions and 245,000 hospitalizations. When multiple comorbidities are present, polypharmacy is common, and in the United States it is nearly inevitable. However, an increased number of medicines used to manage multiple complex diseases amplifies the potential for an inability to follow a medication regimen. Prevention of ineffective treatment as a result of polypharmacy or the nonadherence problems associated with multiple medications is a priority to prevent negative outcomes. End-of-life care needs to provide the older adult with appropriate drug therapy as a part of the overall plan of care. Therefore, health care providers should minimize the number of drugs prescribed but not withhold medications that can prolong survival and preserve quality of life.

REFERENCES

Adelman, A. M., & Daly, M. P. (2001). *20 Common problems: Geriatrics*. New York: McGraw-Hill.

AARP (American Association of Retired Persons). (2001). *Profile of older Americans*. Washington, DC: Author.

American Society of Hospital Pharmacists. (1997). *American hospital formulary service drug information 95*. Bethesda, MD: Author.

Beers, M. (1997). Explicit criteria for determining potentially inappropriate medication by the elderly. *Archives of Internal Medicine, 15*, 1531.

Chrischilles, E. A., Segar, E. T., & Wallace, R. B. (1992). Self-reported adverse drug reactions and related resource use: A study of community-dwelling persons 65 years of age and older. *Annals of Internal Medicine, 117*, 634-640.

Cohen, J. S. (2000). Avoiding adverse reactions: Effective lower-dose drug therapies for older adults. *Geriatrics, 55*(2), 54, 56, 59-60, 63.

Corcoran, M. E. (1997). Polypharmacy in the older patient with cancer. *Cancer Control: JMCC, 4*, 419-428.

Czenis, A. L. (1999). Thyroid disease in the elderly: Not a typical presentation. *Advance for Nurse Practitioners, 7*(9), 38-44.

Deglin, J. H., & Vallerand, A. H. (2001). *Davis's drug guide for nurses* (7th ed.). Philadelphia: Davis.

Field, T. S., Gurwitz, J. H., Avorn, J., McCormick, D., Jain, S., Eckler, M., et al. (2001). Risk factors for adverse drug events among nursing home residents. *Archives of Internal Medicine, 161*, 1629.

Gerety, M. B., Cornell, J. E., Plichta, D. T., & Eimer, M. (1993). Adverse events related to drugs and drug withdrawal in nursing home residents. *Journal of the American Geriatrics Society, 41*, 1326-1332.

Graves, T., Hanlon, J. T., Schmader, K. E., Landsman, P. B., Samsa, B. P., Pieper, C. F., et al. (1997). Adverse events after discontinuing medications in elderly outpatients. *Archives of Internal Medicine, 157*, 2205-2210.

Kane, R. L., Ouslander, J. G., & Abrass, I. B. (1999). *Essentials of clinical geriatrics* (4th ed., pp. 378-409). New York: McGraw-Hill.

Kazanowski, M. K. (2001). Symptom management in palliative care. In M. L. Matzo & D. W. Sherman (Eds.), *Palliative care nursing: Quality care to the end of life* (pp. 327-361), New York: Springer.

Kennedy-Malone, L., Fletcher, K. R., & Plank, L. M. (2000). *Management guidelines for gerontological nurse practitioners*. Philadelphia: Davis.

Ladebauche, P. (1997). Managing asthma: A growth and development approach. *Pediatric Nursing, 23*(1), 37-44.

Lipton, H. L., Bero, L. A., Bird, J. A., & McPhee, S. J. (1992). The impact of clinical pharmacists' consultations on physicians' geriatric drug prescribing: A randomized controlled trial. *Medical Care, 30*, 646-658.

Lubkin, I. M., & Larsen, P. D. (2002). *Chronic illness: Impact and interventions* (5th ed.). Sudbury, MA: Jones and Bartlett.

O'Mahony, S., Coyle, N., & Payne, R. (2001). Current management of opioid-related side effects. *Oncology, 15*(1), 61-73, 77-78, 80-82.

Otto, S. E. (1995). *Oncology nursing: Pocket guide*. St. Louis: Mosby.

Papaioannou, A., Clarke, J., Campbell, G., & Bedard, M. (2000). Assessment of adherence to renal dosing guidelines in long-term care facilities. *Journal of the American Geriatrics Society, 48*, 1470-1473.

Schafer, S. L. (2001). Prescribing for seniors: It's a balancing act. *The Journal of the American Academy of Nurse Practitioners, 13*(3), 108-112.

Semia, T. P., Beizer, J. L., & Gigbee, M. D. (2002). *Geriatric dosage handbook* (6th ed.). Cleveland: Lexi-Comp, Inc.

Springhouse Corporation. (2002). *Better elder care: A nurse's guide to caring for older adults* (pp. 505-513). Springhouse, PA: Author.

Springhouse Corporation. (1994). *Illustrated guide to diagnostic tests* (p. 430). Springhouse, PA: Author.

Stewart, R. B., & Cooper, J. W. (1994). Polypharmacy in the aged: Practical solutions. *Drugs and Aging, 4*, 449-461.

Wynne, A. L., Woo, T. M., & Millard, M. (2002). *Pharmacotherapeutics: For nurse practitioner prescribers*. Philadelphia: Davis.

25

PERI-DEATH NURSING CARE

Marianne L. Matzo

Case Study

When the palliative care nurse pulled up to the house, there was hardly any place to park her car because every available spot was taken by family members' cars. The nurse walked up to the house, where children were playing on the porch, their parents and aunts and uncles talking together. Mrs. J. was in a hospital bed in the living room, surrounded by bustling activity. The Benny Goodman Orchestra played on the radio, and dinner was being cooked in the kitchen. Mr. J. was at the side of his wife, the woman he had met more than 50 years ago. Mrs. J. was actively dying from liver cancer, and it was clear to everyone that she would likely die within the next day. Her skin was darkly jaundiced, and her Foley catheter was draining a small amount of amber-colored urine. She lay with her eyes open and watched the activity around her, but had stopped talking except to answer direct questions. She denied pain or discomfort and looked to be at peace.

At this point, the family was primarily concerned about Mr. J. He had yet to talk about the fact that his wife was dying and would just wander around among his family as though he was lost in his own house. Dealing with their own grief at losing their mother, the family had no idea how to help their father with his pain over the impending death of his wife.

INTRODUCTION

This chapter is intended to assist the nurse caring in providing competent end-of-life care for older adults. The provision of end-of-life care involves flexibility and creativity in order to meet the needs of the elder patient and his or her family as they experience the process of dying and death. The focus of this chapter is on the physiologic changes that occur as death is imminent and the nursing interventions that are appropriate at this time. A body of core knowledge is necessary so that the nurse can help facilitate a "good" death for the older adult. As an experiential process, dying and death for the individual, the family, and the health care provider can be one of the most profound and momentous occurrences of their lives.

PERI-DEATH NURSING CARE

Dying and death should be viewed as a process, just as pregnancy and birth is a process that is described as the perinatal period. The pregnancy and birth process has a series of biologic changes, signs and symptoms, cultural beliefs, and responses that are hallmarks of each stage of the process. So, too, does death. Organizing death into a chronologic series of stages (or phases) each consisting of specific events, conflicts, and changes that occur provides a foundation/framework within which the themes and issues of dying and death can be organized and presented for the nurse (Matzo, Ury, & Sulmasy, in press).

This way of organizing the cycle of death helps the nurse to be better able to recognize and address the specific themes (denial, fear, anger, spiritual concerns, etc.), clinical issues (pain, fatigue, depression, etc.), and needs (home care, spiritual care, caregiver support, etc.) that arise during the cycle of death experienced by the older

Adapted from Matzo, M. L., & Sherman, D. W. (2002). *Palliative Care Nursing: Quality Care to the End of Life*. New York: Springer Publishing Company.

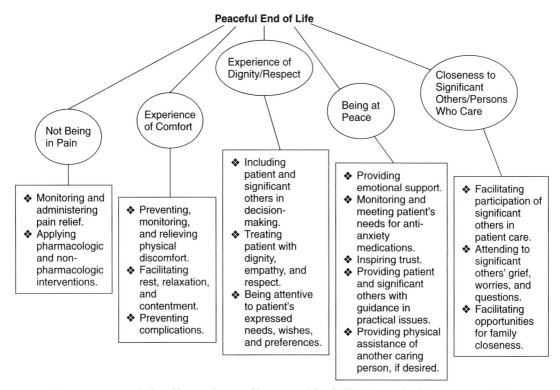

Fig. 25-1 Outcome criteria and interventions to achieve a peaceful end of life. (From Ruland, C., & Moore, S. [1998]. Theory construction based on standards of care: A proposed theory on the peaceful end of life. *Nursing Outlook, 46*(4), 169-175.)

adult patient and his or her family. The last hours of life—specifically the symptoms and experiences right before the death occurs, the actual death, and the care of the body after death—can be conceptualized as the peri-death period, which requires intensive holistic nursing care (Matzo, 2001). Ruland and Moore's (1998) theory for a peaceful end of life identifies five outcome criteria and related interventions. Specifically, the outcome criteria include assuring that the patient is not in pain, experiences comfort, experiences dignity and respect, is at peace, and has closeness with significant others or people who care about the patient. Outcome criteria and nursing interventions are presented in Figure 25-1.

Symptom Assessment and Management in the Last Hours of Life

The first phase of the peri-death period is when death is imminent, comfort care is provided, and the withdrawal of life-preserving interventions occurs. This period extends from the last few weeks to the last hours of life and ends with death and its pronouncement by the nurse or the physician. Any, all, or none of the following symptoms may occur during the final stages of the dying process: pain, weakness, fatigue, immobility, lack of interest in eating or drinking, drowsiness, dyspnea, and delirium. Palliative care nursing interventions for the older adult with advanced disease are detailed in the previous chapters of this book.

Essential to quality care of the older adult at the end of life is the management of symptoms. Few studies have examined the experience of dying (Fields & Cassel, 1997) and those that do exist document high rates of uncontrolled pain and other symptoms (Coyle, Adelhardt, Foley, & Portenoy, 1990; Ng & von Gunten, 1998; Vainio & Auvinen, 1996; Weitzner, Moody, &

Box 25-1 **Principles of Managing Symptoms during the Last 48 Hours of Life**

1. Use problem-solving approach to symptom control.
2. Avoid unnecessary interventions.
3. Review all drugs and symptoms regularly.
4. Maintain effective communication.
5. Ensure support for family and caregivers.

From Adam, J. (1997). ABC of palliative care: The last 48 hours. *British Medical Journal, 315,* 1600-1603.

McMillan, 1997). Hermann and Looney (2001) collected data via retrospective chart reviews (n = 100) to identify the most common symptoms experienced by hospice patients in the last 7 days of life. They also examined interventions to treat the symptoms and the efficacy of these interventions. Their findings (Table 25-1) offer the nurse insight into symptoms that typically are encountered in dying patients as well as potential interventions for management.

As the older adult enters the peri-death phase of life, all drugs should be reviewed with regard to their need and route of administration. Drugs once considered to be essential to maintain life (e.g., antiarrhythmics, diuretics) may no longer be needed or the burden may outweigh the benefit to the patient. Likewise, drugs such as analgesics, sedatives, anticonvulsants, and antiemetics may need to be added to control symptoms the patient is experiencing as he or she approaches death (Adam, 1997). Table 25-2 details the routes and types of drugs typically administered during the last 48 hours of life. Box 25-1 outlines principles of managing symptoms during that time.

Pain (see Chapter 21)

As the body begins to shut down and die, the older adult's need for pain medication may change or decrease. Drugs most often used to manage pain at the end of life are morphine (MS Contin) and morphine sulfate immediate release (MSIR) and oxycodone (OxyContin) (Fields & Cassel, 1997). Long-acting opioids (e.g., transdermal fentanyl, sustained-release morphine) should not be started when the patient is close to death because of a delay in reaching effective blood levels to alleviate the pain and the inability to titrate the drug in situations of uncontrolled pain (Adam, 1997). If the elder is already using fentanyl patches, they should be continued and MSIR should be added to manage breakthrough pain. The liver conjugates these drugs, and the active metabolites remain in the body to exert a pharmacologic effect until metabolized by the kidneys. As the body is dying, renal and hepatic function is compromised and the drugs are very slowly excreted, resulting in increased serum opioid concentrations, increased drowsiness, and mild confusion. A nursing priority should be to keep the elder patient pain free and comfortable, while understanding that the dosage necessary to achieve this goal may be less than what had been previously required for effective pain management (Matzo, 2001).

Older adults and families may need to be educated about the importance and value of pain management during the dying process. The older adult may be accepting of pain relief, but it is not uncommon to hear an elder refuse pain medication because he or she does not want to be "doped up" or may view pain as a way to "atone for sins." Nurses may be concerned that using too high a dose of morphine will result in hastening or causing the death of the patient. Like the nurse, the family members may fear being the person to give the elder the "last dose" of morphine before death (Matzo, 2001).

The role of the nurse in pain management is to assess the level of pain that the older adult is experiencing, as well as the elder's and family's attitudes toward pain, and to assure them that comfort and alleviation of pain are a priority of care. Encouraging patients to report their pain before it becomes intense will prevent unbearable suffering. Determining the adequacy of the pain control and its duration are important assessment factors so that dosages can be appropriately adjusted (Matzo, 2001).

Pain medications frequently cause constipation, so the nurse must be vigilant in assessing bowel function. Caregivers should be encouraged to continue prophylactic bowel regimens to prevent or alleviate constipation and its associated discomfort (Matzo, 2001). Often family members will tell the nurse that, since the patient is not eating, they are not concerned about con-

Table 25-1 **Interventions for Symptoms Documented in Last 7 Days of Life**

Symptom (n)	Intervention	Intervention Used: n (%)	Intervention Effective: n (%)	Intervention Ineffective: n (%)	Effectiveness Not Documented: n (%)
Pain (90)	Morphine concentrate	54 (60%)	39 (72%)	3 (6%)	12 (22%)
	Fentanyl	30 (33%)	17 (57%)	8 (27%)	5 (17%)
	Oxycodone/ acetaminophen	22 (24%)	13 (59%)	7 (32%)	2 (9%)
	OxyContin	18 (20%)	9 (50%)	3 (17%)	6 (33%)
	Morphine SR	11 (12%)	9 (82%)	0 (0%)	2 (18%)
Dyspnea (70)	Oxygen	48 (69%)	6 (13%)	0 (0%)	42 (88%)
	Ativan	17 (24%)	6 (35%)	0 (0%)	11 (65%)
Dysphagia (50)	Change medication route	32 (64%)	1 (3%)	0 (0%)	31 (97%)
	Education	12 (24%)	1 (8%)	0 (0%)	11 (92%)
Terminal congestion (47)	Education	15 (32%)	1 (7%)	1 (7%)	13 (87%)
	Benadryl	13 (28%)	1 (8%)	1 (8%)	11 (85%)
	Change position	7 (15%)	3 (43%)	0 (0%)	4 (57%)
	Suction	6 (13%)	0 (0%)	2 (33%)	4 (67%)
	Elevate HOB	5 (11%)	1 (20%)	0 (0%)	4 (80%)
	Scopolamine	5 (11%)	3 (60%)	1 (20%)	1 (20%)
Constipation (39)	Senokot	16 (41%)	3 (19%)	2 (13%)	11 (69%)
	Bisacodyl	16 (41%)	2 (13%)	1 (6%)	13 (81%)
	Enema	12 (31%)	7 (58%)	1 (8%)	4 (33%)
	Check for impaction	10 (26%)	3 (30%)	2 (20%)	5 (50%)
	Milk of Magnesia	9 (23%)	0 (0%)	2 (22%)	7 (78%)
Bladder incontinence (36)	Insert catheter	15 (42%)	2 (13%)	2 (13%)	11 (73%)
	Diaper	11 (31%)	0 (0%)	0 (0%)	11 (100%)
Terminal restlessness (34)	Ativan	25 (74%)	6 (24%)	0 (0%)	19 (76%)
	Check impaction	6 (18%)	1 (16%)	1 (16%)	4 (67%)
	Check pain	6 (18%)	1 (16%)	0 (0%)	5 (83%)
	Xanax	4 (12%)	0 (0%)	0 (0%)	4 (100%)
Bowel incontinence (31)	Check for impaction	7 (23%)	3 (43%)	2 (29%)	2 (29%)
	Diaper	7 (23%)	0 (0%)	0 (0%)	7 (100%)
	Education	4 (13%)	2 (50%)	0 (0%)	5 (50%)
Nausea/vomiting (22)	Phenergan	8 (36%)	6 (75%)	1 (13%)	1 (13%)
	Compazine	6 (27%)	5 (83%)	1 (17%)	0 (0%)

HOB, head of bed.

From Hermann, C., & Looney, S. (2001). The effectiveness of symptom management in hospice patients during the last 7 days of life. *Journal of Hospice and Palliative Nursing, 3*(3), 88-96.

Table 25-2 **Routes of Administration of Drugs for the Last 48 Hours of Life**

ORAL
All drug types

SUBLINGUAL

Antiemetic	Hyoscine hydrobromide, 0.3 mg/6 hr
	Prochlorperazine, 3-6 mg/12 hr
Sedative or anxiolytic	Lorazepam, 0.5-2 mg/6 hr (fast acting and short duration)

TRANSDERMAL

Opioid	Fentanyl (only if patient already uses patches)
Antiemetic	Hyoscine hydrobromide, 0.5 mg/72 hr (Tranderm Scop)

SUBCUTANEOUS*

Opioid	Morphine (individual dose titration)
Nonsteroidal anti-inflammatory drug	Diclofenac (infusion), 150 mg/24 hr
Antiemetics	Cyclizine, 25-50 mg bolus q8h, up to 150 mg/24 hr
	Metoclopramide,[†] 10 mg bolus q6h, up to 40-80 mg/24 hr
	Hyoscine hydrobromide,[‡] 0.4- to 0.6-mg bolus, up to 2.4 mg/24 hr (also dries secretions)
	Methotrimeprazine,[‡] 25-mg/mL ampule, 6.25- to 25-mg bolus, 6.25 mg titrated up to 250 mg/24 hr (also sedative at higher doses)
Sedative	Haloperidol,[‡] 2.5- to 5-mg bolus, 5-20 mg/24 hr (also useful for confusion with altered sensorium)
	Midazolam,[‡] 2.5- to 10-mg bolus, 5-60 mg/24 hr (anxiolytic at smaller doses, anticonvulsant)
Somatostatin analogue	Octreotide,[‡] 150-600 μg/24 hr (for large-volume vomiting associated with bowel obstruction)

RECTAL

Opioid	Morphine (individual dose every 4 hr)
	Oxycodone, 30-60 mg/8 hr
Nonsteroidal anti-inflammatory drug	Diclofenac, 100 mg once daily
Antiemetic	Prochlorperazine, 25 mg twice daily
	Domperidone, 30-60 mg/6 hr
	Cyclizine, 50 mg/8 hr
	Chlorpromazine, 100 mg/8 hr (equivalent to 50 mg/8 hr orally) (also a sedative)
Sedative	Diazepam (also anxiolytic and anticonvulsant)

*All subcutaneous preparations diluted in sterile water except diclofenac (0.9% saline).
[†]Compatible with morphine but liable to precipitate as concentrations increase.
[‡]Compatible with diamorphine.
Adapted from Adam, J. (1997). ABC of palliative care: The last 48 hours. *British Medical Journal, 315,* 1600-1603.

stipation. Education of the family and professional caregivers regarding the prophylaxis and treatment of constipation cannot be emphasized strongly enough.

Nonpharmacologic interventions that alleviate pain include a calm environment, soothing music, and aromatherapy. Simple human touch or therapeutically intended touch, such as Reiki, can relieve stress, be a source of comfort or support, and help the elder to overcome any fear of abandonment (Matzo, 2001).

Anorexia/Dehydration (see Chapter 23)

As older adults approach the end of life, they may say that they are not hungry, which is a normal predeath finding. Decreased eating results in a metabolic imbalance wherein the energy from nutritional intake does not cover the energy expended, which results in a state of dehydration. Although healthy people experiencing dehydration will report pain, abdominal cramps, nausea, vomiting, and dry mouth, patients who are terminally ill do not report such symptoms. At the end of life, patients typically state that they have a dry mouth, which is often unrelated to hydration status and most often the result of medication side effects, increased respiration, or mouth breathing (Matzo, 2001).

Artificial hydration and nutrition can be construed as nurses and physicians "doing something" at a time when the mistaken perception exists that there is little else that can be done for the older adult. Intravenous fluids given to a person who is actively dying increase urinary output, which may result in the necessity of a Foley catheter. This increased hydration typically will increase respiratory secretions (that may require suctioning), increase cough, and increase gastrointestinal fluids, which can lead to abdominal distention and nausea and/or vomiting (Matzo, 2001).

Increasing the intravascular volume in the presence of decreasing renal function can further result in peripheral edema and increase the incidence of pressure ulcers. Pain can result where the intravenous (IV) line is inserted, and restraints may become necessary to prevent the older adult from removing the tubing. The presence of the IV line may act as a physical barrier to the family and may cause anxiety for them. In summary, artificial nutrition and hydration at the end of life can result in symptoms of congestive heart failure, increased tracheal and bronchial secretions, nausea and vomiting, painful edema, and diarrhea (Gates, 1997) and do little (if anything) to improve symptoms or prolong life (Matzo, 2001).

Conversely, as death nears, there can be many benefits to the older adult in not starting artificial food and fluids. Calorie deprivation results in an increased production of ketones and an elevation of naturally occurring opioid peptides or endorphins that provide analgesia. Electrolyte imbalances, if present, will also result in increased analgesia. Decreased fluid intake reduces pulmonary fluids, which eases respiration, lessens coughing, and alleviates the sensation of drowning. If a tumor is present, it may shrink in the presence of a dehydrated state, decreasing the edematous layer and resulting in less pressure and pain (Matzo, 2001).

Nursing interventions for the older adult related to anorexia and dehydration focus on meticulous mouth care to alleviate mouth dryness and to prevent sores, dental problems, and infections. Meticulous cleaning and ongoing moistening of the mouth can be a vital intervention to prevent suffering in the older adult who is nearing death (IOM, 1997). The mouth and teeth can be cleaned with a soft-bristled toothbrush or sponge-covered oral swabs. To maintain moisture in mucosal membranes, the mouth should be rinsed frequently with water. A spray bottle can be used to mist the mouth often, and a cool mist vaporizer should be run in the elder's room. Commercial salivary substitutes or supplements such as Salivart, Oral Balance, Salagen, and MoiStir can also help keep the patient comfortable. Chamomile tea is very soothing when used to clean the mouth or offered to the patient to sip on. Generously applying lip lubricant can prevent dry, chapped lips and alleviates any associated discomfort (Matzo, 2001).

To treat oral pain, morphine or morphine elixir can be used if the pain is severe, during mouth care, and before meals. Topical agents for mouth pain include lidocaine (Xylocaine Viscous 2% solution), 5 to 15 mL, swish and spit every 2 to 4 hours as needed. KBX solution (Kaopectate, diphenhydramine [Benadryl], and Xylocaine Viscous in equal parts), 5 to 15 mL, swish for 1 minute, then spit or swallow every

EVIDENCE-BASED PRACTICE

Reference: Vig, E. K., Davenport, N. A., & Pearlman, R. A. (2002). Good deaths, bad deaths, and preferences for the end of life: A qualitative study of geriatric outpatients. *Journal of the American Geriatrics Society, 50,* 1541-1548.

Research Problem: Patient involvement in decision making has been advocated to improve the quality of life at the end of life. Although the size of the oldest segment of the population is growing, with greater numbers of older adults facing the end of life, little is known about their preferences for the end of life. This study aimed to explore the attitudes of older adults with medical illness about the end of life, and to investigate whether current values could be extended to end-of-life preferences.

Design: Descriptive study with interviews using open- and closed-ended questions.

Sample and Setting: 16 older men and women attending two university-affiliated geriatric clinics who were identified by their physicians as having nonterminal heart disease or cancer.

Methods: Patients were interviewed in a private conference room near the clinic they attended or in their homes. The interview contained open-ended questions such as: "What are the most important things in your life right now?" and "What would you consider a good/bad death?" The interview also contained closed-ended questions about symptoms, quality of life, and health status. Additional questions elicited preferences for the end of life, such as location of death and the presence of others.

The open-ended questions were tape-recorded, transcribed, and analyzed using qualitative methods. The closed-ended questions were analyzed using descriptive statistics.

Results: Patients with heart disease and cancer provided similar responses. Participants' views about good deaths, bad deaths, and end-of-life scenarios were heterogeneous. Each participant voiced a unique combination of themes in describing good and bad deaths. Because each participant described a multifaceted view of a good death, for instance, no single theme was mentioned by half of the participants. Participants provided differing explanations for why given themes contributed to good deaths. Currently valued aspects of life were not easily translated into end-of-life preferences. For example, although the majority of participants identified their family as being important, many gave reasons why they did not want their family members present when they died.

Implications for Nursing Practice: A thorough understanding of an individual's end-of-life preferences may help health professionals working with older adults develop patient-centered care plans for the end of life.

Conclusion: Because of the heterogeneity of views and the difficulty in inferring end-of-life preferences from current values, older adults should be asked not only questions about general values, but also specific questions about their end-of-life choices and the reasons for these choices.

2 to 4 hours as needed, may also be ordered. The Xylocaine provides topical anesthesia; the Benadryl is a short-acting anesthetic; and the Kaopectate (Mylanta may be substituted) serves as an alkalizing agent (Gates & Fink, 1997; Matzo, 2001).

Swallowing (see Chapter 19)

If the elder is still sipping fluids, he or she should be encouraged to take those fluids that contain salt to help prevent electrolyte imbalance. Fluids such as bouillon, tomato juice, or Pedialyte, or sport drinks such as Gatorade, may be well tolerated. Citrus juices, spicy foods, and extremes of temperature should be avoided because they can irritate the mouth. Families should be told that it is acceptable if the elder does not want to eat or drink and be supported if they have a difficult time accepting this decision on the part of the older adult who is dying.

As death approaches, elder patients may lose their ability to swallow as a result of weakness or a decrease in neurologic function, or secondary to their primary disease process (e.g., Alzheimer's disease). The gag reflex may diminish and secretions will tend to accumulate in the tracheobronchial tree. Positioning with the head of the bed elevated is important to prevent the accumulation of secretions in the back of the throat and upper airways (Ferrell, Virani, & Grant, 1999). Suctioning is usually not recommended because it may result in an increase in secretion production (Ferrell et al., 1999). Anticholinergic medication such as scopolamine transdermal patches, atropine, or hyoscyamine (Levsin, 0.125 mg [1 to 2 tablets] by mouth or sublingually every 6 hours as needed) can be used to decrease secretion production and decrease the occurrence of the "death rattle," which, although it does not distress the patient, can be very upsetting to the family.

Weakness and Fatigue (see Chapter 20)

Fatigue is a primary complaint of patients in the last 4 weeks of life (Gorman, 1998). The tiredness may be a result of both the disease and the treatment for the disease, as well as malnutrition and disrupted sleep patterns. Fatigue may interfere with an elder's ability to move, bathe, or toilet (IOM, 1997).

Skin Care (see Chapter 22)

The nurse should be aware that, although the patient is at high risk for a pressure ulcer, turning and positioning should be done as frequently as possible but only as often as comfort permits. Bony prominences should be padded and supported if this is comfortable for the patient. If any of these interventions results in increased pain or suffering, it should not be implemented. Initially, this may be difficult for the novice nurse to support because it is contrary to the basic nursing skills that he or she has been taught. When a patient is actively dying, intervention goals should focus on comfort; any intervention that compromises this goal should be discontinued (Matzo, 2001).

Dyspnea (see Chapter 17)

Dyspnea is a common symptom experienced at the end of life and results from the lungs' inability to function in proportion to the metabolic demands of the body (IOM, 1997). Shortness of breath is a subjective awareness of being unable to breathe; patients describe the feeling as "agonizing and worse than pain." Terminal dyspnea occurs in as many as 75% of patients in the peri-death period; elders and their families should be warned that changes in respiration are normal prior to death and should be anticipated (LaDuke, 2001, p. 26).

The breathing pattern can become irregular and include shallow breathing alternating with apnea lasting 5 to 60 seconds (Cheyne-Stokes breathing). Cheyne-Stokes respirations are not treated and indicate that death is imminent.

Gasping respirations, or agonal breathing, is the last respiratory pattern prior to terminal apnea. How long this phase lasts varies from elder to elder, but it can be as short as a couple of breaths before death to gasping that lasts minutes or hours (Perkin & Resnik, 2002). This breathing pattern should be considered burdensome to the dying elder and should be treated with opioids. End-stage stridor is treated with anxiolytics and opioids (Adam, 1997).

Nursing interventions for dyspnea include positioning the patient with the head of the bed raised and/or turning the person on one side to optimize breathing. Oxygen is typically only effective if the dyspnea is secondary to hypoxia (e.g., chronic obstructive pulmonary disease, pulmonary fibrosis), although it may provide a placebo effect (Horn, 1992). If the elder has a dry cough or sticky secretions, nebulized 0.9% saline can be helpful (but should be avoided if bronchospasms are present or if the elder is unable to expectorate) (Adam, 1997). A fan blowing a gentle breeze toward the patient's face can relieve feelings of breathlessness. Emotion-focused interventions such as relaxation techniques, prayer and meditation, and distraction may alleviate the anxiety often associated with dyspnea (Horn, 1992; Matzo, 2001). Box 25-2 lists techniques useful for management of breathlessness.

During the last hours of life, opioids are the cornerstone of the management of dyspnea and agonal breathing; benzodiazepines are an appropriate adjuvant therapy if the dyspnea is exacerbated by anxiety (LaDuke, 2001). Morphine alleviates dyspnea by altering the feeling of breathlessness, decreasing anxiety, and therefore decreasing oxygen demand. It also has a dilating effect on the pulmonary vessels, which will

---

Box 25-2 Management of Breathlessness

1. Reverse what is reversible
2. General supportive measures—explanation, position, breathing exercises, fans or cool airflow, relaxation techniques
3. Oxygen therapy
4. Opioid
5. Benzodiazepine
6. Hyoscine
7. Nebulized saline (if no bronchospasm and patient able to expectorate)

From Adam, J. (1997). ABC of palliative care: The last 48 hours. *British Medical Journal, 315*, 1600-1603.

---

increase oxygen supply and decrease lung congestion (LaDuke, 2001). For opioid-naive patients, low-dose opiates such as morphine, 5 mg by mouth or in the buccal cavity every 4 hours, can alleviate the sensation of breathlessness. Nebulized morphine and fentanyl may also be effective. If morphine is already being used for pain, an increase of 2.5 times the regular dose is generally effective (Matzo, 2001).

Multisystem Failure

As the body is shutting down, a decrease in blood perfusion results in shutdown of the major organs (e.g., renal and hepatic). Decreased cardiac output and intravascular volume result in tachycardia and hypotension. The body will attempt to conserve blood volume for the perfusion of vital organs, resulting in peripheral cooling (as the body conserves heat), and peripheral and central cyanosis. The skin may therefore become mottled and discolored, which is normal before death.

Urine output is greatly diminished, and there can be a loss of sphincter control resulting in urinary and/or fecal incontinence. It may be a good idea to insert a urinary catheter to reduce the need for frequent bedding changes and to prevent skin breakdown. The catheter also helps the continent patient conserve energy by removing the need to use a bedpan or urinal.

Neurologic dysfunction is a result of multiple, concurrent, and nonreversible organ failure. Consequently the patient may experience reduced cerebral perfusion, hypoxemia, metabolic imbalances, acidosis, accumulation of toxins from renal and hepatic failure, and sepsis (Ferrell et al., 1999). The net effect of these changes may be a decreased level of consciousness or terminal delirium.

Terminal Delirium (see Chapter 18)

Terminal delirium can be manifested as confusion, anxiety, agitation, or restlessness and occurs in 28% to 83% of patients near the end of life (Casarett & Inouye, 2001). Confusion is a mental state in which a person reacts inappropriately to his or her environment because of being confounded or disoriented. It may be the side effect of medications or be caused by the dying process itself (IOM, 1997). Anxiety is the biologic and emotional reaction to stressful situations, including the approach of death. The patient may experience dread, anger, or tension, with somatic complaints that include shortness of breath, nausea, and diarrhea (IOM, 1997). The nurse may misinterpret moaning, grimacing, agitation, and restlessness as pain (Ferrell et al., 1999). The patient may be restless and make repetitive motions (e.g., pulling on clothing or the sheets) (Matzo, 2001).

According to Casarett and Inouye (2001), delirium impedes good end-of-life care for four primary reasons: (1) it is frightening to patients and can cause as much distress as pain for them; (2) families are distressed when the patient can no longer communicate; (3) delirium is predictive of impending death; and (4) delirium robs the elder of the ability to make final choices. Prompt recognition and management of delirium will improve the elder patient's comfort and enhance the death experience for all who are involved.

Nursing interventions to manage terminal delirium should focus on the treatment of the underlying physical cause if it is practical and possible. Determining the cause of the delirium must be balanced with the elder patient's goals of care, the burden of the evaluation on the elder, and the likelihood that a treatable cause will be found (Casarett & Inouye, 2001). The goal of any intervention for delirium in the peri-death period is to bring the elder close to his or her baseline mental status with as little sedation as possible. Box 25-3 lists usual starting doses for pharmacologic management of delirium, although there are few evidence-based studies to support the use of these drugs (Casarett & Inouye, 2001).

Box 25-3 **Pharmacologic Management of Delirium: Usual Starting Doses***

PREDOMINANTLY NEUROLEPTIC EFFECTS

- Haloperidol, 0.5-1 mg every 30 minutes orally (0.5-1 mg every 30 minutes subcutaneously or intravenously, titrate to effect, usual maximal dose not to exceed 3 mg/24 hr)
- Olanzapine, 2.5-5 mg orally once daily
- Risperidone, 0.5 mg orally twice daily

PREDOMINANTLY SEDATIVE EFFECTS

- Lorazepam, 0.5-1 mg every 4 hr orally, subcutaneously, or intravenously
- Propofol, 10-mg bolus followed by 10 mg/hr intravenously
- Midazolam, 1-2 mg/hr subcutaneously or intravenously

*Titrate dose to effect in all regimens.
Adapted from Casarett, D. J., & Inouye, S. K. (2001). Diagnosis and management of delirium near the end of life. *Annals of Internal Medicine, 135,* 32-40.

Box 25-4 **Causes of Restlessness and Confusion**

1. Drugs—such as opioids, corticosteroids, neuroleptics, alcohol (intoxication and withdrawal)
2. Physical—unrelieved pain, distended bladder or bowel, immobility or exhaustion, cerebral lesions, infection, hematological, major organ failure
3. Metabolic upset—urea, calcium, sodium, glucose, hypoxia
4. Anxiety and distress

From Adam, J. (1997). ABC of palliative care: The last 48 hours. *British Medical Journal, 315,* 1600-1603.

Benzodiazepines are typically not advocated as a first-line treatment in the management of delirium near the end of life; sedation is a typical side effect that is usually unacceptable to elders and their families. Should sedation be the goal, chlorpromazine is a better choice because of its sedative effect with less risk for respiratory depression (Casarett & Inouye, 2002).

In general, haloperidol offers the best balance of effectiveness and toxicity. It has been suggested that imbalance or hyperactivity in the dopaminergic system (Casarett & Inouye, 2002) or opioid toxicity (Adam, 1997) may contribute to delirium (Box 25-4). Therefore, a dopamine-blocking agent such as haloperidol demonstrates beneficial effects for the hallucinations, delusions, paranoia, confusion, restlessness, and agitation that can accompany delirium at the end of life.

The family can be advised to continue to talk to the older adult and calm him or her with their words; familiar faces can be very comforting during this time. Maintaining a calm environment and offering spiritual comfort and emotional support are vital in the peri-death period. Light massage is effective. It may be suggested that the number of people in the room be limited if there is a great deal of activity. Refraining from asking the elder patient many questions can also diminish agitation (Matzo, 2001). Distress or anxiety may be helped by diazepam or midazolam, but the nurse should bear in mind that the elder may be experiencing spiritual or emotional distress that will not be relieved by medications (Adams, 1997).

Eventually the elder's level of consciousness will decrease and he or she may even become unarousable. This can be a very upsetting time for families because the elder patient may seem unresponsive and withdrawn; the fact that this is a normal aspect of the dying process should be reinforced. At this time the older adult is starting to "let go" in preparation for death, detaching from relationships and the physical environment. The dying patient may ask to be with only one person toward the end or seem distant from the family. A dying elder may talk about seeing people who have already died, talk about taking a trip with a long-deceased relative, or describe feeling separate from his or her body. This is a normal experience and is not considered a hallucination (Matzo, 2001).

Even if the elder patient is unresponsive, the nurse should encourage family members to talk with him or her. Assume that the patient hears everything that is said; this is the time for loved ones to say "good-bye," "I'm sorry," "I love you," or "thank you." The patient may have difficulty letting go, and the nurse may need to encourage the family to give the patient "permission" to die. Encourage the family to show affection to the patient, touch the patient, and let the patient know that he or she will be missed (Matzo, 2001).

Terminal Sedation

Sedation for the imminently dying person is an intervention to relieve intractable symptoms of patients who are suffering at the end of their life. It involves the definitive decision to make the dying elder "unconscious to prevent or respond to otherwise unrelievable physical distress" (Quill & Byock, 2000, p. 409), but not to intentionally end his or her life. This intervention should only occur when the symptoms or suffering cannot be relieved in any other way.

Jansen and Sulmasy (2002) differentiated sedation of the imminently dying from "sedation toward death," and see these two practices as morally distinct from each other. Sedation of the imminently dying is a practice in which

1) the patient is close to death (hours, days, or at most a few weeks); 2) the patient has one or more severe symptoms that are refractory to standard palliative care; 3) the patient's physician or advanced practice nurse vigorously treats these symptoms with therapy known to be efficacious; 4) this therapy has a dose-dependent side effect of sedation that is a foreseen but unintended consequence of trying to relieve the patient's symptoms; and 5) this therapy may be coupled with the withholding or withdrawing of life-sustaining treatments that are ineffective or disproportionately burdensome. (p. 845)

This type of sedation fulfills the conditions set forth in the rule of double effect (see Chapter 5) and is considered to be morally justifiable. These authors define sedation toward death as

a practice in which 1) the patient need not be imminently dying; 2) the symptoms believed to be refractory to treatment are simply the consciousness that one is not yet dead; 3) the patient's physician or advanced practice nurse selects therapy intended to render the patient unconscious as a means of treating the refractory symptoms; and 4) other life-sustaining treatments are withdrawn to hasten death. (p. 845)

The aim of the health care practitioner in this case is to cause the patient to be unconscious and to shorten life.

Indications for terminal sedation are uncontrolled physical suffering, such as intractable pain, dyspnea, seizures, or delirium. Table 25-3 offers general guidelines for terminal sedation, and Table 25-4 lists medications and guidelines for their use in sedating an imminently dying patient. The level of sedation that eliminates objective signs of discomfort is maintained until the elder dies; death will typically occur within hours or days of the initiation of sedation (Quill & Byock, 2000). There is no literature to support the belief that imminently dying patients die quicker when sedated to control intractable symptoms. Panke (2002) suggested that patients with unrelieved symptoms may die sooner secondary to "increased physiologic stress, diminished immunocompetence, decreased mobility, increased risk of thromboembolism and pneumonia, increased difficulty breathing, and greater myocardial oxygen requirements" (p. 31).

Terminal sedation requires participation of the entire health care team for monitoring the elder and support of the family. The sedation is maintained by continuous subcutaneous or intravenous infusion. Opioids that have already been initiated for pain and other symptoms should be continued to prevent unobservable pain or opioid withdrawal, but opioids should not be used to maintain the sedation itself (Quill & Byock, 2000).

Affirming Life and Maintaining Hope

Three goals that the palliative care nurse should strive to meet when working with dying older adults are (1) helping them live their lives to the fullest until they die; (2) preventing indignity, and (3) encouraging hope. The nurse can help the patient live until he or she dies by encouraging socialization, listening, being honest, and helping the elder finish any unfinished business. By offering patients choices regarding routines, food, and activities, nurses promote continued independence and the ability to help maintain control over one's life. The elder's degree of independence is contingent upon his or her energy levels, family and social support, and ability. The wishes of the older adult as he or she approaches death should be respected, even if these choices are inconsistent with the family's or health care provider's values (Birchenall & Streight, 1997; Matzo, 2001).

Quality of life is a concept that is often discussed in relation to the experience of dying and

Table 25-3 General Guidelines for Terminal Sedation

Guideline Domain	Terminal Sedation
Palliative care	Must be available, in place, and unable to adequately relieve current suffering.
Usual patient characteristics	Severe, immediate, or otherwise unrelievable symptoms (e.g., pain, shortness of breath nausea, vomiting, seizures, delirium) or to prevent severe suffering (e.g., suffocation sensation when mechanical ventilation is discontinued).
Terminal prognosis	Usually days to weeks.
Patient informed consent	Patient should be competent and fully informed or noncompetent with severe, otherwise irreversible suffering (clinician should use advance directive or consensus about patient wishes and best interests).
Family participation in decision	Clinician should strongly encourage input from and consensus of immediate family members.
Incompetent patient	Can be used for severe, persistent suffering with the informed consent of the patient's designated proxy and family members. If no surrogate is available, team members and consultants should agree that no other acceptable palliative therapies are available.
Second opinion(s)	Should be obtained from an expert in palliative care and a mental health expert (if uncertainty exists about patient's mental capacity).
Health care practitioner participation in decision	Input from staff involved in immediate patient care activities is encouraged; physician and staff consent is required for their own participation.

Adapted from Quill, T. E., & Byock, I. R. (2000). Responding to intractable terminal suffering: The role of terminal sedation and voluntary refusal of food and fluids. *Annals of Internal Medicine, 132,* 408-414.

death. It should be acknowledged, though, that quality of life is a different concept than quality of death. The peri-death period brings with it challenges, and often indignities, that are unique to the actual act of dying. Dignity is considered a personal quality, one that the health care professional can neither give nor take away. What nurses are able to do for their older adult patients who are dying is to ensure that they die without *indignity*—those transgressions that include unrelieved symptoms and pain, or that exclude the elder from decisions regarding his or her own living and dying (Allmark, 2002).

Hope is a vital component in the emotional stages of dying and death and was a factor in helping the elder and his or her family cope during the challenging months and years that led up to death. Hope supports the spirit of each individual older adult and gives him or her the courage and strength to go on. Typically, as the elder reaches the beginning of the dying process, what he or she hopes for may change, but hope does not end. At the beginning of the illness, the elder may have hoped for a "miracle"—that he or she would have been completely cured; it is not acceptable for the nurse to take this hope away or to tell the patient and family to be "realistic." As the disease progressed, the hope may have changed from that of cure to the hope of eating a full meal, a visit from a favorite friend, or less pain (Matzo, 2001).

Persons with hope have been found to live longer and have a better quality of life than those who are hopeless (Birchenall & Streight, 1997). The nurse should be an active participant in the end-of-life experience for the elder patient and

Table 25-4 **Medications Used in Terminal Sedation***

Medication	Type	Usual Starting Dosage	Usual Maintenance Dosage	Route
Midazolam	Rapid, short-acting benzodiazepine	0.5-1.5 mg/hr after bolus of 0.5 mg	30-100 mg/day	Intravenous or subcutaneous
Lorazepam	Benzodiazepine	1-4 mg q4-6h orally or dissolved buccally; infusion of 0.5-1.0 mg/hr intravenously	4-40 mg/day	Oral, buccal, subcutaneous, or intravenous
Propofol	General anesthetic; ultrarapid onset and elimination	5-10 mg/hr; bolus doses of 20-50 mg may be administered for urgent sedation, but continuous infusion is required	10-200 mg/day	Intravenous
Thiopental	Ultrashort-acting barbiturate	5-7 mg/kg of body weight to induce unconsciousness	Initial rate may range from 20 to 80 mg/hr; average maintenance rates range between 70 and 180 mg/hr	Intravenous
Pentobarbital	Long-acting barbiturate	2-3 mg/kg, slow infusion, to induce unconsciousness	1 mg/hr, increasing as needed to maintain sedation	Intravenous
Phenobarbital	Long-acting barbiturate	200-mg loading dose, repeated every 10-15 minutes until patient is comfortable	Approximately 50 mg/hr	Intravenous or subcutaneous

Goal of treatment is to relieve suffering by inducing sedation. Dosage should be increased by approximately 30% every hour until sedation is achieved. Once desired level of sedation is achieved, infusion is usually maintained at that level as long as the patient seems comfortable. If symptoms return, dosages should be increased in 30% increments until sedation is achieved. The ranges above are representative. Individual patients may require lower or higher doses to achieve the desired goal. Previous doses of opioids and other symptom-relieving medications should be continued.

*Adapted from Quill, T. E., & Byock, I. R. (2000). Responding to intractable terminal suffering: The role of terminal sedation and voluntary refusal of food and fluids. *Annals of Internal Medicine, 132*, 408-414.

his or her family. People typically want companionship in the face of death, especially as they face the dualism of trying to maintain hope and accepting that their life is coming to an end (Finucane, 2002). The nursing role includes supporting their feelings as they experience the dying process. Listening and caring for their needs are important nursing functions at this time of life (Matzo, 2001).

Dying in a Nursing Home

Even though 1 in 5 older adults dies in a nursing home, the last hours of life for an older adult whose home is a long-term care facility may not include actually dying in that environment. Hospitalization of terminally ill nursing home residents is common and quite often inappropriate. Miller, Gozalo, and Mor (2001) looked at Minimum Data Set assessments from the Health

Care Financing Administration to determine rates of hospitalization of elders utilizing the Medicare hospice benefit. In the 30 days before death, 24% (n = 2208) of those elders receiving hospice care and 44% (n = 12,100) of the non-hospice group were hospitalized.

In a comparative analysis of deceased nursing home resident records, Happ and colleagues (2002) found that those elders with hospice referrals and palliative care interventions did not receive these services until the week before their death. Most of the elder residents in the sample died without their family present and with little documentation of pain or symptom management.

Family Support during the Last Hours of Life

Supporting the family during the last hours of the patient's life is an important nursing role. When possible, one nurse should be assigned to be with the family through the last phase of life. Enough time with the dying person should be given to the family so that they have the opportunity to resolve any final interpersonal issues. If the death is occurring at home, the family should have access to a Symptom Relief Kit with detailed, easy-to-understand instructions for its use (Fig. 25-2). Depending on cultural and religious considerations, the family should be afforded privacy and clergy support. The primary nurse should communicate with the family regarding what they can expect the dying process to be like and how they will know when the person has died.

Many people have not been with someone who is actively dying and do not know what to expect. Even though no two deaths are alike, it helps to give significant others an idea of what the final stage of life may be like and the symptoms that they may see during this period. Box 25-5 presents an information sheet written for the general public regarding the dying process and is a good source of information for families (Matzo, 2001).

Signs of Death

Objective indications of death include stopping of heartbeat and respiration, release of bowel and bladder, eyelids slightly open and not blinking, pupils fixed and dilated, body temperature falling, the jaw relaxed and slightly open, and no response from the patient. As the blood settles in the body, the color turns to a waxen pallor. These

signs do not occur in any order, and it may take a few minutes for the body to completely shut down. If the death occurs at home, the family should be told that it is not an emergency situation; they should be given a number to call to inform the hospice staff or their physician of the elder's death. The body does not have to be moved immediately; the family should not feel rushed or pressured to act until they are ready to do so (Ferrell et al., 1999; Matzo, 2001).

PERI-DEATH RITUALS AND CUSTOMS

Throughout the dying process, and particularly at the very end of life, the nurse must be aware of cultural and religious values, practices, and traditions of the older adult patient and his or her family. The family's customs and rituals will have an immense significance in the healing process following death, and the grief response is often structured by these rituals. The nurse's role is to ask the family what rituals are important to them and to help the family carry out the rites and practices that provide solace and support. The nurse should be open-minded and accepting of the physical, psychosocial, and spiritual needs of the dying elder patient and his or her family, and offer them respect and privacy (Matzo, 2001; Purnell & Paulanka, 1998).

The following sections regarding religion and culture are meant as a reference for the reader to guide assessment. The nurse should be cautious not to make generalizations about any ethnic or religious group. Many people blend practices or have their own interpretations of traditional rituals. The only way for the health care practitioner to know how best to assist the grieving family is to ask them about their practices and beliefs regarding dying, death, burial, and bereavement.

Religious Practices

Traditions of Christianity

The Western divisions of Christianity are Protestant and Catholic. Protestant funeral practices vary, although most services take place in a church sanctuary. There is a belief in heaven and hell. Catholic priests will give the Sacrament of the Anointing of the Sick, which in the past was called the Last Rites. This sacrament is for those who are seriously ill. The family, friends, and priest gather at the bedside to pray for healing. If it is God's will that the person not recover from illness, then the prayer is that God will accompany the dying person toward the rewards of heaven (Miller, 1993). The priest would hear the patient's confession of sins, make absolution, and offer the Sacrament of the Anointing of the Sick. The nurse can ask the family if they would like the priest to be called. The comfort that this ritual can bring to the dying Catholic and family cannot be underestimated.

Autopsy and organ donations are accepted options. There is no formal preparation of the body; funeral practices vary according to culture and individual preferences. Many Catholics today still believe that the Church forbids cremation. This was true prior to Vatican II; the Judaic roots of Christian tradition carried a long-standing prohibition of cremation as a reaction to equally long-standing attempts to eliminate Jewish traditions (Archdiocese of San Antonio, 2002).

Text continued on p. 517

Health Care Provider Information Sheet—Symptom Relief Kit

- For signs/symptoms of **pain or dyspnea**: Morphine solution,* 0.25–0.5 mL (20-mg/mL solution) PO/SL q2 h PRN. May increase up to 1–2 mL q1–2h PRN as directed by the health care provider.
- For loud, **wet respirations or excessive secretions**: Hyoscyamine (Levsin), 0.125 mg (1–2 tablets) PO/SL q6h PRN.
- For **unrelieved respiratory fluid accumulation**: Furosemide (Lasix), 40 mg IV/IM/PO/SC. May repeat.
- For **nausea or vomiting**: Prochlorperazine, 25-mg suppository PR q8h PRN. If not effective, give ABH† Suppository PR q8h PRN.
- For severe agitation or restlessness:
  - Determine if client is in pain and treat accordingly.
  - Determine if client is constipated or having urinary retention; take appropiate action.
- If agitation persists, administer pentobarbital suppository PR q6h PRN

*Clients taking opioids for pain will need to increase their usual morphine dose (for breakthrough pain) for effective treatment of dyspnea.

†ABH suppository = Ativan (lorazepam), Benadryl (diphenhydramine), and Haldol (haloperidol). Reglan (metoclopramide) may be added by the pharmacist for severe nausea/vomiting; this would become an ABHR suppository.

Information Sheet for Patients and Families—Symptom Relief Kit

The **Symptom Relief Kit** is designed to help you cope with physical problems that might unexpectedly arise. In the kit:

- **Liquid Morphine**: There are 4 syringes with caps for pain or difficulty breathing. It is given by mouth or can be inserted rectally.
  There are 4 kinds of suppositories in 4 differently labeled bags:
- **Prochlorperazine** (which is the active ingredient in **Compazine**). Use this for nausea with or without vomiting.
- **ABH** (this stands for Ativan, Benadryl, and Haldol). This is used for severe nausea and vomiting. It may also be used if the patient is very restless or anxious and may cause the patient to be very sleepy.
- **Pentobarbital** is used for severe agitation or seizures and will make the patient very sleepy.
- **Acetaminophen** is used for high fevers.
- **Levsin** tablets are used for noisy, wet, "gurgly" breathing sounds. They can help to dry up secretions.
- **Furosemide (Lasix)**: There are 2 syringes with caps for severe difficulty breathing because of fluid buildup. The nurse will visit and give this medicine to the patient if you have not been taught how to give "shots."

If you feel that you need to use this kit, call the hospice nurse first. You don't have to do this alone; we are here to help you. Take a moment for yourself, take a deep breath, and then call us.

Fig. 25-2 Health care provider information sheet–symptom relief kit. (Courtesy Elliot Home Health and Hospice, Manchester, NH.)

Continued

Directions for Using the Contents of the Symptom Relief Kit

SYMPTOM	DRUG	HOW TO USE IT
Unrelieved Pain	Morphine solution	1–2 mL in the mouth, under the tongue, every 2–3 hours as needed.
Unrelieved Shortness of Breath	Morphine solution	0.25–0.5 mL in the mouth, under the tongue, every 2 hours as needed.
Nausea & Vomiting	Prochlorperazine suppository	One suppository inserted into the rectum every 8 hours as needed.
Unrelieved Nausea & Vomiting or Restlessness & Anxiety	ABH Suppository	One suppository inserted into the rectum every 8 hours as needed.
Severe Agitation & Restlessness	Pentobarbital suppository	One suppository inserted into the rectum every 4–6 hours as needed.
Wet, "Gurgly" Breathing	Levsin tablets	One or two in the mouth or under the tongue every 4–6 hours as needed.
Unrelieved Accumulation & Respiratory Distress	Furosemide injection	Inject 40–80 mg as instructed by the nurse.
Fever	Acetaminophen suppository	One suppository inserted into the rectum every 4 hours as needed.

Fig. 25-2, cont'd.

Box 25-5 Final Stages–Dying Process

When a person enters the final stage of the dying process, two different dynamics are at work. On the physical plane, the body begins the final process of shutting down, which will end when all the physical systems cease to function. Usually this is an orderly, progressive series of physical changes that are not medical emergencies. These physical changes are the natural way in which the body prepares itself to stop. The most appropriate kinds of responses are comfort-enhancing measures.

The other dynamic of the dying process is emotional and spiritual in nature. The "spirit" of the dying person begins the final process of release from the body, its immediate environment, and all attachments. This release also tends to follow its own priorities, which may include the resolution of whatever is *unfinished* of a practical nature and exercising permission from family members to "let go." The most appropriate kinds of responses to the emotional/spiritual changes are those that support and encourage this release and transition.

When a person's body is ready and wanting to stop, but the person is still unresolved or is not reconciled about some important issue or relationship, the person may tend to linger in order to finish whatever needs finishing. On the other hand, when a person is emotionally/spiritually resolved and ready for this release, but his/her body has not completed its final physical process, the person will continue to live until the physical shutdown is completed.

The experience we call "death" occurs when the body and the spirit complete the natural process of shutting down, reconciling, and finishing. These processes need to happen in a way appropriate and unique to the values, beliefs, and lifestyle of the dying person.

The physical and emotional/spiritual signs and symptoms of impending death that follow are offered

Box 25-5 **Final Stages—Dying Process—cont'd**

to help you understand the natural kinds of things that may happen and how you can respond appropriately. Not all these signs and symptoms will occur with every person, nor will they occur in this particular sequence. Each person is unique and needs your full acceptance, support, and comfort.

PHYSICAL SIGNS AND SYMPTOMS

The following signs and symptoms are indicative of how the body prepares itself for the final stage of life:

Coolness: The person's hands, arms, feet, and legs may be increasingly cool. At the same time, the color of the skin may change. The underside of the body may become darker and the skin mottled or discolored. This is a normal indication that the circulation of blood is decreasing to the body's extremities and being reserved for the most vital organs. Keep the person warm with a nonelectric blanket.

Sleeping: The person may spend an increasing amount of time sleeping and appear to be uncommunicative or unresponsive, at times difficult to arouse. This normal change is due in part to changes in the metabolism of the body. Sit with your loved one, and speak softly and naturally. Plan to spend time when the person seems most alert and awake. Try not to talk as if the person were not there. Speak directly as you normally would, even though there may be no response. Never assume the person cannot hear; hearing is the last of the senses to be lost.

Fluid and Food Decrease: The person may have a decrease in appetite and thirst, wanting little or no food or fluid. The body will naturally begin to conserve energy that would be expended on these tasks. Do not try to force food or drink into the person. To use guilt or manipulation only makes the person more uncomfortable. Small chips of ice, frozen Gatorade, or juice may be refreshing in the mouth. If the person is able to swallow, fluids may be given in small amounts by syringe (ask the hospice nurse for guidance). Swabs moistened with water may help keep the mouth and lips moist and comfortable. A cool, moist washcloth on the forehead may also increase physical comfort.

Incontinence: Control of urine and/or bowels may be lost as the muscles in that area begin to relax. Discuss with your hospice nurse what can be done to protect the bed and keep your loved one clean and comfortable. If it would make the person more comfortable, the nurse may suggest a catheter to drain the bladder into a collection bag. The person's normal urine output may decrease and become dark due to the decrease in circulation through the kidneys.

Congestion: The person may have gurgling sounds coming from the chest as though marbles were rolling around inside. These sounds may become very loud. This normal change is due to the decrease of fluid intake and the inability to cough up normal secretions. The sound of the congestion does not indicate the onset of severe or new pain. Suctioning usually increases the secretions and should be avoided. The nurse or home health aide can show you how to keep the mouth clean with "touthettes" (mouth sponges moistened with water).

Breathing Pattern Change: The person's regular breathing pattern may change and become irregular, e.g., shallow breaths with periods of no breathing for 5 to 30 seconds and up to a full minute. This is called Cheyne-Stokes breathing. The person may also experience periods of rapid, shallow panting. Elevating the head and/or turning the person on one side may bring comfort. Use your hands to touch and soothe. Speak gently.

Disorientation: The person may seem to be confused about the time, place, and identity of people, including those close and familiar. This is due in part to changes in metabolism. Identify yourself by name before you speak rather than asking the person to guess who you are. Speak softly, clearly, and truthfully when you need to communicate something important, such as, "It's time to take your medication," and explain the reason for the communication, such as, "So you won't begin to hurt." Never use this method to try to manipulate the person to meet your own needs or values. It may be difficult to make this distinction.

Restlessness: The person may make restless and repetitive motions, such as pulling at bed linen or clothing. This often happens and is due to the decrease in oxygen circulation to the brain and to metabolism changes. Do not interfere with or try to restrain such motions. Occasionally the person may twitch or make jerking motions. This may have to do with medication or the disease itself. Sometimes other medication helps decrease this twitching. To have a calming effect, speak in a

Continued

Box 25-5 **Final Stages–Dying Process–cont'd**

quiet, natural way, lightly massage the forehead, back or arms, read to the person, or play some soothing music. Try to decrease the number of people around the person. Asking a lot of questions may increase the person's agitation.

EMOTIONAL SYMPTOMS AND RESPONSES

Withdrawal: The person may seem unresponsive, withdrawn, or in a comatose-like state. This indicates preparation for release, a detaching from surroundings and relationships, and a beginning of "letting go." Since hearing remains almost all the way to the end, now is the time to say whatever you need to say that will help the person let go. The person may only want to be with a very few or even just one person. This is another sign of preparation for release. If you are not part of this "inner circle" at the end, it does not mean you are not loved or are unimportant. It means you have already fulfilled your tasks, and it is time for you to say "good-bye."

Vision-like experiences: The person may speak or claim to have spoken to persons who have already died, or to see places not presently accessible or visible to you. This does not indicate hallucinations or a drug reaction. The person is beginning to detach from this life and is preparing for the transition. Do not contradict, explain, belittle, or argue about what the person claims to have seen or heard. Affirm the experiences. They are normal and natural.

Letting Go: The person may continue to perform repetitive and restless tasks. This may indicate that something is still unresolved or unfinished and preventing the letting go. The hospice team can assist you in identifying what may be happening and help the person find release from tension or fear. As hard as it might be, you need to give the person permission to let go.

Saying Good-Bye: When the person is ready to die, and you are able to let go, saying "good-bye" is your final gift of love. It achieves closure and makes the final release possible. It may be helpful to hold or touch the person and say the things you want to say. It may be as simple (or as complicated) as saying, "I love you." It may include recounting favorite memories, places, and activities you shared. It may include saying "I'm sorry for whatever I've done to cause any tensions or difficulty." You may also want to say "Thank you." Tears are a normal and natural part of saying "good-bye."

You don't need to apologize for them or try to hide them. They are a natural expression of your sadness and loss. It is all right to say, "I will miss you so much."

HOW WILL YOU KNOW WHEN DEATH HAS OCCURRED?

Although you may be prepared for the dying process, you may not be prepared for the actual moment. It may be helpful for you and your family to think about and discuss what you would do if you were alone when the death occurs. The death of a hospice patient is expected and is not an emergency. Nothing must be done immediately. The signs of death include such things as

- No heartbeat
- Release of bowel and bladder
- No response
- Eyelids slightly open
- Pupils enlarged
- Eyes fixed on a certain spot
- No blinking
- Jaw relaxed and mouth slightly open

You may now notify a hospice nurse or the on-call nurse as you have been instructed. The nurse will make the pronouncement and notify your physician. The body does not have to be moved until you are ready. The nurse can call the funeral home, but you or a member of your family will probably need to speak with the funeral director.

LATER ON

Hospice staff and volunteers continue to be available to support you and your family through the bereavement program. We will contact you a week or so after the death has occurred, after all the "busyness" is over and the visitors have gone. If you need or want to communicate with us before then, please do not hesitate to call. Even if you just need a place to go for comfort and support, call or stop in.

We salute you for all you have done during this difficult time. We know it has been an enormous commitment and a true act of love. We feel honored to have shared this experience with you in spite of your pain. You accompanied someone you love as far as you could on life's final journey. We hope you feel good about what you've done. We hope this feeling will sustain you, give you courage, and allow you eventually to go on with your life.

Courtesy Elliot Home Health and Hospice, Manchester, NH.

The reforms of the Second Vatican Council touched all areas in the life of the Church, including funeral and burial rites. The first document to be promulgated by Pope Paul VI, after the Council, indicated that the rite for the burial of the dead should be more in keeping with the wishes of the individual and correspond more closely to the circumstances and traditions found in various regions. An instruction of the Holy Office related specifically to cremation modified the Church's position to allow cremation to be requested for any sound reason. Only if the request were motivated by denial of Christian ideology, hatred of the Catholic Church, or a heretic spirit would there be denial from the Church (Archdiocese of San Antonio, 2002).

The Church prefers that the body of the deceased be present for the funeral rites; masses with cremated remains present can be performed. When cremated remains are present, they must be contained in a "worthy vessel," placed on a table or in the place normally occupied by the casket, and must be covered with a pall. The Easter Candle may be present. The words in the blessing and the dismissal would be changed for cremation; the prayer of committal would read "earthly remains" in place of "body" (Archdiocese of San Antonio, 2002).

The cremated remains should be treated with respect and buried in a grave or entombed in a mausoleum or columbarium out of respect for the human body. Scattering at sea, from the air, or from the ground, or keeping the remains at home is not considered reverent disposition. The Church still recommends burial or inurnment in a Catholic cemetery. Throughout the history of the Church, the Catholic cemetery has served as a visible sign of the faith community, attesting to the dignity of the baptized and the promise of the Resurrection (Archdiocese of San Antonio, 2002). Mourning has traditionally been expected to be kept to a minimum with the view that people should "get on with their lives" (Bhungalia & Kemp, 2002).

Hindu Traditions

With respect to end-of-life care, many Hindu patients prefer to die at home because death in the hospital can be very distressing. It is important for elders to complete unfinished business and resolve relationships. Dying full of anger is believed to lead to a lower level of rebirth than dying with love and acceptance. Family members may be present in large numbers near the time of death. Chanting, prayer, and incense are part of the rituals of the dying process. Symptoms may not be reported because it is believed that suffering is inevitable and the result of karma; many seek a conscious dying process without mental clouding from medications.

A Hindu who is dying may request holy rites before death; readings and hymns from holy books are also comforting. Some may wish to lie on the floor to symbolize their closeness to the earth. A Hindu priest (Brahmin) would administer the holy rites, which may include tying a thread around the wrists or neck of the dying person and placing a sacred tulsi leaf in his or her mouth. Sacred ash may be applied to the forehead, and a few drops of water from the Ganges River (or Ganga Ma) may be placed in the dying person's mouth, while a mantra is softly chanted in the patient's right ear. As death approaches, a lamp may be placed near the patient's head. Some Hindus may wish to return to India to die, especially to the holy city of Banaras; many believe that to die here ensures a rebirth in Heaven or even a release from continued rebirth (Matzo, 2001).

After death, the family should be the only one to touch the body, and, ideally, a family member of the same sex should clean the body. If it is necessary for a non-Hindu to touch the deceased, this should be done as little as possible (especially the head) and disposable gloves should be worn (Bhungalia & Kemp, 2002). Sacred threads, jewelry, and other religious objects should not be removed. The body should not be washed but only wrapped in a plain sheet until the funeral (Matzo, 2001).

Washing of the body is a part of the funeral rite and is typically carried out only by family members; a mixture of milk and yogurt is used to cleanse the body. After being cleansed, a cloth is tied under the chin and over the top of the head, and the body is wrapped in red cloth. The thumbs and great toes are tied together and the body is placed with the head facing south (Bhungalia & Kemp, 2002). In India, a funeral would take place within 24 hours; adult Hindus are cremated, although young children and infants may be buried (Green, 1989a). Embalming and organ donation are prohibited (Bhungalia & Kemp, 2002).

Following the death, religious pictures at home are turned toward the wall, and mirrors are covered. It is believed that for 12 days the soul wanders in the home, trying to let go of life and the material world. During this time the family prays and chants, and, on the 12th day, the soul is reincarnated. On the 12th day, the Brahmin is given money, clothing, and food by the family and friends of the deceased to help the soul in the next life. As a symbol of mourning, men and boys shave their heads. The widow no longer wears makeup or excessive jewelry, or the red bindi (dot on forehead between eyebrows) (Bhungalia & Kemp, 2002).

Buddhist Traditions

For the Buddhist, an important consideration is the state of mind at the time of death; dying thoughts and desires are crucial in determining the next rebirth. The dying Buddhist wishes to

---

EVIDENCE-BASED PRACTICE

Reference: Happ, M. B., Capezuti, E., Strumpf, N., Wagner, L., Cunningham, S., Evans, L., et al. (2002). Advance care planning and end-of-life care for hospitalized nursing home residents. *Journal of the American Geriatrics Society, 50,* 829-835.

Research Problem: To describe advance care planning (ACP) and end-of-life care for nursing home residents who are hospitalized in the last 6 weeks of life.

Design: Constant comparative analysis of deceased nursing home resident cases.

Sample and Setting: 43 deceased residents hospitalized within the last 6 weeks of life at a tertiary medical center (a not-for-profit Jewish nursing home).

Methods: Trained nurse reviewers abstracted data from nursing home records and gerontologic advanced practice nurse field notes. Clinical and outcome data from an earlier original study were used to describe the sample. Data were analyzed using the constant comparative method and validated in interviews with a gerontologic advanced practice nurse and social worker.

Results: The analysis revealed distinct characteristics and identifiable transition points in ACP and end-of-life care with frail nursing home residents. ACP was addressed by social workers as part of the nursing home admission process, focused primarily on cardiopulmonary resuscitation preference, and was reviewed only after the crisis of acute illness and hospitalization. Advance directive forms specifying preferences or limitations for life-sustaining treatment contained inconsistent language and vague conditions for implementation. ACP review generally resulted in gradual limitation of life-sustaining treatment. Transition points included nursing home admission, acute illness or hospitalization, and decline toward death. Relatively few nursing home residents received hospice services, with most hospice referrals and palliative care treatment delayed until the week before death. Most residents in this sample died without family present and with little documented evidence of pain or symptom management.

Implications for Nursing Practice: These findings reinforce the need for research and program initiatives in long-term care to improve and facilitate individualized ACP and palliative care at the end of life.

Conclusion: Limiting discussion of advance care plans to cardiopulmonary resuscitation falsely dichotomized and oversimplified the choices about medical treatment and care at the end of life, especially palliative care alternatives, for these older nursing home residents. Formal hospice services were underutilized, and palliative care efforts by nursing home staff were often inconsistent with accepted standards.

maintain consciousness and think "wholesome thoughts"; these thoughts include awareness of the transient nature of existence, thinking about one's past good deeds, and willingly letting go of life (Bhungalia & Kemp, 2002). A Buddhist monk or minister will chant to facilitate a peaceful state of mind, incense is burned, and images of Buddha may be place near the dying elder. The length of time between death and burial can vary between 3 and 7 days depending on the Buddhist tradition. Organ donation and autopsy are acceptable. Anyone can touch the body after death as long as this is done respectfully. Family members plan the burial; the tradition is to wear white to the funeral, and some close relatives may shave their head as a sign of mourning (Bhungalia & Kemp, 2002).

Islamic/Muslim Traditions

The dying (*mutadha*) older adult of the Muslim faith may wish to lie or sit facing Mecca. If it is possible, the bed should be positioned to accommodate this wish. Muslim rituals include confession and repentance of all earthly sins, and reading of verses from the Qur'an (36th surah, Ya Sin) into the ear of the person who is dying by the eldest male in attendance (Kemp & Bhungalia, 2002). Anyone who is menstruating or considered unclean is not permitted in the room of the dying person (Ross, 2001). The *Shahadah* are the first words heard by the ear of a newborn and the last spoken or heard at death, and are considered to be the basic tenet of Islam: "There is no God but Allah and Muhammad is his prophet" (Ross, 2001).

The Muslim believes that the body belongs to God and therefore autopsies are forbidden unless ordered by the coroner. Likewise, organ donation and cremation are not acceptable unless absolutely necessary (Kemp & Bhungalia, 2002). In Iran, a person is immediately placed in a casket if he or she has died during the day. If he or she dies at night, a copy of the Qur'an should be placed on the chest and a lighted candle at the head (Iserson, 2001); the body is watched during the night by a person reading the Qur'an (Matzo, 2001). Many cities have funeral homes associated with mosques to prepare the body and plan the funeral (Ross, 2001).

Following the death, non-Muslims should wear gloves when touching the body. If there is no family available to carry out postmortem care, the nurse may carry out the preparation of the body. The body is not washed and hair and nails are not cut; however, the eyes are closed.

[N]ormal Muslim procedure is that the body is straightened immediately after death. This is done by flexing the elbows, shoulders, knees and hips first before straightening them. This is thought to ensure that the body does not stiffen, thus facilitating the washing and shrouding of it. Turn the head towards the right shoulder. This is so the body can be buried with the face towards Mecca. (Green, 1989b, p. 57)

The body is then covered with a sheet that cloaks the whole body until a Muslim is available to perform the ritual bath. The body is usually washed three times (always an odd number of times), first with lotus water, then camphor water, and last with plain water (Iserson, 2001). This bathing is started on the right side with the hands, arms, mouth, nostrils, and feet (Ross, 2001).

All body orifices are closed and packed with cotton (to prevent body fluid leakage, which is considered unclean). Prayers from the Qur'an are read (especially verses of hope and acceptance), and the body is wrapped in a special cotton shroud. This shroud is made from three pieces of white, unsewn cloth, 9 yards long, that are wrapped above, below, and around the midsection. Muslims are not embalmed and are buried in a Muslim cemetery in a 6-foot-deep brick- or cement-lined grave with their head facing Mecca (Matzo, 2001).

Before the body is lowered into the grave, the mourners approach the body to give instructions for the "trial of the grave." This is the belief that two angels will visit the deceased to question him or her about his or her life. An odd number of the deceased person's relatives will make the final preparations for burial by loosening the shroud, whispering the Shahadah, and placing three handfuls of dirt on the grave. The body may also be covered with flowers and blessed rose water (Ross, 2001). In Iran, the body is buried directly in the earth with the shroud removed from the face and one side of the face turned to be in contact with the earth (Purnell & Paulanka, 1998). Men and women mourn separately (Kemp & Bhungalia, 2002), and women are traditionally not allowed to go to the cemetery (Ross, 2001).

Jewish Traditions

Jakobovits (1959) wrote that "the value of human life is infinite and beyond measure, so that a hundred years and a single second are equally precious" (p. 46); therefore, for the Jew, quality-of-life issues are not raised regarding end-of-life care. According to Jewish tradition, a person who is expected to die in 3 days or less is termed a *goses* (Ross, 1998). The Jew who is dying may want to hear or recite special prayers, such as the *Shema*, which confirms one's belief in one God, or psalms, in particular Psalm 23 ("The Lord is My Shepherd"), as well as holding the written prayer in his or her hand (Green, 1989c). A relative remains with the dying person to ensure that the soul does not leave the body when he or she is alone; it is a sign of disrespect to leave the person alone.

When the person takes his or her last breath, the window is opened to allow the spirit to leave the room. Close family members may tear their clothes as part of the mourning tradition (Ross, 1998). Even after death, the body is not left alone until the funeral, so that the body is not left defenseless (Purnell & Paulanka, 1998). The eyes should be closed after death, preferably by a child of the deceased; the body should be covered and left untouched (Green, 1989c).

Autopsies are not permitted (unless the procedure will have a medical benefit to save someone's life), although organ transplants are becoming more acceptable. Traditional Jewish law proscribes organ donation because the person should be buried with all body parts intact. Some Jews will have an amputated limb buried in their cemetery plot so that that their bodies will be intact when the Messiah comes. This tradition applies to limbs containing bone and muscle, making the heart, lung, cornea, kidneys, and the like not subject to this law. Many rabbis see organ donation as compatible with the Jewish teaching that "to save one life is to save the whole world" and support the practice (Ross, 1998).

Non-Jews should handle the body as little as possible, and burial should take place within 24 hours and be delayed only for the Sabbath. Orthodox Jews are always buried, although more liberal Jews may select cremation. Embalming and cosmetics are not a part of traditional practice. The body is washed by a specially trained group of people in a purification ritual called the *taharah*, and then wrapped in a plain linen shroud (*tachrichim*) and a prayer shawl (*tallit*). The casket is made of wood, so that the body and the casket decay at the same rate. There is no wake or viewing of the body. At the funeral, the prayer for the dead (the *Kaddish*) is said, which praises God and reaffirms faith (Purnell & Paulanka, 1998); this prayer is said three times a day during *Shiva* and for a year following death. The funeral is traditionally held at the graveside; as the casket is lowered into the ground, the mourners throw dirt on it (Ross, 1998). This is called *kevorah*, which is the last physical act for the deceased performed by loved ones to help them reach acceptance and reconciliation.

The week-long mourning period after death is called Shiva; the mourning family is said to be "sitting Shiva." During this period, Jews stay at home, mirrors are covered, men do not shave, and the family sits on backless stools, a low bench, or the floor (Kemp & Bhungalia, 2002). Neighbors and friends will bring food to ease the family's burden (Ross, 1998). It is considered improper to greet the mourner; instead the visitor says in Hebrew: "May you be comforted among the mourners of Zion and Jerusalem" (Kemp & Bhungalia, 2002).

On the anniversary of the death, a ceremony is held to place the name of the deceased in the memorial room of the synagogue. The gravestone is also unveiled, and the friends and family of the deceased gather at the graveside to say the Kaddish (Kemp & Bhungalia, 2002).

Mormon Traditions

Mormons (members of the Church of Jesus Christ of Latter-day Saints [LDS]) believe that, at death, the spirit and the body separate and the spirit goes before God for judgment and moves on to the spirit world. This is a place of learning and preparation. After a time, the body and spirit are reunited, never again to be separated; this is called resurrection. It is believed that resurrection is a gift to every person who ever lived, made possible by the death and resurrection of Jesus Christ. Death is something to mourn, but is also a time of hope because it is seen as a step into the next life and eternal life with God.

Death is not seen as the end of our relationships with loved ones. Mormons believe that the Lord revealed to the Prophet Joseph Smith that the "same sociality which exists among us here will exist among us there [in eternity], only it will be coupled with eternal glory" (Doctrine and Covenants 130:2). Family members who accept the Atonement of Jesus Christ and follow His example can be together forever through sacred sealing ordinances performed in God's holy temples. Family and friends grieve for their loss, but they know that they will be with their loved one again; this understanding brings great comfort (Church of Jesus Christ of Latter-day Saints, 2002).

Church members of the same gender who have permission to be admitted into the temple dress deceased members of the church. The body is dressed in white undergarments that are covered by a robe, cap, and apron. A LDS funeral is similar to traditional Christian funerals in practice; the funeral is usually directed by the ward bishop and held in a LDS chapel or mortuary. The mood of the funeral is generally peaceful, reflecting the religious belief that families can be reunited after this life. Funerals are conducted with a spirit of hope and sometimes joy (Church of Jesus Christ of Latter-day Saints, 2002).

Burial is preferred to cremation because internment in the earth symbolizes the return of dust to dust. Prior to burial, white caps are placed on the men, and women's faces are veiled. The grave site of the deceased is viewed as a sacred spot for the family to visit and tend (Beliefnet.com, 2002; Iserson, 2001; Matzo, 2001).

Cultural Perspectives

Cultural Perspectives of Cuban-Americans

Cuban-Americans who are dying are usually attended by large groups of family and friends. The hospital is the preferred place to die, and the entire family is expected to visit and to be present at all times until death. Depending on their religious affiliation, a Catholic priest, Protestant minister, rabbi, or *santero* may be called to perform death rites. Although Catholicism is the primary religion of Cuba, some Cubans practice an African Voodoo-type religion known as *Santería*. Based on beliefs of the Yoruba African people, *Santería* incorporates Yoruba gods (orishas, or the "seven African deities") and variations on Catholic rituals (Baylor University, 2002). For followers of Santería, these rites may

include animal sacrifice, ceremonial displays, and chants (Purnell & Paulanka, 1998).

After the death, candles are lit to light the path of the spirit to the afterlife. Burial is the common custom, although there is no restriction to cremation. Organ donation and autopsy are not common practices (Matzo, 2001).

Cultural Perspectives of Native Americans

Native Americans have different traditions in each tribe. There is a belief that the spirit of the deceased remains where the person has died; therefore, family may not want the person to die at home. At the same time, it is considered inappropriate for the person to die alone; if the person dies at home, the house must be abandoned or a ceremony is held to cleanse it (Matzo, 2001). Families gather together at the time of death. So that the family can begin its new life without the presence of that person, all material goods of the person are given away (Brokenleg & Middleton, 1993).

When a person dies, a cleansing ceremony is performed or else the spirit of the deceased may try to take over someone's spirit. Those who work with the dead must also have a ceremonial cleansing to protect themselves from the dead person's spirit. Funerals are usually held at home because all members of the community are expected to stay with the mourners. If a funeral home is used, around-the-clock access will be assumed (Brokenleg & Middleton, 1993). No embalming is used; the body lies in state for 3 days, and the clergy of all denominations and medicine men are expected to attend. Christian hymns and tribal songs are sung, interspersed with prayers (Box 25-6), condolences, and reminiscences about the dead person (Brokenleg & Middleton, 1993). The deceased are buried in sacred ground with their shoes on the wrong feet, rings on their index fingers, and many gifts surrounding them, or the body is cremated (Matzo, 2001; Purnell & Paulanka, 1998).

Cultural Perspectives from Appalachia

For people from Appalachia, the hospital may be feared and viewed as a place to go to die. The nurse should be sure to allow time for relatives and friends to visit with the deceased prior to moving the body to the morgue or calling the funeral home (Obermiller & Rappold, 1994). A

Box 25-6 Shawnee Indian Cultural Perspective on Death

"So live your life that the fear of death can never enter your heart. Trouble no one about their religion; respect others in their view, and demand that they respect yours. Love your life, perfect your life, and beautify all things in your life. Seek to make your life long and its purpose in the service of your people. Prepare a noble death song for the day when you go over the great divide. Always give a word or a sign of salute when meeting or passing a friend, even a stranger, when in a lonely place. Show respect to all people and grovel to none. When you arise in the morning, give thanks for the food and for the joy of living. If you see no reason for giving thanks, the fault lies only in yourself. Abuse no one and no thing, for abuse turns the wise ones to fools and robs the spirit of its vision. When it comes your time to die, be not like those whose hearts are filled with the fear of death, so that when their time comes they weep and pray for a little more time to live their lives over again in a different way. Sing your death song and die like a hero going home."

Chief Tecumseh, Shawnee Nation

From Sultzman, L. (1998). *Shawnee history.* Retrieved December 29, 2002, from http://www.tolatsga.org/shaw.html

death is an important event, even for extended family; reactions to the death of a loved one and expressions of grief may seem extreme or exaggerated to non-Appalachians.

The funeral is a significant social occasion, and family and friends will come from long distances to be in attendance. The body is displayed for a long period of time so that all who wish to see the body can do so. The deceased is buried in his or her best clothes, and some people have clothes custom-made for burial (Purnell & Paulanka, 1998). Family and friends may wish to take photographs of the body after it has been dressed as a form of remembrance (Obermiller & Rappold, 1994).

Personal possessions are displayed at the funeral home, and it is common to bury these items with the person. Earth burial is the most common form of interment; cremation is infrequent. Grave sites are typically on hillsides because of the fear that they will be flooded out

in low-lying areas (Matzo, 2001; Purnell & Paulanka, 1998). Appalachians may be very hesitant to consent to autopsies and organ donations.

Cultural Perspectives of the Hmong

Subgroups from China, Vietnam, Laos, Thailand, and Burma together are called the Hmong. The Hmong believe that proper burial and worship of the dead and other ancestors directly affects the safety, health, and prosperity of the family. The belief is that the spiritual world coexists with the physical world and that the spirits are able to influence human life. Typically, the preference is to die at home because of the belief that the soul will wander for all of eternity without a resting place if the person dies elsewhere; however, some groups believe that death should take place in the hospital so that bad luck is not brought into the home. Autopsy and cremation are acceptable practices to some families; for these groups, burial occurs in the afternoon (Matzo, 2001).

The Chinese often desire to die at home, believing that the spirit of the deceased lingers near the place of death and is therefore a comfort to the family. If death occurs any place other than home, prayer and ritual are used to shepherd the soul back home (Kemp & Chang, 2002). After death, the family may want to stay with the deceased for as long as 8 hours with privacy. If the deceased is over age 80, a red (celebratory color) cloth is hung outside the family door. The family is expected to help prepare the body for burial; this ritual washing and dressing is done by the eldest son or daughter of the deceased. Often a coin will be placed in the deceased's mouth so that he or she has money to pay anyone who interferes in his or her journey (Matzo, 2001).

If the family originates from northern China, the practice is to place the body in burial clothes, and an unpadded quilt is used as a shroud. The face is covered with cloth or paper and the feet are tied with colored string. The wife or oldest son wipes the deceased's eyes with cotton floss before the coffin is closed (Iserson, 2001; Matzo, 2001).

The funeral focuses on rituals of remembrance. A part of the ceremony is to burn paper money or other representations of necessities. Burial is more common than cremation. In the native country, the body may be disinterred after 5 years and the remains placed in an urn; these may be kept at home or in a temple or reburied (Kemp & Chang, 2002). Instead of being buried immediately after the funeral, the body may be stored so that a husband and wife can be buried together (Iserson, 2001; Matzo, 2001).

Every 7 days after death, relatives gather to pray to direct the soul to paradise and provide an opportunity for collective mourning. In America, these gatherings may take place on weekends. After 7 days times 7 weeks (49 days), it is believed that the soul is at peace and has departed, and the cycle of collective prayer comes to an end (Kemp & Chang, 2002). There is great respect for ancestors, and funeral and memorial rituals transform ancestors into sources of blessings for the living (DeSpelder & Strickland, 1999).

Cultural Perspectives of Japanese

The Japanese custom in funerals is to invite a Buddhist priest to the house to have him recite a *sutra*. The Japanese bathe their dead, shave some of the hair, and dress the person in white. The corpse wears a ceremonial hat or triangular piece of white paper tied to the forehead. The next evening, family members and close relatives burn incense sticks (called *senko*) in front of the altar all during the night. This is what the Japanese call *otsuya*, meaning "all night long." On the third day, after the otsuya, they burn the body to ashes at a funeral hall and bring the ashes back to the house. Finally, a funeral service is conducted; people burn incense by turns in front of the altar while the priest recites a sutra. After the service is over, family members and close relatives go to the graveyard and lay the ashes to rest (Shioda, 1999).

When attending a Japanese funeral, the visitor should bring something to eat to offer at the family altar (*butsudan*) and burn incense before it for the dead. *Ko-den* (money) should be brought to either the otsuya or the funeral service and handed to the person at the reception. Family members prepare token gifts to be given back to the people who come to mourn the dead (Shioda, 1999).

Cultural Perspectives of Mexican-Americans

Mexican-Americans may take turns sitting vigil over the dying person; dying in a hospital is not desirable because the spirit may become "lost." Spiritual amulets, rosary beads, or other religious artifacts are kept near the older adult. When death occurs, family and friends will often come from long distances for the funeral. Mexico is a predominately Catholic country, and funeral and burial practices are consistent with these beliefs. One difference is that the body laid out in the coffin is covered with a *vidrio* (pane of glass) over the section of the coffin that is open.

A *velorio* is a festive watch over the deceased body before burial. The viewing or velorio begins in the evening and lasts as long as there are people present; some last all night or even until the body is taken to the church for the funeral mass. Traditional families my exhibit hyperkinetic shaking and seizure-like activity called *ataque de nervios*, which is a way to release emotions related to grieving (Matzo, 2001).

Mexicans treat death with a combination of reverence and celebration. Family may erect altars in their homes in honor of the anniversary of their relative's death and may include candles and decorations. They may have the deceased's favorite meal at a graveside picnic (Purnell & Paulanka, 1998). Typically, organ donation and autopsies are not allowed.

Death is treated as a part of life. Mexicans celebrate the memory of deceased family members with cemetery vigils, dancing, and parades in a festival called *el Día de los Muertes* (the Day of the Dead). At the grave site, family members decorate the grave with flowers, have a picnic, and socialize with other family and community members who gather at the cemetery. Modern Mexican families may observe the Day of the Dead with only a special family supper featuring the "Bread of the Dead" (*pan de muerto*), a rich coffee cake decorated with meringues made to look like bones. It is considered to be good luck to bite into the plastic toy skeleton hidden in the bread. Friends and family members give one another gifts consisting of sugar skeletons or other items with a death motif (Salvador, 2002).

Cultural Perspectives of Black Americans

Black Americans generally prefer to have people with terminal illness cared for in the home, but prefer death to occur in the hospital for fear of bad luck being brought to the home. Grief is expressed openly and publicly. Autopsy is acceptable, although organ donation is not. The present-day traditions and customs of death can be traced back to African roots of the Bakongo and LaDogaa tribes. There is usually a 5- to 7-day mourning period before the actual funeral. During this time, a wake is held, which is a time for close friends of the family of the deceased to pay respects to the family and view the body. Most wakes are held at the funeral home, but have been known to take place at the church or in the home of the deceased. This is a time when everyone gathers, eats food cooked by the family members, and shares memories of the deceased. At the cemetery, there are traditions (or superstitions) that may be followed concerning the actual burial of the dead. It is believed that it is important that the dead be buried with their feet facing east to allow rising at Judgment Day; otherwise the person remains in the crossways of the world.

An old belief is that the dead cannot be buried on a rainy day; a shining sun is a sign that the heavens are open and welcoming for the deceased. If it rains while a person is dying, or if lighting strikes near his or her house, the devil has come for the soul. Therefore, the family members often attempt to bury the dead on a sunny day (North by South, 1998).

WHEN DEATH HAS OCCURRED

Postdeath nursing care begins with preparing the body for the morgue or funeral home and helping the family through decisions regarding autopsy and burial. Once death has occurred, the blood will begin to pool in the areas of the body closest to the ground; if the corpse were supine, this would be the back and buttocks. A purple-red discoloration of the skin is evident. The blood is no longer circulating through the body and accumulates in the dependent vessels; this is called *livor mortis*. The body begins to cool; postmortem body temperature declines progressively until it reaches the ambient temperature. This fall in body temperature after death is called *algor mortis* (Kastenbaum & Kastenbaum, 1989; Matzo, 2001).

Initially, at the time of death, the muscles in the body relax, but within 2 to 6 hours *rigor mortis* begins. Rigor mortis is the stiffening of all muscle groups beginning with the eyelids, neck, and jaw. During the next 4 to 6 hours, it will spread to the other muscles, including the internal organs. Maximum rigor mortis occurs in about 12 hours

and lasts between 24 and 48 hours depending on the temperature where the body is; after this time the muscles relax and secondary flaccidity develops (Iserson, 2001).

Temperature and weather affect the decay of the body, which occurs in four stages: fresh, bloating, decaying, and dry (skeletal). A rule of thumb holds that "one week in air equals two weeks in water equals eight weeks buried in the ground" (Quigley, 1996, p. 88). If the body had been exposed to heat or the deceased had a fever, decomposition will progress more rapidly. Warm temperatures will speed the destruction of tissues by the body's natural enzymes.

Care of the Body

Care of the body by the nurse should include closing the eyes, inserting dentures and closing the mouth, and elevating the head of the bed so that the blood does not drain into the face and discolor it. If there is an IV line or a catheter, these should be removed (unless institutional protocol indicates otherwise) and the physical environment should be straightened. The nurse should follow institutional protocol regarding jewelry; if there is a wedding ring, it should be secured on the finger with tape. The body should be bathed in plain water and dried and a bed protector placed under the body. If there are dressings on wounds, they should be replaced with clean ones. The hair should be combed and the extremities straightened, and an identification tag tied on the right great toe (Sorrentino, 1999).

The family should be asked if they would like to participate in the preparation of the deceased for the funeral home; they can bathe and dress the body if they wish. Some people find comfort in giving this last bath, knowing that no one will touch the body in this way again.

When the body and the room have been prepared, family and those close to the patient can be encouraged to say a final good-bye. Within the confines of cultural, personal, and religious practices, the family can be invited to touch or hold the person's body. This time spent with the deceased can help to promote the transition from acute grief to a new stage of the grieving process (Ferrell et al., 1999). The body should not be transported to the morgue or mortuary until the family is prepared and they have given their per-

EVIDENCE-BASED PRACTICE

Reference: Hall, P., Schroder, C., & Weaver, L. (2002). The last 48 hours of life in long-term care: A focused chart audit. *Journal of the American Geriatrics Society, 50*, 501-506.

Research Problem: As a component of palliative care educational program development, the faculty at the University of Ottawa Institute of Palliative Care wished to assess end-of-life care for patients in long-term care (LTC) settings to develop an educational strategy for physicians.

Design: A chart audit, focusing on the last 48 hours of life of residents dying in LTC facilities.

Sample and Setting: Residents who died in five LTC facilities in a Canadian city in a 12-month period. Those who died suddenly (i.e., with no palliation period) or in a hospital were excluded.

Methods: Symptoms highlighted in the literature as commonly found in the terminally ill and the matching treatments were recorded on an audit form created by the authors. Included were pain, dyspnea, noisy breathing, delirium, dysphagia, fever, and myoclonus.

Results: A total of 185 charts were reviewed. A large number of patients were cognitively impaired. Cancer was the final diagnosis in 14% of cases. Respiratory symptoms were the most prevalent symptom, with dyspnea being first and noisy breath-ing third. Pain was second, with prevalence similar to that found in studies of cancer patients. Dyspnea was not treated in 23% of the patients with this symptom; opioids were used in only 27% of cases with dyspnea. Ninety-nine percent of patients who experienced pain were treated for it. Less than one third of patients with noisy breathing were treated. Delirium was not treated in 38% of the cases, and no antidopaminergic medications were administered. Nurses were primarily responsible for documenting end-of-life issues, supporting the families of the dying residents, and communicating with other team members.

Implications for Nursing Practice: Nurses played a crucial role in the care of dying residents through their documentation and communication of end-of-life issues. Appropriate palliative care education can provide knowledge and skills to all health care pro-fessionals, including physicians, and assist them in the control of symptoms and improvement of quality of life for patients dying in LTC facilities.

Conclusion: The focused chart audit identified the high prevalence of cognitive impairment in the patient population, which complicates symptom management. Respiratory symptoms predominated in the last 48 hours of life. This symptom profile differs from that of cancer patients, who, according to the literature, have more pain and less respiratory trouble. Management of symptoms was variable.

mission for the body to be moved. The family's wishes should be respected regarding their pres-ence while the body is removed (Matzo, 2001).

If a person has died at home, and the death is expected, the undertaker is called and will remove the body as it is. In a hospital or nursing home setting, the body is wrapped in a shroud or body bag. The shroud should be secured with safety pins or ties and a second identification tag is attached to the shroud or body bag. The body is then taken to the morgue (Matzo, 2001; Sorrentino, 1999).

The nurse can offer to help the family by notifying others of the death in order to give the family time to become accustomed to the immediate loss. The physician should be notified of the death, and the nurse should be certain to follow institutional protocol regarding the removal of medications and equipment. Clergy or bereavement counseling can be offered (Matzo, 2001).

In many states, the nurse can sign the death certificate if the death occurs in the hospital or nursing home or at the family home if hospice is involved. Once the death certificate is signed, the funeral home can be contacted and the body transported. If the nurse or physician is unwilling to sign the death certificate because of the suspicious nature of the death, the medical examiner is called, and he or she will assume responsibility for the body (Iserson, 2001).

Autopsy

If the death is sudden and unexpected or if it occurs at home, the medical examiner must be notified and will decide if an autopsy is required. The family has no authority to stop an officially mandated autopsy (Lynn & Harrold, 1999). The next of kin may request an autopsy even if the medical examiner declines to do one. The nurse should be available to educate the family about the autopsy and assist them in their decision-making process. An autopsy will help determine the cause of death, but the family may be charged a fee for this service (the cost may be as much as $2000). Autopsies also serve other purposes (Box 25-7).

The word autopsy comes from the Greek *autopsia*, which means "seeing with one's own eyes." Pathologists, who are physicians specializing in human anatomy, perform them. Organs are removed and inspected, and body fluids are analyzed. There are three degrees of autopsy: complete, limited, and selective. A complete autopsy exposes all body cavities (including the head) for examination; limited autopsy usually excludes the head; and selective autopsy involves examination of only one or more organs specific to the nature of the illness (Iserson, 2001).

Organ Donation

If the deceased has filled out documentation indicating that his or her organs be donated, the nurse is often the person responsible for notifying the proper agencies for organ and tissue harvesting. Organ donation is the practice of giving a part of the deceased body for transplantation into another person. Approximately 80,000 Americans are waiting for organ transplants; in 2000, fewer than 23,000 people received a transplant and 56,000 died waiting for one. It is estimated that 12,000 to 15,000 deaths a year generate suitable donor organs, but fewer than half of those deaths result in organ donation (Office of the Inspector General, 2002). The

---

Box 25-7 Uses of Autopsies

BENEFITS TO MEDICAL PRACTICE AND SCIENCE
- Discover or elucidate new diseases
- Explain unknown or unanticipated medical complications
- Assist in the development/quality assurance of new technology, procedures, and therapy
- Educate medical students
- Continue physician education

BENEFITS TO THE JUDICIAL SYSTEM
- Classify and explain sudden, unexpected, and/or unnatural deaths

BENEFITS TO PUBLIC WELFARE
- Identify infectious and contagious diseases
- Identify and monitor occupational and environmental health hazards
- Assist quality control and risk assessment in hospital practices
- Provide a source of organs and tissues for medical and scientific purposes
- Provide materials and hypotheses for research
- Improve accuracy, and therefore usefulness, of vital statistics

BENEFITS TO THE DECEASED'S FAMILY
- Assist in the grief process
- Provide a vehicle for contribution
- Discover contagious diseases within the family
- Assist in genetic counseling and identification of family health risks
- Provide information for insurance/death benefits

From Iserson, K. V. (2001). *Death to dust.* Tucson, AZ: Galen Press.

Department of Health and Human Services is taking steps to increase donations by giving grants and assistance to organ procurement organizations (OPOs). Medicare requires hospitals to notify the OPO in their state about all individuals who are imminently dying or who die in the hospital in an effort to ensure that all potential donors consider organ donation.

A person designates his or her wish to donate organs by signing the back of the driver's license indicating preferences, specifying organ donation in an advance directive, or filling out an organ donor card. Organ donor cards can be ordered from the United Network for Organ Sharing (UNOS) (1-804-782-4800 or *www.unos.org*). Persons less than 18 years of age must have the consent of their parents or guardians to sign an organ donor card. Some states will record the intent to donate an organ in a "donor registry," which is a central repository of information regarding the intent to donate. When the OPO identifies a potential donor, it can then contact the donor registry to determine the person's intent (Office of the Inspector General, 2002).

Even with the proper documentation, the family may refuse to allow a relative's organs to be donated. In the United States, at least 5000 human organs are buried because relatives refuse donation. Conversely, unless the deceased has specified that his or her organs should not be donated, the senior next-of-kin may donate all or part of a relative's body (Iserson, 2001; Matzo, 2001).

In order for the deceased to be an organ donor, a physician (preferably a neurosurgeon or neurologist) must declare brain death in accordance with state law. A person who has a beating heart and is on a respirator but is considered brain dead is an acceptable donor for heart, liver, pancreas, eyes/corneas, kidneys, intestine, heart valves, skin, bone, and lungs. If the death is a result of a cardiac arrest and there is no cardiac or respiratory activity, then this person is an acceptable donor for eyes/corneas, blood vessels, cartilage, skin, bone, pericardium, and soft tissues. Other criteria for potential organ and tissue donors include certain age limits and the absence of unresolved systemic infections or extracerebral malignancies (National Kidney Foundation, 2002). General criteria for organ and tissue donors are found in Box 25-8.

The time for organ removal is variable and is dependent upon which organ is being donated. If the body has been refrigerated within 4 hours of the death, the saphenous veins can be harvested during the following 10 hours, and heart valves within 24 hours. Eyes must be removed within 4 hours of the death, but, once they are in a preservative, they can wait 10 to 14 days to be transplanted. Tissues such as bone, skin, and tendons can wait 12 to 24 hours to be removed from the deceased and can be preserved (depending on the method of preservation) for 3 to 5 years (Iserson, 2001; Matzo, 2001).

Embalming

Once the organs are removed, the body is ready for embalming or cremation. Embalming is the process by which the corpse is preserved and prepared for viewing. "Basically, the embalmer is a creator of illusions—of pleasant illusions which banish the traces of suffering and death and present the deceased in an attitude of normal, restful sleep. In the practice of embalming this illusion is called a 'memory picture'" (Strub & Frederick, 1967, p. 133). There is no legal requirement that the body be embalmed, even if it is going to be viewed. The average cost for embalming is between $400 and $500 (Iserson, 2001).

There are four embalming methods that all involve the injection of chemicals to preserve the body. Arterial embalming injects the chemicals into the blood vessels; cavity embalming injects the chest and abdomen; hypodermic embalming injects under the skin; and surface embalming is the application of chemicals in gel or liquid form onto the body surface (Iserson, 2001). The size of the body, age, water content, temperature, decomposition, condition of the body's blood vessels, and premortem medication regimen (e.g., gentamicin inactivates embalming fluid) will dictate the types, solution strengths, and injection rates of the embalming chemicals.

A gravity embalming tank, located above the body, is filled with preservative chemicals (embalming fluid) consisting of 1 gallon (gal.) isopropyl alcohol; 2 gal. propylene glycol; 1/4 gal. amphyl; 1/2 gal. 10% buffered formalin; and 50 oz. liquefied phenol. These chemicals delay the breakdown of cells to prevent putrefaction. Tubing connected to a centrifugal pump is attached to the gravity tank. Before the embalming fluid is injected, air is removed from the connecting tube to avoid airlocks produced by the vessels of the body during the injection of the fluid. Injection periods vary in each case, taking from 8 to 24 hours for the fluids to be injected into the body under 5 to 10 psi of pressure. At the same time, blood and fluid are drained from the body by gravity or electrical aspirators. The embalmer will look for evidence that the chemicals have reached the hands and face and facili-

Box 25-8 Guidelines for Organ and Tissue Donation

ALL TISSUE AND ORGAN DONORS
DEATH BY BRAIN OR HEART CRITERIA

Many centers only accept organ donation from those dead by brain criteria.

- No malignancy other than a primary brain tumor without a shunt
- No body-wide infection or injury to tissue
- No known neurologic disease or acquired immuno-deficiency syndrome risk factors
- Resuscitated cardiac arrest does not preclude donation

TISSUE SPECIFIC (CAN BE RECOVERED UP TO 24 HOURS AFTER DEATH)
HEART VALVES

- Age 3 months to 55 years with no prior heart surgery
- No disease of heart valves
- No injections into the heart

BONE

- Age 16-65 years
- No steroid or insulin use
- No collagen vascular disease (e.g., lupus, rheumatoid arthritis)
- No neurologic disease

CORNEAS

- Any age with no eye disease
- No leukemia or retinoblastoma

ORGAN SPECIFIC
KIDNEY

- No kidney malfunction or infection
- Generally younger than age 75
- Allowable time from donor to recipient: 15-18 hours

HEART

- Generally younger than 65 years old
- No enlargement of the heart
- Allowable time from donor to recipient: 4-5 hours

LIVER

- No liver malfunction or cirrhosis
- Generally younger than 65 years old
- Allowable time from donor to recipient: 12-18 hours

LUNG

- 10-65 years old
- No lung disease
- No fluid or infection in the lungs
- Allowable time from donor to recipient: 5-6 hours

PANCREAS

- Younger than 60 years old
- No pancreatic malfunction
- Allowable time from donor to recipient: 12-15 hours

Adapted from Iserson, K. V. (2001). *Death to dust* (p. 62). Tucson, AZ: Galen Press; and Scientific Registry of Transplant Recipients. (2002). *Transplant Primer.* Retrieved December 18, 2002, from http://www.ustransplant.org/primer.html

tate this process by massaging and repositioning the corpse. When the embalming fluid reaches the hands, they are placed in their final position over the chest or abdomen and the fingers are held together by using cyanoacrylate (e.g., Superglue). The muscles will gradually harden over the 8- to 12-hour period following the embalming; once they are set, the body's position will not be able to be changed (Iserson, 2001; Matzo, 2001).

Thin people and those who were in good health and died suddenly decompose more slowly than others do. Deep burial also retards decom-

position; bodies that have been buried 3 to 4 feet deep may take years to skeletonize. Bodies that were embalmed may decay more slowly over the first 6 months, depending on the amount of body fat. Embalming also retards larval activity and disintegration (Quigley, 1996).

If there will be a viewing at the funeral home, the body is prepared with the use of cosmetics, hair is styled, and the corpse is dressed. The body is then "casketed" in the coffin; typically the right shoulder is lower than the left so the body does not look like it is flat on its back (Matzo, 2001).

Cremation

An increasingly popular alternative to embalming and burial is cremation. Burning the corpse, as a way to dispose of the dead, dates back to prehistoric times. Our primitive ancestors, who believed that a person could return to his or her corpse and harm the living, feared the dead; destroying the corpse removed that danger. Ancient civilizations believed that cremation would provide the dead with heat and warmth in the next world and protected the body from mutilation by animals or other humans. Native Americans believe that souls are conveyed to paradise by means of fire (Matzo, 2001).

Cremation is a process to reduce the "corpse and its container to ashes and small bone fragments" (Iserson, 2001, p. 236). Intense heat, which evaporates water (70% to 80% of nonbone tissue) and burns soft tissue, is used to burn the body. The body does not have to be embalmed before cremation, nor does the family need to purchase a coffin. The only requirement is that the body is burned in a combustible container (e.g., cardboard or particleboard) (Matzo, 2001). This container or casket must be strong enough to assure the protection of the health and safety of the operator, provide a proper covering for the body, and meet reasonable standards of respect and dignity (Cremation Association of North America, 2002). The body is cremated in the same container in which it arrives at the crematory. The body and container are placed in the cremation chamber, where, through heat and evaporation, the body is reduced to its basic elements, which are referred to as cremated remains. Typically, there is a 24- to 48-hour waiting period after the death before cremation can legally take place.

It takes about an hour and a half to cremate a body, and what is left are grey ash and bone fragments (cremains). Depending upon the size of the body, there are normally 3 to 9 pounds of fragments resulting from this process. Prosthetic devices do not burn (e.g., dental gold, metal plates and screws) and are removed with a magnet from the cremains. Pacemakers with lithium batteries will explode when burned and are removed before cremation (Matzo, 2001). Some crematories process the cremated remains in an electric grinder to pulverize the bone fragments, reducing the space that they require for storage. Others do not alter the condition of the cremains after they are removed from the chamber. After preparation, these elements are placed either in a permanent urn or in a temporary container that is suitable for transport (Cremation Association of North America, 2002).

Crematories are the facilities that contain the oven, or retorts, where the cremation will take place. It is becoming increasingly common for funeral homes to build crematories on site and to offer a wide range of disposal options. The cost for this service ranges from $1000 to $1500.

Some cemeteries will have a columbarium for the internment of the urn containing the cremains. Memorial gardens are also available for the ashes to be scattered or buried and give visitors a place to visit or place a marker. Some people will divide the cremains to bury, scatter, keep in an urn, share among family members, or even wear in specially designed jewelry (Matzo, 2001).

Funerals as a Ceremony of Death

People accept an obligation to care for, respect, and honor their dead in all cultures and religions. The actual process of physically preparing the body for the funeral and burial is most often handled by persons outside of the family. The undertaker, a person who "undertook" the responsibility to keep the body safe and make the funeral arrangements, has been a part of society since ancient times. The general public interchangeably refers to the person who prepares the body for burial and conducts all aspects of the funeral service as the undertaker, mortician, embalmer, or funeral director (Iserson, 2001; Matzo, 2001). This professional provides the means for society to dissociate itself from death (O'Gorman, 1998).

In the United States, the funeral director coordinates all details of the funeral for the family and otherwise facilitates the family's burial decisions. These details include the supervision of the body's preparation for viewing or burial, overseeing embalming procedures (if embalming is desired), coordination of cremation planning, instruction and support of the pallbearers, arrangement for the transportation of the family and the deceased to the cemetery, and placement of death notices in the newspaper. Most funeral directors in the United States have at least a bachelor's degree, and about 87% of the 22,000 funeral homes in this country are family operated (Iserson, 2001). Employed by funeral homes are embalmers, cosmetologists, hairdressers, and hearse and limousine drivers (Matzo, 2001).

Those who work in the funeral industry know that the funeral must be perfectly organized and executed because they will not get a second chance to make things right. The funeral originated from theological roots but has evolved, for many people, to be one of the first steps of successful grieving. The funeral is "*of* the person who has died . . . It is *for* those who survive" (Raether, 1993, p. 211).

Postdeath Rituals

Postdeath rituals include three components: the wake, the funeral, and the committal service. The wake is the first element of postdeath ritual, and may be one of the few times that an entire family comes together at the same time. It is the time for family and friends to view the deceased and to pay their final respects. Seeing the dead body emphasizes the fact that the person is dead; declining to see the body may delay grieving. The second component of postdeath rituals is the funeral. The funeral is a ceremony that typically consists of music, prayers, poetry, and eulogies, and it may be part of a funeral mass where communion is celebrated. Some people plan their funeral before they die; this act is often comforting to both the dying elder and his or her family (Raether, 1993). The funeral fills important needs in our society by providing for the dignified and respectful recognition and tribute of the life of the deceased. The funeral service helps the survivors face the reality of death, a first step in the grieving process. It gives friends and relatives a forum to express their love and respect; seeing this care can be of tremendous psychological help to a bereaved family beginning to adjust to their loss (Matzo, 2001).

The last component is the committal service, and it is the final act of caring for the deceased. This service is held at the grave, tomb, or crematorium. This ceremony is a "symbolic demonstration that the kind of relationship which has existed between the mourner and the deceased is now at an end" (Raether, 1993, p. 212).

Another important aspect of the postdeath experience for the bereaved is the formation of a new identity within their community. The role of widow, no longer having a child, or losing a parent brings with it a change in how the bereaved will interact with and their role within society at large. Social groups may shrink, volunteer opportunities may be lost, or favorite activities may be forfeited secondary to the loss. These role shifts are inherently difficult. Nurses should be knowledgeable about these issues and capable of offering alternatives and community support referrals during this transitional stage (Matzo, 2001).

ANALYSES OF THE PERI-DEATH EXPERIENCE

As with any application of the nursing process, the nurse should evaluate the effectiveness of the interventions utilized. In the case of peri-death nursing, there is no way to obtain objective data from the older adult who has just died to determine the efficacy of care. Although family members can be surveyed regarding their experiences, they can truly only report their perceptions as viewed through their own lens. In reality, guilt, remorse, or grief may cloud this lens.

Ternestedt, Andershed, Eriksson, and Johansson (2002) proposed seven questions that the nurse can use to perform a retrospective analysis of the quality of patient care given at the end of life (Box 25-9). These questions should be asked by the health care practitioner after each person has died to attain knowledge about the care of dying older adults and determine areas where improvements can be made.

Case Study Conclusion

After having assessed Mrs. J., the nurse sat next to her husband, who was at the bedside holding her hand. She said, "You have been married for a long time." "Yes," he said, "50 years last June." "How did you meet?" the nurse asked. And he began to talk, telling the nurse funny stories about their courtship, about how her father did not want her to date him, and about their life together and raising their children. The children and their spouses sat and listened to him reminisce; Mrs. J. would occasionally smile. When he stopped talking, the nurse said that it sounded to her like they had a wonderful time together and

Box 25-9 **Analysis of the Quality of Care**

1. Did the patient receive adequate symptom relief and was the care adequate?
2. Could the patient make his or her own decisions during the final phase of his or her life?
3. Could the patient maintain important social relationships to the end of his or her life?
4. Could the patient maintain an acceptable self-image and feeling of personal worth during the final phase of his or her life?
5. Were there signs of conflict resolution and did the patient sum up his or her life?
6. Did the patient accept the fact that death was near, or did he or she struggle against death?
7. Did the patient have a very good death? A good death? A bad death?

From Ternestedt, B., Andershed, B., Eriksson, M., & Johansson, I. (2002). A good death. *Journal of Hospice and Palliative Nursing, 4*(3), 153-160.

Box 25-10 **The Dying Person's Bill of Rights**

- I have the right to be treated as a living human being until I die.
- I have the right to maintain a sense of hopefulness, however changing its focus may be.
- I have the right to be cared for by those who can maintain a sense of hopefulness, however challenging this might be.
- I have the right to express my feelings and emotions about my approaching death, in my own way.
- I have the right to participate in decisions concerning my care.
- I have the right to expect continuing medical and nursing attention even though "cure" goals must be changed to "comfort" goals.
- I have the right not to die alone.
- I have the right to be free from pain.
- I have the right to have my questions answered honestly.
- I have the right not to be deceived.
- I have the right to have help from and for my family accepting my death.
- I have the right to die in peace and dignity.
- I have the right to retain my individuality and not be judged for my decisions, which may be contrary to the beliefs of others.
- I have the right to discuss and enlarge my religious and/or spiritual experiences, regardless of what they may mean to others.
- I have the right to expect that the sanctity of the human body will be respected after death.
- I have the right to be cared for by caring, sensitive, knowledgeable people who will attempt to understand my needs and will be able to gain some satisfaction in helping me face my death.

From Barbus, A. J. (1975). *American Journal of Nursing, 75*(1), 99.

a good life. He agreed, and hugged his wife. As the nurse left, his daughter thanked her for taking care of her father, and noted that this was more talking than he had done in a quite a while. She felt that they could continue the conversation with him, and help him to process the loss of the bride that he loved so much.

Mrs. J. died that night, surrounded by her loving family and the man whom she had defied her father in order to marry. It was a peaceful death for everyone involved.

CONCLUSION

When the nurse is providing end-of-life care, the focus of care is the dying older adult and his or her family. When the death occurs, the work of the nurse is not over because the family is still in need of nursing care and interventions. The goal of postdeath nursing care is to promote optimal adjustment and to help the family and significant others with the tasks of bereavement (see Chapter 9). Bereavement is an important developmental stage; the nurse should provide interventions that offer the opportunity for healing and growth, a redefinition of self, and opportunities to make new plans (Matzo, 2001). Follow-up with the family is important during the bereavement period. The nurse should encourage memorial rituals commemorating the deceased's life and death. There are unique opportunities in peri-death nursing for the nurse to support the dying elder patient and family. The dying person's bill of rights (Box 25-10) can help guide the nurse toward truly excellent end-of-life care for older adults.

REFERENCES

Adam, J. (1997). ABC of palliative care: The last 48 hours. *British Medical Journal, 315,* 1600-1603.

Allmark, P. (2002). Death with dignity. *Journal of Medical Ethics, 28,* 255-257.

Archdiocese of San Antonio. (2002). Cremation for Catholics? In *Catholic Cemeteries and Mausoleums.* Retrieved December 17, 2002, from http://www.catholiccemeteriesofsa.org/Resources/cremation_for_catholics.htm

Baylor University. (2002). *Cuban refugees.* Retrieved December 22, 2002, from http://www3.baylor.edu/~Charles_Kemp/cuban_refugees.htm

Beliefnet.com. (2002). *Transition rituals: A faith-by-faith guide to rites for the deceased.* Retrieved December 22, 2002, from http://www.beliefnet.com/story/78/story_7894.html

Bhungalia, S., & Kemp, C. (2002). (Asian) Indian health beliefs and practices related to end of life. *Journal of Hospice and Palliative Nursing, 4*(1), 54-58.

Birchenall, J., & Streight, E. (1997). *Home care aide.* St. Louis: Mosby.

Brokenleg, M., & Middleton, D. (1993). Native Americans: Adapting, yet retaining. In D. Irish, K. Lundquist, & V. Nelsen (Eds.), *Ethnic variations in dying, death, and grief* (pp. 101-112). Philadelphia: Taylor & Francis.

Casarett, D. J., & Inouye, S. K. (2001). Diagnosis and management of delirium near the end of life. *Annals of Internal Medicine, 135,* 32-40.

Casarett, D. J., & Inouye, S. K. (2002). Delirium at the end of life. *Annals of Internal Medicine, 137,* 295.

Church of Jesus Christ of Latter-day Saints. (2002). *The Church.* Retrieved December 22, 2002, from http://www.mormon.org/learn/0,8672,794-1,00.htm

Coyle, N., Adelhardt, J., Foley, K., & Portenoy, R. K. (1990). Character of terminal illness in the advanced cancer patient: Pain and other symptoms during the last four weeks of life. *Journal of Pain and Symptom Management, 5,* 83-93.

Cremation Association of North America. (2002). *Cremation explained: Answers to most frequently asked questions.* Retrieved December 17, 2002, from http://www.cremationassociation.org/html/explained.html

DeSpelder, L., & Strickland, A. (1999). *The last dance: Encountering death and dying.* New York: Mayfield Publishing Company.

Ferrell, B. R., Virani, R., & Grant, M. (1999). Analysis of end of life content in nursing textbooks. *Oncology Nursing Forum, 26,* 869-876.

Finucane, T. E. (2002). Care of patients nearing death: Another view. *Journal of the American Geriatrics Society, 50,* 551-553.

Fields, M., & Cassell, C. (1997). *Approaching death: Improving care at the end of life.* Washington, DC: National Academy Press.

Gates, R. A., & Fink, R. M. (1997). *Oncology nursing secrets.* St. Louis: Mosby.

Gorman, L. M. (1998). The psychosocial impact of cancer on the individual, family, and society. In R. M. Carroll-Johnson, L. M. Gorman, & N. J. Bush (Eds.), *Psychosocial nursing care along the cancer continuum* (pp. 3-25). Pittsburgh: Oncology Nursing Press.

Green, J. (1989a). Death with dignity: Hinduism. *Nursing Times, 85*(6), 50-51.

Green, J. (1989b). Death with dignity: Islam. *Nursing Times, 85*(5), 56-57.

Green, J. (1989c). Death with dignity: Judaism. *Nursing Times, 85*(8), 65-65.

Happ, M. B., Capezuti, E., Strumpf, N. E., Wagner, L., Cunningham, S., Evans, L., et al. (2002). Advance care planning and end-of-life care for hospitalized nursing home residents. *Journal of the American Geriatrics Society, 50,* 829-835.

Hermann, C., & Looney, S. (2001). The effectiveness of symptom management in hospice patients during the last 7 days of life. *Journal of Hospice and Palliative Nursing, 3*(3), 88-96.

Horn, L. W. (1992, March/April). Terminal dyspnea: A hospice approach. *American Journal of Hospice & Palliative Care,* pp. 24-32.

Iserson, K. V. (2001). *Death to dust: What happens to dead bodies?* Tucson, AZ: Galen Press.

Jakobovits, I. (1959). *Jewish medical ethics: A comparative and historical study of the Jewish religious attitude to medicine and its practice.* New York: Philosophical Library.

Jansen, L. A., & Sulmasy, D. P. (2002). Sedation, alimentation, hydration, and equivocation: Careful conversation about care at the end of life. *Annals of Internal Medicine, 136,* 845-849.

Kastenbaum, R., & Kastenbaum, B. (Eds.). (1989). *Encyclopedia of death.* Phoenix: Oryx Press.

Kemp, C., & Bhungalia, S. (2002). Culture and the end of life: A review of major world religions. *Journal of Hospice and Palliative Nursing, 4*(4), 235-242.

Kemp, C., & Chang, B. (2002). Culture and the end of life: Chinese. *Journal of Hospice and Palliative Nursing, 4*(3), 173-177.

LaDuke, S. (2001). Terminal dyspnea and palliative care: patient deaths are inevitable. "Bad deaths"—those accompanied by severe suffering—are not. *American Journal of Nursing, 10*(11), 26-31.

Lynn, J., & Harrold, J. (1999). *Handbook for mortals: Guidance for people facing serious illness.* New York: Oxford University Press.

Matzo, M. (2001). Peri-death nursing care. In M. Matzo & D. Sherman (Eds.), *Palliative care nursing: Quality care to the end of life* (pp. 487-522). New York: Springer.

Matzo, M., Ury, & Sulmasy (in press).

Miller, E. J. (1993). A Roman Catholic view of death. In K. Doka & J. D. Morgan (Eds.), *Death and spirituality* (pp. 33-50). Amityville, NY: Baywood Publishing.

Miller, S. C., Gozalo, P., & Mor, V. (2001). Hospice enrollment and hospitalization of dying nursing home patients. *American Journal of Medicine, 111,* 38-44.

National Kidney Foundation. (2002). *Understanding the organ/tissue procurement process*. Retrieved December 18, 2002, from
http://www.kidney.org/general/news/factsheet.cfm?=35

Ng, K., & von Gunten, C. F. (1998). Symptoms and attitude of 100 consecutive patients admitted to an acute hospice/palliative care unit. *Journal of Pain and Symptom Management, 16*, 307-316.

North by South. (1998). *The history of African American death: Superstitions, traditions, and procedures*. Retrieved December 26, 2002, from http://www.northbysouth.kenyon.edu/1998/death/deathhistory.htm,.

Obermiller, P., & Rappold, R. (1994). The sense of place and cultural identity among urban Appalachians: A study in postdeath migration. In K. M. Borman & P. J. Obermiller (Eds.), *From mountain to metropolis: Appalachian migrants in American Cities*. Westport, CT: Bergin & Garvey.

Office of the Inspector General. (2002). *Organ donor registries: A useful, but limited, tool* (Executive Report # OEI-01-01-00350). Retrieved December 18, 2002, from http://oig.hhs.gov/oei/reports/oei-01-01-00350.pdf

O'Gorman, S. M. (1998). Death and dying in contemporary society: An evaluation of current attitudes and the rituals associated with death and dying and their relevance to recent understandings of health and healing. *Journal of Advanced Nursing, 27*, 1127-1135.

Panke, J. T. (2002). Difficulties in managing pain at the end of life. *American Journal of Nursing, 102*(7), 26-31.

Perkin, R. M., & Resnik, D. B. (2002). The agony of agonal respiration: Is the last gasp necessary? *Journal of Medical Ethics, 28*, 164-169.

Purnell, L. D., & Paulanka, B. J. (1998). *Transcultural health care: A culturally competent approach*. Philadelphia: Davis.

Quigley, C. (1996). *The corpse: A history*. Jefferson, NC: McFarland and Co.

Quill, T. E., & Byock, I. R. (2000). Responding to intractable terminal suffering: The role of terminal sedation and voluntary refusal of food and fluids. *Annals of Internal Medicine, 132*, 408-414.

Raether, H. C. (1993). Rituals, beliefs, and grief. In K. Doka & J. D. Morgan (Eds.), *Death and spirituality* (pp. 207-216). Amityville, NY: Baywood Publishing.

Ross, H. M. (1998). Jewish tradition in death and dying. *Medsurg Nursing, 7*(5), 275-279.

Ross, H. M. (2001). Islamic tradition at the end of life. *Medsurg Nursing, 10*(2), 83-87.

Ruland, C., & Moore, S. (1998). Theory construction based on standards of care: A proposed theory on the peaceful end of life. *Nursing Outlook, 46*(4), 169-175.

Salvador, R. J. (2002). *What do Mexicans celebrate on the Day of the Dead?* Retrieved December 31, 2002, from http://www.public.iastate.edu/~rjsalvad/scmfaq/muertos.html

Scientific Registry of Transplant Recipients. (2002). *Transplant primer*. Retrieved December 18, 2002, from http://www.ustransplant.org/primer.html

Shioda, E. (1999). *Japanese customs: Taking a bath*. Retrieved December 31, 2002, from
http://www.kt.rim.or.jp/~etshioda/customs.html#bottom

Sorrentino, S. A. (1999). *Assisting with patient care*. St. Louis: Mosby.

Strub, C. G., & Frederick, L. G. (1967). *The principles and practice of embalming*. Dallas: Frederick.

Sultzman, L. (1998). *Shawnee history*. Retrieved December 29, 2002, from http://www.tolatsga.org/shaw.html

Ternestedt, B., Andershed, B., Eriksson, M., & Johansson, I. (2002). A good death. *Journal of Hospice and Palliative Nursing, 4*(3), 153-160.

Vainio, A., & Auvinen, A. (1996). Prevalence of symptoms among patients with advanced care: An international collaborative study. *Journal of Pain and Symptom Management, 12*, 3-10.

Weitzner, M. A., Moody, L. N., & McMillan, S. C. (1997). Symptom management issues in hospice care. *American Journal of Hospice & Palliative Care, 14*, 190-195.

INDEX

Note: Page numbers followed by the letter b refer to boxes, those followed by the letter f refer to figures, and those followed by the letter t refer to tables.

Rituals and customs, 512-524, 530
cultural perspectives and, 521-524
post-death, 530
religious practices and, 512-521

S

Scenarios, practice. *See* Evidence-based practice scenarios.
Schwartz Cancer Fatigue Scale (SCFS), 411
Schwarz, Judith K., 82-104
SCLC (small cell lung cancer), 193-194
Seamless care creation, 73-74, 74b
Sedation, 433-435, 447, 509-517
overviews and summaries of, 433-435, 434b
terminal, 509, 510t-511t, 513f-514f
total, 446
Seizures, 218
Selective norepinephrine reuptake inhibitors (SNRIs), 332, 332t
Selective serotonin reuptake inhibitors (SSRIs), 321, 321t
Self-hypnosis, 358t
Self-transcendence, 140-141
Sensory changes, 415-416
Settings and locations, health care, 66-81. *See also* Health care settings.
Severe hyperkalemia, 260-261, 261t
Sherman, Deborah Witt, 3-30, 386-411
Short-acting benzodiazepines, 321, 321t
Shoulder-hand syndrome (reflex sympathetic dystrophy), 220-221
Shuttle walking test (SWT), 308
Side effects, medications, 432-435, 493-495
Signs and symptoms. *See also* under individual topics.
of anxiety, 319-320, 320t
of ascites, 378
of bowel obstructions, 372-373, 373t
of breast cancer, 198
of cancers, 204-205
of chronic obstructive pulmonary disease (COPD), 279-281
of colorectal cancer, 196
of constipation, 362b
of delirium, 336
of depression, 327
of dysphagia, 359, 360t
of end-stage heart disease, 171-172, 172b
of end-stage liver disease (ESLD), 294-295
of end-stage renal disease (ESRD), 253-256, 253b
of nausea and vomiting (N&V), 353-354, 354b
of prostate cancer, 200-201
of xerostomia, 381
Simpkins, Lynn H., 251-272
Simplification, regimen and scheduling, 496-497
Singultus (hiccups), 374-377
SIS-Q (Suicidal Ideation Screening Questionnaire), 330
Skin care needs, 452-468
case studies of, 452, 465-466
evidence-based practice scenarios for, 461b, 465b
fecal incontinence and, 465
for fistulas, 462-463

Skin care needs *(Continued)*
management of, 462-463
overviews and summaries of, 462
patient comfort and, 463
pouching for, 462-463
trouches for, 463
tubes and suction for, 463
overviews and summaries of, 452, 466
peri-death care and, 506
for peristomal (ostomy) skin, 460-462
assessments of, 460
certified wound, ostomy, and continence nurses (CWOCNs) and, 460, 462
integrity maintenance of, 460-462
overviews and summaries of, 460
total ostomy care management and, 462
Wound, Ostomy, and Continence Nurses Society and, 460
for pressure ulcers, 453-457
Agency for Health Care Policy and Research (ACHPR) guidelines for, 454-455, 455t
incidence and prevalence of, 453t
locations of, 453t, 454
National Pressure Ulcer Advisory Panel (NPUAP) and, 453, 453b
overviews and summaries of, 453-454
pain management for, 456-457
prevention of, 454-455, 455b
quality-of-life and, 456-457
risk assessments for, 454, 455b
staging of, 454
treatment of, 455-456, 456b
reference resources about, 466-468
for skin tears, 457-460
aging skin effects of, 457
care plans for, 458-460
causes of, 457-458
classification of, 458
incidence and prevalence of, 457
locations of, 457-458
overviews and summaries of, 457
Payne-Martin classification system for, 458
prevention protocols for, 458-460, 458b, 459f, 460b
risk factors for, 458
for tumor necroses, 463-466
management of, 463-464
overviews and summaries of, 463
quality-of-life and, 464
Skin tears, 457-460
Sleep disorders, 243-244
Small cell lung cancer (SCLC), 193-194
Smoking cessation, 276
SNRIs (selective norepinephrine reuptake inhibitors), 332, 332t
Social interaction issues, 43
Social worker and counselor roles, 417
Sociohistorical-cultural factors, 141-142
Softening preparations, 366